Naturopathic Physical Medicine

Publisher: Sarena Wolfaard
Commissioning Editor: Claire Wilson
Associate Editor: Claire Bonnett
Project Manager: Emma Riley
Designer: Charlotte Murray
Illustration Manager: Merlyn Harvey
Illustrator: Amanda Williams

Naturopathic
Physical Medicine
THEORY AND PRACTICE FOR MANUAL THERAPISTS AND NATUROPATHS

Co-authored and edited by
Leon Chaitow ND DO

Registered Osteopath and Naturopath;
Former Senior Lecturer, University of Westminster, London;
Honorary Fellow, School of Integrated Health, University of Westminster, London, UK;
Fellow, British Naturopathic Association

With contributions from
Eric Blake ND
Paul Orrock ND DO
Matthew Wallden ND DO

Co-authors of Chapter 1:
Pamela Snider ND
Jared Zeff ND

Foreword by
Joseph Pizzorno Jr ND

Additional contributions from

Hal Brown ND DC
Nick Buratovich ND
Michael Cronin ND
Brian Isbell PhD ND DO
Douglas C. Lewis ND
Benjamin Lynch ND
Lisa Maeckel MA CHT
Carolyn McMakin DC
Les Moore ND
Dean E. Neary Jr ND
Roger Newman Turner ND DO
David Russ DC
David J. Shipley ND DC
Brian K. Youngs ND DO

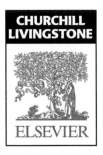

CHURCHILL LIVINGSTONE

ELSEVIER

Edinburgh London New York Oxford Philadelphia St Louis Sydney Toronto 2008

CHURCHILL LIVINGSTONE
ELSEVIER

First published 2008

ISBN: 978-0-443-10390-2

British Library Cataloguing in Publication Data
A catalogue record for this book is available from the British Library

Library of Congress Cataloging in Publication Data
A catalog record for this book is available from the Library of Congress

Notice
Neither the Publisher nor the Editors assume any responsibility for any loss or injury and/or damage to persons or property arising out of or related to any use of the material contained in this book. It is the responsibility of the treating practitioner, relying on independent expertise and knowledge of the patient, to determine the best treatment and method of application for the patient.

The Publisher

Dedication

This book is dedicated to the naturopathic teachers and pioneers who inspired all those involved in writing it, as well as to all students, educators and practitioners of naturopathy, and their patients.

Table of Contents

Authors and Contributors

Eric Blake ND MSOM Dipl Acupuncture
National College of Naturopathic Medicine,
Hydrotherapy Department Coordinating Supervisor and
Academic Adjunct Faculty; Clinical Director, Holistic
Health PC, Portland, Oregon, USA
  3. History of naturopathic physical medicine
     (author)
  4. Naturopathic physical medicine (contributor)
  8. Integrated naturopathic (manual) physical medicine
     protocols (contributor)
  11. Naturopathic hydrotherapy (author)
  12. Electrotherapy modalities (author)

Hal Brown ND DC RAc
Naturopathic Physician and Acupuncturist, Vancouver,
BC; Department Chair and Instructor in Physical
Medicine, Boucher Institute of Naturopathic Medicine,
New Westminster, BC, Canada
  7. Modalities, methods and techniques (contributor)
  10. Naturopathic physical medicine approaches to
     general health enhancement and specific
     conditions (contributor)

Nick Buratovich ND
Professor, Department Chair – Physical Medicine,
Southwest College of Naturopathic Medicine, Tempe,
Arizona, USA
  1. Physical medicine in a naturopathic context
     (contributor)
  7. Modalities, methods and techniques (contributor)
  10. Naturopathic physical medicine approaches to
     general health enhancement and specific
     conditions (contributor)
  12. Electrotherapy modalities (contributor)

Leon Chaitow ND DO
Registered Osteopath and Naturopath, Honorary Fellow,
School of Integrated Health, and former Senior Lecturer
University of Westminster, London, UK
  1. Physical medicine in a naturopathic context
     (co-author)
  2. Adaptation and the evolution of disease and
     dysfunction (author)
  3. History of naturopathic physical medicine
     (contributor)
  4. Naturopathic physical medicine (contributor)
  5. Assessment and palpation: accuracy and reliability
     issues (author)
  6. Assessment/palpation section: skills (author)
  7. Modalities, methods and techniques (author)
  8. Integrated naturopathic (manual) physical medicine
     protocols (author)
  10. Naturopathic physical medicine approaches to
     general health enhancement and specific
     conditions (author)
  11. Naturopathic hydrotherapy (contributor)

Michael Cronin ND DAAPM
Practice specializing in Physical Medicine; Diplomate
American Academy of Pain Management; Founding
President, Southwest College of Naturopathic Medicine;
Residency in Physical Medicine, National College of
Naturopathic Medicine; Board member, Naturopathic
Academy of Therapeutic Injection
  1. Physical medicine in a naturopathic context
     (contributor)

Brian Isbell PhD BSc ND DO
Head of Department, Department of Complementary
Therapies, School of Integrated Health, University of
Westminster, London, UK
  10. Naturopathic physical medicine approaches to
     general health enhancement and specific
     conditions (contributor)

Douglas C. Lewis ND
Naturopathic Physician/Physical Medicine Practitioner,
Seattle; Former Faculty and Chair of the Department of

Physical Medicine, Bastyr University, Kenmore, Washington; President, Washington Association of Naturopathic Physicians, Seattle, Washington, USA

7. *Modalities, methods and techniques* (contributor)
8. *Integrated naturopathic (manual) physical medicine protocols* (contributor)
11. *Naturopathic hydrotherapy* (contributor)
12. *Electrotherapy modalities* (contributor)

Benjamin Lynch ND

Naturopathic Physician; President, Eco-Integration, Inc.

11. *Naturopathic hydrotherapy* (contributor)

Lisa Maeckel MA CHT

Hakomi Therapist, Portland, Oregon, USA

7. *Modalities, methods and techniques* (contributor)
10. *Naturopathic physical medicine approaches to general health enhancement and specific conditions* (contributor)

Carolyn McMakin MA DC

President, Frequency Specific Seminars, Inc, Vancouver, Washington; Clinical Director, Fibromyalgia and Myofascial Pain Clinic, Portland, Oregon, USA

12. *Electrotherapy modalities* (contributor)

Les Moore ND MSOM LAc

Director, Integrative Medicine Department, Clifton Springs Hospital, New York, USA

11. *Naturopathic hydrotherapy* (contributor)

Dean E. Neary Jr ND

Associate Professor Chair, Physical Medicine Department, Bastyr University School of Naturopathic Medicine, Kenmore, WA, USA

7. *Modalities, methods and techniques* (contributor)
10. *Naturopathic physical medicine approaches to general health enhancement and specific conditions* (contributor)
12. *Electrotherapy modalities* (contributor)

Roger Newman Turner ND DO BAc

Newman Turner Clinic, Letchworth Garden City, Herts, and Harley Street, London, UK

4. *Naturopathic physical medicine* (contributor)
7. *Modalities, methods and techniques* (contributor)
10. *Naturopathic physical medicine approaches to general health enhancement and specific conditions* (contributor)

Paul Orrock RN ND DO MAppSc

Senior Lecturer, Director of Clinical Education, Coordinator of Clinical Sciences (Osteopathy), Department of Natural and Complementary Medicine, Southern Cross University, NSW, Australia

1. *Physical medicine in a naturopathic context* (contributor)
4. *Naturopathic physical medicine* (author)

David Russ DC

Chiropractic physician, Portland, Oregon, USA

6. *Assessment/palpation section: skills* (contributor)
10. *Naturopathic physical medicine approaches to general health enhancement and specific conditions* (contributor)

David J. Shipley ND DC

Naturopathic Physician, Tigard, Oregon, USA

6. *Assessment/palpation section: skills* (contributor)

Pamela Snider ND

Executive and Senior Editor, Foundations of Naturopathic Medicine; Associate Professor, National College of Natural Medicine, Portland, Oregon, USA

1. *Physical medicine in a naturopathic context* (co-author)

Matthew Wallden ND DO MSc Ost Med CHEK IV HLC III

CHEK Practitioner/osteopath/naturopath, Sports Orthopaedics Spinal, Weybridge, Surrey, UK

1. *Physical medicine in a naturopathic context* (contributor)
2. *Adaptation and the evolution of disease and dysfunction* (contributor)
5. *Assessment and palpation: accuracy and reliability issues* (contributor)
9. *Rehabilitation and re-education (movement) approaches* (author)

Brian K. Youngs BSc(Lond) ND DO

Practitioner of complementary medicine, Harley Street, London, UK

7. *Modalities, methods and techniques* (contributor)

Jared Zeff ND

Adjunct Professor, Bastyr University of Natural Health Sciences, Seattle, Washington, USA

1. *Physical medicine in a naturopathic context* (co-author)

Foreword

Our modern world suffers a tremendous burden of poor health and disease. The incidence of most chronic degenerative diseases has increased in virtually every age group during almost every decade of the past 50 years. Much of this suffering is unnecessary – as research has now shown that a large body of healing wisdom, long the province of naturopathic medicine, has been missing from the health care system.

We have much to be grateful for in conventional medicine – almost miraculous advances in the treatment of acute illness, trauma and life-threatening disease accomplished through dedication, intense research, and a huge investment of financial resources (unfortunately to the exclusion of most other approaches to health care). Key to this advancement has been standardization of diagnosis, of therapy and, unfortunately, of patients. In addition, the advancement of this disease treatment model has apparently necessitated isolation of diagnosis and treatment to distinct entities separate from the whole person. Conventional medicine has developed standardized therapies for standard diagnoses for specific conditions in generic patients that are sometimes curative, often highly effective in symptom relief, but not very effective in promoting health, ignore the interactive complexity of whole-person systems and are utterly incapable of recognizing how truly different each of us is, starting at the cellular level. Worse, this reductionistic isolation of attention and the lack of recognition of each patient's uniqueness is a primary cause of the huge incidence of adverse drug reactions from *appropriately prescribed* medications. As the number of drugs prescribed per person has increased, so has the incidence of adverse drug reactions and health-damaging interactions.

Widespread public dissatisfaction with the cost, side effects and limited health advancement that characterize the dominant medical system has led to the search for a new medicine. Patients are looking for health care professionals who integrate the best of conventional and natural medicine and treat them as a whole, complex person, not as isolated parts. This search has led to renewed appreciation of naturopathic medicine and the healing wisdom it offers.

The growth and increasing sophistication of naturopathic medicine over the past few decades has been phenomenal. The naturopathic precepts of the causes of ill health and rules for healthful living, which were once dismissed as faddism (and worse), are now becoming mainstream wisdom. Eating a whole foods, organically grown diet; avoiding endogenous and exogenous toxins; physical exercise and balance; stress reduction; healthy social relationships – all once dismissed – are now known as necessary for health.

Over the past century, physical medicine has been foundational to the formation and evolution of naturopathic thought and practice. The huge expansion of research into nutrition, lifestyle and physiology has inspired in modern naturopathic medicine a much greater orientation to metabolic approaches for the promotion of health and treatment of disease. While this approach has much to offer, prescribing supplements and changing a patient's diet do not correct the neurological, muscular and vascular dysfunctions caused by musculoskeletal problems. Problems can range from mechanically impaired joints chronically releasing pro-inflammatory chemical mediators that cause health-damaging effects throughout the body to tissues being so poorly vascularized or their lymphatic drainage sufficiently compromised that no amount of detoxification or supplementation can restore normal function.

When we assert that we treat the whole person – mind, body and spirit – we need to remember that the body includes more than just biochemical reactions. Its physical structures can have as much impact on bodily health as nutrients and toxins. And, happily, they are amenable to intervention.

Physical medicine is perhaps the most whole-person of all our therapies. Thinking back to my days as a student, I remember one of Dr Bastyr's wise admonitions, 'Always touch your patients; let them know you care.' The application of physical medicine is in many ways the most intimate of our therapies, where we as physical beings interact personally with our patients with healing intent. In this era of increasing depersonalization and social isolation, this closeness to our patients is a welcome contrast to the 7-minute office call.

In addition to the importance of this textbook in advancing our understanding of physical medicine is its role as another example of the emerging sophistication of academic natural medicine. This excellent textbook was written by experts in all schools of natural medicine from all over the world. Osteopaths, naturopaths, chiropractors, acupuncturists and physical therapists have all contributed their expertise without being limited by the boundaries of their professions and united by their passion for this healing wisdom. Dr Chaitow is to be congratulated for bringing together such an outstanding group of leaders in physical medicine to create such a valuable resource for clinicians.

Joseph Pizzorno Jr ND
Author, *Textbook of Natural Medicine*
Editor-in-Chief, *Integrative Medicine,*
A Clinician's Journal

Preface

Naturopathic physical medicine incorporates a wide array of methods, techniques and modalities, many of which are explored in this text, along with the evidence and rationale for their use in health care. As explained in depth in this book, the use of physical medicine in a naturopathic context may focus on the treatment and rehabilitation of musculoskeletal dysfunction, or it may be employed in treatment of both major and minor health problems in order to enhance and encourage self-regulatory functions.

It is important to note that naturopathic practitioners in different states, provinces and countries practice physical medicine as part of their clinical care of patients, in accordance with local laws and licensing regulations which are anything but uniform. For example, in North America and Canada naturopathic education results in qualification as licensed primary care naturopathic physicians through state or provincial boards of medical examiners.

In contrast, in Europe and Australia (as examples), a naturopathic qualification leads to a more limited scope of practice, unless additional qualifications (DO, DC, PT, MD, etc.) are also held. To an extent these differences are reflected in the physical medicine (and other) methods utilized and, in some instances, to the conditions treated.

The continuum of manual methods employed in naturopathic clinical practice may (depending on licensing variations) incorporate both static and motion palpation, as well as a wide variety of soft tissue techniques, joint articulation, mobilization without impulse (joint play), as well as mobilization with impulse. Mobilization with impulse is also referred to as high velocity, low amplitude (HVLA) thrust technique and, because of concerns as to safety, this modality is deserving of some explanation (Hurwitz et al 2005).

Naturopathic manipulation (including HVLA) is directed towards correcting imbalances in structural integrity, commonly manifested as joint fixation/restriction and/or malposition, by means of mechanical/manual stimulation, delivered by physician/practitioner controlled soft-tissue, spinal and extremity mobilization. Evidence is offered in the book of the ways in which such treatment approaches can beneficially influence neurological, circulatory and biomechanical functions, as well as having positive effects on the individual's psychological/emotional status.

In keeping with the naturopathic principle of *first do no harm,* when mobilization with impulse (HVLA) is applied, it is with an appropriate (to the patient's needs and current health status) degree of force, designed to produce just sufficient impulse to overcome articular restriction and/or malposition. It is the application of such an extrinsically applied thrusting impulse that has attracted concern regarding safety and competency.

It is worth emphasizing that, by definition, HVLA impulse, or thrust, involves *high velocity,* not *high force,* delivered over a very small distance. This use of velocity rather than force is an essential skill in HVLA delivery, only employed once an appropriate diagnosis has been made. Once a dysfunctional segment or joint has been identified, specific HVLA techniques *may* be selected to achieve mobilization. The mechanics of such applications include the use of long or short levers, focused tissue tension with joint locking, appropriate line of drive, and physician and patient positioning, all achieved with balance and control (see Chapter 7).

The efficacy of mobilization with impulse (HVLA thrusting) has longstanding and current validation from both the osteopathic and chiropractic professions (see Chapters 7 and 10, in particular). HVLA issues relating to safety are commonly directed to cervical spine manipulation, and these safety concerns, in naturopathic practice, are covered in some detail in Chapter 7. Safety concerns exist in the realm of the knowledge of potential risk, precautions, complications, reactions and contraindications, as much as in the realm of technique application. In naturopathic educational programs that provide instruction in naturopathic physical medicine and naturopathic manipulation, including HVLA usage, the topics of risk, precautions, complications, reactions and contra-indications are studied in depth. These topics are not only covered in specific classes on naturopathic manipulation but are also included in other aspects of the curriculum which deal with pathology and dysfunctional conditions involving the musculoskeletal system and general systemic function, including classes in diagnostic imaging. The naturopathic student, practitioner and practicing physician usually focuses on whole body issues and restoration of health, and so the training in physical medicine, including naturopathic manipulation, is taught within that context. Naturopathic manipulation using HVLA techniques is seldom employed in isolation but as part of a process designed to restore maximal pain-free movement of articulations, restoration of postural balance, systemic functionality and facilitation of the self-regulatory mechanisms of the body.

In a recent study of licensed Canadian naturopathic physicians there was a strong indication that core naturopathic manipulation skills were adequate and thorough (Verhoef et al 2006).

Similarly, a recent American Association of Naturopathic Physicians (AANP) Position Paper reminds us that naturopathic manipulative treatment, as part of naturopathic physical medicine, has historically been an integral part of the practice of naturopathic medicine, and has been included in naturopathic medical education and licensure since the early 1900s. That Position Paper states that naturopathic medical education prepares naturopathic physicians to safely and competently perform and practice naturopathic physical medicine and naturopathic manipulation (Buratovich et al 2006).

It is worth re-emphasizing that HVLA is not a part of the training of naturopathic practitioners in Europe or Australia, and is employed by naturopathic practitioners in those countries only if the ND also holds a qualification as an osteopath, chiropractor or physical therapist, or as an appropriately trained medical practitioner.

Over and above the issue of safe HVLA usage, naturopathic physical medicine employs a wide range of methods, modalities and techniques, including hydrotherapy and electrotherapy, and a plethora of manual, movement, rehabilitation and re-education approaches, all designed and employed to achieve one of three objectives:

- To reduce adaptive demands via, as examples, modifying patterns of use including improved mobility, stability, balance, posture and/or respiratory function

- To improve the body's capacity to cope with adaptive demands via, as examples, enhanced biomechanical, circulatory and/or neurological functions

- To safely modulate the patient's presenting symptoms – without adding to existing adaptive overload.

Naturopathy considers that the body heals itself, unless damage, dysfunction and degeneration are too advanced. Even then, functional improvement, or a delaying of further decline, may be possible. In all these objectives, use of naturopathic physical medicine methods rely for efficacy on intrinsic, endogenous, innate, homeostatic, self-regulatory forces.

All naturopathic therapeutic interventions, including naturopathic physical medicine methods, are therefore focused on encouraging these processes.

Nick Buratovich, Paul Orrock, Leon Chaitow – and all the other co-authors, contributors and internal reviewers responsible for this book.

References

Buratovich N, Cronin M, Perry A et al 2006 AANP Position Paper on Naturopathic Manipulative Therapy. American Association of Naturopathic Physicians, Washington DC

Hurwitz E, Morgenstern H, Vassilaki M, Chiang L 2005 Frequency and clinical predictors of adverse reactions to chiropractic care in the UCLA neck pain study. Spine 30:1477–1484

Verhoef M, Boon H, Mutasingwa D 2006 The scope of naturopathic medicine in Canada: an emerging profession. Social Science and Medicine 63(2):409–417

Acknowledgments

My profound thanks go to those who were active in the compilation of this book. Thanks to my co-authors – Eric Blake, Paul Orrock, Pam Snider, Matt Wallden and Jared Zeff; to the contributors and internal reviewers – Hal Brown, Nick Buratovich, Michael Cronin, Brian Isbell, Doug Lewis, Ben Lynch, Lisa Maeckel, Carolyn McMakin, Les Moore, Dean Neary, Roger Newman Turner, David Russ, David Shipley and Brian Youngs . . . and of course to the author of the Foreword, Joseph Pizzorno, whose inspirational work over the past 25 years has helped to launch and sustain naturopathic medicine's renaissance in North America.

Sincere thanks also to the editorial team at Elsevier, particularly Claire Bonnett and Claire Wilson for their consistent and good natured help; and not forgetting Sarena Wolfaard, who embraced the concept of this book from the outset, and provided support throughout its evolution.

On a personal level, as so often in the past, my gratitude goes to Alkmini, for creating a warm, supportive and loving environment in which to write, on the beautiful island of Corfu.

**Leon Chaitow ND DO,
Jared Zeff ND, Pamela Snider ND**

With contributions from:
Nick Buratovich ND
Michael Cronin ND
Paul Orrock ND DO
Matthew Wallden ND DO

Physical Medicine in a Naturopathic Context

In order to appreciate the meaning of the term naturopathic physical medicine (NPM), it is first necessary to have an understanding of just what naturopathic medicine is (Lindlahr 1913); see Box 1.1.

The naturopathic profession

Naturopathic medicine is a worldwide profession with concentrations in the USA, Germany, Canada, UK, Australia and India. In these countries, naturopathic medicine functions, or is legally defined, as a primary health care profession whose practice incorporates health promotion and the prevention, diagnosis and treatment of acute and chronic disease. There are marked scope of practice and training differences among various regional and global traditions (Standish et al 2005).

In the USA and Canada naturopathic doctors (NDs) are trained as general practice family physicians. This is intentional and consistent with naturopathic principles of practice. Naturopathic doctors (and practitioners in countries where licensing and scope of practice are not as full as in the USA where a broad medical scope of practice prevails in many states) are trained to assess and treat disease from a whole person perspective, taking into account not only the presenting pathology but also deeper causes and collateral relationships with other systems of the body (Standish et al 2005).

Boon et al (2004) report that:

Naturopathic medicine is a licensed health care profession in twelve US states (Alaska, Arizona, Connecticut, Hawaii, Maine, Montana, New Hampshire, Oregon, Utah, Vermont, Washington, California), Puerto Rico and four Canadian provinces (British Columbia, Manitoba, Ontario and Saskatchewan) (Hough et al 2001, American Association of Naturopathic Physicians 2007). In most states and provinces where naturopathic medicine is not regulated, individuals call themselves naturopaths (whether or not they have been trained at a school for naturopathic medicine) because the term naturopathic medicine is not a restricted term in all jurisdictions. The number of individuals practicing in unregulated jurisdictions is unknown. All licensed states require standardized training and board examinations to obtain a license.

Naturopathic medicine

Naturopathic medicine encompasses treatment and diagnostic modalities whose use is guided by the principles and theory of naturopathic medicine that are critical to the practice's identity and effectiveness. Clinical application of naturopathic theory influences case management; selection, sequencing and integration of therapies; patient diagnoses; healing practices, and lifestyle and wellness approaches (Standish et al 2005). Both effectiveness and safety can be influenced by theory. Leading ethicists such as Edmund Pellegrino have observed that all health care systems have an inherent theory which influences clinical decision-making, whether explicitly described or not, and a system of thinking is implied by the pattern of clinical decisions in each discipline (Pellegrino 1979).

The *vis*

Naturopathic medicine is based upon principles that are abstracted from observations of health and healing. Although to some extent these principles are consis-

tent with all branches of the healing arts, the key principle in naturopathic medicine is a major distinguishing element. That first principle is *vis medicatrix naturae* ('the healing power of nature'), which establishes naturopathic medicine as a vitalistic medicine, a modern inheritor of the vitalistic tradition. This fundamental principle identifies naturopathy as being focused on the natural tendency of the body to heal itself. This tendency is intelligent, always acting in the best interest of the body. It can be seen in Hans Selye's work (1946, 1975), expressed there as 'homeostasis' and the 'adaptation response', described as 'a relative constancy in the internal environment, naturally obtained by adaptive responses that promote healthy survival'. (See Chapter 2 for a discussion of Selye's *General Adaptation Syndrome* model that has both permeated much medical thinking over the last half century and which many take as a conceptual scientific validation of traditional naturopathic thinking.)

Between 1986 and 1989 the American naturopathic profession undertook a 3-year national consensus process, after which it adopted the following definition of naturopathic medicine, based on principles of practice, rather than modalities. This definition (Box 1.1) has been widely accepted throughout the international naturopathic community (Snider & Zeff 1989, American Association of Naturopathic Physicians 2006).

Box 1.1 Definition of naturopathic medicine

Naturopathic medicine is a distinct system of primary health care – an art, science, philosophy and practice of diagnosis, treatment and prevention of illness. Naturopathic medicine is distinguished by the principles that underlie and determine its practice. These principles are based upon the objective observation of the nature of health and disease, and are continually re-examined in the light of scientific advances.

Methods used are consistent with these principles and are chosen on the basis of patient individuality. Naturopathic physicians and practitioners are primary health care providers, whose diverse techniques include modern and traditional, scientific and empirical methods. The following principles are the foundation for the practice of naturopathic medicine.

Principles

I. The healing power of nature *(Vis medicatrix naturae)*

The healing power of nature is the inherent, self-organizing and healing process of living systems that establishes, maintains and restores health. Naturopathic medicine recognizes this healing process to be ordered

and intelligent. It is the naturopathic practitioner's role to support, facilitate and augment this process by identifying and removing obstacles to health and recovery, and by supporting the creation of a healthy internal and external environment.

II. Identify and treat the causes *(Tolle causam)*

Illness does not occur without cause. Causes may originate in many areas. Underlying causes of illness and disease must be identified and removed before complete recovery can occur. Symptoms can be expressions of the body's attempt to defend itself, to adapt and recover, to heal itself, or may be results of the causes of disease. The naturopathic physician/ practitioner seeks to treat the causes of disease, rather than to merely eliminate or suppress symptoms.

III. First do no harm *(Primum non nocere)*

Naturopathic physicians and practitioners follow three precepts to avoid harming the patient:

1. Naturopathic physicians/practitioners utilize methods and medicinal substances that minimize the risk of harmful effects and apply the least possible force or intervention necessary to diagnose illness and restore health.

Box 1.1 Definition of naturopathic medicine continued

2. Whenever possible the suppression of symptoms is avoided, as suppression is generally considered to interfere with the healing process.
3. Naturopathic physicians respect and work with the *vis medicatrix naturae* in diagnosis, treatment and counseling, for if this self-regulating process is not respected the patient may be harmed.

IV. Doctor as teacher *(Docere)*

The original meaning of the word 'doctor' is teacher. A principal objective of naturopathic medicine is to educate the patient and emphasize self-responsibility for health. Naturopathic physicians and practitioners also recognize and employ the therapeutic potential of the doctor–patient relationship.

V. Treat the whole person *(Tolle totum)*

Health and disease result from a complex of physical, mental, emotional, genetic, environmental, social and other factors. Since total health also includes spiritual health, naturopathic physicians and practitioners encourage individuals to pursue their personal spiritual development. Naturopathic medicine recognizes the harmonious functioning of all aspects of the individual as being essential to health. The multifactorial nature of health and disease requires a personalized and comprehensive approach to diagnosis and treatment. Naturopathic physicians and practitioners attempt to treat the whole person, taking all of these factors into account.

VI. Prevention *(Preventare)*

Naturopathic colleges and universities emphasize the study of health as well as disease. The prevention of disease and the attainment of optimal health in patients are primary objectives of naturopathic medicine. In practice, these objectives are seen to be best accomplished through education and the promotion of healthy ways of living. Naturopathic physicians and practitioners assess risk factors, heredity and susceptibility to disease, and make appropriate interventions in partnership with their patients to prevent illness. Naturopathic medicine asserts that one cannot be healthy in an unhealthy environment and is committed to the creation of a world in which humanity may thrive.

Practice

Naturopathic methods

Naturopathic medicine is defined primarily by its fundamental principles. Methods and modalities are selected and applied, based upon these principles in relationship to the individual needs of each patient. Diagnostic and therapeutic methods are selected from various sources and systems, and will continue to evolve with the progress of knowledge.

Naturopathic practice

Depending on local licensing laws and scopes of practice, naturopathic practice may include the following diagnostic and treatment modalities: utilization of all methods of clinical and laboratory diagnostic testing including diagnostic radiology and other imaging techniques; nutritional medicine, dietetics and therapeutic fasting; medicines of mineral, animal and botanical origin; hygiene and public health measures; naturopathic physical medicine including naturopathic manipulative therapies; the use of water, heat, cold, light, electricity, air, earth, electromagnetic and mechanical devices, ultrasound and therapeutic exercise; homeopathy; acupuncture; psychotherapy and counseling; minor surgery and naturopathic obstetrics (natural childbirth).

Naturopathic practice excludes major surgery and the use of most synthetic drugs (Snider & Zeff 1989, American Association of Naturopathic Physicians).

International perspective

International perspectives on naturopathic practice and principles demonstrate increasing coherence and consistency between North America, Australia and the United Kingdom, as evidenced by a recent publication on naturopathic medicine that included naturopathic physician authors from several countries (Myers et al 2003). In this, naturopathic medicine is described as the eclectic and integrative practice of health care, united by the core underlying principles (and their applied clinical theory) described above.

Central to these principles is the healing power of nature (*vis medicatrix naturae*), a concept that is ascribed to Hippocrates, and which is as old as the healing arts. The healing power of nature refers to the inherent self-organizing and healing process of living systems that establishes, maintains and restores health (Myers et al 2003).

In the words of Newman Turner (1984): 'Naturopathy is based on the recognition that the body possesses not only a natural ability to resist disease, but inherent mechanisms of recovery and self-regulation.'

Naturopathic medicine bases its clinical theories and reasoning, as evidenced by its therapeutic choices, on assisting the self-regulation processes by means of removing obstacles to recovery and/or enhancing the functionality of systems, organs and tissues.

Allopathic medicine – a comparison

In contrast, the defining features of allopathic medicine have been summarized by a number of naturopathic theorists and clinicians (Pizzorno & Snider 2004, Zeff 1997).

For example, Zeff et al (2006) have advanced four underlying assumptions of standard allopathic medicine, the fundamental basis of which is generally characterized as 'the diagnosis and treatment of disease'.

In allopathic medicine:

1. diseases are commonly regarded as entities (e.g. measles, smallpox, cancer, diabetes, etc.)
2. diseases are seen as entities that can be identified ('diagnosis')
3. treatment is directed against disease entities (the diabetes is treated, rather than the person with the diabetes)
4. appropriate allopathic medical treatment is the evidence-based application of drugs, surgery and other methods.

In distinction, naturopathic medicine can be characterized by a different model from one that 'diagnoses and treats disease': the 'restoration of health' would be a better characterization of the naturopathic approach.

In 1989 naturopathic physicians and practitioners adopted the following brief statement, characterizing naturopathic medicine: 'Naturopathic physicians treat disease by restoring health' (Snider & Zeff 1989).

It should be possible to recognize a distinct difference: mainstream medicine is disease-based; naturopathic medicine is health-based. In naturopathic medicine disease is seen much more as a *process* than as an *entity*.

Rather than seeing the ill patient as suffering from a 'disease', the naturopathic practitioner views the ill person as functioning within a process of disturbance and recovery, in which disease and ill-health can be seen to involve an adaptive state – a response to disturbances, changes, adaptations and stresses within the system. In this perspective equal weight is given to biochemical, structural and psychosocial influences interacting with the unique genetic and acquired characteristics of the individual.

Psychoneuroimmunology – towards a broader allopathic model?

The description of core features of allopathic medicine as it is most commonly practiced, as listed above, is by no means the only model operating, as some branches of mainstream medicine evolve from its current biomedical focus.

There are strands within current medical thinking that mirror naturopathic ideas, offering a hopeful prospect for the future. An example can be observed in the concepts promoted by the study of psychoneuroimmunology (as expounded by Engel 1977) as a major feature of what has come to be called the biopsychosocial model of medicine. The main theme of biopsychosocial medicine is that mechanistic biological explanations, as proposed by biomedicine, are unable to account for many health outcomes, and that the etiology and progress of many conditions demand an understanding of the interaction between biological, psychological and social factors (Borrell-Carrio et al 2004).

Alford (2007) has observed that:

One of Engel's main criticisms was that the biomedical model encouraged separation of mind and body. In the biomedical model the body is viewed as a machine to be fixed and is separate from emotions. Engel and his colleagues considered that this was leading to the dehumanization of medicine. They considered that patients were being seen as objects to be fixed, and [that] their subjective experiences were of no relevance to assessment and management decisions.

Were structural, biomechanical influences more closely incorporated into this perspective, alongside psychosocial and biochemical/biological factors, the model would start to resemble a naturopathic appreciation of health and disease.

It has been suggested by some that the psychosocial aspect of this new paradigm has tilted it too far, as it attempts to counterbalance the biomedical approach of most mainstream medical practitioners. Waddell (2004), for one, has concluded that this is so, particularly in relation to musculoskeletal conditions such as low back pain where, he maintains, the emphasis has swung excessively towards consideration of psychosocial issues, to the neglect of structural and physical aspects of dysfunction.

Figure 1.1, reproduced from a review of psychoneuroimmunology by Lutgendorf & Costanzo (2003), allows us to appreciate the progress medicine has made via this broader understanding of health and disease, and how this resembles much traditional naturopathic thinking. It is easy to observe the interacting systems, coping with adaptation processes, within this model, as described in detail in Box 1.2. Chapter 2 provides a deeper discussion of adaptation and health.

Examples of ill-health involving clear evidence of a process of adaptation might include the following.

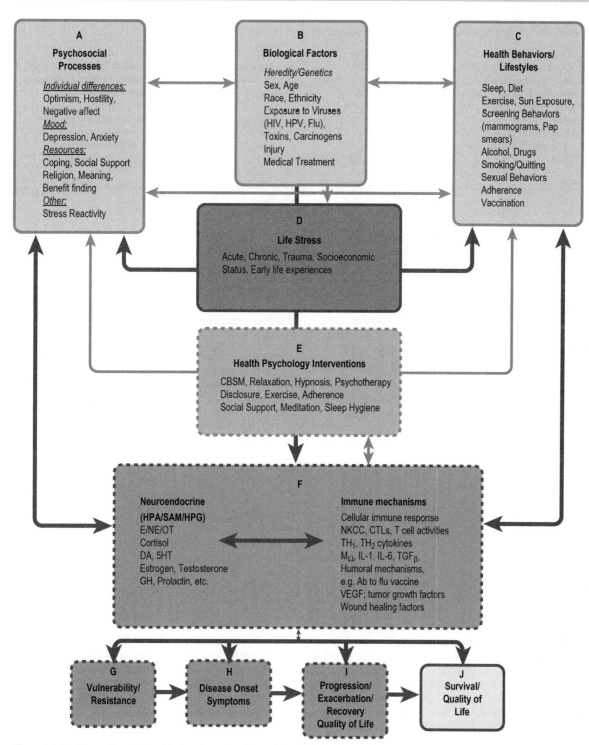

Figure 1.1 The biopsychosocial model of medicine. See Box 1.2 for a full description of the interacting systems within this model. 5HT, serotonin; Ab, antibody; CTLs, cytotoxic lymphocytes; DA, dopamine; E, endocrine; GH, growth hormone; HPA, hypothalamic pituitary adrenocortical axis; HPG, hypophyseal pituitary gonadal axis; HPV, human papilloma virus, IL-1, interleukin 1; IL-6, interleukin 6; M$_\Omega$, macrophage; NE, neuroendocrine; NKCC: natural killer cell cytotoxicity; OT, oxytocin; SAM, sympathoadrenomedullary axis; TGF$_\beta$, transforming growth factor beta; TH, T-helper; VEGF, vascular endothelial growth factor. Reproduced with permission from Lutgendorf & Costanzo (2003)

Box 1.2 Interacting systems within the biopsychosocial model of medicine (Fig. 1.1)

The interaction between psychosocial processes (Box A), biological factors (Box B), and health behaviors (Box C) leads to a vulnerability (or resistance) to illness (Box G), disease onset and symptoms (Box H), progression, exacerbation, recovery, with concomitant quality of life (Box I), and survival with concomitant quality of life (Box J) via processes involving neuroendocrine and immune mechanisms (Box F). Effects of life stress (Box D) are filtered through psychosocial processes (Box A) and health behaviors (Box C) in their resultant effects on downstream mechanisms. Health psychology interventions (Box E) can modulate effects of psychosocial processes and health behaviors on neuroendocrine and immune mechanisms and on resultant health outcomes. There are also pathways between biobehavioral factors and disease outcomes not involving neuroendocrine or immune mechanisms, but other pathways are not included in this figure.

Psychosocial processes (A) encompass psychological and social factors, particularly those that involve interpretation of and response to life stressors. These include personality variables (e.g. optimism, hostility and negative affect), mental health and mood variables (e.g. depression and anxiety), coping, social support, spirituality and sense of meaning. Health behaviors (C) include drug and alcohol use, smoking, sleep, nutrition, exercise, adherence to medical regimens, physical examinations, risk screenings and risky sexual behaviors, among others. Health psychology interventions (E) can

be used to alter psychosocial processes (A: e.g. decrease depression, increase coping) or improve health behaviors (C: e.g. smoking cessation) to provide a more positive influence on neuroendocrine and immune factors and perhaps slow disease progression/exacerbation. Interventions include cognitive-behavioral stress management (CBSM), relaxation, hypnosis, meditation, emotional disclosure, adherence-based interventions, sleep hygiene, exercise, social support groups, psychotherapy, imagery, distraction, behavioral pain management, yoga, massage, biofeedback, drug/alcohol prevention/rehabilitation, psychotherapy and behavioral conditioning. These interventions can be used at all points of the trajectory of the disease or condition. Box F shows selected mechanisms involved in the bidirectional interactions between neuroendocrine and immune axes that mediate the relationships between biobehavioral factors (A–D) and disease outcomes (G–J).

This is by no means an all-inclusive list of mechanisms, but it represents some of the commonly studied factors in this literature. Once vulnerability (G) has been established, continued interaction with positive or negative psychosocial factors (A: e.g. depression/social support), disease factors (B), adaptive/maladaptive health behaviors (C) and stress (D) will contribute to expression (or lack thereof) of disease symptoms (H), disease-free intervals/progression/exacerbation, and quality of life (e.g. functional, physical, emotional, and social well-being) (I), and survival (J).

Example 1

Gastrointestinal irritation and/or inflammation may be caused by dietary imbalances, allergy, stress factors, local bowel flora changes due to use of medication (e.g. antibiotics) (Vanderhoof et al 1999), environmental pollution or other factors, resulting in altered gut ecology (McCourtie & Douglas 1984). This process involves depleted beneficial bacterial function (Valeur et al 2004), reduced protective secretory IgA levels (Crago & Tomasi 1987) and increased gut permeability (Crissinger et al 1990).

This sequence of adaptations to previous or ongoing events results in larger than desirable molecules being absorbed from the gut, potentially triggering allergic reactions (Heyman 2005), as well as overloading liver function, with the possibility of autoimmune implications (Peltonen et al 1994).

A host of symptoms might be anticipated, ranging from fatigue to palpitations, skin disturbances, head-

aches, nausea, joint pain and more (Bengtsson et al 1996).

A virtual domino-effect cascade is observed as symptoms progress from initially acute, through chronic phases, many of which are anxiety-provoking, so adding to the distress of the individual and further aggravating normal gut function (Tache et al 2001).

Restoration of normal gut ecology (Hickman 1998, Perdigon et al 1990, Verhoef et al 1998) and permeability (Alverdy 1990) would be one aspect of the therapeutic plan, rather than focusing on obvious symptoms and secondary effects (allergic symptoms, fatigue, arthritis, etc.).

In addition to normalizing the gut flora and reducing inappropriate permeability, enhancing stress management could be another primary focus (Brosschot 2002).

Naturopathic care has an excellent record in such situations, even where autoimmune conditions such as rheumatoid arthritis coexist with food allergy, increased gut permeability, increased circulating immune complexes, excessive inflammatory processes and increased oxidative stress (Dunn & Wilkinson 2005).

Example 2

An emotionally stressful period might initiate an altered breathing pattern (Lum 1984), in which diaphragmatic function is reduced and an anxiety-linked upper chest respiratory pattern evolves (Perri & Halford 2004).

Initially this response is a physiologically normal adaptation to an acute/alarm situation ('fight/flight'). However, if prolonged and/or repetitive, the changes engendered may become chronic as the adaptation phase of the general adaptation syndrome (GAS) develops (Selye 1975). See Chapter 2 for more detail of GAS.

Excessive, physiologically undesirable and ultimately unsustainably high levels of CO_2 exhalation occur, resulting in respiratory alkalosis (Foster et al 2001). This, in turn, induces smooth muscle constriction (Litchfield 2003), reducing the diameter of blood vessels (impeding normal circulation) (Neill et al 1981) as well as the intestines, so altering normal peristaltic function (Ford et al 1995).

Respiratory alkalosis also induces the *Bohr* effect in which hemoglobin's attachment to oxygen increases, reducing delivery of O_2 to tissues such as brain and muscles (Fried 1987, Pryor & Prasad 2002), resulting in fatigue and a variety of cognitive and emotional repercussions (Nixon & Andrews 1996).

Neural function is impaired by these changes, and neural sensitization, with heightened pain awareness as one consequence, is common (Charney & Deutch 1996, Sergi et al 1999).

Homeostatic adaptation to these changes involves increased bicarbonate excretion via the kidneys in an effort to return pH to normal (~7.4), so disturbing calcium and magnesium balance (George 1964, Macefield & Burke 1991) and further interfering with already unbalanced neural and muscular function.

The hyperventilating individual's symptoms might therefore include irritable bowel, short-term memory loss, perception of a variety of areas of increased head, neck, shoulder, chest and back pain (commonly associated with overuse of accessory breathing muscles), feelings of sympathetic arousal, anxiety, panic and general fatigue (Abelson et al 2001). Many other symptoms might evolve as this cycle of compensation, adaptation, decompensation and possible illness behavior advances (Vlaeyen & Crombez 1999).

Ultimately, in a state of chronic pain and fatigue, and with minimal likelihood of adequate aerobic activity, the deconditioned individual's ATP production will come to rely on anaerobic glycolysis – resulting in lactic and other acid waste production that further stimulates hyperventilation tendencies – accelerating and exacerbating the processes described above (Nixon & Andrews 1996).

Should such an adaptive process occur in a woman between the ages of 15 and 50 (chances are 7 : 1 that this will be the case rather than the individual being male), where progesterone levels rise following ovulation, the respiratory rate will accelerate, further aggravating all these symptoms during the premenstrual phase (Damas-Mora et al 1980, Ott et al 2006).

All these symptoms will also be exaggerated if this pattern of breathing coincides with periods of hypoglycemia (Timmons & Ley 1994).

This kaleidoscope of interacting influences, synchronicities, compensations and adaptations offers a clear picture of biochemical, biomechanical and psychosocial effects – deriving from an initial adaptation to stress – leading to complex chronic ill-health.

Resolution demands, among other things, breathing rehabilitation (Mehling et al 2005), which has been shown to be best achieved by a combination of relearning diaphragmatic respiration, structural mobilization of the thorax, stress management (DeGuire et al 1996) and a lifestyle that encourages nutritional excellence, adequate exercise and sleep (Gardner 1996).

Example 3

Matthew Wallden ND DO

It is well documented that, when exposed to a sensitizing food such as gluten, there may initially be a non-specific immune response resulting in increased mucus production and swelling of the body's mucous membranes and tissues, such as tonsils and adenoids (Brostoff & Gamlin 1998, Tortora & Grabowski 1993). These two factors (the tissue swelling more than the mucus) result in a decreased patency of the nasal airway. When there is a decreased nasal patency this induces an increased respiratory rate with multiple sequelae (Chaitow 2004), including forward head posture (Hiyama et al 2002, Roithmann et al 2005) and anterior translation of the mandible (Shikata et al 2004).

Anterior translation of the mandible creates shear at the highly innervated temporomandibular joint (TMJ) that interferes with the forward head posture already driven by the food allergy, contributing to an upper crossed syndrome postural imbalance (Janda 1982) (see description in Chapter 6 and Fig. 6.33 for detail of crossed syndromes).

In forward head posture, the tone of the suboccipital group is reflexively upregulated to keep the eyes on the optic plane (in line with the horizon). The resulting increase in tone in the suboccipital group (rectus capitis posterior minor in particular) invokes the tonic neck reflex, meaning that the tone of the hamstrings automatically becomes upregulated (Fukuda 1984, McPartland et al 1997). If this hypothetical individual then sprints or plays a sport, a hamstring strain is likely to occur due to excessive or inappropriate tone. Any injury resulting in pain – including a hamstring strain – induces a stress response, which increases forward head posture (the fetal or 'red-light' posture), reinforcing shear at the TMJ, adverse tone in the suboccipitals, increased tone in the hamstrings and a modified respiratory pattern. Such additional stress on the bodily systems as a whole increases adrenal output (Selye 1956) and automatically increases cardiorespiratory rate that, if sustained, is likely to result in respiratory alkalosis, relative tissue hypoxia and ischemia, and increased formation of trigger points (Chaitow 2004), which – in tandem with forward head posture – involves the upper fibers of trapezius, sternocleidomastoid (SCM), levator scapula and/or the suboccipitals with tracking of the disc within the TMJ. This shear increases afferent drive to the trigeminal nucleus and this afferent bombardment causes increased neural drive to the SCM and upper portion of trapezius, via the trigemino-accessory reflex (Di Lazzaro et al 1996).

Increased tone in these two muscle (SCM and upper trapezius) groups reinforces forward head posture, leading to further loading through this muscle group. Forward head posture creates an incremental load on these neck extensors by a factor of 1 for each inch (2.5 cm) the head migrates forward (Chek & Curl 1994). This means that if the normal load on the neck extensors was, say, 7 lb (~3 kg) (the center of gravity of the head is anterior to the spine, meaning that even in optimal posture there is a load on the neck extensors), then a forward head posture of 2 inches (5 cm) – which is extremely common clinically – would result in a load of 21 lb (~9 kg) through the neck extensors. Since it only takes a contraction of 10% of the maximum voluntary contraction to induce ischemia in a muscle (Chek & Curl 1994), a forward head posture of 2 inches not only triples the load on the neck extensors, but also increases metabolic demand, while concurrently causing ischemic changes in the muscles concerned. As a result, metabolic waste such as lactic acid and pyruvate will accumulate in, and damage, the working muscles (Chaitow 2004). This process is likely to cause muscle and joint distress as well as contributing to the formation of myofascial trigger points.

This scenario illustrates how simply applying soft tissue techniques or ultrasound to a hamstring strain, or using ischemic pressure or spray and stretch techniques to deactivate a trigger point in the trapezius, may be, at best, a temporary solution, or, at worst, futile, unless underlying dysfunctional patterns and causative factors (including nutritional ones) are also addressed.

Complexity

The three examples outlined above illustrate complexity and synchronous processes that inevitably result in symptoms. Understanding the underlying etiological influences allows the practitioner – naturopathic or other – to advise appropriately and/or intervene therapeutically to enhance the self-regulating processes. Inappropriate interventions may well modify or suppress symptoms, but not necessarily to the advantage of ultimate well-being.

Identifying what is and what is not appropriate in any given situation depends on information gathering and assessment skills, as well as an awareness of the probable natural evolutionary order of events in relation to the particular patient, with idiosyncratic characteristics. Part of that understanding involves what has become known in naturopathic medicine as the 'hierarchy of healing' or 'therapeutic order' seen within the context of a broader theory, encompassing naturopathic principles and tenets such as the naturopathic model of healing, the determinants of health, and other tenets defining the processes in the disease and healing process. This theory is described by Zeff and others as 'the process of healing' and is discussed below. It is important to be aware that this 'order' remains a work in progress as the naturopathic profession evolves its understanding of the complex processes involved.

Figures 1.2 and 1.3 offer relatively simplistic pictorial representations of the complex interactions associated with the progression from health towards ill-health and dysfunction (see also Figs 9.1 and 9.2 in Chapter 9).

The healing power of nature and a therapeutic order

These three examples offer pictures of normal health being disturbed by a variety of factors, where a virtual

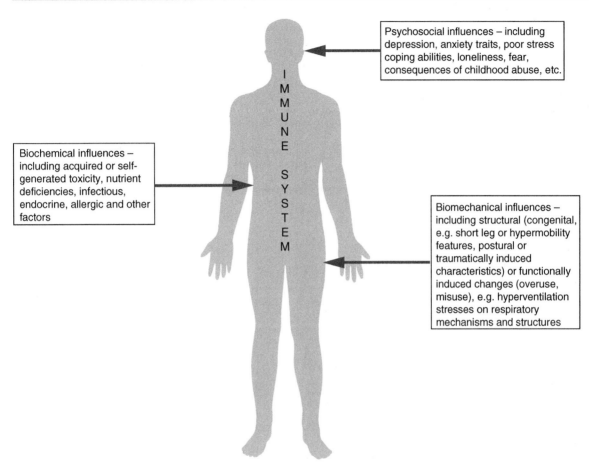

Psychosocial influences – including depression, anxiety traits, poor stress coping abilities, loneliness, fear, consequences of childhood abuse, etc.

Biochemical influences – including acquired or self-generated toxicity, nutrient deficiencies, infectious, endocrine, allergic and other factors

Biomechanical influences – including structural (congenital, e.g. short leg or hypermobility features, postural or traumatically induced characteristics) or functionally induced changes (overuse, misuse), e.g. hyperventilation stresses on respiratory mechanisms and structures

IMMUNE SYSTEM

Figure 1.2 The interacting influences of a biochemical, biomechanical and psychosocial nature produce complex changes. For example, a negative emotional state produces specific biochemical changes, modifies immune response and alters muscle tone. A biomechanical function such as breathing, when dysfunction (hyperventilation) modifies blood pH, alters neural function, creates feelings of apprehension and anxiety, and causes smooth muscle constriction, so altering circulatory and digestive efficiency. Nutritional imbalances, or acquired or self-generated toxicity, modify biochemical status, affecting mood, which can modify respiratory function, with all the changes listed above. Reproduced with permission from Chaitow (2003)

chain reaction of symptom-inducing events follows logically, as the human system attempts to maintain functionality in the face of adaptive demands that seem to be overwhelming.

The task of the naturopathic physician/practitioner is to identify and understand these disturbances and to then assist the patient to remove or moderate them (or some of them) and/or to improve the ability to cope with the imposed stressors. In doing so, the cascade of adaptive changes should reduce sufficiently to allow self-regulation to restore health and optimal function. This process has been referred to as 'the naturopathic model of healing' and is intimately related to functions described within a 'hierarchy of healing' or the 'therapeutic order'. One can dissect health disturbance into a number of identifiable categories, based upon those that determine health, and these can be listed as such (Standish et al 2005, Zeff et al 2006).

In facilitating the process of healing, the naturopathic physician/practitioner seeks to use those therapies that are most efficient and that have the least

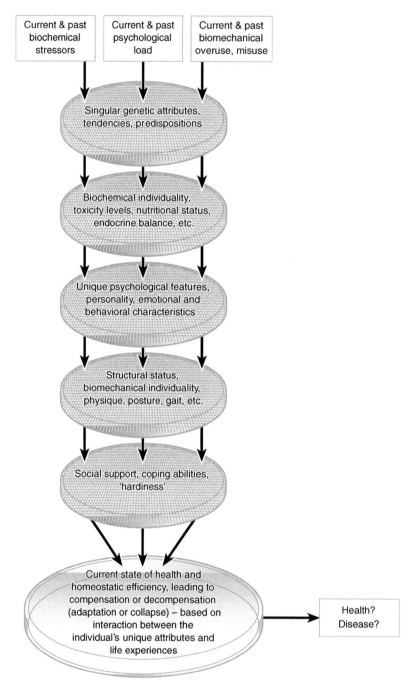

Figure 1.3 Schematic 'life-grid' representing many of the multiple interactions – both acquired and genetic – involved in an individual's progression from health to ill-health. Reproduced with permission from Chaitow (2003)

potential to harm the patient. The concept of 'harm' includes the effects of suppression, or exhaustion, of natural healing processes, including inflammation and fever. These precepts, coupled to an understanding of the process of healing, have resulted in an appreciation of a therapeutic hierarchy.

This hierarchy (or therapeutic order) appears to be a natural consequence of how the organism heals itself. This 'order' also calls for therapeutic modalities to be applied in a rational sequence, determined by the nature of the healing process, partly determined by, and balanced with, the individual needs of the patient for safe and effective care.

It is important at this juncture to state that the 'therapeutic order', as currently expressed (see below), is under constant review and debate by the naturopathic profession, its educators and leading clinicians, and is not by any means fixed in stone. It is to be anticipated, therefore, that aspects of the sequencing, as described below, will modify and change as these ideas are explored in coming years.

Zeff et al (2006) have offered one perspective of a natural order of appropriate therapeutic interventions, embracing the principles outlined above, suggesting that in treating people who are ill it is (or may be) necessary to follow a model of care as laid out in Box 1.3.

Underlying principles of the therapeutic order

The concepts expressed in the naturopathic therapeutic order are derived from Hippocrates' writings and those of medical scholars, nature doctors and naturopathic physicians concerning the function and activation of the self-healing process. The recognition of a sense of order in the healing processes, and in the selection of therapeutic and restorative practices, has permeated the modern dialogue on naturopathic clinical theory, and has evolved to recognize the dynamic interface and balance between a natural therapeutic order and its accommodation to patient individuality.

The therapeutic order proceeds from least to most force, although all modalities can be found within the various steps and stages, depending on their application. The spiritual aspect of the patient's health is considered to begin with Step 1 (Pizzorno & Snider 2004).

The philosophy represented in the naturopathic therapeutic order does not determine what modalities are 'good or bad', useful or useless. Rather, it provides a clinical framework for all modalities, used in the order consistent with that of the natural self-healing process. It respects the origins of disease, as well as

---

Box 1.3 The therapeutic order (modified from Zeff et al 2006)

1. **Address acute concerns**
2. **Re-establish the basis for health**
   Identify and remove causes of disease and obstacles to healing:
   • establish a healthy regime
   • identify and modify or eliminate adaptive demands (biochemical, biomechanical, psychosocial) and initiate enhancement of adaptive capacity of tissues, systems, and the individual.
3. **Stimulate the *vis medicatrix naturae*** (healing power of nature)
   Many systems and modalities incorporate methods that have the potential to stimulate the inherent self-regulating processes. Examples include botanical, homeopathic and/or nutritional approaches; physical/structural methods including therapeutic exercise, manipulation, massage, etc.; hydrotherapy, psychological–spiritual medicine, Ayurvedic, Tibetan, Traditional Chinese Medicine, acupuncture.
4. **Tonify weakened systems**
   Many systems and modalities have system-specific strategies (botanical, homeopathic and/or nutritional approaches; physical/structural methods including therapeutic exercise, manipulation, massage, etc.; hydrotherapy, psychological–spiritual medicine, Ayurvedic, Tibetan, Traditional Chinese Medicine, acupuncture and others). Examples of objectives are to:
   • strengthen the immune system
   • decrease toxicity
   • normalize inflammatory processes
   • optimize metabolic function
   • balance regulatory systems
   • enhance regeneration
   • harmonize with the life force.
5. **Prescribe specific natural substances**: Appropriate modalities or interventions.
6. **Prescribe specific pharmacological or synthetic substances**: Appropriate modalities or interventions.
7. **Use higher force interventions**: Examples are surgery, suppressive drugs, radiation, chemotherapy and other approaches.

Note: The actual therapeutic order may change depending on the individual patient's needs and unique characteristics.

the applications of care and interventions necessary for health and healing with the least force.

The therapeutic order schematically directs the naturopathic practitioner's therapeutic choices in an efficient order, based on individual patient needs and priorities for safe and effective care, rather than using a 'shotgun' approach. It is this common philosophy and theory that both distinguishes the field of modern naturopathic medicine and enables it to consider and incorporate new therapies (Pizzorno & Snider 2004).

Practical example

To express these theories in practical form, a simple example may be illustrative:

- A fall or strain results in tissue damage.
- The damage (tear, break, sprain) may have been 'caused' by the fall or strain, but the scale of damage will be dependent on many other factors, including age, degree of fitness, relative stability/instability/vulnerability of the area and tissues affected, the individual's nutritional status, the surface onto which the fall occurred – and more.
- In simple cases, addressing the acute strain or break would probably be sufficient – immobilizing and possibly compressing the damaged tissues, use of ice, elevation, etc.
- However, in cases of recurrent strains or breaks, or where such an injury does not heal as rapidly as expected, a naturopath would be expected to look more deeply into all of the determining factors and make a variety of corrections and suggestions (possibly involving nutritional, stability, flexibility, balance, postural, ergonomic, psychosocial and other factors) following the therapeutic order.

The words synchronicity or 'simultaneity' (Jung 1973) can be used to describe this way of viewing patterns and events. Such spatial thinking – which mirrors much naturopathic clinical decision-making – may represent the most effective way of evaluating health problems, avoiding naive cause–effect (and 'cure') considerations. It may be useful to now examine these considerations with specific reference to naturopathic physical medicine (which is explained in greater detail in Chapter 4).

Derivation – naturopathy's antecedents

'The bulk of professional naturopathic clinical theory' in the USA, subsequent to the establishment of natu-

ropathic medicine in the USA, 'was to be found in Benedict Lust's magazines: *Herald of Health* and *The Naturopath*' (Zeff et al 2006). These publications displayed the prodigious writings of Lust, but did not contain a comprehensive and definitive statement of either philosophy or clinical theory. Lust often stated that all natural therapies fell under the purview of naturopathy.

He stated for example:

Naturopathy is the mother, all inclusive, of natural therapy. It is the basic platform of all methods of healing . . . (Lust 1925)

and

Naturopathy is a distinct school of healing, employing the beneficent agency of Nature's forces, of water, air, sunlight, earthpower, electricity, magnetism, exercise, rest, proper diet, various kinds of mechanical treatments, such as massage, osteopathy, and chiropractic, mental and moral science . . . As none of these agents of rejuvenation can cure every disease, the Naturopath rightly employs the combination that is best adapted to each individual case . . . (Lust 1918, Kirchfeld & Boyle 1994)

There were also several other defining texts used by the emerging profession. These included:

- Henry Lindlahr MD's seven volume *Natural Therapeutics*, published in the 1910s and 1920s.
- *Nature Cure* (1913) by Lindlahr is considered a seminal work in naturopathic theory, laying the groundwork for a systematic approach to naturopathic treatment and diagnosis.
- Lindlahr ultimately presented the most coherent naturopathic theory extant, summarized in his *Catechism of Naturopathy* (1913), which presented a five-part therapeutic progression:
    1. 'Return to Nature' – which meant paying attention to the basics of diet, dress, exercise, rest, etc.
    2. Elementary remedies – water, air, light, electricity
    3. Chemical remedies – botanicals, homeopathy, etc.
    4. Mechanical remedies – manipulations, massage, etc.
    5. Mental/spiritual remedies – prayer, positive thinking, doing good works, etc. (Zeff et al 2006).

Early 20th century texts that influenced naturopathic thinking also included Macfadden's five volume *Encyclopedia of Physical Culture* published in 1918.

Additional literature emerged:

- In the US, Spitler wrote *Basic Naturopathy, a Textbook* (1948), and Wendel, *Standardized Naturopathy* (1951). These books presented the somewhat opposing perspectives of the more science-based, or 'green allopathic', and the purist 'nature cure' camps.
- Kutts-Cheraux's *Naturopathic Materia Medica* (1953) was produced to satisfy a statutory demand by the Arizona legislature, but as one of the few extant guides persists.
- A number of earlier texts have been relied upon, many of which arose from the German hydrotherapy practitioners (Kneipp 1889, 1891, 1894, Rausse 1838, Rikli 1869, Trall 1851) or the Eclectic school of medicine (a refinement and expansion of the earlier 'Thomsonian' system of medicine; Beach 1848, Boyle 1988, Ellingwood 1919, Felter 1922, Thomson 1821) that predated the formal American naturopathic profession (1896).

The history of naturopathic medicine in general and naturopathic physical medicine in particular are described more fully in Chapter 3.

It is out of this background that current concepts and practices have emerged, including identification by the North American naturopathic profession of the principles and therapeutic order, as discussed above.

Naturopathic physical medicine
(see Chapter 4)

Naturopathic physical medicine:

- is the practice of physical medicine, in the context of naturopathic medicine
- integrates both scientific knowledge in physical medicine and the principles of naturopathic medicine into a distinct approach to physical medicine practice.

Core components

1. A respect for the traditional and empirical naturopathic approach to knowledge of the physical aspect of the human being in health and disease.
2. Recognition of the value of individualization of therapy and constitutional needs.
3. A concentration on holistic diagnosis and the interaction of all bodily systems.

4. Having the general therapeutic goal of enhancement of self-regulating systems and mechanisms (*vis medicatrix naturae*).

Features of naturopathic physical medicine

A central concept that distinguishes naturopathic physical medicine from other forms of manual medicine is the perception of a vitalistic organism, seen to be adapting to inherited and acquired stressors, ultimately becoming symptomatic as a result of failure to manage this load, and then requiring holistic assessment and diagnosis, followed by sensitive, minimal, physical medicine (and other naturopathic) interventions to stimulate self-regulation (*vis medicatrix naturae*) in order to restore or enhance functionality and well-being.

The variety of eclectic modalities and methods used by NPM to achieve these ends are summarized and discussed in some detail in Chapter 4 (Introduction to NPM), Chapter 5 (Assessment and palpation approaches), Chapter 7 (NPM modalities), Chapter 8 (Constitutional approaches), Chapter 9 (Rehabilitation and re-education), Chapter 10 (Specific conditions), Chapter 11 (Hydrotherapy) and Chapter 12 (Electrotherapy).

Each of the modalities/methods incorporated into NPM has been shown to be effective and safe when utilized appropriately. Even when degenerative processes have progressed beyond a stage where realistic anticipation exists for the restoration of normal function, the authors suggest that clinical experience has demonstrated that NPM has the potential to alleviate pain, modulate dysfunction and encourage functionality.

For example, an individualized protocol combining – as appropriate to the person involved and their current condition – mind–body approaches/stress management (Berman & Singh 1997, Lundgren & Stenstrom 1999, Stevens 2005), nutritional strategies (Egger et al 1983, Gottlieb 1997, Maheu et al 1998), use of botanical substances (Ernst & Chrubasik 2000, Mills et al 1996), manual methods (Bonfort 1999, Brattberg 1999, Garfinkel et al 1994; see Chapters 7 and 8), exercise and education (Fitzcharles et al 2006, Gowans et al 1998; see Chapter 9), acupuncture and/or moxibustion (Berman et al 1999, Ernst & White 1998), hydrotherapy (Evcik et al 2002, Faull 2005, Mannerkorpi et al 2000; see Chapter 11) and/or electrotherapy (McMakin 1998, 2004; see Chapter 12) can be significantly beneficial in treatment of patients with conditions as diverse as low back pain, migraine, fibromyalgia and degenerative joint disease.

As will become clear, particularly in Chapters 7, 8, 9 and 10, a wide range of general health problems, often of a severe life-threatening nature, ranging from acute pneumonia in the hospitalized elderly (Noll et al 2000) to pancreatitis (Radjieski et al 1998) and postsurgical recovery problems, can all be shown to benefit from a variety of physical medicine interventions that encourage self-regulatory functions (O-Yurvati et al 2005).

It is worth reflecting on the potential for patient benefit of this wide range of approaches, all of which are selectively employed in naturopathic physical medicine, within a context that treats the person not the disease, and which relies on inherent, endogenous, self-healing potentials for health enhancement.

As mentioned above, treatment approaches for specific conditions are discussed in Chapter 10.

The meaning of symptoms

Within the framework of naturopathic thinking there exists an appreciation that symptoms are frequently evidence of self-regulation in action – to be understood, respected, assisted and possibly modulated if excessive (inflammation is a clear example) – and ideally not to be suppressed (Lindlahr 1913).

Pain, arguably the most common symptom of all, epitomizes the need to understand the sources and mechanisms involved, and the processes associated with its origin and maintenance. Merely suppressing pain without such understanding, and where possible the taking of appropriate action to relieve symptoms and remove causes, is a prescription for chronicity.

Pain may represent:

- a warning (hand touches a flame)
- a caution not to move the area (due to a tear, a break or a process of degeneration)
- part of a protective process
- a signal that repair is underway (inflammation, etc.)
- a remnant of past trauma or dysfunction that has little current relevance (e.g. post-herpes pain)
- evidence of neural sensitization or other forms of neurologically mediated distress or pathology
- reflexogenic activity (viscerosomatic, somaticovisceral, myofascial trigger point, etc.).

Pain and the mind

Pain may also have many other possible (e.g. psychogenic) meanings.

Understanding the processes involved in the production and maintenance of pain (or other symptoms) is clearly desirable in making clinical choices; however, if naturopathic principles are to be applied these should always go beyond the obvious and should include not only the structural/physical aspects of the problem but also biochemical and psychosocial contextual ramifications and influences.

A comprehensive review (Linton 2000) of over 900 studies involving back and neck pain concluded that psychological factors play a significant role, not only in chronic pain but also in the etiology of acute pain – particularly in the process of transition to chronicity:

Stress, distress or anxiety as well as mood and emotions, cognitive functioning, and pain behaviour all were found to be significant in the analysis of 913 potentially relevant articles.

In an athletic (or any other) injury setting the need to consider both the context and all aspects of the individual and the injury event becomes obvious. Crown et al (1997) have observed:

Both extrinsic and intrinsic factors can increase the risk of injury. Extrinsic factors include training errors, faulty technique, poor environmental conditions, incorrect equipment and surfaces. Intrinsic factors include biomechanical deficiencies including malalignment of limbs, muscular imbalances, degenerative processes, and other anatomical factors.

A fuller list of additional factors might also include nutritional imbalances, past and present pathological processes, adaptive changes to previous injury or repetitive microtrauma, etc.

Specific examples will be offered in later chapters, emphasizing the naturopathic approaches to such common features as restriction and pain, as well as the wider range of conditions that are treated using naturopathic physical medicine approaches.

Beyond biomechanical dysfunction

Naturopathic physical medicine is also employed in the treatment of patients with a wide range of diseases, unrelated to obvious biomechanical problems.

As in other manual medicine settings, NPM commonly focuses on obvious structural, physical, biomechanical pain and dysfunction; however, the modalities and methods used can – as in physiotherapy, osteopathy and chiropractic – also be beneficially used in the treatment of patients presenting with a variety of general health problems.

Massage and general health

Amongst the most widely beneficial manual methods of treatment commonly incorporated into naturopathic care is traditional massage therapy, which has been shown in numerous research studies to have value in the care of conditions as diverse as pregnancy, prematurity, ADHD, autism, stroke, leukemia and low back pain – offering as it does relief from psychological distress, stress modulation, enhanced sleep, mood and behavior, improved circulation and lymphatic flow, better bowel and breathing function, and raised immunity – among many other benefits (Field 2000, Rich 2002).

The studies listed and/or discussed in Chapters 7 and 8 provide a small selection from those described in *Massage Therapy Research* (2006) by Tiffany Field PhD, of the Touch Research Institute, University of Miami Medical School.

Osteopathic and chiropractic treatment and general health

Modalities deriving from osteopathic medicine have demonstrated the value of osteopathic manipulative therapy (OMT) in a wide range of pathological settings (see discussions in Chapters 7 and 8).

As will become evident in subsequent chapters, particularly Chapters 4 and 7, the soft tissue modalities that are discussed as being appropriate and useful in NPM settings include those employed in the osteopathic studies listed in Chapter 7. These include muscle energy technique (MET), positional release technique (PRT) and myofascial release (MFR), as well as general joint mobilization and high velocity, low amplitude (HVLA) thrust methods, where appropriate. A number of well-conducted studies have also shown the benefit of HVLA thrust in chiropractic practice in the treatment of conditions such as infantile colic and pyloric stenosis (Fallon 1994).

Some of the many studies in which OMT and chiropractic manipulation methods have been employed with benefit in the treatment of patients with serious pathological conditions are discussed in Chapters 7 and 8.

In addition, methods developed in physical therapy, such as mobilization with movement (MWM), McKenzie rehabilitation exercises and supportive ('unloading') taping methods, are all suitable for use in a naturopathic practice (see Chapter 7).

All or any of the methods used in these and numerous other studies would be appropriate in a naturopathic setting, as part of a comprehensive therapeutic approach.

Are all 'natural' modalities necessarily naturopathic?

In general health settings a person may effectively reduce digestive distress by using, say, peppermint or chamomile infusions, or by taking mastic capsules or probiotics. However, unless the reasons for the digestive distress are also evaluated and addressed, such methods could be described as 'green allopathy', where 'natural' substances are used in a symptom-focused manner.

While it is true that taking these substances would probably carry less risk of side-effects than use of over-the-counter pharmacological medication, such treatment approaches would nevertheless fail to meet basic naturopathic requirements. The concept of *tolle causum* (identify and treat the cause, as discussed earlier in this chapter) requires further evaluation if a naturopathic approach is to be true to its principles. Examination from a naturopathic physical medicine perspective may reveal facilitated mid-thoracic spinal segments (see Box 2.2 for discussion of segmental facilitation) contributing significantly to digestive distress, or poor posture might be contributing to crowding of the abdominal organs (see notes under the subheading 'Postural adaptation influences on visceral and somatic function' on page 42 for discussion of the influence of posture on visceral function).

Additionally or alternatively, emotional distress might be a key feature in the etiology of digestive distress, or an unbalanced dietary pattern may be implicated. Whichever of these (or other) factors is identified as being part of the etiology, the use of peppermint or chamomile infusions to ease the symptoms would not be dealing with cause.

Objectives and methods

Naturopathic physical medicine can be defined by its comprehensive objectives, as well as by the context in which it employs safe and effective modalities. Such approaches demand focus on the processes involved, and the context and etiology of the presenting symptoms.

Essential requirements need to be considered and, if possible, met in naturopathic patient management:

- Causes need to be comprehensively addressed. It is worth emphasizing at this point that the causes of disease and dysfunction, as perceived by naturopathic medicine, might include a variety of constitutional features such as toxicity, organ dysfunction, endocrine imbalance, lowered general vitality, nutritional deficiencies and more. The broad scope of 'causes' will be more fully outlined in relation to specific conditions in Chapter 10.
- An inclusive assessment should be made of, and selective attention given to, those components of dysfunction that best meet the patient's current needs.

- A preventive educational and/or rehabilitative element needs to be incorporated as a standard aspect of naturopathic physical medicine.

Note: There is no suggestion implied that other health care disciplines do not also seek causes; however, the principles of naturopathic medicine demand a primary attention to context and the processes involved in symptom manifestation (e.g. lowered vitality, organ dysfunction, nutritional imbalance, toxicity), as well as the more obvious etiological features of any given condition.

Non-naturopathic manual methods

Examples of manual medicine approaches that offer short-term gain, without consideration of the context out of which the symptoms have emerged, can be described for almost all modalities. This is the case when they are applied in isolation, outside of a comprehensive contextual evaluation of the patient's broader symptoms and needs.

Massage therapy for example (or forms of hydrotherapy or aromatherapy) might well represent safe, effective, non-specific interventions that reduce feelings of anxiety, enhance sleep and reduce sympathetic arousal – encouraging self-regulation. However, these methods will not be being employed naturopathically unless the causes of the individual's health problems are also addressed, and preventive methods considered and discussed. Simple examples might include cases of anxiety, treated by means of massage and/or aromatherapy, without recourse to attention to the underlying causes of the anxiety state (Cooke & Ernst 2000, Field et al 1996).

This suggests that much that is currently done in massage therapy, chiropractic, osteopathic and physical therapy settings may fail to meet the basic naturopathic requirements of dealing with the whole person and the causes of their problems. If naturopaths mimic symptom-oriented approaches in dealing with musculoskeletal dysfunction they are not living up to the core principles on which their profession is based. Box 1.4 compares and contrasts the major health professions using physical medicine.

What methods and modalities form naturopathic physical medicine?

Most of the treatment and rehabilitation methods and techniques employed in physiotherapy (physical therapy), osteopathy and chiropractic, as well as massage and the wide range of other soft tissue and movement methods and modalities (including hydro-

therapy and electrotherapy), are commonly used in naturopathic practice, although few of the methods used in NPM actually originated in naturopathic settings. An exception is neuromuscular technique (NMT) which is described and illustrated in Chapters 5, 7 and 8.

A method or modality is seen to be 'naturopathic', less by its *form* than by its *intent*, mode of operation and the *context* in which it is applied, i.e. the general state of health of the patient and the nature of the pathology or dysfunction, as well as the state of the tissues requiring attention – are they inflamed, hypertonic, in spasm, edematous, etc.?

This points to the fact that the same modality may be used either allopathically or naturopathically – depending largely on the context in which it is employed, the intent behind its use and the condition of the person to whom (as well as the tissues to which) it is being applied.

A structural example will suffice at this stage (see Chapters 4, 7, 8 and 9 for more detailed analysis of this topic):

- High velocity, low amplitude (HVLA) thrust is a major tool in chiropractic and osteopathic medicine, as well as increasingly in physical (physio) therapy (see Box 1.5 for a detailed statement as to what constitutes manipulative therapy as viewed from a naturopathic perspective).
- In the context of an intra-articular restriction that has failed to respond to gentler soft tissue and movement therapy approaches, and in the absence of contraindications to its use, an HVLA thrust may be an effective means of restoring functionality to a joint. This would be seen as offering a naturopathic solution to a problem if used as part of a comprehensive approach to the needs of the tissues and the person.
- The same thrust, utilized without recourse to prior soft tissue treatment (which may well make the thrust redundant), used in a setting contraindicated for a forceful thrust (possibly due to age or state of the tissues) or as an end in itself (i.e. mobilize ('adjust') the joint and nothing else), or where careful analysis of risk/benefit factors has not been considered or the patient was fearful of the procedure, would not be considered naturopathic.
- The use of an HVLA thrust to successfully mobilize a restricted joint, where no attempt was made to identify and remedy etiological features, would equally not fully match naturopathic requirements.

Box 1.4 Comparison and contrast between the major health professions using physical medicine

Paul Orrock ND DO

- **Biomedicine**
- **Chiropractic medicine**
- **Naturopathic medicine**
- **Osteopathic medicine**
- **Physiotherapy/physical therapy**
- **Traditional Chinese Medicine**
- **Ayurvedic medicine**

Preamble

What is 'medicine'? Medicine is:

- *the science of diagnosing, treating, or preventing disease and other damage to the body or mind* (www.thefreedictionary.com/medicine)
- *the art and science of the diagnosis, treatment, and prevention of disease and the maintenance of good health* (Mosby's Medical Dictionary 1998).

Practicing a system of medicine (as opposed to a therapy, modality or technique) requires an established diagnostic and therapeutic methodology, and core training in that identifiable style of medicine.

Therapies and techniques are open for all practitioners to use unless:

- limited by law in a jurisdiction (e.g. Australian States limit spinal manipulation to registered medical practitioners, osteopaths, chiropractors and physiotherapists)
- there is no evidence of having trained in the safe and appropriate use of the therapy/technique (Jonas & Levin 1999).

Biomedicine

Features of the biomedical profession:

- Specific therapy is employed that is antagonistic to a specific condition/disease.
- Clinical practice attempts to be evidence based in a biomedical science foundation.

The use of many physical medicine techniques by a practitioner of biomedicine may be limited by the uncertain answers to the questions:

- What is the condition? *and*
- What is the evidence base for certain therapies (e.g. spinal manipulation) for that condition?

Chiropractic medicine

Traditional features of this profession are as follows (Redwood 1997):

- The diagnosis of subluxation – at a specific spinal segment
- Diagnosed by plain radiographs and palpation

- The neurological model of compression and dysfunction
- The goal of treatment is to balance neural function by correcting subluxation.

There are modern developments in chiropractic that are more complex, subtle, 'reprogramming' approaches (e.g. bio-energetic synchronization technique, BEST).

Naturopathic medicine

- Identifies individual maladaptive response, failing adaptation (i.e. suboptimal system/organ function; reduced self-regulatory potential)
- Leading to acute and chronic illnesses, toxicity.

Therapeutic approach is to support self-regulation via nutrition, botanical substances, homeopathy, lifestyle and holistic physical therapies.

Osteopathic medicine

- Diagnoses somatic dysfunction – circulatory/neural/lymph effects.

Manual treatment/strategies to encourage normal function = decrease somatic dysfunction. Treatment of immune and organ dysfunction.

Physiotherapy/physical therapy

- Physiotherapy is concerned with human function and movement, maximizing potential.

Uses science-based physical approaches to promote, maintain and restore well-being, and to speed healing, rehabilitation and prevent recurrence.

Traditional Chinese Medicine and Ayurvedic medicine

- Identify constitutional types with imbalanced energy as a feature of ill-health.

Therapeutic interventions aim to balance flow and distribution of energy by natural methods.

Case example

A 42-year-old male presented with mid-thoracic pain and stiffness following increased manual labor. Most of the seven practitioners from the listed professions utilized spinal manipulation of the T6/7 segment. What was their rationale for this use, and what else might they do?

- *Biomedicine*: Anti-inflammatory and/or analgesic medication for pain relief, and/or referral to physiotherapist or (increasingly) a chiropractor or osteopath.
- *Chiropractic medicine*: The straight/traditional approach would treat a radiologically defined subluxation – manipulated for all related T6/7 functions to be healthy and to prevent disease. Modern chiropractic approaches

Continued

Box 1.4 Comparison and contrast between the major health professions using physical medicine *continued*

would include rehabilitation and postural soft tissue-based therapies (Liebenson 2006).

- *Naturopathic medicine*: Manipulation to relieve regional muscle spasm and immobility that is seen to be negatively influencing physical vitality and adaptive energy. All appropriate areas would be treated using massage, manipulation, physical methods including hydrotherapy and/or electrotherapy – with attention to ergonomics, posture and use patterns. Attention would be offered to lifestyle and occupational activities that might be stressing the area, including respiratory function. Considerations would be given to possible nutritional influences.
- *Osteopathic medicine* (Ward 1996): Focus would be on segmental/articulation and soft tissue-based dysfunction, with altered range of motion and tender tissue changes, treated with multiple manual and exercise methods to influence function at a circulatory, neural (visceral and somatic – viscerosomatic facilitation concepts) and lymphatic level, aimed to enhance function = optimal health.

- *Physiotherapy/physical therapy* (The Physiotherapy Site Network): Soft tissue and joint diagnosis and general identified stiffness, treated with application of evidence-based manual exercise (e.g. Maitland (Maitland et al 2001), Mulligan (1999) and/or McKenzie (1981) methods) and electrotherapies (e.g. ultrasound), in order to change local findings and pain. Exercise prescription to stabilize and mobilize.
- *Traditional Chinese Medicine* and *Ayurvedic medicine* (incorporating yoga therapy): Diagnosis of constitutional and energy imbalances, with treatment to balance these, some local manual massage and manipulation and/or acupuncture to remove obstacles to flow of energy; balanced flow = health and prevention of disease.

All or any of the professions listed might incorporate or refer aspects of Pilates methodology, yoga, Alexander technique and other movement-based modalities, techniques and systems.

Avoiding adaptive overload

Almost all modalities and techniques used in NPM (ranging from massage to specific soft tissue methods, exercise, movement, hydrotherapy or electrotherapy) can be shown, in particular situations, contexts and patients, to be undesirable, to be imposing undue adaptive demands or to carry unnecessary risks of 'doing harm' – the avoidance of which is one of the defining features of naturopathic medicine.

Needless to say, almost all other disciplines also express a desire to avoid harm; however, the definition as to what constitutes harm is likely to differ from that of naturopathy, where 'harm' is seen to embrace failure to comprehensively deal with underlying causative features including nutrition, lifestyle and emotion. Treating symptoms, and possibly relieving or removing these short term, without due attention to etiology, is tantamount to doing harm.

Reference back to basic principles, as outlined earlier in this chapter, can usually determine just how naturopathic, or non-naturopathic, a treatment approach is.

Is the therapeutic method being used likely to achieve any of the following key objectives?:

1. To reduce adaptive load (e.g. deactivation of a pain-producing, active trigger point, together with attention as to its cause).

2. To enhance functionality (better posture, enhanced breathing function, greater mobility, etc.).
3. To ease symptoms without adding to the patient's adaptive burden (how sensitive and vulnerable, and how far along the road to decompensation, is this individual?).
4. To be working with self-repair, self-regeneration, self-healing processes (see items 1, 2 and 3 above).
5. To be taking account of the whole person, the context, and not just the symptoms (see item 6 below).
6. To be cognisant of where the individual is in the spectrum of adaptation – judging as best possible the current degree of exhaustion and susceptibility (see notes on the Zink & Lawson assessments on page 138), with a rule-of-thumb guideline that the more complicated the condition, the more vulnerable the individual, the less that should be done therapeutically at any given time.
7. To deal with causes where possible – for example, symptomatic headache relief by means of gentle release of suboccipital muscles, and/or trigger point deactivation, and/or mobilization of upper cervical restrictions, would be followed by addressing

Box 1.5 Position Paper of AANP (Buratovich et al 2006)

Nick Buratovich ND, Michael Cronin ND,
MA Perry ND et al

Extracts from a Position Paper on Naturopathic
Manipulative Therapy, by the American Association of
Naturopathic Physicians (AANP), have been listed
below.

These extracts demonstrate how the naturopathic
profession in North America perceives physical
medicine, in the context of its broader scope of practice.
The Position statement notes that:

• 'Naturopathic physical medicine', including
  'naturopathic manipulative treatment' (NMT), has
  historically been an integral part of the practice of
  naturopathic medicine and has been included in
  naturopathic medical education and licensure since
  the first naturopathic college (1902).

• Naturopathic physicians use appropriate diagnostic
  and imaging methods with physical medicine
  modalities and procedures as part of an integrated
  approach to the diagnosis and treatment of the full
  spectrum of health disorders, and the optimization of
  structure and function in healthy individuals, including
  but not limited to the musculoskeletal/postural,
  nervous, circulatory, respiratory, metabolic,
  psychosocial and bioenergetic systems.

• Naturopathic physical medicine is the therapeutic use
  by naturopathic physicians of the physical agents of
  air, water, heat, cold, sound, light and the physical
  modalities/procedures including but not limited to
  hydrotherapy, electrotherapy, diathermy, ultrasound,

ultraviolet, infrared and low level laser light, therapeutic
exercise, naturopathic manipulative treatment and the
use of needling and injection therapies, including dry
needling, regenerative injection therapy (prolotherapy),
mesotherapy, neural therapy and myofascial trigger
point therapy.

• Naturopathic manipulative treatment (NMT) is
  treatment by manual and other mechanical means
  of all body tissues and structures, including bones,
  fascia, muscles, tendons, ligaments, joint capsules,
  bursa, tendon sheaths, visceral organs located in
  the spine, cranium, thoraco-abdominal cavity and
  extremities by naturopathic physicians. These manual
  and mechanical techniques involve the use of
  oscillation, thrust and sustained tension including but
  not limited to high and low velocity techniques, high
  and low amplitude techniques, traction, mobilization
  through physiological and extra-physiological ranges of
  motion, including passive intrinsic mobility of all body
  joints, and repositioning of displaced body tissues and
  organs.

• Naturopathic medical education includes naturopathic
  physical medicine and manipulative treatment in
  courses devoted specifically to NPM and NMT and
  integrated with other courses and clinical experience
  and prepares NDs to competently perform NPM and
  NMT, to recognize the limits of their skills, understand
  the risks, contraindications and limitations of the
  modality and to refer patients to specialists when
  appropriate.

postural and use patterns (aspects of the
adaptive demands) that may have produced or
contributed to these changes. In addition,
possible nutritional, toxicity, lifestyle (e.g.
inadequate sleep or exercise) and psychological
influences would be considered.

8. To do no harm.

These objectives represent the major principles on
which naturopathic physical medicine is based.

The processes of adaptation, maladaptation, compensation and decompensation are described and
discussed in Chapter 2, with the intention of providing insights into naturopathic thinking in terms
of the contextual evolution of dysfunction and disease,
and to therefore reflect on clinical reasoning and
choice of therapeutic options that should naturally
follow.

References

Abelson J, Weg JG, Nesse RM, Curtis GC 2001
Persistent respiratory irregularity in patients with panic
disorder. Biological Psychiatry 49(7):588–595

Alford L 2007 Findings of interest from immunology
and psychoneuroimmunology. Manual Therapy
12(2):176–180

Alverdy J 1990 Effects of glutamine-supplemented diets
on immunology of the gut. Journal of Parenteral
Nutrition 14(4):1095–1135

American Association of Naturopathic Physicians 2006.
www.naturopathic.org

American Association of Naturopathic Physicians 2007.
www.naturopathic.org

Beach W 1848 A treatise on anatomy, physiology and
health. Baker & Scribner, New York

Bengtsson U, Hanson LA, Ahlstedt S 1996 Survey of gastrointestinal reaction to foods in adults in relation to atopy, presence of mucus in the stools, swelling of joints and arthralgia in patients with gastrointestinal reactions in foods. Clinical and Experimental Allergy 26(12):1387–1394

Berman BM, Singh BB 1997 Chronic low back pain: an outcome analysis of a mind–body intervention. Complementary Therapies in Medicine 5:29–35

Berman BM, Singh BB, Lao L et al 1999 A randomized trial of acupuncture as an adjunctive therapy in osteoarthritis of the knee. Rheumatology 38:346–354

Bonfort G 1999 Spinal manipulation, current state of research and its indications. Neurological Clinics of North America 17(1):91–111

Boon HC, Cherkin D, Erro J 2004 Practice patterns of naturopathic physicians: results from a random survey of licensed practitioners in two US States. BMC Complementary and Alternative Medicine 4:14

Borrell-Carrio F, Suchman A, Epstein R 2004 The biopsychosocial model 25 years later: principles, practice, and scientific inquiry. Annals of Family Medicine 2(6):576–582

Boyle W 1988 The herb doctors. Buckeye Naturopathic Press, East Palestine, Ohio

Brattberg G 1999 Connective tissue massage in the treatment of fibromyalgia. European Journal of Pain 3:235–245

Brosschot J 2002 Cognitive–emotional sensitization and somatic health complaints. Scandinavian Journal of Psychology 43:113–121

Brostoff J, Gamlin L 1998 The complete guide to food allergy and intolerance. Bloomsbury, London

Buratovich N, Cronin M, Perry A et al 2006 AANP Position Paper on Naturopathic Manipulative Therapy. American Association of Naturopathic Physicians, Washington DC

Chaitow L 2003 Fibromyalgia syndrome: a practitioner's guide to treatment. Churchill Livingstone, Edinburgh

Chaitow L 2004 Breathing pattern disorders, motor control and low back pain. Journal of Osteopathic Medicine 7(1):33–40

Charney D, Deutch A 1996 Functional neuroanatomy of anxiety and fear. Critical Reviews in Neurobiology 10(3–4):419–446

Chek P, Curl DD 1994 Posture and craniofacial pain. In: Curl DD (ed) Chiropractic approach to head pain. Williams & Wilkins, Baltimore, p 121–162

Cooke B, Ernst E 2000 Aromatherapy for anxiety: a systematic review. British Journal of General Practice 50:493–496

Crago S, Tomasi T 1987 Mucosal antibodies, food allergy and intolerance. Baillière Tindall/WB Saunders, London, p 167–189

Crissinger K, Kvietys P, Granger D 1990 Pathophysiology of gastrointestinal permeability. Journal of Internal Medicine 228:145–154

Crown L, Hizon J, Rodney W 1997 Musculoskeletal injuries in sports: the team physician's handbook. Mosby, St Louis, p 361–370

Damas-Mora J, Davies L, Taylor W, Jenner FA 1980 Menstrual respiratory changes and symptoms. British Journal of Psychiatry 136:492–497

DeGuire S, Gevirtz R, Hawkinson D, Dixon K 1996 Breathing retraining: a three-year follow-up study of treatment for hyperventilation syndrome and associated functional cardiac symptoms. Biofeedback and Self-Regulation 21(2):191–198

Di Lazzaro V, Restuccia D, Nardone R et al 1996 Preliminary clinical observations on a new trigeminal reflex: the trigemino-cervical reflex. Neurology 46(2):479–485

Dunn J, Wilkinson J 2005 Naturopathic management of rheumatoid arthritis. Modern Rheumatology 15(2):87–90

Egger J, Carter CM, Wilson J, Turner MW, Soothill JF 1983 Is migraine food allergy? A double-blind controlled trial of oligoantigenic diet treatment. Lancet 2:865–869

Ellingwood F 1919 Materia medica, therapeutics, and pharmacognosy. Ellingwood's Therapeutist, Evanston, IL

Engel G 1977 The need for a new medical model: a challenge for biomedicine. Science 196:129–136

Ernst E, Chrubasik S 2000 Phyto-anti-inflammatories: a systematic review of randomized, placebo-controlled, double-blind trials. Rheumatic Diseases Clinics of North America 26(1):13–27

Ernst E, White AR 1998 Acupuncture for back pain, metaanalysis. Archives of Internal Medicine 158:2235–2241

Evcik D, Kizilay B, Gokcen E 2002 The effects of balneotherapy on fibromyalgia patients. Rheumatology International 22(2):56–59

Fallon J 1994 Assessing the efficacy of chiropractic care in pediatric cases of pyloric stenosis. International Chiropractic Association: Proceedings of National Conference of Chiropractic and Pediatrics, Arlington VA, p 72

Faull K 2005 Comparison of the effectiveness of Watsu and Aix massage for those with fibromyalgia syndrome: a pilot study. Journal of Bodywork and Movement Therapies 9(3):202–210

Felter H 1922 The eclectic materia medica, pharmacology, and therapeutics. John K Scudder, Cincinnati

Field T 2000 Touch therapy. Churchill Livingstone, Edinburgh

Field T 2006 Massage therapy research. Churchill Livingstone, Edinburgh

Field T, Grizzle N, Scafidi F, Schanberg S 1996 Massage and relaxation therapies' effects on depressed adolescent mothers. Adolescence 31:903–911

Fitzcharles M-A, Almahrezi A, Shir Y 2006 New insights into pain mechanisms. Practical advice on pain management – pain: understanding the challenges for the rheumatologist. Arthritis & Rheumatism Research News Alerts. Posted 01/05/2006 www.interscience.wiley.com/journal/arthritis

Ford MJ, Camilleri MJ, Hanson RB 1995 Hyperventilation, central autonomic control, and colonic tone in humans. Gut 37:499–504

Foster G, Vaziri N, Sassoon C 2001 Respiratory alkalosis. Respiratory Care 46(4):384–391

Fried R 1987 Hyperventilation syndrome. Johns Hopkins University Press, Baltimore

Fukuda T 1984 Statokinetic reflexes in equilibrium and movement. University of Tokyo Press, Tokyo, p 5

Gardner WN 1996 The pathophysiology of hyperventilation disorders. Chest 109:516–534

Garfinkel MS, Schumacher HR, Husain A, Levy M, Reshetar RA 1994 Evaluation of a yoga based regimen for treatment of osteoarthritis of the hands. Journal of Rheumatology 21:2341–2343

George S 1964 Changes in serum calcium, serum phosphate and red cell phosphate during hyperventilation. New England Journal of Medicine 270:726–728

Gottlieb MS 1997 Conservative management of spinal osteoarthritis with glucosamine and chiropractic treatment. Journal of Manipulative and Physiological Therapeutics 20:400–414

Gowans SE, deHueck A, Voss S, Richardson M 1998 A randomized, controlled trial of exercise for fibromyalgia syndrome. Arthritis Care and Research 11:196–209

Heyman M 2005 Gut barrier dysfunction in food allergy. European Journal of Gastroenterology and Hepatology 17(12):1279–1285

Hickman MA 1998 Interventional nutrition for gastrointestinal disease. Clinical Techniques in Small Animal Practice 13(4):211–216

Hiyama S, Ono T, Ishiwata Y, Kuroda T 2002 Effects of mandibular position and body posture on nasal patency in normal awake subjects. Angle Orthodontist 72(6):547–553

Hough HJ, Dower C, O'Neil E 2001 Profile of a profession: naturopathic practice. Center for the Health Professions, San Francisco. University of California, San Francisco

Janda V 1982 Introduction to functional pathology of the motor system. Proceedings of the VII Commonwealth and International Conference on Sport. Physiotherapy in Sport 3:39

Jonas WB, Levin JS (eds) 1999 Essentials of complementary and alternative medicine. Lippincott, Williams and Wilkins, Philadelphia

Jung C-G 1973 Synchronicity: an acausal connecting principle. Princeton University Press, Princeton, NJ

Kirchfeld F, Boyle W 1994 The nature doctors: pioneers in naturopathic medicine. Medicina Biologica, Milan, p 194

Kneipp S 1889 Thus shalt thou live. Kosel, Kempten, Bavaria

Kneipp S 1891 My water-cure. Translation and preface by A deF. Thorsons, Wellingborough (1979 reprint of the 1891 edition)

Kneipp S 1894 My will. Kosel, Kempten, Bavaria

Kutts-Cheraux A (ed) 1953 Naturae medicina and naturopathic dispensatory. American Naturopathic Physicians and Surgeons Association, Washington DC

Liebenson C 2006 Rehabilitation of the spine, 2nd edn. Williams & Wilkins, Baltimore

Lindlahr H 1913 Nature cure: philosophy and practice based on the unity of disease and cure. The Nature Cure Series, Vol. 1. Nature Cure Publishing, Chicago

Linton S 2000 Review of psychological risk factors in back and neck pain. Spine 25:1148–1156

Litchfield PA 2003 Brief overview of the chemistry of respiration and the breathing heart wave. California Biofeedback 19:1

Lum L 1984 Hyperventilation and anxiety states [editorial]. Journal of the Royal Society of Medicine January: 1–4

Lundgren S, Stenstrom CH 1999 Muscle relaxation training and quality of life in rheumatoid arthritis. A randomized controlled clinical trial. Scandinavian Journal of Rheumatology 28:47–53

Lust B 1918 Universal naturopathic encyclopedia, directory and buyers' guide: year book of drugless therapy for 1918–1919. Benedict Lust, Butler, NJ

Lust B 1925 The naturopath. Naturopathic News 30:368

Lutgendorf S, Costanzo E 2003 Psychoneuroimmunology and health psychology: an integrative model. Brain, Behavior and Immunity 17:225–232

Macefield G, Burke D 1991 Paraesthesiae and tetany induced by voluntary hyperventilation. Brain 114:527–540

Maheu E, Mazieres B, Valat J P et al 1998 Symptomatic efficacy of avocado/soybean unsaponifiables in the treatment of osteoarthritis of the knee and hip. Arthritis and Rheumatism 41:81–91

Maitland GP, Hengeveld E, Banks K, English K 2001 Maitland's vertebral manipulation, 6th edn. Butterworth-Heinemann, Oxford

Mannerkorpi K, Nyberg B, Ahlmen M, Ekdahl C 2000 Pool exercise combined with an education program for patients with FMS. A prospective, randomized study. Journal of Rheumatology 10:2473–2481

McCourtie J, Douglas L 1984 Relationship between cell surface composition, adherence, and virulence of Candida albicans. Infection and Immunity 45:6–12

McKenzie R 1981 The lumbar spine: mechanical diagnosis and therapy. Spinal Publications, Waikanae, New Zealand

McMakin C 1998 Microcurrent treatment of myofascial pain in the head, neck and face. Topics in Clinical Chiropractic 5(1):29–35

McMakin C 2004 Microcurrent therapy: a novel treatment method for chronic low back myofascial pain. Journal of Bodywork and Movement Therapies 8:143–153

McPartland J, Brodeur R, Hallgren R 1997 Chronic neck pain, standing balance and suboccipital muscle atrophy – a pilot study. Journal of Manipulative and Physiological Therapeutics 20(1):24–29

Mehling WE, Hamel KA, Acree M et al 2005 Randomized, controlled trial of breath therapy for patients with chronic low-back pain. Alternative Therapies in Health and Medicine 11(4):44–52. See: www.breathexperience.com

Mills SM, Jacoby RK, Chacksfield M et al 1996 Effect of a proprietary herbal medicine on the relief of chronic arthritic pain: a double-blind study. British Journal of Rheumatology 35:874–878

Mosby's medical, nursing and allied health dictionary, 5th edn, 1998. Mosby, St Louis

Mulligan BR 1999 Manual therapy: nags, snags, MWMs, etc., 4th edn. Plane View Services, Wellington, New Zealand

Myers SP, Hunter A, Snider P, Zeff JL 2003 Naturopathic medicine. In: Robson T (ed) An introduction to complementary medicine. Allen & Unwin, Sydney

Neill W, Pantley GA, Nakornchai V 1981 Respiratory alkalemia during exercise reduces angina threshold. Chest 80(2):149–153

Newman Turner R 1984 Naturopathic medicine. Thorsons, Wellingborough

Nixon P, Andrews J 1996 A study of anaerobic threshold in chronic fatigue syndrome (CFS). Biological Psychology 43(3):264

Noll D, Shores J, Gamber R et al 2000 Benefits of osteopathic manipulative treatment for hospitalized elderly patients with pneumonia. Journal of the American Osteopathic Association 100(12):776–782

Ott H et al 2006 Symptoms of premenstrual syndrome may be caused by hyperventilation. Fertility and Sterility 86(4):1001e17–19.

O-Yurvati AH, Carnes MS, Clearfield MB et al 2005 Hemodynamic effects of osteopathic manipulative treatment immediately after coronary artery bypass graft surgery. Journal of the American Osteopathic Association 105(10):475–481

Pellegrino E 1979 Medicine, science, art: an old controversy revisited. Man and Medicine 4(1):43–52

Peltonen R, Kjeldsen-Kragh J, Haugen M et al 1994 Changes of faecal flora in rheumatoid arthritis during fasting and one-year vegetarian diet. British Journal of Rheumatology 33:638–643

Perdigon G, Alvarez S, Nader M et al 1990 The oral administration of lactic acid bacteria increases the mucosal intestinal immunity in response to enteropathogens. Journal of Food Protection 53:404–410

Perri M, Halford E 2004 Pain and faulty breathing. Journal of Bodywork and Movement Therapies 8(4):237–312

Pizzorno JE, Snider P 2004 Naturopathic medicine. In: Micozzi MS (ed) Fundamentals of complementary and alternative medicine. Churchill Livingstone, Philadelphia, p 159–192

Pryor J, Prasad S 2002 Physiotherapy for respiratory and cardiac problems, 3rd edn. Churchill Livingstone, Edinburgh, p 81

Radjieski J, Lumley M, Cantieri M 1998 Effect of osteopathic manipulative treatment on length of stay for pancreatitis: a randomized pilot study. Journal of the American Osteopathic Association 98(5):264–272

Rausse JH 1838 Der Geist der Graffenberger Wasserkur. Schieferdecker, Zeitz

Redwood D (ed) 1997 Contemporary chiropractic. Churchill Livingstone, Edinburgh

Rich G 2002 Massage therapy: the evidence for practice. Mosby, St Louis

Rikli A 1869 Die Thermodiatetik oder das tagliche thermoelectrische Licht und Luftbad in Verbindung mit naturfemasser Diat als zukunftige Heilmethode. Braumueller, Vienna

Roithmann R, Demeneghi P, Faggiano R, Cury A 2005 Effects of posture change on nasal patency. Revista Brasileira de Otorrinolaringologia (English ed.) 71(4):478

Selye H 1946 The general adaptation syndrome and the diseases of adaptation. Journal of Clinical Endocrinology 6:117–231

Selye H 1956 The stress of life. McGraw-Hill, New York

Selye H 1975 Confusion and controversy in the stress field. Stress 1(2):37–44

Sergi M, Rizzi M, Braghiroli A et al 1999 Periodic breathing during sleep in patients affected by fibromyalgia syndrome. European Respiratory Journal 14(1):203–208

Shikata N, Ueda HM, Kato M et al 2004 Association between nasal respiratory obstruction and vertical mandibular position. Journal of Oral Rehabilitation 10:957–962

Snider P, Zeff JL 1989 Definition of naturopathic medicine. American Association of Naturopathic Physicians (AANP) Position Paper. Select Committee on the Definition of Naturopathic Medicine. AANP House of Delegates, Rippling River, Oregon. Online. Available: www.naturopathic.org

Spitler H 1948 (ed) Basic naturopathy, a textbook. American Naturopathic Association

Standish L, Calabrese C, Snider P et al 2005 The future and foundations of naturopathic medical science. The naturopathic medical research agenda. Bastyr University Press, Kenmore, Washington

Stevens A 2005 The two million-year-old self. Texas A&M University Press, College Station, TX, p 118

Tache Y, Martinez V, Million M, Wang L 2001 Stress and the gastrointestinal tract III. Stress-related alterations of gut motor function: role of brain corticotropin-releasing factor receptors American Journal of Physiology. Gastrointestinal and Liver Physiology 280(2): G173–G177

The Physiotherapy Site Network: www. thephysiotherapysite.co.uk/physio/physiotherapy.html

Thomson S 1821 A brief sketch of the causes and treatment of disease. EG House, Boston

Timmons B, Ley R (eds) 1994 Behavioural and psychological approaches to breathing disorders Plenum Press, New York, p 118–119

Tortora G, Grabowski S 1993 Principles of anatomy and physiology, 7th edn. HarperCollins, New York, p 69

Trall RT 1851 Hydropathic encyclopedia: a system of hydropathy and hygiene. Fowler & Wells, New York

Valeur N, Engel P, Carbajal N, Connolly E, Ladefoged K 2004 Colonization and immunomodulation by Lactobacillus reuteri ATCC 55730 in the human gastrointestinal tract. Applied Environmental Microbiology 70(2):1176–1181

Vanderhoof JA, Whitney DB, Antonson D et al 1999 Lactobacillus GG in the prevention of antibiotic-associated diarrhea in children. Journal of Pediatrics 135:564–568

Verhoef MJ, Scott CM, Hilsden RJ 1998 A multimethod research study on the use of complementary therapies among patients with inflammatory bowel disease. Alternative Therapies in Health and Medicine 4:68–71

Vlaeyen J, Crombez G 1999 Fear of movement, (re)injury, avoidance and pain disability in chronic low back pain patients. Manual Therapy 4:187–195

Waddell G 2004 The back pain revolution, 2nd edn. Churchill Livingstone, Edinburgh, p 457–459

Ward R (ed) 1996 Foundations for osteopathic medicine. Williams & Wilkins, Baltimore

Wendel P 1951 Standardized naturopathy (published by the author)

Zeff JL 1997 The process of healing: a unifying theory of naturopathic medicine. Journal of Naturopathic Medicine 7(1):122–125 (submitted to the Journal in 1993; presented as Hierarchy of Therapeutics)

Zeff J, Snider P, Myers S 2006 A hierarchy of healing: the therapeutic order. The unifying theory of naturopathic medicine. In: Pizzorno J, Murray M (eds) Textbook of natural medicine, 3rd edn. Churchill Livingstone, Edinburgh

2

Leon Chaitow ND DO

With contributions from:
Matthew Wallden ND DO

Adaptation and the Evolution of Disease and Dysfunction

Adaptation processes

One significant way of understanding the processes involved in the evolution of disease and dysfunction requires an appreciation of Selye's general adaptation syndrome (GAS) (Selye 1946, 1952). Selye described stages in which an initial defensive/protective ('fight/flight') alarm phase occurs in response to a stressor (Rosch 1999) (see Fig. 2.1 and also Box 2.1), followed, if the stressor (or multiple stressors) continues to be operative, by a phase of adaptation ('resistance') which, when exhausted, results in collapse, frank illness and death.

Selye defined the basic, inborn, endogenous, self-regulating process as *homeostasis* (Fig. 2.2A), which eventually failed when overloaded, at which time a stage of *heterostasis* was reached, where 'something' – treatment in this context – is required to restore health and the self-regulating (adaptive) potential.

Heterostasis (Fig. 2.2B) calls for appropriate treatment to reduce adaptive load or to enhance adaptive capacity in order to avoid adaptation exhaustion, i.e. to avoid the

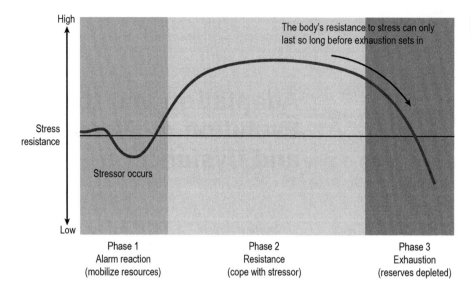

Figure 2.1 Selye's general adaptation syndrome

Box 2.1 Understanding Selye's use of the word 'stress'

The material in this box derives from the writings of Selye's close colleague Paul Rosch MD (2003). Rosch attempts to explain the choice by Selye of the word 'stress' that he used to describe the background to adaptation.

Rosch points out that although Selye was fluent in many languages, including English, his choice of the word 'stress' to describe the non-specific response syndrome he discovered was probably an error of judgment. He had used the word 'stress' in his initial letter to the Editor of *Nature* in 1936, who suggested that it be deleted since this word implied nervous strain, recommending that he use the term 'alarm reaction' instead.

Selye was unaware that the word 'stress' had been used for centuries in physics to explain elasticity, the property of a material that allows it to resume its original size and shape after being compressed or stretched by an external force. As expressed in Hooke's Law, the magnitude of an external force, or *stress*, produces a

proportional amount of deformation, or *strain*. Selye apparently expressed the view that had his knowledge of English been better he would have gone down in history as the father of the 'strain' concept.

Finding an acceptable definition of stress was a problem that exercised Selye for the rest of his life. He noted to Rosch that 24 centuries previously Hippocrates had written that disease was not only *pathos* (suffering), but also *ponos* (toil), as the body fought to restore normalcy.

Ultimately, because many people viewed stress as an unpleasant threat, Selye created a new word, 'stressor', in order to distinguish between stimulus and response. Even Selye had difficulties when he tried to extrapolate his laboratory research to humans. In helping to prepare the *First Annual Report on Stress* in 1951, Rosch included the comments of one critic, who, using verbatim citations from Selye's own writings concluded: 'Stress, in addition to being itself, was also the cause of itself, and the result of itself.'

---

point at which the 'stretched elastic' of the individual's adaptive potential snaps.

An evolution of these models has included recognition of an altered version of homeostasis – *allostasis* – that produces exaggerated, or insufficient, responses to stressors (Fig. 2.2C) (McEwan 1994, Sapolsky 1990, 1994).

Stress defined

Stress is defined by Selye in his writings (1976) as the non-specific response of the body to any demand, whether it is caused by, or results in, pleasant or unpleasant conditions.

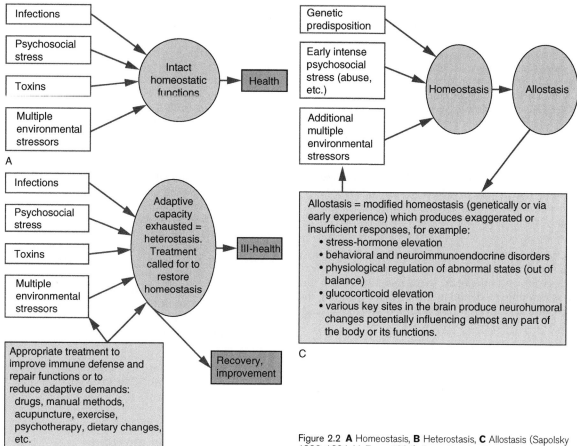

Figure 2.2 A Homeostasis, **B** Heterostasis, **C** Allostasis (Sapolsky 1990, 1994, McEwan 1994). Reproduced with permission from Chaitow (2003a)

Many of Selye's findings and concepts fit intimately with naturopathic thought, as outlined in Chapter 1 (Selye 1976):

The fact that the state of stress, even if due to the same agent, can cause different effects in different individuals, has been traced to 'conditioning factors' that can selectively enhance or inhibit one or the other stress effect. This conditioning may be endogenous (genetic predisposition, age or sex) or exogenous (treatment with certain hormones, drugs or dietary factors). Under the influence of such conditioning factors, a normally well-tolerated degree of stress can even become pathogenic, selectively affecting those parts of the body that are particularly sensitized both by those conditioning factors and by the specific effects of the eliciting agent, just as physical tensions of equal strength in different chains will break the particular link that is the weakest, as a result of internal or external factors.

In this model, a spectrum of adaptive changes – many of which produce symptoms, some benign and others serious or sinister – is seen to emerge from a background of the interaction of variable (in degree, variety and chronicity) idiosyncratic adaptive demands, superimposed on the individual's unique acquired and inherited biochemical, biomechanical and psychosocial characteristics, qualities and attributes – sometimes called polymorphism (Williams 1956).

Stress explained

A close colleague of Selye, Istvan Berczi, provides insights into Selye's thinking regarding disease causation, from the perspective of the general adaptation syndrome (Berczi 2005):

The prediction by Dr. Selye of the pluricausal nature of most diseases is really the recognition that living organisms have evolved multiple mechanisms to defend themselves against harmful agents. For this reason, in most cases, it is necessary to interfere with these defense mechanisms at more than one point to cause disease. The redundancy of immune effector mechanisms (Berczi & Nagy 1994, Clark & Kamen 1987) or the recent recognition that it is necessary to deregulate more than one gene to cause cancer (Berczi & Nagy 1991) certainly supports this view. In his last years he turned his attention to the protective power of certain hormones against various toxins and other noxious stimuli and created the term 'catatoxic steroids' for those hormones that have protective effect (Selye 1969, 1971). That hormones are important in immunological and other forms of resistance, is the subject of current scientific inquiry (Berczi 1986, 1994).

The schematic representation in Figure 2.3 suggests many of the events and pathways related to the way stress influences the body. In the mid-1940s when this was first presented, and in 1955, when explaining the progress his research had achieved and how much more was unknown, Selye noted:

Non-specific damage, again through unknown pathways, also acts upon the hypophysis and causes it to increase corticotropic hormone production at the expense of a decreased gonadotropic, lactogenic and growth hormones. The resulting corticotropic hormone excess causes enlargement of the adrenal cortex with signs of increased corticoid hormone production. These corticoids in turn cause changes in the carbohydrate (sugar active corticoids) and electrolyte metabolism (salt-active corticoids) as well as atrophy of the thymus and the other lymphatic organs. It is probable that the cardiovascular, renal, blood pressure and arthritic changes are secondary to the disturbances in electrolyte metabolism since their production and prevention are largely dependent upon the salt intake . . . We do not know as yet, whether the hypertension is secondary to the nephrosclerosis or whether it is a direct result of the disturbance in electrolyte metabolism caused by the corticoids. Similarly, it is not quite clear, as yet, whether corticoids destroy the circulating lymphocytes directly, or whether they influence the lymphocyte count merely by diminishing lymphocyte formation in the lymphatic organs. Probably both these mechanisms are operative.

In 2005, Berczi brought Selye's original observations closer to present times by observing:

Today we know that a variety of insults, including trauma and infection, stimulate the release of chemotaxic, proinflammatory cytokines, and a whole host of other mediators from a variety of cells in the damaged area that include mast cells, endothelial cells, platelets. The released mediators attract blood borne leucocytes, such as neutrophilic granulocytes, monocytes/macrophages, lymphocytes, eosinophils and basophils that release additional mediators, and thus contribute to the inflammatory response. In some cases certain cytokines, such as interleukin-1 (IL-1), tumor necrosis factor-α (TNF-alpha) and interleukin-6 (IL-6), become detectable in the blood and function as acute phase hormones. They act on the brain causing fever and other functional modifications (IL-1, TNF-alpha), release certain pituitary hormones and inhibit others, promote general catabolism (mediated primarily by TNF-alpha, also known as cachectin), stimulate the production of new serum proteins known as acute phase reactants in the liver (the joint action of IL-6, glucocorticoids and catecholamines), and also elevate the production of leucocytes in the bone marrow, the mechanism of which is not fully elucidated (Berczi & Nagy 1994). Thus, with the recent discovery of cytokines and our increasing recognition of their functions, we have begun to fill in the gaps in Dr. Selye's adaptation syndrome outlined nearly half a century ago.

Huether (1996) has further outlined the ways in which Selye's original work has evolved.

Selye's observation regarding GAS and LAS

Reviewing the topic of the so-called 'pluricausal causes' of disease, Selye et al (1968) noted:

The characteristic response of the body to systemic stress is the General Adaptation Syndrome (GAS), characterized by manifold morphologic and functional changes throughout the organism, whereas topical stress elicits a Local Adaptation Syndrome (LAS) whose principal repercussions are confined to the immediate vicinity of the eliciting injury. The term 'stress' implies only non-specificity of causation; it does not presume to distinguish between manifestations of damage and of defense. Also, depending upon the simultaneous application of certain 'conditioning agents', both systemic stress and local stress can produce vastly different and highly specific reactions The pluricausal causes of disease are due to complex pathogenic constellations . . .

A patient in traumatic shock furnishes a characteristic example of the GAS and, in particular in its earliest stage, the 'shock phase' of the general alarm reaction.

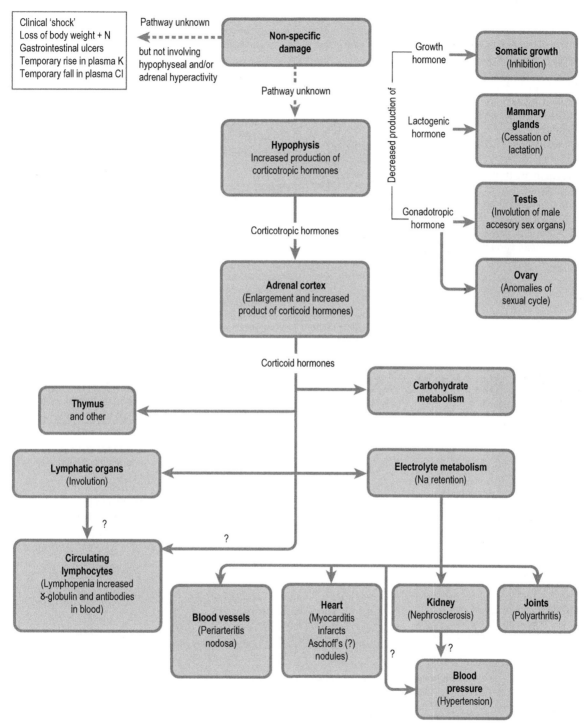

Figure 2.3 Functional interrelations during general adaptation syndrome. Schematized drawing indicating that non-specific damage causes clinical shock, loss of body weight and nitrogen, gastrointestinal ulcers, temporary rise in plasma potassium with fall in plasma Cl, through unknown pathways (nervous stimulus?, deficiency?, toxic metabolites?) but manifestly not through the stimulation of the hypophyseoadrenal mechanism. This is proven by the fact that the above manifestations are not prevented either by hypophysectomy or by adrenalectomy; they even tend to be more severe in the absence of either or both of these glands (Selye 1946)

An abscess, formed around a splinter of wood, represents a typical instance of the LAS, and, in particular, of its 'stage of resistance' during which the defensive, inflammatory phenomena predominate. On the surface, these two conditions [traumatic shock and the abscess] reveal no obvious similarities; however, more careful studies show them to be closely related.

The GAS and the LAS are thought to be interrelated because:

(1) Both are nonspecific reactions comprising damage and defense.

(2) Both are triphasic [stages of alarm, resistance, exhaustion] with typical signs of 'cross-resistance' during the 'stage of resistance'.

(3) Both are singularly sensitive to the so-called 'adaptive hormones' (ACTH, corticoids, STH [growth hormone]).

(4) If the two reactions develop simultaneously, they greatly influence one another: systemic stress markedly alters reactivity to local stress and vice versa (Selye 1953).

Selye's observations speak to the recognition of multicausal ('pluricausal'), contextual sequences of events that underlie ill-health, and of self-regulating, protective endogenous substances and functions (Fig. 2.4). These concepts are at the very heart of naturopathic thinking and practice.

Differing responses to adaptation

Illness and dysfunction can be seen in this model to represent either a partial or total failure of adaptation, or adaptation in progress.

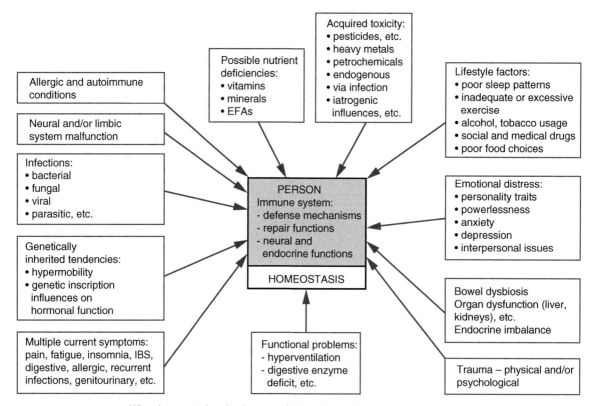

Figure 2.4 Multiple stressors in fibromyalgia. EFAs, essential fatty acids; IBS, irritable bowel syndrome. Reproduced with permission from Chaitow (2003a)

Although many such adaptive changes manifest as symptoms, these [symptoms] may at times be no more than evidence of processes of repair (e.g. inflammation following trauma) or attempts at restoration of the status quo.

Within this framework it becomes clear that responses to apparently similar stressors (adaptive load) will produce different responses in severity and degree, dependent on the unique characteristics of the individual or of the tissues affected.

Rosch (1999) reports that:

Selye observed that patients suffering from different diseases often exhibited identical signs and symptoms. They just 'looked sick'. This observation may have been the first step in his recognition of 'stress'. He later discovered and described the General Adaptation Syndrome, a response of the body to demands placed upon it. The Syndrome details how stress induces hormonal autonomic responses and, over time, these hormonal changes can lead to ulcers, high blood pressure, arteriosclerosis, arthritis, kidney disease, and allergic reactions.

It is also evident that similar symptoms might emerge from a background of very different stressors, interacting with the idiosyncratically distinctive biomechanical, biochemical and psychosocial features of the individual.

This highlights and underscores a basic requirement in naturopathic medicine – the need to consider the individual features, attributes and qualities of each person and condition, when considering therapeutic interventions.

Local adaptation syndrome – an example and a naturopathic solution

The discussion above of the general adaptation syndrome (GAS) can easily be refined to a more local, regional focus – a local adaptation syndrome (LAS).

A painful, restricted, shoulder problem might be seen to be responding (adapting) variously to postural imbalances, possible spinal restrictions and overuse, in which symptoms have evolved over time, as adaptation to the imposed demands has gradually exhausted the elastic and dynamic self-repair potential of the tissues involved.

For example, the anterior glenohumeral capsule is structurally stronger than the posterior joint capsule, though functionally it is exposed to greater cumulative trauma, particularly in those who use their arms in an overhead position – for example, racket sports players, baseball pitchers (Wilk et al 1993), volleyball players, painters and decorators, window cleaners. Hence, the anterior joint capsule will undergo creep,

become unstable and inflamed and commonly, in time, would become restricted in flexion.

This can be seen in terms of the local adaptation syndrome as follows.

- An acute (alarm) phase would follow initial stress (excessive throwing action perhaps)
- During this phase, repair activity would be carried out, almost certainly involving some inflammation and discomfort.
- Compensatory recruitment patterns would operate to minimize stress on the anterior capsule region.
- A combination of repetitive microtrauma due to continued throwing activity, overlaid on a modified recruitment pattern, possibly overlaid on long-term postural stressors (forward head position, inhibited lower fixators of the scapula, excessive activity of some of the rotator cuff muscles, etc.), together with possible nutritional imbalances, leads to a situation where *the damage rate exceeds the repair rate*.
- Pain and greater restriction of movement become the dominant symptoms leading to underuse of the arm and psychological distress, as well as further compensation/adaptation demands on other tissues and structures.
- Thus wear and tear eventually produce a stage of virtual decompensation – the final phase of Selye's local adaptation syndrome.
- The potential for further functional adaptation in that shoulder to the imposed demands would have been exhausted, and other dysfunctional adaptations, involving overuse of the unaffected shoulder and more widespread postural changes, become increasingly likely.
- Solutions to such symptom-producing situations do not lie in local treatment of the painful and restricted area (anterior capsular strain), where little more than symptomatic – short-term – relief would be possible.
- For the manual therapist to attempt to locally mobilize the glenohumeral joint into greater ease in flexion, without understanding the biomechanical rationale for the original local stress to the anterior glenohumeral capsule, would most probably prove both futile and detrimental.
- A naturopathic physical medicine approach would ideally give attention to the larger picture, including whole body postural considerations, potential thoracic spinal

restrictions and improved use patterns, as well as normalization, if possible, of the shortened, and the inhibited, muscles and other soft tissues including deactivation of trigger points and mobilization of the shoulder joint.

- In this broader clinical approach, consideration would also be given to nutritional features as well as to rehabilitation, including aspects of pain behavior and altered patterns of use resulting from the condition.
- Therapeutically it is important to incorporate appropriately focused use patterns into a rehabilitation process, building on the re-education and retraining potential of imposed demand, and so minimizing the likelihood of further symptom-producing adaptational changes.

Thoughts on specific adaptation from a professional baseball trainer

Based on specific adaptation to imposed demands (SAID), athletes adapt to the imposed demands of their particular sport, the physical requirements of the activities demanded within the sport and specific exercise regimes. Failure to adapt leads to proneness to injury or inadequate performance (Kraemer & Gomez 2001). For example, generalized patterns of adaptation are recognized in the overhead throwing athlete. Various experts (Crockett et al 2002, Osbahr et al 2002, Reagan et al 2002) have described a variety of adaptation possibilities in the throwing shoulder, and the ability to adapt adequately seems to be what allows the athlete to compete at the top levels of the chosen sport (Fig. 2.5).

As such adaptations to sporting activities occur, the athlete's general habits also become important. Green-field et al (1995) demonstrated that posture degradation, such as forward head position, can affect the shoulder of the throwing athlete, making assessment of postural adaptations important in order to maintain optimal function of the athlete. (For deeper consideration of adaptation issues in relation to trauma and rehabilitation, see Chapter 9.)

Crenshaw (2006), a senior athletic trainer for a major league baseball team, insightfully notes:

Not only are athletes challenged physically, they must adapt to many other stressors as well. Mental, social, environmental, nutritional stressors combined with aging, competition requirements, travel, and sleep pattern disruption, all add to the athlete's adaptation burden. General health depends on more than the absence of disease. It is critical to keep stressors to a minimum and/or to use mechanisms such as recovery and relaxation techniques to improve stress-coping potentials.

'Slow' adaptation examples from Juhl, Janda and Grieve

How do structural features adapt?

There are few more common structural imbalances than leg-length inequality. Juhl et al (2004) report that:

Asymmetry within the pelvic structure can lead to a cascade of postural compensations throughout the axial spine, predisposing persons to recurrent somatic dysfunction and decreased functionality. Numerous

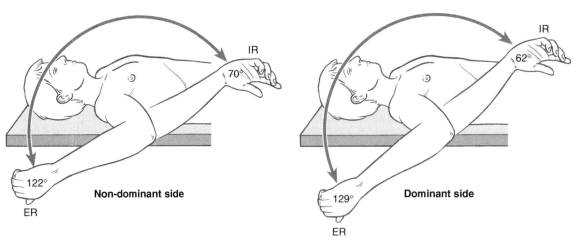

Figure 2.5 The total motion concept discussed by Wilk (2004) shows the adaptation of the throwing shoulder in the professional baseball pitcher. ER, external rotation; IR, internal rotation. Reproduced with permission from Chaitow (2006)

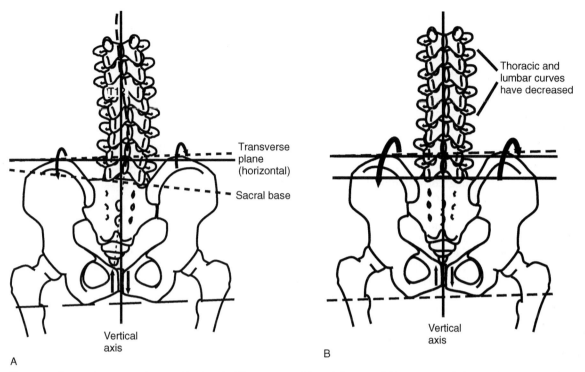

Figure 2.6 Sacral adjustment to functional leg-length difference caused by malalignment. **A** Uncompensated: the sacral base and iliac crest are oblique, and there is an accentuated compensatory scoliosis. **B** Compensated: although the obliquity of iliac crests persists, the sacral base is now level and the degree of scoliosis decreased. Reproduced with permission from Schamberger (2002)

authors have found a correlation between leg length inequality and low back pain (LBP).

(See Fig. 2.6.)

How common is anatomic leg-length discrepancy?

Using data on leg-length inequality, obtained by accurate and reliable x-ray methods, Knutson (2005) found the prevalence of anatomic leg-length inequality to be 90%, the mean magnitude being 5.2 mm (SD 4.1). The evidence suggested that, for most people, anatomic leg-length inequality does not appear to be clinically significant until the magnitude reaches ~20 mm (~¾"). This finding supports the supposition that *the degree of 'load'* (leg-length inequality in this example) along temporal features and multiple other factors determines whether and when adaptation ultimately fails, allowing dysfunctional symptoms to emerge.

Most schools of manual therapy hold to the concept of considering the body as a whole, and yet in reality attention to local features still seems to be the dominant clinical approach. Janda (1988) offers examples

as to why this is extremely clinically short sighted. He describes the adaptive changes resulting from the presence of a significant degree of leg shortness, as follows.

- A short leg inevitably requires an altered pelvic position.
- This unlevels the sacral base and leads to scoliosis.
- As the spine adapts, a sequence of compensations is likely to lead to joint dysfunction at the cervicocranial junction.
- This inevitably results in compensatory activity of the small cervico-occipital muscles and a modified head position.
- Further compensation occurs concerning most of the neck musculature, some of which will involve increased muscle tone and possibly muscle spasm.
- A sequence follows of compensation and adaptation responses in many muscles, ligaments and joints of the region, followed by the development of a variety of possible syndromes and symptoms involving the head,

neck, temporomandibular joint, shoulder and/ or the arm.

Janda's point is that after all the adaptation that has taken place, treatment of the most obvious cervical restrictions, where the person might be aware of pain and restriction, would offer only limited benefit. Whether the short leg is anatomic or functional (i.e. where there is a primary sacroiliac dysfunction that alters the position on the innominate and therefore creates an apparent change in leg length), the changes described by Janda will occur. The difference is that with a functional change, correction of the sacroiliac joint problem should correct the chain reaction of adaptational modifications, whereas with a true anatomic short leg, choices would be far more limited – for example, a heel and sole lift, or possibly surgery.

Janda also points to the existence of oculopelvic and pelviocular reflexes, which indicate that any change in pelvic orientation alters the position of the eyes and vice versa, and to the fact that eye position modifies muscle tone – visual synkinesis (Komendatov 1945) – particularly involving the suboccipital muscles (look up and extensors tone, look down and flexors prepare for activity, etc.). The implication of modified eye position, due to altered pelvic position, therefore becomes yet another factor to be considered when unraveling chain reactions of interacting adaptive elements.

'These examples,' Janda says, 'serve to emphasize that one should not limit consideration to local clinical symptomatology . . . but [that we] should always maintain a general view'. This approach is profoundly naturopathic.

Grieve (1986) echoes this viewpoint. He has explained how a patient presenting with pain, loss of functional movement or altered patterns of strength, power or endurance, will probably either have suffered a major trauma, which has overwhelmed the physiological limits of relatively healthy tissues, or will be displaying 'gradual decompensation demonstrating slow exhaustion of the tissue's adaptive potential, with or without trauma'.

As this process of decompensation progresses, postural adaptation, influenced by time factors and possibly by further trauma, leads to exhaustion of the body's adaptive potential and results in dysfunction and symptoms.

Grieve reminds us of Hooke's Law, which states that within the elastic limits of any substance, the ratio of the stress applied to the strain produced is constant (Bennet 1952). In simple terms, this means that tissue capable of deformation will absorb or adapt to forces applied to it within its elastic limits, beyond which it will break down or fail to compensate (leading to decompensation).

Grieve rightly reminds us that while attention to specific tissues incriminated in producing symptoms often gives excellent short-term results, 'Unless treatment is also focused towards restoring function in asymptomatic tissues responsible for the original postural adaptation and subsequent decompensation, the symptoms will recur'. This description of attention to causes is a clear naturopathic position.

Adaptation to breathing imbalance

Just as poor posture, or the presence of a structural imbalance such as a short leg, can result in widespread dysfunction, a breathing pattern disorder (BPD) – the extreme of which is hyperventilation – can produce an astonishing array of adaptive changes creating biomechanical, biochemical and psychological compensations as summarized in Figure 2.7. Solutions may involve a variety of rehabilitation and structural approaches, as discussed in Chapters 7, 8 and 10 (Chaitow et al 2002).

It is possible to see in the sequence illustrated in Figure 2.7 (and discussed more fully in later chapters) that symptoms as diverse as neck and head pain, chronic fatigue, anxiety and panic attacks, cardiovascular distress, gastrointestinal dysfunction, lowered pain threshold, spinal instability and hypertension (and this is not a comprehensive listing) might be directly caused, or more commonly aggravated and maintained, by breathing pattern disorders such as hyperventilation (Timmons & Ley 1994).

The complex sequences of biochemical, psychological and structural adaptations and compensatory changes involved in this example highlight the absolute requirement for attention to cause. Part of that attention also needs to focus on the causes of breathing pattern disorders, which are themselves, after all, symptoms.

Neurophysiological responses to trauma (Patterson & Wurster 1997)

There is a neurophysiological dimension to trauma adaptation, including what can be termed peripheral and central (adaptive) changes.

An initial response to injury usually involves local changes in the affected tissues, possibly including swelling, inflammation and pain (Bevan 1999, Johansson 1993).

Pain receptors (nociceptors) will be stimulated and transmit their distress to the dorsal horn of the spinal cord, and, if the intensity of this stimulation from the periphery is great enough, pain will be registered in the brain. Additionally, stimulation of motor neurons at the ventral horn will ensure an increase in muscular tone (He et al 1988) and sympathetic responses will

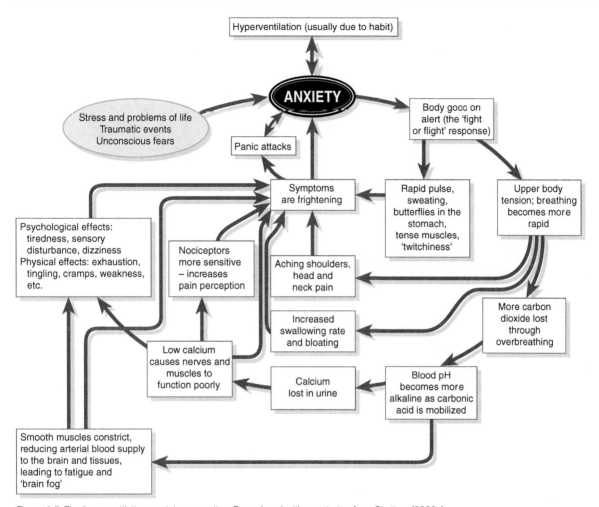

Figure 2.7 The hyperventilation–anxiety connection. Reproduced with permission from Chaitow (2003a)

cause increased circulatory perfusion of the muscles (Sato & Schmidt 1973).

While all these adaptive responses have protective value, if they are prolonged or repetitive a 'neurological footprint of abnormal patterning' (Brookes & Pusey 2006) may remain, with pain circuits inappropriately maintaining their post-injury activity.

The nervous system will effectively have become sensitized, and therefore more vulnerable to being far more easily triggered into a similar series of responses by relatively mild stimuli. This process of the *facilitation* of neural responses has been widely studied in osteopathic medicine (Korr 1976) and is discussed in greater detail in Box 2.2 along with consideration of localized areas of facilitation (sensitization) and myofascial trigger points (Box 2.3). Areas that have become adaptively sensitized are more vulnerable to the influence of subsequent stressors, and

increased vulnerability – as part of an adaptive process – has important implications in many chronic health situations such as, for example, fibromyalgia (see Chapter 10).

Naturopathic physical medicine approaches would focus on reducing adaptive demands while attempting simultaneously to enhance integration of neurological and physiological function, modulating the sensitized tissues.

Korr and axonal transportation of trophic substances

Korr – the premier osteopathic researcher of the second half of the 20th century – summarizes another vital implication of soft tissue dysfunction – interference with axonal transport mechanisms evolving out

Box 2.2 Facilitation and sensitization

Spinal (segmental) facilitation

Adaptational changes to neural structures are a central feature of understanding the effects of viscerosomatic reflex effects.

In osteopathic terminology, when these changes occur spinally, the term 'segmental facilitation' is used (Korr 1976).

A similar local phenomenon occurs throughout the myofascial tissues of the body, where the term 'myofascial trigger points' is used to describe the resulting dysfunction (see below).

Beal (1985) has described the segmental phenomenon as resulting from afferent stimuli arising from dysfunction of a visceral nature. An adaptational progression is readily noted in this sequence.

- The reflex is initiated by afferent impulses arising from visceral receptors, transmitted to the dorsal horn of the spinal cord, where they synapse with interconnecting neurons.
- The stimuli are then conveyed to sympathetic and motor efferents, resulting in changes in the somatic tissues, such as skeletal muscle, skin and blood vessels.
- Abnormal stimulation of the visceral efferent neurons may result in hyperesthesia of the skin and associated vasomotor, pilomotor and sudomotor changes.
- Similar stimuli of the ventral horn cells may result in reflex rigidity of the somatic (usually paraspinal) musculature.
- Pain may result from such changes.
- The degree of stimulus required, in any given case, to produce such changes will differ, because factors such as prior facilitation (sensitization) of the particular segment, as well as the response of higher centers, will vary from person to person (Fig. 2.8).

In many cases the viscerosomatic reflex activity may be noted before any symptoms of visceral change are evident and this phenomenon is therefore of potential diagnostic and prognostic value (Korr 1976).

The first signs of viscerosomatic reflexive influences are vasomotor (increased skin temperature) and sudomotor (increased moisture of the skin) reactions, skin textural changes (e.g. thickening), increased subcutaneous fluid and increased contraction of muscle. The value of light skin palpation in identifying areas of facilitation cannot be too strongly emphasized (Lewit 1999) (see Chapter 6). These signs usually disappear if the visceral cause improves.

When such changes become chronic, however, trophic alterations/adaptations are noted, with increased thickening of the skin and subcutaneous tissue, and localized muscular contraction. Deep musculature may

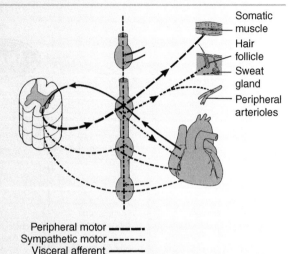

Somatic muscle
Hair follicle
Sweat gland
Peripheral arterioles

Peripheral motor ▬ ▬ ▬ ▪
Sympathetic motor - - - - - - -
Visceral afferent ▬▬▬▬

Figure 2.8 Schematic representation of viscerosomatic reflex. Reproduced with permission from Chaitow & DeLany (2000)

become hard, tense and hypersensitive. This may result in deep splinting contractions, involving two or more segments of the spine, with associated restriction of spinal motion. In the thoracic spine the costotransverse articulations may be significantly involved in such changes.

Beal (1983) notes that, when the voluminous research into segmental associations with organ dysfunction is compounded, three distinct groups of visceral involvement are found in respect of particular sites:

- T1–T5: heart and lungs
- T5–T10: esophagus, stomach, small intestine, liver, gall bladder, spleen, pancreas and adrenal cortex
- T10–L2: large bowel, appendix, kidney, ureter, adrenal medulla, testes, ovaries, urinary bladder, prostate gland and uterus.

Kelso (1971) reports that in one 5-year study involving more than 5000 hospitalized patients, it was found that most visceral disease appeared to influence more than one spinal region, and that the number of spinal segments involved seemed to be related to the duration of the disease. This study showed that there was an increase in the number of palpatory findings in the cervical region, relating to patients with sinusitis, tonsillitis, diseases of the esophagus and liver complaints, whereas soft tissue changes were noted in patients with gastritis, duodenal ulceration, pyelonephritis, chronic appendicitis and cholecystitis, in the region of T5–T12.

Research (Bendtsen et al 1996) suggests that there exists:

Box 2.2 Facilitation and sensitization continued

. . . a pathophysiological model for tension-type headache [resulting from] central sensitization [facilitation] at the level of the spinal dorsal horn/ trigeminal nucleus due to prolonged nociceptive inputs from pericranial myofascial tissues. The increased nociceptive input to supraspinal structures may in turn result in supraspinal sensitization. The central neuroplastic changes may affect the regulation of peripheral mechanisms and thereby lead to, for example, increased pericranial muscle activity, or sensitization may be maintained even after the initial eliciting factors have been normalized, resulting in conversion of episodic into chronic tension-type headache.

This research demonstrates the need to understand how, over time, a reversible problem may become entrenched and chronic.

Areas of facilitation appear to be irritated by stressors of all types which create adaptive demands on any aspect of the individual – physical, chemical or psychological – even if there is no direct or obvious impact on the area of facilitation.

• From a naturopathic perspective this fits directly into the contextual model of understanding ill-health and dysfunction.
• It also offers explanations for the influence of a wide array of stressors (climatic, emotional, postural, nutritional, etc.) on the health of individuals who are somewhere on the road towards decompensation/ adaptation exhaustion, exacerbating symptoms, despite apparently not directly impacting the involved tissues, systems or structures.

of a background of compensatory and adaptation-induced changes (Korr 1981):

Any factor that causes derangement of transport mechanisms in the axon, or that chronically alters the quality or quantity of the axonally transported substances, could cause trophic influences to become detrimental. This alteration in turn would produce aberrations of structure, function and metabolism, thereby contributing to dysfunction and disease. Almost certainly to be included among these harmful factors are the deformation of nerves and roots, such as compression, stretching, angulation and torsion that are known to occur all too commonly in humans, and that are likely to disturb the interaxonal transport mechanisms, intraneural microcirculation and the blood–nerve barrier. Neural structures are especially vulnerable in their passage over highly mobile joints, through bony canals, intervertebral foramina, fascial layers and tonically contracted muscles.

Many of such biomechanically induced deformations are, of course, capable of amelioration and correction by means of appropriate manipulative and soft tissue treatment (Korr 1967, 1970).

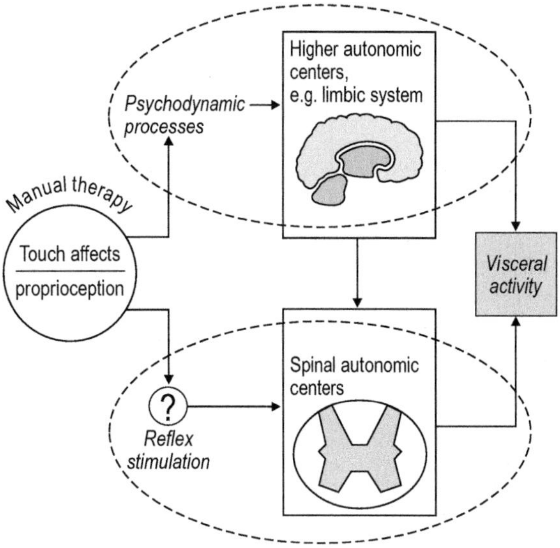

Simons et al and the trigger point phenomenon

Simons et al (1999) have detailed somatovisceral responses arising from abdominal musculature, influencing internal visceral organs and functions (see Box 2.2 and Fig. 2.12).

This is not meant to suggest that local adaptation-induced changes (such as trigger points) are necessar-

Figure 2.9 The effect of manual therapy on visceral activity is unlikely to occur via reflex stimulation of spinal autonomic centers. Most manual influences are related to the psychodynamics of touch and its effect on the limbic system. Reproduced with permission from Lederman (2005)

ily the *cause* of such dysfunctions and diseases (see list below), but that there exists a strong possibility, in any given case, that the condition/disease may be being aggravated and/or maintained by reflexogenic activity associated with myofascial trigger points, and that attempts to treat such conditions without a primary

Box 2.3 More on local facilitation – myofascial trigger points

Wall & Melzack (1990), in their exhaustive investigation of pain, are clear that all chronic pain has myofascial trigger point activity as at least a part of its etiology, and that in many instances trigger points are the major contributors to the pain (Figs 2.10–2.12).

- Trigger points are localized, palpable areas of deep tenderness and increased resistance, and digital pressure on such a trigger will often produce twitching and fasciculation.

- Trigger points are located either close to the motor endpoint of a muscle or near the attachments.
- Pressure maintained on such a point will produce referred pain in a predictable area.
- If there are a number of active trigger points, the reference areas may overlap.
- What is distinctive about trigger points (myofascial trigger points) is that, when active, they are not only painful but also refer sensations or symptoms to a precise target area; this target area is more or less

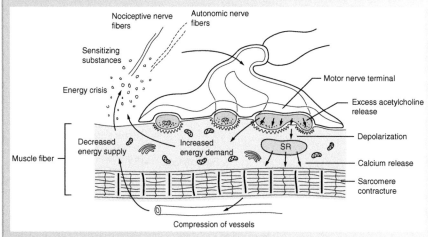

Figure 2.10 Integrated trigger point hypothesis (after Simons et al 1999). Reproduced with permission from Chaitow (2003a)

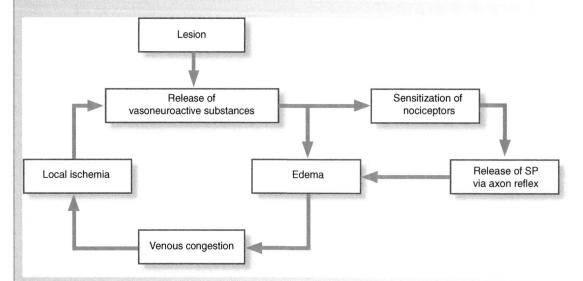

Figure 2.11 Schematic diagram showing hypothesized mechanism for sustained tenderness in trigger points. SP, substance P. Reproduced with permission from Chaitow (2003b)

Box 2.3 More on local facilitation – myofascial trigger points continued

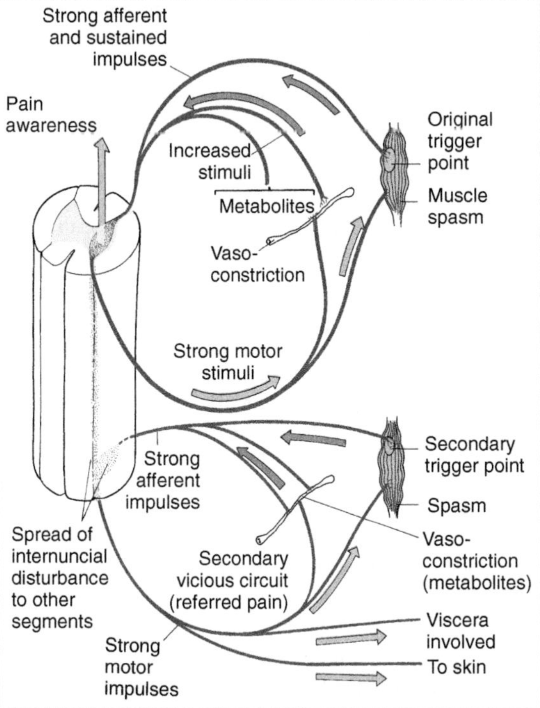

Figure 2.12 Schematic representation of the secondary spread of neurologically induced influences deriving from acute or chronic soft tissue dysfunction and involving trigger point activity and/or spasm. Reproduced with permission from Chaitow (2003b)

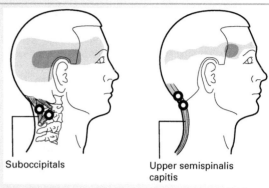

Figure 2.13 The referral patterns of the suboccipital muscles and the upper semispinalis capitis are similar. Reproduced with permission from Chaitow & DeLany (2000)

reproducible in other individuals, when trigger points are located in similar positions (Fig. 2.13). No other soft tissue dysfunction has this particular attribute.

- Before an active trigger point exists there needs to be a period of evolution that involves the development of soft tissue changes that are palpable and probably sensitive or painful, but that, until sufficient localized stress has been involved, will not refer symptoms onwards.
- In other words, many localized muscular areas of sensitivity or pain, which do not refer pain or other symptoms, may be considered to be embryonic or evolutionary trigger points.
- A trigger point is a localized, palpable area of soft tissue that is painful on pressure, and that refers symptoms, usually including pain, to a predictable target area some distance from itself.
- It is an area of local facilitation that has developed following a very similar etiological pathway to that occurring in segmental (spinal) facilitated areas (possibly involving overuse, reflexogenic influences, ischemia or trauma).

Much research and clinical work has been done in recent years in this field by Simons et al (1999) who maintain that if a pain is severe enough to cause a patient to seek professional advice (in the absence of organic disease), referred pain is likely to be a factor and therefore a trigger point is probably involved.

To be defined as 'active' (ideal for treatment) rather than 'latent', a trigger point should refer symptoms or sensations that are familiar to the patient as part of their symptom picture.

A single trigger may refer pain to several reference sites and can give rise to embryonic, or satellite, triggers in those target areas.

While pain is the commonest symptom arising from the activity of trigger points, other symptoms may be noted (Travell & Simons 1983, 1992), including:

- lymphatic stasis and reduced mobility of joints
- vasoconstriction (blanching)
- coldness
- sweating
- pilomotor response
- ptosis
- hypersecretion.

Analysis of substances surrounding trigger points

The degree of pathophysiological change associated with trigger points is now clear following National Institutes of Health sponsored research into the local tissue state surrounding the trigger point. The biochemistry has been evaluated in a prospective, controlled trial, using a remarkable microanalytical technique (Shah et al 2003). This showed that a novel microdialysis needle can successfully sample the biochemical milieu of myofascial trigger points (MTrP).

Continued

Box 2.3 More on local facilitation – myofascial trigger points continued

Pressure algometry was performed to determine pain pressure threshold (PPT) in individuals with active trigger points, latent trigger points and no trigger points. Samples were obtained continuously from normal tissue (controls) as well as from tissues where latent and active trigger points had been identified, using the microdialysis needle.

This technique recovered extremely small quantities (<0.5 μL) of very small substances (molecular weight <100 kD) directly from soft tissue. There were significant differences in the levels of pH, substance P, calcitonin gene-related peptide, bradykinin, norepinephrine, tumor necrosis factor and interleukin-1 in those subjects with an active MTrP (symptoms, MTrP present) compared with subjects with a latent MTrP (no symptoms, MTrP present) and normal subjects (no symptoms, no MTrP).

Trigger points can be deactivated manually or by chilling, injection (procaine etc.), acupuncture or dry needling. However, removal of the stressor features (postural, overuse, misuse, etc.) is the most effective means of removing trigger point activity.

Assessment and treatment approaches are discussed in later chapters, with manual protocols described in Chapter 7.

Naturopathic considerations

From a naturopathic perspective, trigger points can most commonly be seen to represent focal areas of dysfunctional adaptation. For this reason it is obvious that the context out of which trigger points emerge requires evaluation and, if possible, correcting – better posture, breathing, nutrition (deficiencies of iron, vitamin B complex and/or vitamin C, as well as hypothyroidism, have been reported as predisposing factors by Travell & Simons (1992), the main researchers into this phenomenon), sleep, stress and lifestyle modification, etc., as well as enhanced muscle tone and flexibility.

At times it may be noted that trigger points represent a functional adaptation, a means whereby increased stability may be being maintained in an economical manner. Examples can be seen in an unstable joint or an individual who is hypermobile.

- *Protection of an unstable sacroiliac joint*: Trigger points in the hamstrings would increase tone in the muscle, producing tension via the sacrotuberous ligament that would stabilize the sacroiliac joint. Removal/deactivation of the MTrP, or stretching of the tight hamstring, would probably destabilize the joint (Chaitow & DeLany 2003, Hong & Simons 1998).
- *Hypermobility*: Individuals who are hypermobile tend to have a higher incidence of musculoskeletal pain (Goldenberg 1991) and to have soft tissues that contain a high level of active myofascial trigger points. The question arises as to whether there is increased functionality as a result, involving greater stability.

In such settings trigger points may be seen as alarm signals and to be creating stabilizing influences, and so should not be deactivated unless the stability they offer is replaced by other means. Instead, the reason for their presence should be addressed – for example by means of improved core stability involving enhanced balance, tone, flexibility and stability, or other means of support such as a sacroiliac support or prolotherapy.

---

focus on the reflexogenic activities of trigger points are likely to be less than optimally successful:

- projectile vomiting
- anorexia
- nausea
- intestinal colic
- diarrhea
- urinary bladder and sphincter spasm
- dysmenorrhea
- pain symptoms mimicking those of appendicitis and cholelithiasis
- symptoms of burning, fullness, bloating, swelling or gas
- heartburn and other symptoms of hiatal hernia
- urinary frequency (interstitial cystitis – see below)
- groin pain
- chronic diarrhea
- pain when coughing
- belching
- chest pain that is not cardiac in origin
- abdominal cramping
- colic in infants as well as adults.

Baldry's perspective

Baldry (1999) details a huge amount of research that validates the link (a somatovisceral reflex) that Simons et al have made between trigger points and symptoms as diverse as anorexia, flatulence, nausea, vomiting, diarrhea, colic, dysmenorrhea and dysuria.

Pain of a deep aching nature, or sometimes of a sharp or burning type, is reported as being associated with this range of symptoms, which mimic organ disease or dysfunction (Hoyt 1953, Ranger 1971, Travell & Simons 1991).

Baldry emphasizes the importance of the abdominal region as a source of considerable pain and distress involving pelvic, abdominal and gynecological symptoms. He states:

Pain in the abdomen and pelvis most likely to be helped by acupuncture is that which occurs as a result of activation of trigger points in the muscles, fascia, tendons and ligaments of the anterior and lateral abdominal wall, the lower back, the floor of the pelvis and the upper anterior part of the thigh. Such pain, however, is all too often erroneously assumed to be due to some intra-abdominal lesion, and as a consequence of being inappropriately treated is often allowed to persist for much longer than is necessary.

What activates these triggers?

Similar factors that produce 'stress' and adaptation load anywhere else in the musculoskeletal system: postural faults, trauma, environmental stressors such as cold and damp, surgery (another form of trauma), nutritional imbalances and psychogenic factors. Differential diagnosis is obviously important in a region housing so many vital organs, as is attention to the overall pattern of symptom presentation and the etiological context.

If the word *acupuncture* is replaced by the term *appropriate manual methods*, it is possible to appreciate that a large amount of abdominal and pelvic distress – much of it mimicking pathology – is remediable manually (see below).

Example: Interstitial cystitis and chronic pelvic pain

- Between September 1995 and November 2000, 45 women and 7 men, including 10 with interstitial cystitis and 42 with the urgency-frequency syndrome, were treated once or twice weekly for 8–12 weeks, using manual therapy applied to the pelvic floor, aimed at decreasing pelvic floor hypertonus and deactivating trigger points (Weiss 2001).
- Of the 42 patients with the urgency-frequency syndrome, 35 (83%) had moderate to marked improvement or complete resolution, while 7 of the 10 with interstitial cystitis had moderate to marked improvement.
- In 10 cases the subjective results (symptom score sheet) were confirmed by measuring resting pelvic floor tension by electromyography before and after the treatment course.

Conclusion

Whether structural influences on function, on a cellular or whole body level, are being considered, the examples outlined above offer evidence that in many instances biomechanical, structural, factors are of primary importance in restoration of a situation in which self-regulation can operate efficiently.

Specifically relevant is the evidence that in situations where cells are unable to process and metabolize nutrients, due to being in a distorted state, there seems little advantage in attempting to assist function by nutritional manipulation.

This does not negate nutritional intervention, but it strongly questions the automatic primacy of such an intervention.

Identifying vulnerability

Defeo & Hicks (1993) note that:

Osteopathic physicians Zink and Lawson have observed clinically that a significant percentage of the population assumes a consistently predictable postural adaptation, arising from nonspecific mechanical forces such as gravity, gross and micro-trauma, and other physiological stressors. These forces appear to have their greatest impact on the articular facets in the transitional areas of the vertebral column.

It is clearly important for the naturopathic practitioner to have an awareness, as best this can be ascertained, as to the patient's current level of vitality and vulnerability – both of which can be considered as reflections of the degree to which the person (or the local tissues) have adapted. The principle this reflects, in naturopathic terms, would be the desire to avoid interfering with self-regulation (*'vis'*) by further overloading adaptation mechanisms.

Zink & Lawson (1979) described methods for testing tissue preference in these transitional areas where fascial and other tensions and restrictions can most easily be noted, i.e. the occipitoatlantal (OA), cervicothoracic (CT), thoracolumbar (TL) and lumbosacral (LS) levels of the spine. These sites are tested for rotation and side-flexion preference.

Zink & Lawson's research showed that most people display (assessing the occipitoatlantal pattern first) alternating patterns of rotatory preference, with about 80% of people showing a common pattern of left-right-left-right (L-R-L-R) compensation, termed the 'common compensatory pattern' (CCP).

In a hospital-based study involving over 1000 patients they also observed that the approximately 20% of people whose compensatory pattern did not alternate in the CCP manner had poor health histories, low levels of 'wellness' and poor stress-coping abilities.

Methods for evaluation of the CCP and the accompanying imbalances are given in Chapter 6. See also Chapter 9 (Rehabilitation) which contains ways of addressing problems associated with such imbalances and asymmetries.

The Zink–Lawson sequence is described more fully, and illustrated, in Chapter 6.

Postural adaptation influences on visceral and somatic function

The first comprehensive discussion of how biomechanical alignment influences visceral function was described by the orthopedic surgeon Joel E. Goldthwaite in his book *Essentials of Body Mechanics* (1934). The concepts first described by Goldthwaite and subsequently developed by others (see below) are extremely relevant to naturopathic practice. They demonstrate the normal progression as tissues adapt to postural imbalance, with the added influences of aging and gravity adding to the picture.

The main factors which determine the maintenance of the abdominal viscera in position are the diaphragm and the abdominal muscles, both of which are relaxed and cease to support in faulty posture. The disturbances of circulation resulting from a low diaphragm and ptosis may give rise to chronic passive congestion in one or all of the organs of the abdomen and pelvis, since the local as well as general venous drainage may be impeded by the failure of the diaphragmatic pump to do its full work in the drooped body. Furthermore, the drag of these congested organs on their nerve supply, as well as the pressure on the sympathetic ganglia and plexuses, probably causes many irregularities in their function, varying from partial paralysis to overstimulation. All these organs receive fibers from both the vagus and sympathetic systems, either one of which may be disturbed. It is probable that one or all of these factors are active at various times in both the stocky and the slender anatomic types, and are responsible for many functional digestive disturbances. These disturbances, if continued long enough, may lead to diseases later in life. Faulty body mechanics in early life, then, becomes a vital factor in the production of the vicious cycle of chronic diseases and presents a chief point of attack in its prevention . . . In this upright position, as one becomes older, the tendency is for the abdomen to relax and sag more and more, allowing a ptosic condition of the abdominal and pelvic organs unless the supporting lower abdominal muscles are taught to contract properly. As the abdomen relaxes, there is a great tendency towards a drooped chest, with narrow rib

angle, forward shoulders, prominent shoulder blades, a forward position of the head, and probably pronated feet. When the human machine is out of balance, physiological function cannot be perfect; muscles and ligaments are in an abnormal state of tension and strain. A well-poised body means a machine working perfectly, with the least amount of muscular effort, and therefore better health and strength for daily life.

Schamberger's malalignment model

Some 70 years later Schamberger's malalignment model (2002) has offered important messages for naturopathic consideration, as he follows Goldthwaite and takes the discussion of postural imbalance beyond the biomechanical towards body-wide adaptational influences. He describes some of the inevitable changes that are associated with common asymmetries, as follows.

*Malalignment of the pelvis, spine and extremities remains one of the frontiers of medicine . . . the associated biomechanical changes – especially the shift in weight-bearing and asymmetries of muscle tension, strength, joint ranges of motion – affect soft tissues, joints **and organ systems throughout the body** and therefore have implications for general practice and most medical sub-speciality areas. [Emphasis added]*

Schamberger offers examples of visceral problems emerging from malalignment of the pelvis, resulting in pelvic floor dysfunction:

Typical visceral problems that have been attributed to pelvic floor dysfunction include:

- *Incontinence of bowel and bladder attributed to a lax floor*
- *Constipation and incomplete voiding with excessive tension*
- *Dysmenorrhoea, dyspareunia, impotence and sexual dysfunction*
- *Recurrent cystitis and urinary tract infection.*

He continues:

Distortion of the vagina and uterus may account for problems of dyspareunia and dysmenorrhoea, which can sometimes disappear just as miraculously with realignment (Barral & Mercier 1989, Costello 1998, Herman 1988).

Naturopathic physical medicine should be able to offer biomechanical solutions, or at least help and support, for such problems, and these issues will be discussed in greater detail in Chapter 10.

Beyond dysfunction towards pathology

Over time, adaptational changes, as listed by Goldthwaite and Schamberger, may progress from the production of dysfunction (e.g. low back pain) to the development of actual pathological changes. Staying with the same anatomic short leg example discussed earlier, Gofton & Trueman (1971) found a strong association between leg length and unilateral osteoarthritis on the side of the anatomically long leg.

They noted that all subjects with this type of OA 'had led healthy active lives prior to the onset of hip pain', and few subjects were aware of any difference in leg length. They also point out that this form of OA has its onset around the age of 53, but acknowledge that many people with precisely this anatomic asymmetry failed to develop an arthritic hip, *suggesting that factors other than the leg-length disparity are also important.*

This underscores the importance of the context in which this mechanical adaptation was being processed by the tissues under stress – with some joints becoming arthritic and others not.

What were the other variables? Nutritional? Genetic? Gender? Weight? Occupation? Other . . . ?

A naturopathic perspective should involve evaluation of the obvious anatomic and biomechanical, as well as identifiable contextual (e.g. environmental, psychological, nutritional, etc.) etiological features. These issues will be covered more fully in Chapters 4, 9 and 10.

A question

The onset of arthritic changes in the hip as a (partial) result of adaptation to a leg-length discrepancy leads logically to the question: Might surgery such as hip replacement ever be a naturopathic option? Clearly the answer here would depend upon the degree of pathology and its impact on the individual's life and lifestyle.

Naturopathic options might include ergonomic and postural advice, altered footwear (incorporation of cushioned insoles to reduce jarring); physical therapy and home stretching advice to enhance muscular function in the pelvic and lower limb regions; nutritional interventions to assist in weight control, reduced pro-inflammatory arachidonic acid-rich food intake (i.e. low animal fat and high fish oil content); enhanced intake of anti-inflammatory nutrients and potential cartilage-enhancing substances (glucosamine, chondroitin); pain-relieving strategies including hydrotherapy and acupuncture; pain-relieving botanical products; pain management methods including cognitive-behavioral and relaxation methods, etc.

However, if despite such efforts – in cases where pain has become constant, pathology extensive, function (walking etc.) extremely limited, and the potential for recovery without surgery extremely doubtful or impossible – the conclusion that hip replacement surgery may be the least worst option would be obvious. At that point this would be the best way of restoring function and reducing adaptive demands on the rest of the body. Therefore at times surgery could be considered to be a naturopathic choice.

Adaptation following trauma

Patterns of adaptation-induced dysfunction that emerge from habitual use patterns (poor posture, upper chest breathing, etc.) or from an anatomic anomaly (short leg, small hemi-pelvis, etc.) appear to differ from those that result from injury.

Lederman (1997) points out that following actual traumatically induced structural damage, tissue repair may lead to compensating patterns of use, with reduction in muscle force and possible wasting, often observed in backache patients. If uncorrected, such altered patterns of use inevitably lead to the development of habitual motor patterns and eventually to structural modifications.

The possible adaptational sequelae to trauma may include the following:

- Modified proprioceptive function due to alteration in mechanoreceptor behavior.
- If joint damage has occurred there may be inhibition of joint afferents influencing local muscle function, possibly involving the build-up of metabolic by-products (Lederman 1997).
- Altered motor patterns result from higher center responses to injury. These psychomotor changes may involve a sense of insecurity and the development of protective behavior patterns, resulting in actual structural modification such as muscle wasting.
- There may be non-painful reflexogenic responses to pain and also to injury (Hurley 1991).

Naturopathic physical medicine treatment of the patterns of imbalance that result from trauma, or from habitually stressful patterns of use, needs to address the causes of residual pain, as well as aiming to improve these patterns of voluntary use, with a focus on rehabilitation towards normal proprioceptive function.

Active, dynamic rehabilitation processes that re-educate the individual and which enhance neurological organization may usefully be assisted by passive manual methods, including basic massage and soft tissue approaches (see Chapter 9 for rehabilitation options in a naturopathic setting). Such methods fit with naturopathic concepts of assisting self-regulation, reducing adaptive demands and enhancing functionality.

A naturopathic approach

Wallden (2000) has explained how a biomechanical adaptation sequence calls for a comprehensive (i.e. naturopathic) therapeutic intervention:

Across the life-span of an organism, or of a tissue, the rate of repair slowly declines, whilst the rate of cumulative micro-trauma to the organism/tissue increases. The point at which the rate of trauma exceeds the rate of repair is the point at which the organism/tissue fails. If repair mechanisms are optimal, the organism or tissue should realize its genetic potential. If repair mechanisms are impaired or overloaded, potential is not realized, and adaptation will fail.

(See Fig. 9.1.)

Quite simply, in order to reduce microtrauma, there is a requirement for better patterns of use. However, for tissue repair to occur in an optimal manner, there is also a requirement for an optimal anabolic environment – which may be influenced by nutrition, breathing patterns, sleep patterns, hydration levels and modification of other potential stressors to the system or the organism (when unbalanced).

A naturopathic therapeutic formula that focuses on lightening the adaptive load, as well as on enhancing functionality (the ability to handle 'the load'), may be initiated by drawing on all or any of the requirements for health – whether these involve biomechanical, biochemical or psychosocial factors.

Can adaptation be used to restore optimal function?

The processes of adaptation have been used with great refinement in athletic and sport training.

Methods and principles devised in those settings can help guide therapeutic and rehabilitation choices in naturopathic practice, since they involve employment of sound physiological principles that do not conflict with basic naturopathic concepts.

The acronym SAID describes how a process of *specific adaptation to imposed demand* occurs. This is a familiar 'training' approach that employs structured adaptation principles that can offer athletic (and therapeutic) benefits (Norris 1995).

Take, for example, rehabilitation of the injured ankle, where therapeutic goals that are in tune with naturopathic principles might include encouragement of decreased swelling, pain and initial inflammatory response, without suppressing the essential healing process, using a combination of protection, rest, ice, compression and elevation (acronym = PRICE) (Andrews et al 1998).

In addition there would need to be protection of the joint, so that secondary inflammatory responses did not develop as a result of overly aggressive rehabilitation (Mattacola & Dwyer 2002).

In such cases – following the healing of damaged tissues – strategies need to be introduced to restore range of motion, muscular strength, power and endurance (as well as proprioceptive efficiency) to pre-injury levels, so that full, asymptomatic functional activities can be performed.

In this recovery and rehabilitation process the application of specific functional exercises is important to 'stress' the healing tissue, with SAID principles being helpful in the design of functional progression (Kegerreis 1983). Such stress will lead to the formation of collagen cross-bridges along the lines of stress, resulting in the development of 'functional scar tissue'. Injured tissues that are fully immobilized without functional stress applied to the healing tissue will form dysfunctional scar tissue that may go on to cause further symptoms (Croft 1995).

It is ironic that SAID principles can work to rehabilitate and add functionality just as effectively as they can to create dysfunction, depending on the appropriateness or otherwise of the imposed demands.

The use of SAID methods are directly in tune with naturopathic thinking when used therapeutically, representing as they do a means for reducing the adaptive load at the same time as enhancing functionality, while respecting and working with self-repair mechanisms.

Maladaptation

Adaptation is not necessarily beneficial and can substantially reduce efficiency. Take for example the processes involved in what is known as stimulus–fatigue–recovery–adaptation (SFRA).

Verkhoshansky (1986, 1988) noted that several weeks of a unidirectional concentrated load of strength, or strength-endurance training in track and field athletes, commonly resulted in a diminished speed–strength (power) capability. Put simply this means that adaptation to one demand (strength) caused reduced efficiency in another function (speed).

It has been found that a return to more comprehensive (less specialized) training reversed this trend – which is not surprising since removal of an unbalanced training approach would reduce an excessive degree of adaptive load.

Interestingly, the changes that occur during such unbalanced training are not just a matter of learned responses, but seem to involve endocrine imbalances (as Selye predicted) as observed when young weight lifters introduced just such a modified training (Fry et al 2000).

Stone et al (1991) noted that adaptation – or maladaptation – is the summation of all stressors that an athlete may encounter (a contextual rather than a linear perspective), with recovery–adaptation being viewed as involving a long-term interplay between various stressors.

'We are all athletes, but not all of us are in training!' (Vaughan 1998)

Substitute the word 'patient' for 'athlete', and we can easily see how specialized knowledge in relation to sport and adaptation can translate into an understanding of use patterns completely divorced from athletics.

- How does the individual sit, stand, bend, breathe?
- What are the positions adopted for frequently performed tasks?
- What work or leisure postures are regular features of the individual's life?
- What aspects of the individual's close environment (chair, bed, desk, shoes, car seat, etc.) add contextual stressors to the picture?
- What are the individual's age, gender, health history and record of adaptation to past trauma, occupational and leisure activities?
- What nutritional, endocrine, neurological and/or psychosocial factors may be influencing this situation?

These are the potential stressors that could impose adaptive demands on each of us, overlaid on our unique inherited and acquired characteristics, the summation of our past and ongoing adaptations.

The questions that need to be asked in a naturopathic setting are to what extent any of these factors have contributed to the patient's presenting symptoms, and/or may be acting to aggravate or maintain dysfunction?

Safe adaptation

In both training and rehabilitation settings, common sense and clinical experience suggest that injury is less likely (i.e. recovery and prevention are both optimal) when:

- muscle and joint structures are coordinated, balanced, flexible and stable and are free of mechanical dysfunction
- appropriate movement(s) are used for exercise
- there is an opportunity for complete recovery between training/exercise periods
- overtraining is avoided
- light (and in home-based settings – pleasurable) training periods are scheduled
- increases of intensity or volume of exercise are progressive, and only modest increases of intensity are introduced between adaptations
- dietary and sleep factors are balanced.

In contrast, injury is more likely to occur if biomechanical structures have not adapted well to previously imposed demands or if features of the list above are not operating.

Bakker et al (2003) remark that musculoskeletal tissues not only weaken from overuse or disuse but also that the actual shape of the vertebrae and the intervertebral discs, as well as the ligaments, adapts and adjusts to the type of load imposed. This is clearly an example of a specific adaptation to imposed demand (Conroy & Earle 2000).

The quality of this physiological musculoskeletal adaptation – that alters function as well as structure – is largely determined by the magnitude of the load, the use, or misuse, to which the spine is put.

Choice of therapeutic approaches

In naturopathic thinking the ideal selection of therapeutic methods and modalities, in any given case, can be seen to require a need for choices that match that individual's current levels of decompensation/maladaptation, vitality and vulnerability.

Treatment approaches should have as objectives a necessity to either reduce adaptive load or enhance functionality (or both), so allowing self-regulation to operate more effectively. The only other therapeutic choice would be to focus attention mainly on symptomatic relief, with little or no immediate attention as to cause. Indeed, symptom-oriented treatment may at times be the only choice initially available; however, in a naturopathic setting, objectives that incorporate the possibility of assisting self-regulation ('lighten the load/enhance functionality') would usually be the primary choices.

Treatment as a potential further stressor

As previously noted, Selye defined stress as anything to which the organism is obliged to respond, to adapt to, good or bad, meaning that stress and stressors are not by definition 'negative' or necessarily undesirable.

Selye (1978) further observed that:

The stress of failure, humiliation, or infection is detrimental; but that of exhilarating, creative, successful work is beneficial. The stress reaction, like energy consumption, may have good or bad effects.

Since all therapeutic interventions, by their very nature, impose *adaptive demands*, these can be seen, in the absolute sense, to be *stressors*.

In naturopathic terms this imposes an obligation on the practitioner to select methods and modalities that achieve the maximum benefit accompanied by the least cost, in terms of demands for further adaptation, on the part of an already distressed system.

Whether an individual receives treatment involving insertion of a needle, a manipulative maneuver, an exercise regime, a change of diet, a hydrotherapy procedure, or anything else, the method involved demands physiological responses – further adaptation.

It is not difficult to imagine how a susceptible, poorly compensated individual, with multiple symptoms and a background of adaptive overload, could be quite unable to adapt to particular therapeutic demands, leading to exacerbation of symptoms – or worse.

Mennell (1964) points out what should be obvious – that imposing adaptive demands needs to consider not only the local tissues but also those at a distance that may be affected. He gives the example of the use of an orthotic device, or a heel lift, that can produce side-effects such as back pain if the structures required to adapt to the altered leg length are incapable of compensating to absorb the imposed changes. In such a case, new symptoms become likely – for example if the lumbar spine of the individual happens to be rigid or arthritic.

Chapter 9 provides exercise-based examples.

Genetic influences

Fibromyalgia syndrome (FMS) and adaptation as an example

FMS involves chronic body-wide pain, fatigue, disturbed sleep and usually a variety of other symptoms, including irritable bowel syndrome (Clauw 1995).

Some studies show clear indications of familial tendencies/genetic components in the development of FMS in a subset of people affected (Buskila & Neumann 1997, Pellegrino et al 1989).

- Mitral valve prolapse has been reported in 75% of patients with FMS, a far higher rate than that noted in the general population (Schneider & Brady 2001).
- When HLA typing was carried out involving four multicase families (in which at least two members of the same family had FMS), statistically significant genetic linkage was established (Yunus et al 1999).

Researchers at the University of Miami (Klimas 1995) have evolved a model that attempts to explain the evolution and perpetuation of fibromyalgia (FMS) and chronic fatigue syndromes (CFS). This suggests that there is an initial predisposition followed by an 'etiological event' (i.e. major adaptation demand) which might involve a single trauma, a reactivation of dormant viral activity or a one-off infection (Fig. 2.14).

One or other such event seems to lead to a major ongoing immunological response which is perpetuated either by further activation of infectious agents – viral as a rule, it is suggested (Keller & Klimas 1994) – or by a dysfunctional hypothalamic–pituitary–adrenal axis related to stress influence (Lowe & Honeyman-Lowe 2003). This hypothesized explanation has strong echoes of Selye's multiple stressor-influence model.

Klimas (1995) further suggests that:

Treatment is basically symptomatic. Our concept is to treat anything we can. If someone has sleep disturbance we treat it. If we can take 20% of the miseries away by giving someone restorative sleep and we can eliminate 20% of the symptoms by treating their allergy overlay, then they are 40% better and that's significant.

These thoughts support the suggestions, expressed earlier, that one aspect of comprehensive care should be 'to lessen the [adaptive] load' and this is probably what any naturopathic practitioner would also do (although the methods employed might differ considerably from those that Klimas might suggest).

A genetic predisposition to FMS – for some patients at least – seems to be a probability, based on the evidence available, and were there nothing to be done about such a predisposition, the approach suggested by Klimas would seem reasonable.

But is there really nothing that can be done to influence genetic predispositions? In other words, is gene expression 'hard-wired'?

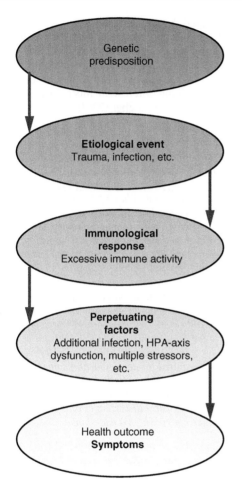

Figure 2.14 Genetic predisposition hypothesis for fibromyalgia. HPA, hypothalamic pituitary adrenocortical [axis]. Reproduced with permission from Chaitow (2003a)

Evidence exists that gene expression can indeed (at least sometimes) be modified or influenced, not only by tinkering with the genes themselves as researchers are currently attempting to do but also by encouraging them to express themselves more normally.

There are at least two approaches that might do so – one a great deal less obvious than the other – involving nutritional (biochemical) and structural considerations.

Environmental risk factors interacting with genetic predisposition leading to disease

Masi (2000) has presented an integrative physiopathogenetic perspective of hormonal and immunological risk factors leading to such diseases as rheumatoid arthritis and fibromyalgia. This model, which reso-

nates strongly with the concepts of adaptation and decompensation discussed above, outlines a multilayer preclinical phase in which, during a long interval of symptomatically silent disease incubation, multiple genetic, somatic, behavioral and environmental risk factors (stressors) perturb the normal homeostasis of the core systems (i.e. the neuroendocrine, immunological and microvascular compartments).

When physiological homeostasis is sufficiently disturbed by such stressors (i.e. when adaptation fails), inflammatory and clinical manifestations appear or progress. Conversely, regulatory mechanisms controlling the homeostasis of perturbed core systems may also become normalized to a point that favors clinical improvements. Such amelioration of disease activity may occur in persons with less strong genetic loading predisposing towards particular disease processes, and with fewer accumulated non-genomic risk factors, something that naturopathic care would aim to encourage (Masi & Chang 1999).

Biochemical and structural factors that modify gene expression

Gene expression (also known as protein expression) is the process by which a gene's information is converted into the structures and functions of a cell. This is a multistep process which involves a sequence of transcription, post-transcriptional modification (involving messenger RNA) and translation, followed by folding, post-translational modification and targeting.

The amount of protein that a cell expresses depends on the tissue, the developmental stage of the organism, and the metabolic or physiological state of the cell (Araujo et al 2006).

Regulation of gene expression is the cellular control of the amount and timing of appearance of the functional product of a gene. Any step of gene expression may be modulated, from the DNA–RNA transcription step to post-translational modification of a protein. Gene regulation gives the cell control over structure and function, and is the basis for cellular differentiation, morphogenesis and the versatility and adaptability of any organism.

Genes may be regarded as nodes in a network, with inputs being proteins such as transcription factors, and outputs being the level of gene expression. The node itself performs a function, and the operation of this function has been interpreted as performing a kind of information processing within the cell that determines cellular behavior.

Hard wired?

Bland has discussed the biochemical possibility for such modification as follows (Bland 1999, Martin 2001):

Functional genomics derived out of the human genome project, in which it was thought that by dissecting the code of life in our 23 pairs of chromosomes people would be able to understand how they were going to die. They would see locked in their genes heart disease, cancer, diabetes, arthritis, whatever it might be, and they would tell from these genetic imperfections what day, and what disease, they would finally fall prey to . . . the discovery of the code of life through the dissection of the encyclopedia of our chromosomes has not told us how we're going to die, but told us how we're going to live. Mendelian determinism . . . said that locked into our genes, when the sperm met the egg, were these strengths and weaknesses that we call the recessive and dominant characteristics of inheritance that we could not get out from under. That basically if we had the genes for cancer we would die of cancer. If we had the genes for heart disease we would die of heart disease. It turns out that the human genome project has discovered that the genes that we thought were hard-wired to produce these diseases, are not hard-wired at all. Within our genes are multiple messages, and the message that is expressed at any moment – that's in our phenotype – is a consequence of the environmental messages including diet, lifestyle, environment, that wash over our genes to give rise to different expression paths of the genes . . . some may be healthy, some may be unhealthy, depending upon the experiences that are washing over our genes . . . what we're really seeing is that the major determinants for the expression of genetic patterns, over decades of living, are the decisions that we make, either consciously or subconsciously, every day. How we exercise, how we work, what our stress patterns are.

Research by Ames et al (2002) has now shown that these concepts are indeed accurate, and that gene expression can often be dramatically modified by nutritional strategies. Ames and colleagues have listed more than 50 genetic diseases, successfully treated with high doses of vitamins and other nutrients, most of them rare inborn metabolic diseases due to defective enzymes.

Modifying gene expression biomechanically

But there exists another – possibly surprising to some – factor that can modify gene expression: the state of structural adaptation of the cells themselves.

These structural adaptations can be seen to influence, and indeed determine, the way cells express themselves genetically. Put at its simplest, structural modification to cell shape, warping or distortion of the cytoskeleton, and the environment in which the

cell is located have been shown unequivocally to modify its ability to process nutrients normally, or to express itself genetically (Ingber 2003). This has profound implications for physical medicine in general, and for naturopathic physical medicine in particular.

There is growing interest in mechanical forces as biological regulators. Ingber (2003) reports:

Clinicians have come to recognize the importance of mechanical forces for the development and function of the heart and lung, the growth of skin and muscle, the maintenance of cartilage and bone, and the etiology of many debilitating diseases, including hypertension, osteoporosis, asthma and heart failure. Exploration of basic physiological mechanisms, such as sound sensation, motion recognition and gravity detection, has also demanded explanation in mechanical terms. At the same time, the introduction of new techniques for manipulating and probing individual molecules and cells has revealed the importance of the physical nature of the biochemical world. Enzymes such as RNA polymerase generate as much force as molecular motors (Mehta et al 1999); cells exert tractional forces on micro-particles greater than those that can be applied by optical tweezers (Schmidt et al 1993); and behaviours required for developmental control, including growth, differentiation, polarity, motility, contractility and programmed cell death, are all influenced by physical distortion of cells through their extracellular matrix (ECM) adhesions.

It is reasonable to ask how a physical force applied to the extracellular matrix, creating cell distortion, can change chemical activities inside the cell and control tissue development. The answer, says Ingber, lies in molecular biophysics and to a large extent in the tensegrity format on which cellular architecture is based (Chen & Ingber 1999, Ingber 1991, 1997, 1999).

It seems that when a distending force is applied to cell surface adhesion receptors, the mechanical load is transferred to linked cytoskeletal elements that form the tensegrity framework of the cell. These may either distort or break (Wang & Stamenovic 2000).

If the cytoskeletal filaments and associated regulatory molecules distort, without breaking, then some or all of the molecules that make up these structures effectively change shape, and when the *shape* of a molecule is altered, its *biophysical properties* change. The resulting changes affect intracellular biochemistry by altering thermodynamic parameters locally in living cells (Ingber & Jamieson 1985).

Ingber (2000) explains further:

In contrast to existing paradigms that look for explanations in terms of specific soluble and insoluble factors and linear signaling pathways, the functional state of the cell appears to 'self-organize' as a result of the architecture and dynamics of its underlying regulatory network.

In this context, tensegrity-based changes in cytoskeletal structure may influence cell phenotype, switching on the basis of their ability simultaneously to alter the biochemical activities of multiple cytoskeleton-associated signaling components throughout the cell. Because it provides a structural basis for the formation of functionally integrated molecular hierarchies, tensegrity might also have played a central role in the origin of cellular life.

It may be of interest to note that Ingber's research into bone density loss in astronauts (on behalf of NASA) demonstrated that the collapse of the cytoskeleton's tensegrity struts in zero gravity warped the cells and was the primary reason for the cells' inability to process calcium and other nutrients normally, leading to the loss of bone density (Ingber 1999). Here we see a picture of complex structural adaptations and modification determining the efficiency of metabolic function and gene expression, at the cellular level.

As mentioned above, the implications for physical medicine in general, and naturopathic physical medicine in particular, are colossal, although as yet difficult to fully comprehend.

What seems clear is that given a structurally modified context (tissues that are, for example, fibrotic, contracted, distorted, hypertonic or even in spasm), the best nutrition in the world would have difficulty being utilized adequately.

The osteopathic dictum 'structure governs function' would seem to be validated by Ingber's research – and this clearly places structural normalization at the forefront of naturopathic therapeutic requirements.

The corollary to this is, of course, that – as described earlier – functional factors such as overuse and misuse, imposed on tissues, will modify structure (shortening, fibrosis, etc.), making the structure–function equation a two-way process.

Structure and function: the adaptation cycle

Leaving aside the obvious link between structure and function on the musculoskeletal (muscle, joint, back pain, etc.) level, it is reasonable to ask what evidence is there for systemic, constitutional, whole-body influences of structural (biomechanical) changes that emerge from a background of adaptation and compensation.

What impact on general health – including gene expression as suggested by Ingber's (1993) studies –

derives from the processes of structural compensation and adaptation that occur in response to aging, environmental influences, overuse, misuse, abuse and disuse and the resulting acquired deviations from the structural norm?

Different areas of recent research offer glimpses of the reality of the scale of structure/function influences on cellular metabolism, gene expression and internal signaling mechanisms. Box 2.4 provides a glimpse of the larger picture of how climate helped to determine the very shape of the human body via a process of adaptation, achieved through evolution.

Langevin's research

Ingber's research – outlined above – suggests that, in the short term, normalizing distorted, crowded, bunched and generally abnormally structured tissues (e.g. through exercise, stretching, massage and manipulation) should enhance metabolic function, health and gene expression (Ingber 2003).

Langevin et al (2002), at the University of Vermont, have added greatly to our understanding of biomechanical force, as exerted on connective tissue by acupuncture, building on Ingber's findings:

We have demonstrated that acupuncture needle rotation results in a measurable deformation of connective tissue. Pulling of collagen and/or elastic fibers and deformation of extracellular matrix during needle manipulation may have powerful and long-lasting effects on local cells, including synthesis and release of extracellular matrix components and modification of interstitial connective tissue composition (Langevin et al 2001). Such changes in matrix composition in turn potentially can modulate the effect of future mechanical signal transduction in connective tissue cells (Brand 1997).

By providing evidence of subcutaneous connective tissue involvement in needle grasp, Langevin et al's research suggests that the mechanism of action of acupuncture also involves extraneural tissues and paves the way for further investigation.

The results of this research highlight the potentially important role of interstitial connective tissue in neuromodulation:

Subcutaneous connective tissue forms a continuous tissue plane throughout the body. This tissue plane is itself continuous with dermis, with interstitial planes separating muscles, bones, and tendons and with intramuscular connective tissue. These connective tissue planes also constitute the 'milieu' surrounding a wide variety of sensory mechanoreceptors and nociceptors (Willis & Coggeshall 1991). Techniques such as acupuncture may act not simply via neural

Box 2.4 How have human body characteristics been affected by adaptation to historical climatic influences?

In 1991, Ruff described how the colder the climate, the wider the body structure appeared to be. He explained that:

The very broad pelvis of small early hominids has previously been interpreted in obstetrical and biomechanical terms. However, neither of these considerations can explain the subsequent decrease in maximum pelvic breadth relative to stature in larger more recent hominids. [This] increase in relative linearity of the body, with an increase in body size, is consistent with basic thermoregulatory principles. Specifically, to maintain a constant surface area/body mass ratio, absolute body breadth should remain constant despite differences in body height. Variation among modern humans supports the prediction: populations living in the tropics vary greatly in stature, but show little variation in body breadth. In contrast, populations living in colder climates have absolutely wider bodies, and thus lower surface area/body mass, regardless of stature.

Ruff also suggested that thermoregulatory constraints on absolute body breadth, together with obstetric and biomechanical factors, have probably contributed to the evolution of the rotational birth process and secondary altriciality [relative underdevelopment of the human newborn infant compared to other primates], associated with increased body and brain size in *Homo erectus*.

Additionally, Stock (2004) has demonstrated that the relative strength of distal limb bones, such as the tibia, shows a stronger correlation with habitual activity patterns than does the relative strength of proximal limb bones, such as the femur, which shows a stronger correlation with climate.

More recently, Ruff et al (2006) pointed out that another way to explain these same features is that the structure of proximal limb bones is influenced by body shape, which itself is in large part determined by adaptation to climatic demands (Ruff 1994). In contrast, it seems that the structure of distal limb bones is probably more influenced by adaptation to activity, rather than climate (or general body type).

Langevin's more recent research (Langevin et al 2005) has profound implications for manual methods:

Cytoskeleton-dependent changes in cell shape are well-established factors regulating a wide range of cellular functions including signal transduction, gene expression and matrix adhesion. Although the importance of mechanical forces on cell shape and function is well established in cultured cells, very little is known about these effects in whole tissues or in vivo. In this study we have used ex vivo and in vivo models to investigate the effect of tissue stretch on mouse subcutaneous tissue fibroblast morphology.

Tissue stretch ex vivo (average 25% tissue elongation from 10 minutes to 2 hours) caused a significant time-dependent increase in fibroblast cell body perimeter and cross-sectional area (ANOVA $p < 0.01$) . . . Tissue stretch in vivo for 30 minutes had effects that paralleled those ex vivo.

*The dynamic, cytoskeleton-dependent responses of fibroblasts to changes in tissue length have important implications for our understanding of normal movement and posture, **as well as therapies using mechanical stimulation of connective tissue including physical therapy, massage and acupuncture**. [Emphasis added]*

Summary

To summarize the research of Ingber, and that of Langevin, insofar as their findings impact this particular discussion:

- Cell behavior – including metabolic functions, handling of nutrients, gene expression and even cell death – is 'shape dependent', powerfully influenced by structural changes (resulting from the adaptational effects of the influence of gravity, environment, aging, etc.).

- Amongst its many other functions, connective tissue acts as an important signaling mechanism with body-wide influences, the efficiency of which is also 'shape dependent', being positively affected by methods such as acupuncture needling and manual methods.

Stating the obvious

At first glance the naturopathic concepts as outlined in this chapter – of attention to cause, doing no harm, encouraging self-regulation, etc. – would seem to state the obvious, to represent no more than common sense, and to possibly be indistinguishable from the primary beliefs and practices of many other health care systems.

stimulation, but also by producing changes in the connective tissue milieu surrounding sensory afferent nerve fibers. These connective tissue changes may be long lasting, which may explain claims that acupuncture can have prolonged effects.

However, on closer examination, differences should become apparent, most notably the incorporation into clinical reasoning of all of these features, overlaid onto a perspective that observes whatever symptoms are evident to be part of ongoing (often adaptational) processes, rather than seeing them as stand-alone entities.

In truth, much that is now done in responsible and evidence-based osteopathic, chiropractic, physical therapy, massage and other 'bodywork and movement therapy' settings conforms to many of these naturopathic principles – but as will become clear in discussions in later chapters, by no means always.

Mainstream ('allopathic') medical approaches to pain, for example, would often seem to have a far less searching focus on enhancing homeostatic mechanisms – with symptom relief to the fore. Analgesic and anti-inflammatory medication – while useful in extreme conditions – hardly deals with cause or encourages self-regulation.

In the next chapter an historical overview of naturopathic physical medicine is presented to allow the context out of which modern naturopathic physical medicine has emerged to be better understood.

References

Ames B, Elson-Schwab I, Silver E 2002 High-dose vitamin therapy stimulates variant enzymes with decreased coenzyme binding affinity (increased Km): relevance to genetic disease and polymorphisms. American Journal of Clinical Nutrition 75(4):616–658

Andrews J, Harrelson G, Wilk K 1998 Physical rehabilitation of the injured athlete, 2nd edn. WB Saunders, Philadelphia

Araujo A, Ribeiroa MFM, Enzveiler A et al 2006 Myocardial antioxidant enzyme activities and concentration and glutathione metabolism in experimental hyperthyroidism. Molecular and Cellular Endocrinology 249(1–2):133–139

Bakker E, Koning H, Verhagen A 2003 Interobserver reliability of the 24-hour schedule in patients with low back pain: a questionnaire measuring the daily use and loading of the spine. Journal of Manipulative and Physiological Therapeutics 26(4):226–232

Baldry P 1999 Acupuncture, trigger points and musculoskeletal pain, 3rd edn. Churchill Livingstone, London

Barral J-P, Mercier P 1989 Visceral manipulation. Eastland Press, Seattle

Beal M 1983 Palpatory testing of somatic dysfunction in patients with cardiovascular disease. Journal of the American Osteopathic Association 82(11): 73–82

Beal M 1985 Viscerosomatic reflexes review. Journal of the American Osteopathic Association 85:786–800

Bendtsen L, Jensen R, Olesen J 1996 Qualitatively altered nociception in chronic myofascial pain. Pain 65:259–264

Bennet C 1952 Physics. Barnes & Noble, New York

Berczi I 1986 Immunoregulation by pituitary hormones. In: Berczi I (ed) Pituitary function and immunity. CRC Press, Boca Raton, FL

Berczi I 1994 The role of the growth and lactogenic hormone family in immune function. Neuroimmunomodulation 1:201–216

Berczi I 2005 Stress and disease: the contributions of Hans Selye to neuroimmune biology. Department of Immunology, Faculty of Medicine, University of Manitoba, Winnipeg

Berczi I, Nagy E 1991 Effects of hypophysectomy on immune function. In: Ader R, Felten DL, Cohen N (eds) Psychoneuroimmunology II. Academic Press, San Diego

Berczi I, Nagy E 1994 Neurohormonal control of cytokines during injury. In: Rothwell NJ, Berkenbosch F (eds) Brain control of responses to trauma. Cambridge University Press, Cambridge

Bevan S 1999 Nociceptive peripheral neurones: cellular properties. In: Wall P, Melzack R (eds) Textbook of pain, 4th edn. Harcourt, Edinburgh, p 85–103

Bland J 1999 Genetic nutritioneering. Keats Publishing, Los Angeles, p 116–118

Brand R 1997 What do tissues and cells know of mechanics? Annals of Medicine 29:267–269

Brookes J, Pusey A 2006 Application of positional techniques in the treatment of animals. In: Chaitow L (ed) Positional release techniques, 3rd edn. Churchill Livingstone, Edinburgh

Buskila D, Neumann L 1997 Fibromyalgia syndrome and nonarticular tenderness in relatives of patients with FMS. Journal of Rheumatology 24:941–944

Chaitow L 2003a Fibromyalgia syndrome: a practitioner's guide to treatment. Churchill Livingstone, Edinburgh

Chaitow L 2003b Modern neuromuscular techniques, 2nd edn. Churchill Livingstone, Edinburgh

Chaitow L 2006 Muscle energy techniques, 3rd edn. Churchill Livingstone, Edinburgh

Chaitow L, DeLany J 2000 Clinical application of neuromuscular techniques: the upper body. Churchill Livingstone, Edinburgh

Chaitow L, DeLany J 2003 Neuromuscular techniques in orthopaedics. Techniques in Orthopaedics 18(1):74–86

Chaitow L, Bradley D, Gilbert C 2002 Multidisciplinary approaches to breathing pattern disorders. Churchill Livingstone, Edinburgh

Chen C, Ingber D 1999 Tensegrity and mechanoregulation: from skeleton to cytoskeleton. Osteoarthritis and Cartilage 7:81–94

Clark SC, Kamen K 1987 The human hematopoietic colony-stimulating factors. Science 236:1229

Clauw D 1995 Fibromyalgia: more than just a musculoskeletal disease. American Family Physician 52(3):843–851

Conroy B, Earle R 2000 Bone, muscle and connective tissue adaptations to physical activity. In: Baechle TR, Earle R (eds)/National Strength & Conditioning Association. Essentials of strength training and conditioning, 2nd edn. Human Kinetics, Champaign, IL, p 57–72

Costello K 1998 Myofascial syndromes. In: Steege J, Metzger D, Levy B (eds) Chronic pelvic pain: an integrated approach. WB Saunders, Philadelphia, p 251–266

Crenshaw K 2006 Use of MET in athletic training. In: Chaitow L (ed) Muscle energy techniques, 3rd edn. Churchill Livingstone, Edinburgh

Crockett HC, Gross LB, Wilk KE et al 2002 Osseous adaptation and range of motion at the gleno-humeral joint in professional baseball pitchers. American Journal of Sports Medicine 30(1):20–26

Croft A 1995 Management of soft tissue injuries. In: Foreman SM, Croft AC (eds) Whiplash injuries: cervical acceleration/deceleration syndrome, 2nd edn. Lippincott Williams & Wilkins, Baltimore

Defeo G, Hicks L 1993 A description of the common compensatory pattern in relationship to the osteopathic postural examination. Dynamic Chiropractic 24:11

Fry A, Kraemer W, Stone M 2000 Relationships between serum testosterone, cortisol and weightlifting performance. Journal of Strength and Conditioning Research 14:338–343

Gofton J, Trueman G 1971 Studies in osteoarthritis of the hip: Part II. Osteoarthritis of the hip and leg-length disparity. CMA Journal 104:791–799

Goldenberg D 1991 Fibromyalgia, chronic fatigue syndrome, and myofascial pain syndrome. Current Opinion in Rheumatology 3:247–258

Goldthwaite J 1934 Essentials of body mechanics. Lippincott, Philadelphia

Greenfield B, Catlin PA, Coats PW et al 1995 Posture in patients with shoulder overuse injuries and healthy individuals. Journal of Orthopedic Sports Physical Therapy 21(5):287–295

Grieve G 1986 Modern manual therapy. Churchill Livingstone, London

He X, Proske U, Schaible H, Schmidt R 1988 Acute inflammation of the knee joint in the cat alters flexor motor neurones to leg movement. Journal of Neurophysiology 59:326–340

Herman H 1988 Urogenital dysfunction. In: Wilder E (ed) Obstetric and gynaecological physical therapy. Churchill Livingstone, New York, p 83–111

Hong C, Simons D 1998 Pathophysiologic and electrophysiologic mechanisms of myofascial trigger points. Archives of Physical and Medical Rehabilitation 79:863–872

Hoyt H 1953 Segmental nerve lesions as a cause of trigonitis syndrome. Stanford Medical Bulletin 11:61–64

Huether G 1996 The central adaptation syndrome: psychosocial stress as a trigger for adaptive modifications of brain structure and brain function. Progress in Neurobiology 48:569–612

Hurley M 1991 Isokinetic and isometric muscle strength and inhibition after elbow arthroplasty. Journal of Orthopedic Rheumatology 4:83–95

Ingber D 1991 Integrins as mechanochemical transducers. Current Opinion in Cell Biology 3:841–848

Ingber D 1993 The riddle of morphogenesis: a question of solution chemistry or molecular cell engineering? Cell 75:1249–1252

Ingber D 1997 Tensegrity: the architectural basis of cellular mechanotransduction. Annual Review of Physiology 59:575–599

Ingber D 1999 How cells (might) sense microgravity. FASEB Journal S1:3–15

Ingber D 2000 Cancer as a disease of epithelial–mesenchymal interactions and extracellular matrix regulation. Differentiation 70:547–560

Ingber D 2003 Tensegrity II. How structural networks influence cellular information processing networks. Journal of Cell Science 116:1397–1408

Ingber D, Jamieson J 1985 Cells as tensegrity structures: architectural regulation of histo-differentiation by physical forces transduced over basement membrane. In: Andersson LC, Gahmberg CG, Ekblom P (eds) Gene expression during normal and malignant differentiation. Academic Press, Orlando, FL, p 13–32

Janda V 1988 Muscles and cervicogenic pain syndromes. In: Grant R (ed) Physical therapy in the cervical and thoracic spine. Churchill Livingstone, New York

Johansson H 1993 Influence on gamma-muscle spindle system from muscle afferents stimulated by KCl and lactic acid. Neuroscience Research 16(1):49–57

Juhl J, Ippolito Cremin T, Russell G 2004 Prevalence of frontal plane pelvic postural asymmetry – Part 1. Journal of the American Osteopathic Association 104(10):411–421

Kegerreis S 1983 The construction and implementation of functional progression as a component of athletic rehabilitation. Journal of Orthopaedic and Sports Physical Therapy 5:14–19

Keller R, Klimas N 1994 Association between HLA class II antigens and CFS. Clinical Infectious Diseases 18(Suppl):S154–S156

Kelso A 1971 A double-blind clinical study of osteopathic findings in hospital patients. Journal of the American Osteopathic Association 70:570–592

Klimas N 1995 Report to CFS patient conference. Charlotte, North Carolina, September 23. In: Fibromyalgia Network Newsletter, January, p 12

Knutson G 2005 Anatomic and functional leg-length inequality: a review and recommendation for clinical decision-making. Part I, anatomic leg-length inequality: prevalence, magnitude, effects and clinical significance. Chiropractic and Osteopathy 13:11

Komendatov G 1945 Proprioceptivnije reflexi glaza i golovy u krolikov. Fiziologiceskij Zurnal 31:62

Korr IM 1967 Axonal delivery of neuroplasmic components to muscle cells. Science 155:342–345

Korr IM 1970 The physiological basis of osteopathic medicine. Postgraduate Institute of Osteopathic Medicine and Surgery, New York

Korr IM 1976 Spinal cord as organiser of disease process. Academy of Applied Osteopathy Yearbook, Newark, OH

Korr IM 1981 Axonal transport and neurotrophic functions. In: Korr IM (ed) Spinal cord as organiser of disease process, part 4. Academy of Applied Osteopathy Yearbook, Newark, OH, p 451–458

Kraemer WJ, Gomez AL 2001 Establishing a solid fitness base. In: Foran B (ed) High performance sports conditioning. Human Kinetics, Champaign, IL, p 3–17

Langevin H, Churchill D, Cipolla M 2001 Mechanical signaling through connective tissue: a mechanism for the therapeutic effect of acupuncture. FASEB Journal 15:2275–2282

Langevin H, Churchill D, Wu J et al 2002 Evidence of connective tissue involvement in acupuncture. FASEB Journal 16:872–874. Online. Available: www.fasebj.org/cgi/content/full/16/8/872

Langevin H, Bouffard N, Badger G et al 2005 Dynamic fibroblast cytoskeletal response to subcutaneous tissue stretch ex vivo and in vivo. American Journal of Physiology. Cell Physiology 288:C747–756

Lederman E 1997 Fundamentals of manual therapy. Churchill Livingstone, Edinburgh

Lederman E 2005 Science and practice of manual therapy. Churchill Livingstone, Oxford

Lewit K 1999 Manipulation in rehabilitation of the motor system, 3rd edn. Butterworths, London

Lowe JC, Honeyman-Lowe G 2003 The metabolic rehabilitation of fibromyalgia patients. In: Chaitow L (ed) Fibromyalgia syndrome: a practitioner's guide to treatment, 2nd edn. Churchill Livingstone, Edinburgh

Martin S 2001 Interview with Jeff Bland: lessons from the genome. CAM November 2001

Masi A 2000 Hormonal and immunologic risk factors for the development of rheumatoid arthritis: an integrative physiopathogenetic perspective. Rheumatic Disease Clinics of North America 26:775–804

Masi A, Chang H 1999 Cigarette smoking and other acquired risk factors for rheumatoid arthritis. In: Kaufman LD, Varga J (eds) Rheumatic diseases and the environment. Chapman & Hall, New York, p 111

Mattacola C, Dwyer M 2002 Rehabilitation of the ankle after acute sprain or chronic instability. Journal of Athletic Training 37(4):413

McEwan N 1994 The plasticity of the hippocampus is the reason for its vulnerability. Seminars in Neuroscience 6:197–204

Mehta A, Rief M, Spudich J 1999 Single-molecule biomechanics with optical methods. Science 283:1689–1695

Mennell J 1964 Joint pain. Churchill, Boston, MA

Norris C 1995 An exercise programme to enhance lumbar stabilisation. Physiotherapy 81(3):138–146

Osbahr DC, Cannon DL, Speer KP 2002 Retroversion of the humerus in the throwing shoulder of college baseball pitchers. American Journal of Sports Medicine 30:347–353

Patterson M, Wurster R 1997 Neurophysiologic system. In: Ward R (ed) Foundations for osteopathic medicine. Williams & Wilkins, Baltimore, p 137–151

Pellegrino M, Waylonis G, Sommer A 1989 Familial occurrence of primary fibromyalgia. Archives of Physical Medicine and Rehabilitation 70(1):61–63

Ranger I 1971 Abdominal wall pain due to nerve entrapment. Practitioner 206:791–792

Reagan KM, Meister K, Horodyski MB et al 2002 Humeral retroversion and its relationship to gleno-humeral rotation in the shoulder of college baseball players. American Journal of Sports Medicine 30(3):354–360

Rosch P 1999 Reminiscences of Hans Selye, and the birth of 'stress'. International Journal of Emergency Mental Health 1(1):59–66

Rosch P 2003 How it all began. International Congress on Stress. The American Institute of Stress. Online. Available: www.stress.org/cong.htm.

Ruff C 1991 Climate and body shape in hominid evolution. Journal of Human Evolution 21:81–105

Ruff CB 1994 Morphological adaptation to climate in modern and fossil hominids. Yearbook of Physical Anthropology 37:65–107

Ruff CB, Holt B, Sladek V et al 2006 Body size, body proportions, and mobility in the Tyrolean 'Iceman'. Journal of Human Evolution 51:91–101

Sapolsky R 1990 Hippocampal damage associated with prolonged glucocorticoid exposure in primates. Journal of Neuroscience 10:2897–2902

Sapolsky R 1994 Individual differences and the stress response. Seminars in Neuroscience 6:261–269

Sato A, Schmidt R 1973 Somatosympathetic reflexes. Physiological Reviews 53:916–947

Schamberger W 2002 The malalignment syndrome. Churchill Livingstone, Edinburgh, p 238–239

Schmidt C, Horwitz A, Lauffenburger D 1993 Integrin–cytoskeletal interactions in migrating fibroblasts are dynamic, asymmetric, and regulated. Journal of Cell Biology 123:977–991

Schneider MJ, Brady D 2001 Fibromyalgia syndrome: a new paradigm for differential diagnosis and treatment. Journal of Manipulative and Physiological Therapeutics 24(8):529–539

Selye H 1946 The general adaptation syndrome and the diseases of adaptation. Journal of Clinical Endocrinology 6:117–230

Selye H 1952 The story of the adaptation syndrome. Acta, Montreal, Canada

Selye H 1953 The part of inflammation in the local adaptation syndrome. In: The mechanism of inflammation. Acta, Montreal, Canada, p 53

Selye H 1955 The stress concept in 1955. Journal of Chronic Diseases 2(5):583–592

Selye H 1969 Catatoxic steroids. Canadian Medical Association Journal 1:51

Selye H 1971 Hormones and resistance. Journal of Pharmaceutical Sciences 60:1

Selye H 1976 Stress in health and disease. Butterworths, Reading, MA

Selye H 1978 The stress of life, revised edn. McGraw Hill, New York

Selye H, Somogyi A, Vegh P 1968 Inflammation, topical stress and the concept of pluricausal diseases. Biochemical Pharmacology Supplement:107–122

Shah J, Phillips T, Danoff J, Gerber L 2003 A novel microanalytical technique for assaying soft tissue demonstrates significant quantitative biochemical differences in three clinically distinct groups: normal, latent, and active. Archives of Physical Medicine 84:9

Simons D, Travell J, Simons L 1999 Myofascial pain and dysfunction: the trigger point manual, vol 1: upper half of body, 2nd edn. Williams & Wilkins, Baltimore

Stock JT 2004 Differential constraints on the pattern of skeletal robusticity in human limbs relative to climatic and behavioral influences on morphology. American Journal of Physical Anthropology 38(Suppl):188–189

Stone M, Keith R, Kearney J 1991 Overtraining: a review of the signs and symptoms and possible causes of overtraining. Journal of Applied Sports Science Research 5(1):35–50

Timmons B, Ley R (eds) 1994 Behavioral and psychological approaches to breathing disorders. Plenum Press, New York

Travell J, Simons D 1983 Low back pain (pt 2). Postgraduate Medicine 73(2):81–92

Travell J, Simons D 1991 Myofascial pain and dysfunction: the trigger point manual, vol 2: lower half of body. Williams & Wilkins, Baltimore

Travell J, Simons D 1992 Myofascial pain and dysfunction: the trigger point manual, vol 2: the lower extremities. Williams & Wilkins, Baltimore

Vaughan B 1998 Presentation: Journal of Bodywork and Movement Therapies 1st North American Conference, Berkeley, CA

Verkhoshansky YV 1986 Fundamentals of special strength-training in sport. Fizkultura i Spovt 1977. Livonia MI: Sportivny Press, Moscow

Verkhoshansky YV 1988 Programming and organization of training. Fizkultura i Spovt 1985. Livonia Sportivny Press, Moscow

Wall P, Melzack R 1990 The textbook of pain, 2nd edn. Churchill Livingstone, Edinburgh

Wallden M 2000 Lumbopelvic associations with hamstring strain in professional footballers. MSc Thesis, British College of Osteopathic Medicine, London

Wang N, Stamenovic D 2000 Contribution of intermediate filaments to cell stiffness, stiffening, and growth. American Journal of Physiology. Cell Physiology 279:C188–C194

Weiss J 2001 Pelvic floor myofascial trigger points: manual therapy for interstitial cystitis and the urgency–frequency syndrome. Journal of Urology 166:2226–2231

Wilk KE 2004 Rehabilitation guidelines for the thrower with internal impingement. Presentation, American Sports Medicine Institute Injuries in Baseball Course, 23 January 2004

Wilk K, Andrews J, Arrigo C et al 1993 The strength characteristics of internal and external rotator muscles in professional baseball pitchers. American Journal of Sports Medicine 21:61–66

Williams R 1956 Biochemical individuality. University of Texas Press, Austin, TX

Willis W, Coggeshall R 1991 Sensory mechanisms of the spinal cord. Plenum Press, New York

Yunus M, Khan M, Rawlings KK 1999 Genetic linkage analysis of multicase families with fibromyalgia syndrome. Journal of Rheumatology 26:408–412

Zink G, Lawson W 1979 An osteopathic structural examination and functional interpretation of the soma. Osteopathic Annals 7(12):433–440

3

Eric Blake ND

With contributions from:

Leon Chaitow ND DO

History of Naturopathic Physical Medicine

There is evidence of physical medicine and manual therapy in almost all healing systems, past and present. It is present in the founding systematization of Chinese therapeutics as documented in the *Nei Jing*, in the Sanskrit texts, described by Greek and Roman physicians, and written about by the European doctors of the Middle Ages (Juhan 1987). Naturopathic physical medicine is a multifaceted branch of the naturopathic healing arts. Since the 1902 founding of the naturopathic profession, naturopathic practitioners have advocated a wide variety of physiotherapy and manual therapy techniques. This includes, but is not limited to, Ling massage techniques (Hewlett-Parsons 1968, Thirion 1913), mechanotherapy (Bureau of Economic Business Research 1958, Juettner 1910, Thiel 2001), zone therapy/reflexology (Lust *c.*1980, Marquardt 1983), spondylotherapy (Abrams 1918, Gregory 1922), neurotherapy (Lake 1946, Lindlahr 1975), manual therapy techniques of physical culture (Macfadden 1914), neuromuscular technique (Chaitow 1987), high velocity, low amplitude (HVLA) mobilization (Lust 1936), graded mobilization (Lust 1936), lymphatic drainage (Lake 1942) and 'bloodless surgery' (Fielder & Pyott 1953, Wendel 1945) or the more modern approaches of visceral manipulation, specific endonasal techniques (Gillett 1931), hydrotherapy, various electrotherapies (Post-Graduate Study of Naturotherapy 1938a) and more.

Contemporary overview of manual therapy approaches

There are currently a large number of health care professions that incorporate manual therapy techniques. While most naturopathic and many osteopathic physicians utilize a variety of manual techniques, allied health care practitioners such as physical therapists, chiropractors, naprapaths, acupuncturists and massage therapists also utilize various manual modalities. The techniques and approaches employed by these different groups are dependent upon historical factors, scope of practice limitations, skills training, educational degree and theoretical orientation.

One of the earliest naturopathic textbooks, *Principles and Practice of Naturopathy* (Cordingley 1925a), categorizes naturopathic manual therapy as 'mechanical naturopathy' according to the tripartite mechanical, psychological and material model proposed by Blumer (1914):

> Mechanical Naturopathy will include all manual methods of overcoming lesions . . . What is now known as osteopathy was really practiced before the name osteopathy was known, in parts of Scandinavia; what are now called chiropractic and naprapathy were practiced a hundred and fifty years before these names were heard of, in Bohemia; and what is now known as mechano-therapy today has been practiced in China, Japan, Egypt, the South Sea Islands and other parts of the earth since long before the dawn of the Christian Era.

The 'mechano-therapy' to which Cordingley refers was an early 20th century manual therapy method. The only US state that ever licensed mechanotherapists was Ohio. The graduates of Dr Spitler's Eaton College of Physiatrics, in Columbus, Ohio, were given a degree as a mechanotherapist if they were to practice in Ohio, or as a naturopathic doctor if they planned to leave the state (Broadwell 2001). The College essentially closed in the 1960s, though it may exist in some form today, and the license may still be obtainable in Ohio. The methods of mechanotherapy involved what are today known as proprioceptive neuromuscular facilitated (PNF) stretching and muscle energy technique (MET) (Neil 1960). A 1929 bill that passed in the US House of Representatives that defined naturopathy specifically includes mechanotherapy as part of the practice of naturopathy. Also included were articular manipulation (HVLA technique), corrective orthopedic gymnastics (exercise therapy) and neurotherapy. The bill did not pass the United States Senate and was never made law (Thiel 2001). Early naturopathic literature considered osteopathy and chiropractic to be single branches of the larger naturopathic profession (Lust 1918). In 1924 the California State Supreme Court adjudicated a decision that determined that chiropractic was a branch of naturopathy (Millsap v Anderson et al 1924).

As we explore the development of naturopathic manual therapy we find that it was consistently centered around 'whole-body' constitutional approaches in conjunction with specific lesion approaches. We also find that manual therapy and physical medicine were applied in naturopathic practice for a variety of acute and chronic conditions, as well as in the treatment of musculoskeletal dysfunction (Chaitow 1980, Lindlahr 1981, Rice 1954, Wendel 1945, 1950).

Naturopathic timeline of physical modalities

In the late 19th century in North America, particularly in New York and New Jersey, a variety of German nature cure adherents and doctors practiced their healing arts. This heterogeneous group, composed of both physicians and patients, self-identified with predecessor American populist health and natural health care movements such as the hygieopaths, Trall water curists, Grahamites, the Turner movement, etc. To a certain extent those earlier movements had created a social foundation, left remnants of a physical infrastructure, and laid the groundwork for a cultural acceptance of the ideas of the German immigrant nature curists in the late 19th century. Benedict Lust was one of those immigrants.

These German nature curists were strongly influenced by the work of Father Kneipp, the German natural healer of Bad Worishofen. Benedict Lust published the German/American journal *Kneipp Blatter*. Many of these nature curists were organized into mutual aid societies, self-help societies, practitioner groups, etc. Some doctors operated both outpatient and inpatient clinics, such as August Reinhold's Institute of Water Cure on Lexington Avenue in New York City, Dr Carl Strueh's Water Cure Sanitarium in Chicago, Illinois, Dr Walter Selfertt and Dr Minna Kupper's Quisisana Nature Cure Sanitarium in Asheville, North Carolina, Dr Ledoux's New Orleans Kneipp Water Cure, and Dr Benedict Lust and Dr Regeniter's New York Naturopathic Institute (*Kneipp Blatter* 1896–1901).

The New York nature cure societies called for a Kneipp convention in the summer of 1901 to enlarge and expand the Kneipp treatment. A commission was established to survey the various nature cure and 'drugless healing' practices at the time. Benedict Lust was the head of the commission. Ultimately the commission decided that all methods of drugless healing should be incorporated into a singular professional field and the title for this field should be determined. At the time the term 'drugless' was used in a fashion similar to the contemporary terminology 'natural'. Box 3.1 lists the professional areas encompassing drugless healing that the commission identified.

Benedict Lust and the word 'naturopathy'

In 1900 Benedict Lust had purchased the rights to the name 'naturopathy' from Dr John Scheel, a German

Box 3.1 1901 Nature Cure Commission founding definition of naturopathy

Metaphysical

Psychotherapy, Psychoanalysis, Mental-Therapy, Suggestive Therapy, Hypnotic Therapy, Mesmeric-Therapy, Magnetic-Therapy, New Thought, Higher Thought

Nature medica

Herbal Therapy, Bio-Therapy, Bio-Chemistry, Homeopathy, Pneumatotherapy

Manipulative therapy

Massotherapy, Massage, Bonesetting, Mechanotherapy, Osteopathy, Chiropractic, Respirotherapy, Medical Gymnastics, Physical Culture

Naturo-therapy

Naturopathy, Natural Therapeutics, Hydrotherapy, Dietetics, Kneipp Methods, Bilz's Methods, Kuhne Methods, Schroth Methods, Just Methods

Light and air treatment

Electrotherapy, Ray Therapy, Heliotherapy, Chromotherapy, Phonotherapy, Phototherapy

Spiritual

Occult Healing, Divine Healing

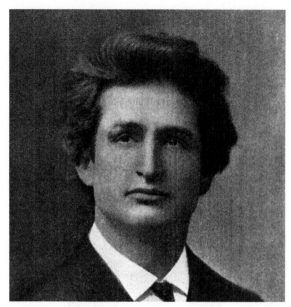

Figure 3.1 Bernarr Macfadden ND, Foundational Leader of the Physical Culture Movement

homeopath and Kneipp and Kuhne practitioner in New York City. The 1901 Kneipp Nature Cure Commission decided that the new name that would be used to describe all methods of natural or 'drugless' healing would be 'naturopathy'.

This 'new' professional title was announced to the world in January of 1902 in the first edition of the *Naturopath and Herald of Health*, the new name for Benedict Lust's *Kneipp Blatter* which had been published since 1896 (Wendel 1951). Thus, the naturopathic profession was officially founded in 1901 and announced to the world through the *Naturopath and Herald of Health* in January of 1902.

Lust wrote in his announcement of the new profession that naturopathy is the 'embodiment of all natural healing methods' (Lust 1902). The naturopathic professional literature of the time *clearly* articulates an understanding that natural therapeutics arose with the dawn of humanity and that different societies around the world had all used systems of natural therapy. The term 'naturopathy' was nothing less and nothing more than the first modern term to differentiate the field of natural medicine – i.e. natural therapy or natural therapeutics – as a distinct practice. While

the word was new, the field and profession were as old as humanity.

Bernarr Macfadden's influence

A 'sister field' of naturopathy in this time period was the Physcultopathy of Bernarr Macfadden (Fig. 3.1). Physcultopathy was the treatment of disease through 'physical culture'. Physical Culture was the period's terminology for the modern trilogy of 'diet, lifestyle and exercise'. Macfadden was most influential in pioneering today's exercise industry and much of today's fitness movement descends directly from his influence. However, Macfadden went far beyond diet and exercise into hydrotherapy and manual therapy as well. Lust and Macfadden were colleagues and collaborators.

Lust claimed to have opened the first health food store in North America, in New York City (Fig. 3.2). Today health food stores, fitness clubs and an extensive sports and fitness culture are testament to the tremendous impact these two individuals have had in making basic naturopathy so common in the world today.

Case management

The 1901 Kneipp Nature Cure Committee included homeopathy and Schussler cell salts as branches of

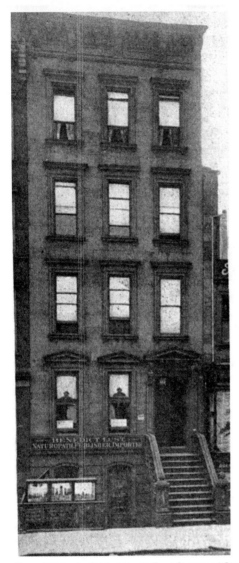

Figure 3.2 Lust's Original Health Food Center and Store at 111 E. 59th Street, New York City

ropathic physician centered around what was known as 'physical-dietetic therapy' (Lust 1909).

What was taught in naturopathic schools?

We can see from a perusal of the prospectus at Lust and Regeniter's Naturopathic College, later renamed the American School of Naturopathy and the first school that provided a diploma as a naturopathic doctor, that the 10-subject program (see Figs 3.3 and 3.5) included primarily physical medicine:

1. Hydro-Therapy (Kneipp)
2. Massage, Osteopathy and Gymnastics
3. Thure-Brandt Massage
4. Electrical Massage
5. Vibratory and Membranous Massage
6. Other Factors of Natural Healing System (Dietetics, Hypnosis, Suggestion)
7. Anatomy
8. Physiology and Hygiene
9. Pathology
10. Diagnosis (Inspection, Palpation, Percussion, Auscultation) (Lust 1901).

In the article 'What is Naturopathy?' in the January 1902 inaugural edition of the *Naturopath and Herald of Health*, the naturopath Ludwig Staden differentiates allopathy, homeopathy and naturopathy. He writes that naturopathy is 'the method of healing all diseases without medicines, drugs, poisons, and almost without any operations' and that 'Naturopathy's materia medica consists of the principal elements derived from nature: light, air, water, heat, and clay, beside non-stimulating diet, exercise and rest, electricity, magnetism and massage, calisthenics, physical culture, mental culture, etc.' (Staden 1902a).

Dr Carl Schultz opened the second significant naturopathic educational institution in Los Angeles, California, in 1905 – The Naturopathic College of California. Dr Schultz was a very well-respected pioneer of the profession. A European-trained physician practicing the nature cure, he arrived in California and opened a practice in Los Angeles in 1885 (Lust 1919a). He wrote and led the fight for the bill that became the first law to license naturopathic doctors in the United States in 1907. The 1910 *Naturopath and Herald of Health* advertisement for the college includes a more expansive curriculum:

. . . fall term begins on the first Tuesday in October, 1909, the following Branches are taught: Anatomy, Physiology, Chemistry, Pathology, Botany, Bacteriology, Hygiene, Dietetics, etc., Electricity,

what came to be called naturopathy. However, in the *Naturopath and Herald of Health*, the primary professional journal of the period, we are afforded insight into the actual case practices common at the time. In practical application and case history the first two decades of the naturopathic professional literature reflects a small focus on non-poisonous botanical remedies, a consistent position that homeopathy is a compatible yet distinct system from naturopathy (Rudolf 1908), and a much larger focus on the physical and dietetic methods of the day. The early 20th century practice of the natu-

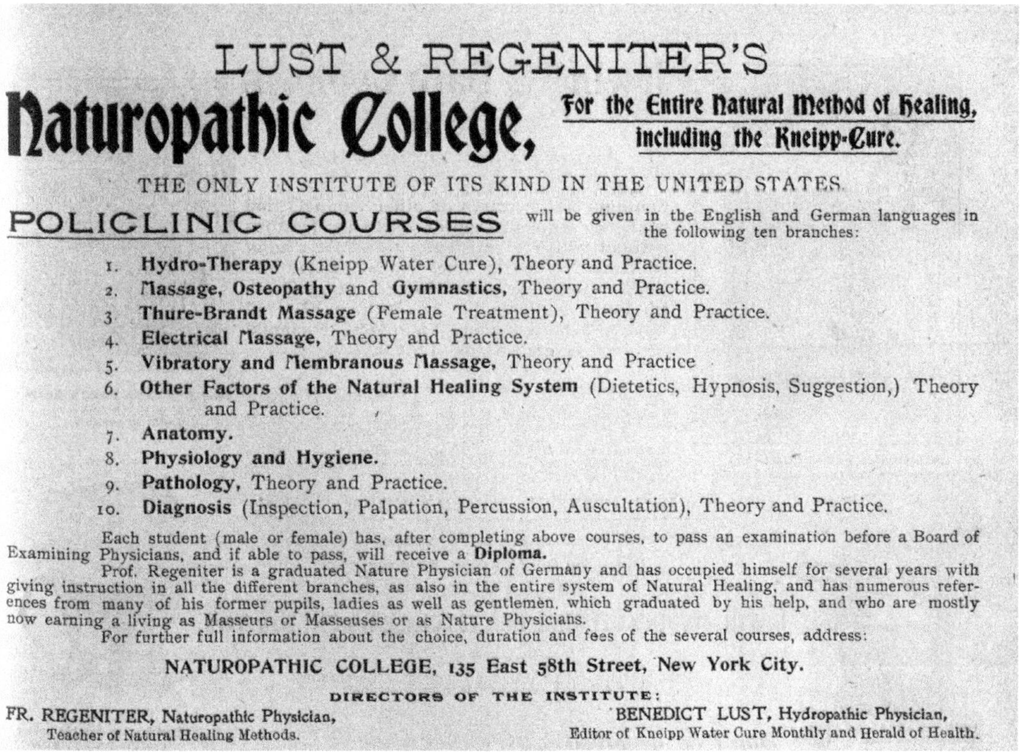

LUST & REGENITER'S
Naturopathic College,
For the Entire Natural Method of Healing, including the Kneipp-Cure.

THE ONLY INSTITUTE OF ITS KIND IN THE UNITED STATES.

POLICLINIC COURSES
will be given in the English and German languages in the following ten branches:

1. **Hydro-Therapy** (Kneipp Water Cure), Theory and Practice.
2. **Massage, Osteopathy** and **Gymnastics**, Theory and Practice.
3. **Thure-Brandt Massage** (Female Treatment), Theory and Practice.
4. **Electrical Massage**, Theory and Practice.
5. **Vibratory and Membranous Massage**, Theory and Practice.
6. **Other Factors of the Natural Healing System** (Dietetics, Hypnosis, Suggestion,) Theory and Practice.
7. **Anatomy.**
8. **Physiology and Hygiene.**
9. **Pathology,** Theory and Practice.
10. **Diagnosis** (Inspection, Palpation, Percussion, Auscultation), Theory and Practice.

Each student (male or female) has, after completing above courses, to pass an examination before a Board of Examining Physicians, and if able to pass, will receive a **Diploma.**

Prof. Regeniter is a graduated Nature Physician of Germany and has occupied himself for several years with giving instruction in all the different branches, as also in the entire system of Natural Healing, and has numerous references from many of his former pupils, ladies as well as gentlemen, which graduated by his help, and who are mostly now earning a living as Masseurs or Masseuses or as Nature Physicians.

For further full information about the choice, duration and fees of the several courses, address:

NATUROPATHIC COLLEGE, 135 East 58th Street, New York City.

DIRECTORS OF THE INSTITUTE:

FR. REGENITER, Naturopathic Physician,
Teacher of Natural Healing Methods.

BENEDICT LUST, Hydropathic Physician,
Editor of Kneipp Water Cure Monthly and Herald of Health.

Figure 3.3 Original naturopathic curriculum

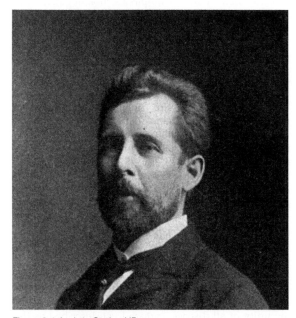

Figure 3.4 Ludwig Staden ND

Hydropathy, Mechano-Therapy, including Massage, Osteopathy, Chiro-Practic, and Orthopedic Surgery, Obstetrics, Minor-Surgery, Fractures, and Dislocations.

The Naturopaths are legalized in California and in some other states, the rest will follow. We not only endeavor to make our students competent to pass any Medical or Osteopathic Board of Examiners, but make them competent and practical Physicians. The Naturopath is the Physician of the future, write for prospectus.

Dr. Carl Schultz, President.

The college was closed in 1951 when it merged with Emerson University.

While the college curriculum includes minor and orthopedic surgery and botany, the thrust of the advertisement for the services of Dr Carl Schultz's Naturopathic Institute and Sanitarium, immediately above the college advertisement in the journal, involves various modalities of physical medicine (Schultz 1910):

All acute and chronic diseases are treated. Electric Light, Hot Air, Vapor, Sun, Electric, Herbal, Needle,

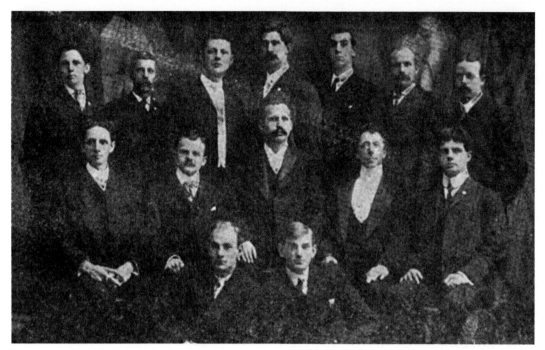

Figure 3.5 1902 Graduating Class of American School of Naturopathy, New York City, Benedict Lust seated center

Sitz, Friction, and Shower Baths, as well as Massage, Swedish, and Other Movements. Osteopathy, Chiropractic, Orthopedic Surgery, and all Hydropathic treatments are given.

'Drugless healing'

In the interest of our current subject – the history of physical medicine in naturopathic practice – it behooves us to consider our Dr Staden (Fig. 3.4) as a representative source of information on early opinions in the profession, rather than attempting to evaluate the relative merits of this perspective. For example, when he states that naturopathy is the larger branch of drugless healing he is using the terminology of the period. Drugless healing was used to differentiate a general category of practice, not only in relation to non-allopathic systems of healing at the time but also to differentiate the category from homeopathic practice and from the botanical practices of the time such as eclecticism.

Early in the naturopathic profession's evolution, the contradiction of the phrase 'drugless healing' quicky becomes self-evident. For example, Dr Staden describes two cases of cancer treated with topical application of rye and fenugreek seed (Staden 1902b). The word drug is derived from an older word 'droog', which was a trading term for 'dried herb'.

Modern research shows that topical application of fenugreek seed has potent antineoplastic activity (Sur et al 2001). The evolution of a modern naturopathic medical field that encompasses homeopathy and extensive botanical practice is a complex and interesting story.

Naturopathy and nature cure

Dr Lust argued early on that naturopathy and nature cure are two distinct entities. In a 1902 article entitled 'Naturopathy vs Nature Cure', Dr Lust articulates that while the two are 'distant relatives, it is true – so are the pussy and tiger'. The thrust of the article is that naturopathy is not a limited patent system of proscriptive natural therapeutics – for example prescribing sitz baths and wet sheet packs for all patients. Instead, naturopathy individualizes treatment in an eclectic and progressively minded fashion. The approach of universal prescription was an early trend derived from the influence of Louis Kuhne who advocated the unity of all disease and hence the unity (relatively so) of all therapeutics. In the 1902 article Lust argues for expansion of the therapeutic worldview of the naturopath beyond universally applied systems for all disease. He did, however, continue to argue for Kuhne's idea of the unity of all diseases, which Lust described as the 'cornerstone of naturopathic pathology' (Lust 1919b).

Lust argued that naturopathy is a larger inclusive field that expands beyond its nature cure foundations. So what was naturopathic practice like during the first quarter of the 20th century?

The role of physical modalities in early naturopathy

If the case histories and disease treatment articles are used as an indication, it is quite clear that hydrotherapy, manual therapy and dietetic prescriptions play the largest role, particularly in relation to acute diseases. Other modalities such as sunlight, breathing therapy and electricity play a supplemental role, as do botanical teas, steam baths and injections. There is scant reference to naturopaths prescribing homeopathic or allopathic medications. Prior scholarship was also used to demonstrate historical antecedents. For example, in 1902 Lust republished an article from the first half of the 19th century, 'The Sweating Cure for Hydrophobia', in which Richard Metcalfe relates five successful case histories of rabies transmitted from animal to human that were treated with Turkish steam cabinet baths (Metcalfe 1902).

In the 1902 article 'How Naturopathy Cures', Dr Staden provides several case histories. These include a 10-month-old paralyzed boy originally diagnosed by allopathic doctors as a case of spinal meningitis, a case of acute peritonitis with a swollen abdomen, cancer of the jaw, and pneumonia with 'brain fever' (presumably meningitis). These cases were treated with various Kneipp wet packs, herbal baths, topical herbal applications and dietetic prescriptions. The cancer case also utilized electric light baths as part of the therapy. Staden (1902c) reported positive outcomes in each case.

That physical therapeutics was paramount to the early naturopathic practice is self-evident to those who take the time to explore the early professional literature. The naturopathic treatment procedures in this period for various conditions such as gonorrhea, syphilis, diphtheria, infantile paralysis, meningitis and other infectious diseases detail what are primarily physical methods of treatment allied with diet. In a 1909 article on spinal meningitis, Dr Lust refers to the naturopathic approach to treatment as 'physical-dietetic' therapy. One of the earliest textbooks on naturopathic practice published by Lust was by Otto Juettner, MD. Originally entitled *Physical Therapeutic Methods: A Handbook of Drugless Medical Practice* when published in 1910, Lust republished the book in 1916 as *A Treatise on Naturopathic Treatment: Based on the Principles and Therapeutic Applications of the Physical Modes and Methods of Treatment (Non-Medicinal Therapy)*.

The renaming of the title and Lust's choice of this text as a textbook of practice indicates the early orientation of the profession's leadership. Dr Juettner also authored *Modern-Physiotherapy* (1906) and *Physical Therapeutic Methods* (1910) and was a member of the American Medical Association. He did not claim an ND as a title.

Early naturopathic legislation

In 1914 the New York State Society of Naturopaths proposed a state naturopathic licensure law (Naturopathic Legislation Series 1914). In their statement to the legislature they declared that the practice of naturopathic therapeutics consists of:

- Dietetics
- Hydrotherapy
- Physical Culture
- Dynamic Breathing
- Massage
- Swedish Movements
- Structural Adjustments
- Sun
- Light
- Air Baths
- Kneipp Cure
- Just Cure
- Fasting
- And other simple natural agencies as Rest, Work, Recreation, Suggestion, Vibration, etc.

The bill was not successful.

Aside from the non-poisonous herbal remedies utilized in the Kneipp cure, the therapeutic means listed are all physical dietetic methods. The leadership of the early naturopathic profession in North America was primarily in New York, New Jersey, and Connecticut and for that reason this bill is particularly insightful.

Eclectic naturopathy

While the early naturopathic profession included internal medication such as botanical medicine and homeopathic medicine in its larger conception of naturopathic practice, it would not be until the demise of the physician level botanical (e.g. eclectic) and homeopathic professions in the 1920s and 1930s, and their disenfranchisement from conventional practice, that those individuals, professional groups and ideas would be absorbed into the naturopathic profession. The professional literature of the 1930s and 1940s documents the naturopathic professional absorption of those withering professions with articles that focus more and more on the use of these internal medications.

Cordingley (1925a) provides an early definition of naturopathy written by Benedict Lust:

Naturopathy is a distinct school of healing, employing the beneficent agency of Nature's forces, or water, air, sunlight, earthpower, electricity, magnetism, exercise, rest, proper diet, various kinds of mechanical treatment, mental and moral science. As none of these agents of rejuvenation can cure every disease (alone) the Naturopath rightly employs the combination that is best adapted to each individual case. The result of such ministrations is wholly beneficent. The prophylactic power of Nature's finer forces, mechanical and occult, removes foreign matter from the system, restores nerve and blood vitality, invigorates organs and tissues, and regenerates the entire organism.

This eclectic view was also translated into a perspective that all individual natural healing arts – including osteopathy and chiropractic and eventually eclectic botanical practices and homeopathy – were single branches of the larger tree of naturopathy. It was mentioned earlier that in 1924 the California State Supreme Court determined that chiropractic was a branch of naturopathy.

Naturopathy, osteopathy and massage

The early naturopathic professional view was also historical and cross-cultural. Naturopathic professional literature did not claim to have discovered natural therapeutics, rather to be carrying on and developing an ancient and universal tradition. Claims by individuals to have discovered one of the fields of drugless therapy, rather than to be elaborating upon an ancient and evolving art, were regularly challenged. For example, in the 1913 article 'Osteopathy Not a New Science of Healing' the author Dr Thirion takes issue with the claim of osteopathy's 'discovery by Andrew Still'. Dr Thirion relates the use of early massage techniques by Herodicus, Hippocrates, Asclepiades, Celsus and Galen, as well as the contemporary practices of the day of Amma-Amma of the Japanese, Toogi-Toogie in the Tonga Islands, Pidjetten in Malaysia, and the Turkish bath massage practices. He differentiates those folk traditions from the scientific approach published 12 years prior to Still and expounds on the extensive and even earlier (1806) work of the Swede Ling. Finally, he lists extensive references prior to Dr Still such as Therapeutic Manipulation by De Betou (1840), Kinesipathy by Dr Georgii (1850), Cases of Scrofula, Habitual Constipation, etc., successfully treated by the Swedish mode of practice (1856) and several others. Interesting is Thirion's reference to Henrik Kellgren, a pupil of Ling, who had great success in treating infectious diseases such as pneumonia, diphtheria, typhoid, and scarlet and rheumatic fever with manual methods.

The 'Physio-Therapists' and naturopathy

In an interesting article 'The Two Brands of Naturopathy' by E.W. Cordingley (1925b) he describes one of the earliest divisions within the naturopathic profession. While one group at the time practiced orthodox 'nature cure' the other was what he called the 'physiotherapist' group that incorporated various physical therapy modalities. This categorization is somewhat analogous to the chiropractic division between 'straights' and 'mixers'. The former group advocates limiting practice to adjustment of the spine and the latter integrated various physical therapy and other modalities. The naturopathic division was between one group that would limit themselves to fundamental nature cure techniques and the other that would implement appliances such as sine wave, diathermy, galvanic, etc., as part of the office treatment protocol. By the 1930s and 1940s the ideas of the naturopathic physiotherapist or mixers of the naturopathic profession were far more prominent. Theirs were also ideas compatible with this period of integration of expanded homeopathy and botanical pactice. However, it should be pointed out that these methods were utilized in a fashion consistent with the naturopathic and nature cure theories that predominated in the profession at the time.

In a 1927 editorial Dr Lust complained that:

Medical Doctors have even taken the name of our science, 'Naturopathy', and translated it into its Greek synonym 'Physiotherapy'. Then they have so arranged it with the powers that be that a 'Naturopath' cannot any longer practice his art – in this Commonwealth anyhow [referring to New York] he must be a 'Physiotherapist'. And he must have learned his physiotherapy at some institute stipulated by the medical doctors as the original and sole source of such a science . . . Fight for your rights, for you will never get them in any other way.

It should be pointed out here that in 1945 the Australian Physiotherapy Association changed its name to the Australian Naturopathic Association (*Journal of the Australian Naturopathic Association* 1945).

Naturopathic physical medicine emerges

We can make several conclusions regarding naturopathic physical medicine and the first three decades of 20th century naturopathic practice. The first is that physical medicine played a tremendously large role in practice. The second is that physical methods were being employed not only for musculoskeletal ailments (the restricted field commonly encountered with modern-day physical therapy) but also for the rehabilitation of chronic disease and for acute infectious processes. These modalities of physical medicine included hydrotherapy, electrotherapy, exercise, reflexology, massage, spinal adjustment, cupping (vacuum therapy), and various other derivatives and combinations of physical means.

While contemporary physical therapy and physical medicine approaches are commonly prescribed for musculoskeletal dysfunction, physical fitness and physical rehabilitation, the early naturopathic physical medicine approach did not limit itself to these conditions. Infectious diseases were also treated with physical methods. Case reports of meningitis, diphtheria, scarlet fever, influenza, pneumonia, polio, measles and all manner of infectious diseases can be found in the naturopathic literature.

The great flu pandemic and other infectious diseases

For example, during the 1918–1919 influenza epidemic, 290 'drugless doctors' using naturopathic methods reported managing 14 841 cases with 18 deaths. This mortality rate of about 12 per 10 000 is compared to the reported mortality rate for medical methods in New York City of 640 per 10 000. The overall mortality rate for the epidemic is generally conceded to be approximately 2.5%. Dr B. Claunch reported working at one of the largest naturopathic sanitariums in Chicago where 300 cases were managed without a single mortality. The Cook County Hospital, two blocks away, lost 54 of every 300 cases (Clements 1926).

While we can be certain that some degree of individualization was applied in each case, published case reports and therapeutic strategies of the day that were utilized for infectious disease can be relied upon as a guide to how management was instituted. In the case of Dr Claunch we can be relatively confident that he is describing the Lindlahr Sanitarium and Lindlahr has described his methods of handling acute or infectious diseases in *Natural Therapeutic: Practice*. The methods of Lindlahr are quite similar to the treatments outlined by Dr Lust (1930) in his book *The Naturopathic Treatment of Disease*:

1. *Produce elimination from the bowels.*
2. *Stop all food intake.*
3. *Take orange juice at 8, 12, 4, and 8 o'clock. For variety take grapefruit, or diluted lemon juice may be used.*
4. *Use body packs.*
5. *Rest in bed with wide open windows.*

The body packs to which Dr Lust refers are the cold wet packs of Kneipp, a very commonly prescribed method at the time. Lindlahr describes his approach to the application of wet packs considerably in *Natural Therapeutics*. The cold towel application in constitutional hydrotherapy and the modern-day warming sock are examples of variations of the wet pack. The body pack would be a modified Kneipp short pack – wrapping the torso, under the arms, with cotton cloth, linen or flannel sheeting that had been wetted with cold water. A second dry layer most commonly of wool is then wrapped over the sheeting, the second layer acting as an insulator.

Naturopathic management of poliomyelitis

How confident were the naturopaths in managing acute infectious diseases through the methods of the period which were primarily 'physical therapy techniques'? In the 1934 article 'Infantile Paralysis Controlled by Naturopathic Physicians', Dr Carl Frischkorn reports that his state association (Virginia) would draft a bill to present in the legislature to 'make it unlawful for a medical doctor to take a case of Infantile Paralysis [polio] unless it is found impossible to get a Naturopathic physician'.

If we examine the methods outlined in the book *Poliomyelitis* by the osteopath Millard (1918) we will discover at least two important insights, aside from the description of a successful method of managing both acute and chronic cases of polio and related viral diseases. The first insight we will discover is that while individual cults of the time were supposedly claiming a unitary method of disease treatment regardless of the condition (e.g. for chiropractic the subluxation interfering with the nervous system need be corrected, for osteopathy the subluxation interfering with the arterial blood flow need be corrected), we will see in this osteopathic text an eclectic method being used. The second insight we will discover is that this therapeutic eclecticism is essentially a *naturopathic* approach by any standard, quite similar to the naturopathic treatment of influenza. It is highly likely that the methods Millard describes were similar to the Virginia naturopaths who attempted to legislate primary access to polio cases in 1934. Indeed, the outlined methods are remarkably similar to the methods described by the naturopath Dr Shakur for the treatment of acute and chronic polio in the 1948 *Alberta Journal of Drugless Healing* and comparable to the management of all acute infections advocated by Lindlahr (1918) in 'Acute Disease and Its Uniform Treatment According to Natural Methods'.

Poliomyelitis by Millard (1918) is a compilation of the polio case experiences of various osteopaths. There are a number of contributing doctors, 39 in all, with details of 56 case histories as well as descriptions of the different doctors' general experience with the disease. The general opinion was that 'osteopathic' intervention in chronic cases, after the acute stage had passed, was uniformly helpful and significant progress could always be made. The opinion was also that if the treatments were started early the likelihood of sequelae was lessened and the likelihood of complete resolution most likely. As for acute cases, the general consensus amongst the contributors was that 'osteopathic' treatment applied at the outset had a high likelihood of aborting the case or minimizing the negative sequelae. So what was the 'osteopathic treatment of poliomyelitis' as detailed in this book? Essentially it is eclectic naturopathy:

1. *Isolate the case in the coolest room.*
2. *Stop all food, except water, until the temperature is below 100 F. Break the fast with fruit juices and gradually integrating a regular diet.*
3. *Give plenty of water.*
4. *Hydrotherapy – hot compresses along the spine, or cool compresses with a fever. Patient lying on the abdomen to promote venous drainage of the spine.*
5. *Irrigate the colon.*
6. *Keep the nose and throat clean.*
7. *Keep the feet warm.*

During this time period osteopathy was still very much centered upon manipulative procedures. Millard advocates waiting until the tenderness of the spinal segments has diminished before applying osteopathic manipulation. Their omission from the initial treatment approach for acute poliomyelitis is enlightening. These general supportive measures were the hallmark of successful natural treatment of acute infectious disease management of the period. It should be also be pointed out that the osteopathic manipulative methods of that time were general constitutional treatments (see more on this topic below, and in Chapter 7) as well as specific joint restriction/dysfunction mobilization.

A standardized approach – the 'Universal Naturopathic Tonic Treatment'

In 1923 Dr Cordingley authored an article in the *Naturopath and Herald of Health*, 'Let Us Standardize the Practice of Naturopathy'. In the article he proposes this office treatment as a standard naturopathic visit:

1. The universal or general naturopathic tonic treatment
2. Correction of active spinal, rib, and pelvic lesions

3. Concussion at nerve centers
4. Common sense advice on hygiene and diet.

The universal naturopathic tonic treatment (UNTT) was developed by F.W. Collins in the early 1920s and a good deal more will be discussed on that topic later in this work (see Chapter 7). For now suffice to say that it was a 5- to 7-minute series of movements that were designed to mobilize most of the major joints and articulations of the body. The correction of lesions (specific joint restrictions, now known as areas of *somatic dysfunction* in osteopathic medicine, as *subluxations* in chiropractic terminology and as *restricted segments* in naturopathic medicine) refers to HVLA thrusting techniques as well as graded mobilization and what would be considered soft tissue techniques today. Concussion at nerve centers is a reference to the spondylotherapy of Abrams.

Cordingley's views on spinal joint dysfunction

Dr Cordingley (Fig. 3.6) was a frequent and regular contributor to the naturopathic literature in the 1920s and 1930s. In an article entitled 'Naturopathic Spinal Treatment' (1929), he elaborates upon the definition of

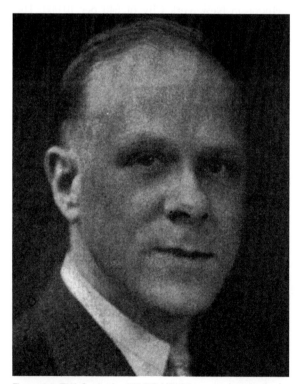

Figure 3.6 E.W. Cordingley ND DO MD DC

a naturopathic spinal lesion. He criticizes the chiropractic subluxation theory that a vertebra 'slips out of place and pinches spinal nerves' as unscientific and undemonstrable, 'because when a so-called spinal lesion exists it is found that a bone is not out of place but that it is simply held in some part of its normal range of movement by muscular contraction ... that then is the naturopathic spinal lesion'.

He goes on to clarify that the lesion may be due to organic disturbance and its reflex influence upon tissues at the associated levels of innervation. Cordingley's statements foreshadow the modern osteopathic view (Korr 1976) of the spinal lesion as facilitated segments with restricted motion due to patterns of muscular tonus.

Eclectic naturopathy advances

By the third decade of the North American naturopathic profession an eclectic approach to naturopathic practice began to predominate in the naturopathic literature. Infrared, diathermy, galvanic, faradic, high frequency, vacuum 'cupping' devices, color therapy appliances, the oscilloclast and other devices are prominent in case reports and articles. These methods were also applied for surgical procedures, as in the case of diathermy and galvanic treatment of hemorrhoids (see Chapter 12 for more on these modalities). Manipulative methods continued to be used and we see during the 1930s the initial development of manipulative surgery, also known as bloodless surgery, and today referred to as visceral manipulation.

A most informative reference from this period is the Post-Graduate Study of Naturotherapy (PGSN). The PGSN was one of several courses delivered in a series of lessons in the monthly issues of the *Naturopath and Herald of Health*. Spanning the time of several years of the journal, the 100-lesson PGSN provides insight into therapeutics and case management of the period. Techniques include reflexology, physical therapy modalities, hydrotherapy and manual therapies such as vibration, massage and joint mobilization. Lesson 44 in the section on examination of patients ends with this statement: 'No diagnosis should be made, however, before the spine is examined carefully for existing lesions' (PGSN 1937).

In the management of acute otitis media the PGSN recommends this course of treatment:

1. Cleansing sprays to the nasopharynx.
2. A few minutes of vibrator treatment around the outer portion of the ear.
3. The ear is sponged.
4. Insertion of the 4th finger to manipulate the passage.

5. Manipulation of the middle cervicals.
6. Stretching of the lower mandible.

The treatment of emphysema recommended in the PGSN in 1938 encourages an individualized but systematic plan incorporating some of the following:

1. Hot pack or the electric light bath every 2 or 3 days to induce diaphoresis without circulatory depression.
2. Intervening days alternating hot and cold spinal douches. (Several months of application are recommended to improve overall health and well-being. In the case of cardiac weakness hot foot baths or cold applications to the precordium may be indicated. Nauheim baths are strongly recommended.)
3. Mechano-therapy of the chest.
4. Whole body massage, particularly the chest and cervical area.
5. Positive galvanism to the chest, negative pad over the nape of neck.
6. High frequency to the spine. (PGSN 1938b)

Manipulative methods continued to be central to naturopathic practice and we see during the 1930s the development of surgery or visceral manipulation. The 1940s and 1950s was a blossoming period for the work of visceral manipulation. At the time, visceral manipulation was referred to as bloodless surgery or manipulative surgery. Drs Fielder and Pyott authored an extensive work on the subject entitled *Manipulative Surgery*, Dr Paul Wendel authored *Bloodless Surgery* (1945) and Major DeJarnette authored multiple works on the subject of bloodless surgery as well as conducting annual courses.

A time of change

Several parallel circumstances began to influence the profession during the 1930s. One was the incorporation of members of the declining organized homeopathic and botanic professions.[1] The other was the solidification of physical therapy as an allied health profession that increasingly required medical referral for services rather than direct or primary access (Lust 1937). Another was the growing predominance of multiple degree institutions that offered both chiropractic and naturopathic training. The first would influence naturopathic therapeutics, clinical theory

---

[1] During this period the literature reflects a new incorporation of homeopathic case management as well as botanical prescribing that reflected the ideas of Thomsonianism, eclectic, physiomedical ideas, etc. (see Brinker 1998).

and clinical practice; the second would alienate the physical therapy profession from the naturopathic political organizations, and the last would influence professional orientation and clinical approaches to manipulation.

Naturopathic political infighting and factional dismemberment initiated in the 1940s – led by Washington State and Colorado naturopaths and involving California and Oregon State naturopaths – crippled the organized naturopathic profession and reduced its politically organized presence to relative obscurity by the mid 20th century (Kirchfeld 1994).

Naturopathic revival and emerging professional divisions

The modern resurrection of the self-identified naturopathic professions has generated multiple subsets of self-identified naturopathic practitioners. Academically and professionally the legitimate scope of naturopathy is the entire field of natural medicine. The two are essentially synonymous. The scope and titles of different types of naturopathic practitioner is, of course, a professional and legal matter. For example, the Profile of a Profession generated through the University of California San Francisco articulates two large categories of naturopathic practitioners: one group practices naturopathic medicine and trains practitioners regulated as naturopathic doctors and physicians, while the other group practices naturopathy and provides allied practitioners of naturopathic health promotion trained in a varied and non-uniform fashion (Hough et al 2001). A larger historical perspective will help to elucidate this breadth of practice.

The resurgence of naturopathic medicine and the training of naturopathic physicians in the second half of the 20th century was heavily influenced by naturopathic doctors located in the Northwest United States and Western Canada. It was in the Northwest, particularly Oregon, Washington and British Columbia, where relatively stable naturopathic associations, license laws and schools were maintained throughout the 20th century. In large part this was due to the relatively favorable legislative environment and the longevity of the naturopathic license laws. While other states licensing naturopathic doctors in the United States repealed license laws, such as in Tennessee, Florida, Texas, Georgia and South Carolina, the legal environment in the Northwest was more hospitable. Most assuredly this was in part due to the larger, more tolerant cultural environment that supported simultaneous acceptance of widely divergent social groups.

For example, in some geographic regions of the Northwest, culturally conservative religious groups predominated through the 20th century as today, and in others culturally progressive groups dominate the landscape. Consumer research data on users of natural medicine identify these two subsets as the largest users of natural medicine. The naturopathic professional literature also reflects this apparently contradictory dichotomy. For example, while Christian religious beliefs dominate the early naturopathic literature, Dr John Bastyr preceptored with a doctor previously a member of the International Workers of the World (IWW). The IWW was the largest revolutionary anarcho-syndicalist trade union in the history of the United States. Its strongest base of support was in the Northwest United States logging industry.

The IWW of the time was antagonistic to Christian religious beliefs. Of course this is no reflection on Dr Bastyr or the doctor he preceptored with, just an historical curiosity reflecting the diversity of opinion that naturopathy would unite in common cause.

Manipulation and naturopathy

While the early naturopathic approaches to manipulation were whole-body constitutional approaches, the lesion-specific approach began to predominate in the second half of the 20th century. The political realities of the 20th century American medical wars are most certainly implicated in the eventual focusing of manipulative therapies to the lesion-specific approach. For example, the chiropractic legal strategy of 'spinal adjustment only' was an effort to survive their persecution in the mid to late 20th century. On the other hand, the American osteopathic strategy of medical integration permitted lesion-specific manipulation embedded within the developing osteopathic medical paradigm, and somewhat limited to musculoskeletal dysfunction.

While several legitimate colleges of naturopathic medicine existed well into the 1960s in the United States, with several others briefly surfacing throughout the 1970s and 1980s, in the Northwest United States the last naturopathic degree available prior to the founding of the National College of Naturopathic Medicine was through a chiropractic institution (Western States College of Chiropractic). According to the late Dr Boucher, this program was essentially a chiropractic degree plus three courses to receive an ND – Herbology, Endocrinology and Naturopathic Philosophy (Boucher 1981). Many of the individuals involved in the resurgent subset of the larger naturopathic profession had been trained at chiropractic/naturopathy dual degree programs. These naturopaths utilized a wide variety of lesion-specific approaches to manual therapy. Beyond spinal adjustment, other areas of the body were specifically mobilized. This included methods such as the Nasal Specific developed but not invented by the late Dr Stoebner (Dr Gillette, DC, published a post-graduate correspondence course in 1931 including a lesson on the Gillette Nasal Specific), the abdominal and extremity techniques of Drs White, Failor and Jacob, and the manipulative surgery of Fielder and Pyott.

Comparatively, the 'east coast' naturopaths continued to focus upon constitutional manual therapies and soft tissue work more akin to massage techniques as evidenced in the work of Paul Wendel. Emphasis on lesion-specific HVLA techniques within the 'west coast' branch of the naturopathic profession is less a demonstration of the scientific development of naturopathic ideas, and more a demonstration of the influence of politics on professional development. Regardless, the late 19th and early 20th century United States osteopathic, naturopathic and chiropractic professions utilized a paradigm of general treatments in addition to specific lesion resolution.

While there is a great deal of deserved elaboration, research and literature in the modern era regarding lesion-specific HVLA manipulation and individual soft tissue paradigms, general constitutional approaches currently receive less attention. This trend is most probably a cultural artifact rather than a scientific conclusion, i.e. the predominant focus upon lesion-specific manipulation is a product of the priorities of larger social forces at play rather than conclusions reached through investigation and research.

Naturopathic approaches to manual therapy

The universal naturopathic tonic treatment was developed in the 1920s primarily by Frederick Collins, MD, ND, DO, DC, and is an example of the constitutional approach. The treatment incorporates a variety of movements from the soft tissue armamentarium. What is uniquely naturopathic about the treatment is the theoretical precept and goal of the therapy.

The early professional theoretical paradigm of naturopathic treatment was to restore tissue function to a normal state of affairs, free of 'morbid encumbrance'. Morbid encumbrance was an early naturopathic concept that human tissues may accumulate products that are inimical to cell function. In modern terminology these products may be exogenous substances such as chemical pollutants or endogenous by-products of normal cellular function such as free radical species. The unexcreted wastes (endogenous) and exogenous toxins could accumulate for a shorter or longer period of time dependent upon pathways of detoxication and elimination. This is the hallmark of the 'unity of disease' advanced by Kuhne – that all

disease processes involved the accumulation of waste matter of some type. An example of this perspective is seen in the 1927 Maine Naturopathic Bill which defines naturopathy as the:

'Science and Art' of using such natural and vital and purifying therapeutic agencies as will enable the body to cleanse itself of abnormal conditions and set up such inherent healing processes as will restore and maintain the highest degrees of health, employing among other agencies . . . Corrective Movements, Swedish Movements, Mechanotherapy . . . (Cordingley 1927)

Dr Cordingley more succinctly states (1925a) that: 'Whatever system we employ, we produce results only as we purify the blood of poisonous encumbrances.' We would be remiss to reduce this theoretical cornerstone to the toxemia theories of Tilden (1926). More accurately, the early naturopathic theoretical paradigm was that the particular constitution (i.e. genetics) of the individual, in interaction with their environment, would, in an overwhelmed or maladapted state, create functional disorders that would produce dysfunction (phenotypic expression), such that processes of elimination were hindered generally and specifically, this common process leading to accumulation of waste products inimical to normal organism functioning.

The naturopathic understanding was that by restoring the function of nerve, blood, lymphatic and somatic tissue, the body would be able to most effectively eliminate impurities via the depurative organs. The result would be a restoration of health to the degree possible within the limits of the individual (genetic) endowment relative to the degree of tissue destruction that had occurred.

The role of manual therapy in the naturopathic method also includes lesion-specific musculoskeletal joint correction. Just as importantly, however, it includes techniques that restore structural function to normalize circulatory and lymphatic flow, normalize adequate respiration, remove impediment to nerve function in the spine and extremities, restore prolapsed organs to a more appropriate location to optimize function by reducing strain on those organs, stimulation or inhibition of nerve and reflex zones as indicated, and stretching tissues to maintain plasticity and mobility. The goal of these techniques is broadly that of physiological regulation.

Naturopathic manipulative therapy includes all manual methods of overcoming somatic dysfunction. Somatic dysfunction includes any mechanical lesion that impedes normal homeostatic function. Alleviation of lesions, i.e. mechanical obstructions that interfere with joint articulation, nerve conduction, lymphatic flow, blood circulation, organ motility and reflex mapping systems, will restore the organism to a more fully functioning adaptive state. This adaptive state prevents the accumulation of disease-producing substances that may be due to internal generation or external exposure. It does this in part by enabling the organs of depuration in their elimination of substances injurious to life. It is the goal of the manual therapy that makes it distinctly naturopathic.

The modern landscape of naturopathic therapeutics is quite wide. The broad application of manual and physiotherapy treatments as understood and developed by the profession throughout the 20th century enlarges that landscape considerably. We will now examine the general naturopathic tonic treatment (GNTT), one of those many methods. The GNTT is a representative technique of the profession that has survived to this day. As a representative technique we will see that in fact it comprises a variety of manual therapy movements in use today, combined in a novel fashion that embraces naturopathic theory on many levels.

General naturopathic tonic treatment

Early osteopathic and naturopathic manipulation literature indicates a strong bias towards constitutional manual therapy. Early texts almost always include a thorough general treatment, in addition to more specific manipulations. Indeed, these general treatments were primarily a combination of a series of movements that were in and of themselves considered to be specific. Modern manual therapies that incorporate a constitutional paradigm include, but are not limited to, Bowen therapy, foot reflexology and neuromuscular technique (NMT) after Lief and Chaitow (see Box 3.2).

Dr Collins was a 1907 graduate of Lusts' American School of Naturopathy and the founder of the First National University of Naturopathy. The University was founded in 1912 and to some extent still exists. The tonic treatment evolved out of a round table discussion group of prominent manual therapy practitioners. There was a contention that the general osteopathic treatment included too many moves and caused hyper-reflex reactions. This group reviewed the movements employed in manual therapy of the day. This included the works of Barber, Still, Murray and Macfadden, and German texts on massage and manual therapy. These texts represent hundreds of movements.

Out of this review, this group of doctors evolved a specific set of movements that constituted a comprehensive general treatment. This set of movements became known as the universal naturopathic tonic treatment. The term universal is perhaps anachronis-

tic, and we will refer to the treatment as the general naturopathic tonic treatment. This treatment then represents a distilled perspective on the manual therapy techniques that were in widespread use throughout the professions at the time. It is then the tip of the iceberg.

The general naturopathic tonic treatment (GNTT) includes a representative variety of manual therapy methods. Methods represented include graded mobilization, HVLA manipulation, passive stretching, the massage movements of stroking, kneading, effleurage and petrissage, neurotherapy inhibition via heavy direct pressure, vibration, fascial mobilization, lymphatic drainage, visceral manipulation and passive mobilization (Fig. 3.7). The GNTT takes approximately 6–8 minutes to perform once the movements are learned.

The early manual therapy practitioners acknowledged the tremendous role that somatic dysfunction had on disease processes. Manual therapy was a primary aspect of patient management in early osteopathic literature. Similar attention to manual therapy is found in early naturopathic literature in addition to hygiene, dietetics and hydrotherapy.

The repercussions of somatic dysfunction have far-reaching consequences beyond simple musculoskeletal disorder. Dr Collins (Fig. 3.8) made the boastful

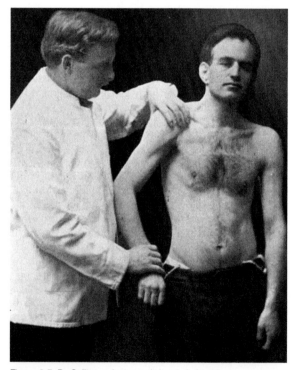

Figure 3.7 Dr Collins reducing a dislocated shoulder

Box 3.2 Naturopathic physical medicine in the UK

Leon Chaitow ND DO

The history of naturopathic physical medicine in the UK cannot be fully appreciated without reference to the work of Stanley Lief DC ND (1892–1963) who studied with both Macfadden and Lindlahr before the 1st World War (Kirchfield 1994, page 277), in which he served as a physical training instructor with the British forces. After the war, Lief practiced as a naturopath ('nature cure'), and established a reputation as a gifted healer. He utilized fasting as his main treatment tool, but almost always employed manual techniques derived from his training in early chiropractic and osteopathy, as well as Macfadden's 'physical culture'.

In 1925 Lief founded Champney's a residential 'Nature Cure Clinic' that became the foremost natural health retreat in Europe, outside of Germany. It was in the 1930s that Lief became aware of the work of an Ayurvedic physician working in France, Dewanchand Varma, whose work he studied, and, assisted by his cousin Boris Chaitow ND DC DO (1907–1995), which he adapted to create what became known as the neuromuscular technique (Chaitow 1980).

In addition, Lief strongly promoted the regular use of general mobilization and visceral techniques on most patients, along with exercise, lifestyle change, 'dietary reform', and hydrotherapy. In the 1930s he founded the British College of Naturopathy, which subsequently changed its name to The British College of Naturopathy and Osteopathy, and in the 1990s to The British College of Osteopathic Medicine – where NMT is still taught as part of the osteopathic degree course. Neuromuscular technique is also taught at the University of Westminster, London, as a 3-year undergraduate degree subject, alongside a naturopathic degree course. (See Chapter 7, page 241, and Chapter 8, page 310, for more on NMT.)

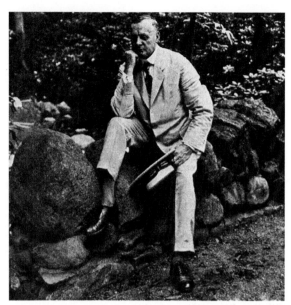

Figure 3.8 Frederick W. Collins. Birthplace: Paterson, NJ. Date of birth: January 18, 1873. Hour: 4° 57′ 53″. Sidereal time: 0° 51′ 22″. Latitude: 40° 54′ N, Longitude: 74° 12′ W, C.L. 3841

opment. The approach of the tonic treatment is constitutional by its nature. The manner of delivery of the GNTT provides simultaneous diagnosis and treatment. A practitioner who employs the GNTT in practice in addition to correction of specific lesions will be treating the whole body within which the lesion is manifest (Box 3.2).

References

Abrams A 1918 Spondylotherapy: physio- and pharmaco-therapy and diagnostic methods based on a study of clinical physiology. Philopolis Press, San Francisco. 6th edition enlarged to include progressive spondylotherapy for the years 1913 and 1914

Blumer 1914 Revolution in medical practice. Naturopath and Herald of Health. Benedict Lust Publications, New York

Boucher JA 1981 History of NCNM to 1973 [sound recording]. National College of Naturopathic Medicine, Portland, OR

Brinker F 1998 The role of botanical medicine in 100 years of naturopathy. Herbalgram 42:49–59. American Botanical Council

Broadwell R 2001 Interview with Dr Robert Broadwell, personal communication, regarding previous experience from the era. Additional documentation in the National Association of Naturopathic Physicians

claim that in conjunction with hygiene, hydrotherapy and proper diet, the GNTT could alleviate 95% of human disease. While this is most certainly an overstatement, it is a testament to the importance given to constitutional manual therapy approaches at the time.

The total time for the treatment, beginning to end, is approximately 6–8 minutes. In that time almost every portion of the body has, in some manner, been treated. The type of manual therapy applied to particular tissues can be seen to be relevant to the type of tissue affected.

The GNTT is a relevant clinical treatment developed in an early period of naturopathic professional devel-

archives stored at the National College of Naturopathic Medicine in Portland, OR

Bureau of Economic and Business Research 1958 Survey of naturopathic school/prepared by the Bureau of Economic and Business Research, University of Utah, Salt Lake City

Chaitow L 1980 Neuromuscular technique: a practitioner's guide to soft tissue manipulation. Thorsons, Wellingborough, p 90–179

Chaitow L 1987 Soft tissue manipulation. Healing Arts Press, Rochester, VT

Clements JR 1926 True science of naturopathy. Nature's Path. Benedict Lust Publications, New York, p 74–76

Cordingley EW 1923 Let us standardize the practice of naturopathy. Naturopath and Herald of Health. Benedict Lust Publications, New York, p 687

Cordingley EW 1925a Principles and practice of naturopathy: a compendium of natural healing. O'Fallon, Bazan, CA

Cordingley EW 1925b The two brands of naturopathy. Naturopath and Herald of Health. Benedict Lust Publications, New York

Cordingley EW 1927 Naturopath and Herald of Health. Benedict Lust Publications, New York, p 191

Cordingley EW 1929 Naturopathic spinal treatment. Natures Path. Benedict Lust Publications, New York, p 448–449

Fielder SL, Pyott WH 1953 The science and art of manipulative surgery. American Institute of Manipulative Surgery Inc. Carr Printing, Bountiful, UT

Frischkorn C 1934 Infantile paralysis controlled by naturopathic physicians. Natures Path. Benedict Lust Publications, New York, p 294

Gillett C 1931 The Gillett course in eye, ear, nose, and throat technique. Hollywood, CA

Gregory A 1922 Spondylotherapy simplified: a compendium of the science of spinal concussion and sinusoidalization. Online. Available: www. meridianinstitute.com/eamt/files/gregory/gregcont. htm

Hewlett-Parsons J 1968 Naturopathic practice: a valuable guide to students and others in the principles and practice of naturopathy. Arco Publishing, New York

Hough HJ, Dower C, O'Neil EH 2001 Profile of a profession: naturopathic practice. Center for the Health Professions, University of California, San Francisco

Journal of the Australian Naturopathic Association. Sydney, Australia, 1945

Juettner O 1910 Physical therapeutic methods: a handbook of drugless medical practice. Harvey Publishing, Cincinnati, OH

Juhan D 1987 Job's body: a handbook for bodywork. Station Hill Press, New York, p xxi–23

Kirchfeld F 1994 Nature doctors: pioneers in naturopathic medicine. Buckeye Naturopathic Press, East Palestine, OH, p 185–219

Kneipp Blatter 1896–1901 See editions of Kneipp Blatter from the era. Benedict Lust Publications, New York

Korr IM 1976 Spinal cord as organiser of disease process. Academy of Applied Osteopathy Yearbook

Lake TT 1942 Endo-nasal, aural and allied techniques – a manual of manipulative techniques for conditions of anoxia and anoxemia, 3rd edn. Self-published manuscript, Philadelphia

Lake TT 1946 Treatment by neuropathy and the encyclopedia of physical and manipulative therapeutics. Online. Available: www.meridianinstitute. com/eamt/files/lake/lakecont.html

Lindlahr H 1918 Acute disease and its uniform treatment according to natural methods. Lindlahr Publishing, Chicago

Lindlahr H 1975 Philosophy of natural therapeutics: the classic nature cure guide to health and healing. Edited and revised by JCP Proby. Vermillion, London, p 248–252

Lindlahr H 1981 Natural therapeutics, vol 2: practice. Edited and revised by JCP Proby. CW Daniel, Saffron Walden, Essex

Lust B 1901 Kneipp Water Cure Monthly. Benedict Lust Publications, New York, p 164

Lust B 1902 Naturopath and Herald of Health. Benedict Lust Publications, New York, p 14

Lust B 1909 How to protect ourselves against cerebro-spinal meningitis. Naturopath and Herald of Health. Benedict Lust Publications, New York

Lust B 1918 Universal naturopathic encyclopedia, directory and buyers' guide: year book of drugless therapy for 1918–1919. Benedict Lust, Butler, NJ, p 64

Lust B 1919a Universal naturopathic encyclopedia, directory, and buyers guide. Benedict Lust Publications, Butler, NJ

Lust B 1919b Universal naturopathic encyclopedia, directory, and buyers guide. Benedict Lust Publications, Butler, NJ, p 27

Lust B 1927 Is this justice? Naturopath and Herald of Health. Benedict Lust Publications, New York, p 369–371

Lust B 1930 Naturopathic treatment of disease. Benedict Lust Publications, New York, p 55–56

Lust B 1936 Post-graduate study of naturotherapy. Naturopath and Herald of Health. Benedict Lust Publications, New York

Lust B 1937 Naturopath and Herald of Health. Benedict Lust Publications, New York, p 282

Lust B c.1980 Zone therapy: relieving pain and sickness by nerve pressure. Benedict Lust Publications, New York

Macfadden B 1914 Macfadden's encyclopedia of physical culture, vols I–VIII. Physical Culture Publishing, New York

Marquardt H 1983 Reflex zone therapy of the feet: a textbook for therapists. Thorsons, New York, 1st US edition

Metcalfe R 1902 The sweating cure for hydrophobia. Naturopath and Herald of Health. Benedict Lust Publications, New York, p 172

Millard FP 1918 Poliomyelitis. Journal Printing Company, Kirksville, MO

Millsap v Anderson et al 1924 California State Supreme Court ruling

Naturopathic Legislation Series 1914 Naturopath and Herald of Health. Benedict Lust Publications, New York, p 144–148

Neil JB 1960 Course in naturopathy and drugless therapy leading to ND Diploma. Anglo-American Institute of Drugless Therapy, Bournemouth

Post-Graduate Study of Naturotherapy 1937 Naturopath and Herald of Health. Benedict Lust Publications, New York, p 333

Post-Graduate Study of Naturotherapy 1938a Naturopath and Herald of Health. Benedict Lust Publications, New York

Post-Graduate Study of Naturotherapy 1938b Naturopath and Herald of Health. Benedict Lust Publications, New York, p 144

Rice G 1954 Angina pectoris. Naturopath 59:183

Rudolf W 1908 Homeopathy and its relation to naturopathy. Naturopath and Herald of Health. Benedict Lust Publications, New York

Schultz C 1910 Advertisement in the Naturopath and Herald of Health. Naturopath and Herald of Health. Benedict Lust Publications, New York

Staden L 1902a Acute and chronic disease. Naturopath and Herald of Health. Benedict Lust Publications, New York, p 16

Staden L 1902b Naturopathic adviser. Naturopath and Herald of Health. Benedict Lust Publications, New York, p 46

Staden L 1902c How naturopathy cures. Naturopath and Herald of Health. Benedict Lust Publications, New York, p 190–193

Sur P, Das M, Gomes A et al 2001 Trigonella foenum graecum (fenugreek) seed extract as an antineoplastic agent. Phytotherapy Research 15(3):257–259

Thiel RJ 2001 Naturopathy for the 21st century: combining old and new. Whitman Publications, Warsaw, IN

Thirion R 1913 Osteopathy not a new science of healing. Naturopath and Herald of Health. Benedict Lust Publications, New York, p 574–578

Tilden JH 1926 Toxemia explained. Life Science, Yorktown, TX

Wendel P 1945 Bloodless surgery: with technique and treatments. Wendel, Brooklyn, NY

Wendel P c.1950 Naturopathic spinal manipulative technique. Wendel, Brooklyn, NY, p 1–15

Wendel P 1951 Standardized naturopathy: the science and art of natural healing. Wendel, Brooklyn, NY

4

Paul Orrock ND DO

With contributions from:
Eric Blake ND
Leon Chaitow ND DO
Roger Newman Turner ND DO

Naturopathic Physical Medicine

Introduction

This chapter presents a conceptual overview of naturopathic physical medicine. For an evaluation of the evidence basis from which this medicine draws its clinical modalities, a study should be made of Chapters 7, 8, 9 and 10 in this text.

Naturopathic physical medicine utilizes modalities from a broad variety of origins which fit its philosophical concept, and whilst naturopathy has not developed original physical modalities of its own, apart from European (or Lief's) neuromuscular technique (Chaitow & DeLany 2000) (see Chapter 7), it has evolved unique modifications and combinations of methods and modalities traditionally used by osteopaths, chiropractors and massage therapists (Cordingley 1925), as detailed in Chapters 7 and 10 in particular. Chapter 8 outlines naturopathic constitutional physical methods, which are also discussed in historical terms in Chapter 3.

Definition of naturopathic physical medicine

Naturopathic physical medicine (NPM):

- is the practice of physical medicine in the context of naturopathic medicine (NM)
- integrates both scientific knowledge in physical medicine and the principles of naturopathic medicine into a distinct approach to physical medicine practice.

Core components comprise:

- a respect for the traditional and empirical naturopathic approach to knowledge of the physical (structural and biomechanical) aspect of the human being in health and disease
- the value of individualization of therapy and constitutional needs

- a concentration on holistic diagnosis and the interaction of all systems
- the general therapeutic goal of stimulation, or modulation, of the body's self-regulating systems and mechanisms (*vis medicatrix naturae*) as well as reduction of adaptive demands
- education, self-care and prevention.

This definition of NPM is based on a template developed by a broad group of naturopathic educators exploring the features that identified a naturopathic modality (Southern Cross University 2003). It gives a broad outline of the context of its practice, and this chapter aims to deepen and expand on these ideas to consolidate the characteristic naturopathic approach to physical medicine. Many professions utilize similar methods and techniques, and a few have similar naturalistic and holistic principles underpinning their practice. The naturopathic approach needs to be identifiable in order for the profession to progress and claim its unique position in health care provision.

NM, as mentioned, is most strongly driven by the principles outlined in Chapter 1:

- The healing power of nature
- The need to identify and remove or modulate the cause of disease
- The need to do no harm
- Perceiving the doctor as teacher,

all of which have a direct impact on the clinical practice of NPM that clearly makes it different.

The following sections explore elements of how these principles affect the practice of NPM. Some sections are conceptual and build on treatises on the philosophy and practice of NPM, whilst others review the literature, where it exists, that provides supporting evidence for the mechanisms of effects of NPM.

Self-healing and regulation (*vis medicatrix naturae*)

How this is expressed in physical terms

In naturopathic medicine, the primary diagnostic question concerns the potency and efficiency of the self-regulating and adaptive 'energy' (i.e. potential) of the individual, its strength and vitality, and an evaluation of any obstacles or hindrances to its action. In physical terms, this assessment/diagnosis is clarified by close analysis of the case history, physical examination findings and diagnostic test results to analyze a number of functional domains, including:

- mobility/flexibility of the whole and part(s) – for example, having full range of motion of the hip and pelvic region in order to walk briskly without discomfort
- tissue and cellular perfusion – for example, having well-oxygenated cardiac and skeletal muscle to allow optimal physical activity
- lymphatic and venous drainage – for example, in efficient recovery from injury or infection
- efficiency of respiratory function, where increased demand is easily met and gas exchange is optimal
- aerobic status
- strength, stability and stamina of the somatic tissues
- tissue healing potential after injury, evidenced by personal history, circulatory status and general immune health
- tissue response to stress (e.g. postural, inflammatory, pain) evidenced by personal history and provocative physical examination
- adaptation efficiency, evidenced by personal history and physical examination
- neuromuscular control of movement, posture and balance
- normal digestive, absorption and eliminative functions
- positive indicators of nutritional and toxicity status
- balanced hormonal status
- indications of harmonious psychosocial/ emotional influences on somatic structures.

When each of these domains is functioning optimally for any individual, the naturopathic medical diagnosis should be relatively straightforward. It is important to establish the current level of wellness, firstly in order to guide an individual in management and self-directed activities, secondly in being able to accurately set goals and limits, and finally in order to establish a reasonable prognosis. Since, by definition, those individuals who seek professional health assistance already have established problems, optimal health is unlikely to be identified in clinical practice. Although the principles of NM set these optimal goals, no experimental research has tested the incidence of such higher-order health markers in the normal asymptomatic population. There is in all probability a high degree of variability in these functional activities across the population, and the skill in NPM lies in assessing each patient in the context of his or her idiosyncratic uniqueness, involving inherited tendencies, personal history, acquired characteristics and lifestyle habits and behavior.

The place of symptoms – the avoidance of suppression

The approach of NM in diagnosis is to assess how the individual is responding and adapting to the various stressors in their life. This includes considering whether the symptoms being experienced might represent positive expressions of self-regulation in-process, with the probability of a healing outcome. This is often referred to as the 'intelligence' of the *vis medicatrix naturae*. Symptoms such as pain, inflammation/heat, stiffness and fatigue may all contribute to the individual taking rest, which may be the best medicine at that time. On the other hand, in some cases, reduced activity may be what these symptoms are requesting as their remedy. However, if these symptoms are excessive or prolonged, therapeutic modalities might be called for to assist self-regulation.

Foremost in the mind of the practitioner of NM should be how to assist in the self-healing of the individual, without interrupting or suppressing positive symptoms that may be contributing to the healing process. The practitioner of NM has to consider what effect any therapeutic action might have on outcomes, as it may at times be best to:

- leave the symptoms to let them progress naturally, while observing closely
- leave the symptoms, but add supportive therapy discrete from the symptomatic region – for example, lymphatic drainage of the limbs in a patient recovering from respiratory infection
- mildly palliate the symptoms in order to comfort the individual, enhancing recuperation
- give symptomatic therapy in order to effectively treat the cause – for example, reducing muscle spasm and joint stiffness locally in order to increase comfortable aerobic exercise with a detoxifying goal
- treat symptoms as a first step in management, increasing patient compliance for additional therapy later
- identify aggravating and maintaining features and modulate or remove these.

These are amongst many therapeutic options, and they demonstrate the quandary of NM diagnosis in general – when to treat and when to leave alone? The answers to this question lie in the analysis of the condition, in the total context of the patient, and require a thorough grounding in physiological pathology – especially with regard to the effect of tissue trauma and inflammation.

Tissue inflammation has many causes:

- physical (micro- or macrotrauma, heat or cold, radiation)
- chemical (poisons)
- infective (bacteria, viruses, parasites)
- immunological (antigen–antibody, cell mediated).

The body sets up inflammation in order to reach the goal of resolution, repair and reorganization (Govan & MacFarlane 2004). In the practice of NPM, this resolution to optimal function is seen as the most important clinical outcome. Lindlahr (an early naturopathic pioneer – see Chapter 3) himself thought that manipulation was useful in infections because it 'hastened the normal development of the inflammatory process' (Lindlahr 1918a). Thus aspects of NPM might be employed to increase the speed and degree of inflammation, based on the fact that it is an essential component of optimal healing. This runs counter to many symptomatic treatments in other forms of medicine, and requires a brief discussion. This discussion also has relevance in the context of the hyperthermic measures in naturopathic hydrotherapy and electrotherapy discussed in Chapters 11 and 12.

In order to avoid interference with the healing processes associated with acute inflammation it is usual to:

- immobilize the part
- rest the system
- enhance circulation locally (chemotaxis/scar formation)
- enhance drainage (resolution).

The stage following the acute stage is termed regeneration, and is where collagen synthesis occurs and new collagen fibers are laid down. Hunter (1998) suggests that this is a key time for initiating constructive treatment: 'The tendency for the formation of randomly oriented collagen fibers that restore structure but not function can be reduced by careful tensioning of the healing tissue during the regeneration phase.' The key objective during this stage is the encouragement of enhanced tensile strength and stability, involving improved functional alignment of collagen fibers.

During the remodeling stage that follows, as collagen cross-linkage increases, stability returns but often at the expense of mobility. An understanding of the properties of connective tissue and fascia allows for the selection of appropriate treatment strategies. Slow deliberate movements that localize tension to the injury site, as precisely as possible, are considered useful early at this stage. In order to prevent undue loss of pliability during this phase, treatment that carefully encourages full range of movement is helpful. Eventually, functional movements, such as those encountered in daily life, are encouraged. Pain-avoidance behaviors should be recognized and attempts made to reassure the patient to continue movement therapies even in the face of some types of discomfort (see Chapter 9 for more on the topic of rehabilitation).

A failure within any of these stages can lead to chronic inflammation, which may lead to increased fibrosis and scarring, ischemia, loss of function and repeated microtrauma. The focus of NPM is to establish the optimal conditions for a concise and effective acute inflammation, with full resolution and return to normal function, and prevention of progression to chronic inflammation.

Many patients attending clinics have already reached the chronic stages of inflammation, so the task of NPM is to return the system towards health and to rejuvenate the tissue within the context of the prevailing structural limitations. This requires management, and stimulation in some cases, of the inflammatory process in order to achieve resolution. The process in NPM is to treat and make decisions based on whether the symptoms suggest positive or negative consequences resulting from the inflammatory process.

What are the features of positive symptoms from this perspective? They have characteristics that are:

- understandable, from a functional viewpoint (i.e. increased function necessary to heal)
- short lived
- predictable

and the patient states that, despite the local symptoms, there is a sense of enhanced well-being, and that general and local symptoms are improving.

First do no harm

Assessment of harm

One of the paramount principles of all Hippocratic-influenced medicine is to at least do no harm to the patient. Following this principle, the therapeutic initiatives that are chosen should have the best interests of the patient at the core of the decision, and have no side-effects or long-term consequences that decrease the wellness and vitality of the system. NM takes this principle seriously, and in turn this drives the search for minimum doses of remedies deriving from nature, and the avoidance of, or limits on, the use of processed and synthetic substances.

The assessment of harm in NM is also based on a careful consideration of the principles that underlie its application. Having a goal of self-healing means that the practitioner will wait and observe symptomatic reactions for clues that the system is self-regulating, when other forms of medicine may observe the same symptoms as suffering, and attempt to modify or suppress them. This careful observation of individual reactions in NM, using physiological knowledge and an understanding of adaptive potential, can lead to an interpretation of symptoms that arise after treatment as positive signs of a long-term beneficial outcome, rather than a simple aggravation. It also creates the platform for decision-making that seeks to avoid suppression of symptoms. Therefore, defining what is harmful for each individual is highly context driven, and should be understandable in functional terms. An example in physical medicine is the ache that may arise when mobility and blood supply are increased in a region that had been functioning suboptimally before treatment.

Dosage

In the realm of physical medicine, modalities of treatment span a continuum of high to low provocation of the system. Vigorous manipulative end of range of motion techniques undoubtedly offer greater risk to the tissues, and the patient, than do gentle within range unwinding techniques (Ernst 2001).

In Chapter 7 Hal Brown discusses the evidence for and against the safety of the high velocity, low amplitude (HVLA) thrust method, where he argues strongly that, when appropriate to the patient's needs, and skillfully applied, this method is safe.

Undoubtedly any technique can provoke a reaction when poorly performed or inappropriate to the patient's needs. For example, the more robust drainage techniques (such as those described in Chapter 7), whilst being gentle, can nevertheless stimulate a dysfunctional system beyond its adaptive capacity, and so cause an untoward reaction (Kasseroller 1998). The goal of remedy or modality selection in NM is to use the lowest dose that provides the required stimulus to self-healing. In physical medicine terms, this *dose* is related to:

- vigor of touch and pressure applied to tissue
- velocity of technique application
- amplitude of technique application
- duration of application (or combination of applications) in a single consultation
- nature of applied force (compression, shearing, traction, torsion, etc.)

- whether force is applied actively (by the patient) or passively (to the patient)
- frequency of consultations over time.

The amount of stimulus to a sensory-based system can be measured in both quantity of pressure and its speed of application. These are vital features in all modalities, as the sensory–motor reflex mechanism is highly individual, a factor that needs to be addressed at the commencement of therapy. The patient who has been involved in major trauma can be highly sensitive to touch, and can require a very slow and gentle initial contact, and progression of technique.

Velocity can range from low to high, as can amplitude (see technique chapters, particularly Chapters 7, 8 and 10). The lower ends of the spectrum are gentler and less likely to cause reaction. Techniques can be applied for as little as a few seconds, up to hours in a single consultation. For example, in myofascial release therapy, as soon as the tissue softens, the goal has been reached. This might take just 5 seconds – or minutes. In hydrotherapy, the temperature required might take 30–60 minutes to be slowly reached. Within each modality, there is a sliding scale of low to high application of degree and duration, with ultimate responses depending on complex interactions between the biomechanical influences being applied, and the unique features of the tissues and the individual.

The frequency of repetition of consultation is also an important feature of dose and is often matched with length of application to achieve the dose that does least harm, but achieves the greatest healing. For instance, 10 minutes three times a week is quite different in dosage compared to 30 minutes once a week. This is because the system reacts to the applied dose over time, before the next increment of dose is given. This 'divided dose' approach is known in pharmacy in terms of absorption and therapeutic serum levels, and can be translated into physical medicine in this way. Another benefit of dividing the dose over a number of consultations is that the effect of the previous reaction is observed and considered before the next application, and a decision to steadily increase or decrease the dose can be made to obtain the desired effect.

Another way of considering repetitive exposure to incremental 'doses' of physical treatment (e.g. manual pressure or hydrotherapy) is that these repetitively applied stimuli offer a virtual training effect, as the body or local tissues adapt to the treatment, in much the same way as weight training or athletic activity requires the body to gradually adapt to the training efforts involved.

Identifying the level of therapeutic stimulus appropriate for an individual, at any given time, is as much an art as a science, since it is all too easy to overwhelm an already relatively exhausted adaptive capacity.

This discussion would not be complete without the description of modalities in physical medicine being categorized as either *direct* or *indirect*. These terms can relate to an identified restriction in motion, and whether the technique addresses the 'barrier' of restriction directly, to take it into a bind (as in preparation for a high velocity thrust or a stretch), or whether the tissue is taken away from the barrier into ease (Greenman 1997). Indirect techniques, by their nature, reduce stress in the tissues during their application, require less pressure and velocity, and are less risky in terms of tissue reaction. For these reasons, they suit the methodology of naturopathic physical medicine (refer to Chapter 7 where such methods are described in detail, for example under the heading 'Positional release techniques').

Constitutional issues

The interaction between treatment and patient is a critical one. Too much of any treatment, applied too quickly, too forcefully or for too long – or inappropriately to the needs of the patient – will unsurprisingly have negative (or at least no positive) effects. The make-up of the patient and the underlying constitutional influences are equally important. The same degree and dosage of physical treatment will have quite different effects in varying situations and patients. The notes on constitutional considerations in Box 4.1 offer some insights into the patient's side of this equation.

For further discussion of the use of constitutional typology, see later in this chapter – 'Practicing whole body physical medicine'.

Patient education

Another area of therapy in NPM that illustrates this principle, and reduces risk, is the use of patient education and self-directed activities. These are commonly mainstream, evidence-based approaches to many acute and chronic conditions, and their use in NM is vital to ensure practice is based on naturopathy's foundational principles. When patients understand their condition, its causes and remedies, their compliance and motivation to change are enhanced (Prochaska et al 1992). The individual needs to gain an understanding of the multifactorial influences associated with the onset, the aggravations and ameliorating factors of the condition, in order to prevent relapses and to heal appropriately. The diagnostic process in NPM comes to the fore here, where an analysis of pre-existing and maintaining factors in a holistic context should result in a better understand-

Box 4.1 Constitutional considerations

Roger Newman Turner ND DO BAc

One of the important determinants of the degree of stimulus applied in treatment is the physique of the patient. From the earliest times, attempts have been made to classify physical and temperamental characteristics and to correlate these with disease susceptibilities. Hippocrates (460–400 BC) distinguished between the Habitus apoplecticus, with a short, thickset physique, and the Habitus phthisicus, who was long and thin.

In the early 20th century, a number of systems of anthropometric classification were put forward, most notably by Draper (1924), Kretchmer (1921), Sheldon (1940) and others, which sought to draw parallels between body composition and metabolic and behavioral traits. Although they reached broadly similar conclusions, many are now regarded as outmoded but the most systematic of them provide useful guides to the intensity of treatment. In addition, calculation of the cardiovascular index (CVI) and observation of the structure of the irids of the eye can provide useful information about the resilience and vitality of the patient.

ing of the individual's patterns of dysfunction, allowing informed decision-making regarding therapeutic and self-management strategies.

In summary, the approach to minimization of harm in NPM is of primary importance and drives the choices of therapy in this field. The positive and negative effects following treatment need to be managed skillfully, within the context of a global aim of optimal healing. The process of healing should, if possible, be:

- gentle
- individualized
- patient regulated
- abiding (i.e. long lasting)

and the effects of treatment should be understood and professionally managed to ensure that Hippocrates' words are not forgotten or ignored.

Clinical goals of NPM

The proposed *therapeutic order*, as described in Chapter 1, outlines a useful order of therapeutics that identifies the multiple layers and levels of healing. The model suggests that there is a need for 'correcting structural integrity', but this is just one aspect of the NPM effect.

It is also necessary to stimulate the *vis medicatrix naturae* (VMN), for instance, with the suggestion that constitutional hydrotherapy, exercise and enhancing immune function should all form part of the NPM approach. Utilizing modalities from NPM to improve function in any aspect of *physical expressions of the VMN* (see subheading 'How this is expressed in physical terms' earlier in this chapter) can be seen to be directly stimulating the healing power of nature.

Physical medicine is also helpful in addressing the acute needs of the patient, particularly when there is pain and/or anxiety/agitation. This assertion is validated by evidence provided in Chapter 10 of benefit from a variety of modalities used in NPM, involving a huge range of acute and chronic conditions.

NPM is therefore an essential aspect of naturopathic care, at least in regard to the first four steps in this proposed therapeutic order, which appears to make it a core practice from both the principles of naturopathic medicine (Chapter 1) and historical experience (Chapter 3). NPM is also valuable in this *hierarchy of healing* that prioritizes minimal intervention – it is an aspect of patient care that, when applied by a sensitive practitioner, is very low dose and generally without side-effects.

Utilizing this set of abiding principles, as established in Chapter 1, a clear set of clinical goals can be set out for specific NPM practice. These goals are not in any order, and each is reviewed and discussed in the context of the principles of NM and any supportive evidence that exists for NPM effectiveness in reaching each goal.

Detoxification

A major goal in the general practice of naturopathic medicine is 'detoxification' of the individual. This concept requires a review of the physiology of this process and how this applies to physical medicine (Box 4.2).

Immune enhancement

The complex activities that comprise immunity are of special interest to the practitioner of naturopathic medicine. How an individual responds to initial, acute challenge from antigenic stressors is a direct marker of their immunity. If an individual is in optimal health, it is considered that these initial provocations can be dealt with and fully resolved. The immune system, by specific or non-specific methods, enables the system to interact with antigens in an efficient manner should they re-present over time, and thereby minimizes the risk to healthy life.

Box 4.2 Detoxification

Roger Newman Turner ND DO BAc

To maintain optimal physical and mental functions, the body has a complex network of enzyme reactions and mechanisms to prevent the accumulation of the waste products of metabolism (endotoxins) and xenobiotic compounds (exogenous toxins) derived from food and the environment to a level that may prove deleterious to health.

The toxemia theories have long been a central tenet of naturopathic medicine. Nineteenth century physicians emphasized the importance of promoting eliminative functions and, in the early 20th century, Dr Henry Lindlahr described 'the accumulation of waste matter, morbid materials, and poisons' as the basis of many illnesses (Lindlahr 1918b). In the 20th century, advances in the understanding of free radical biochemistry have done much to substantiate the views of those early pioneers (Newman Turner 1996).

The flow equilibrium

The balance between the processes of assimilation and elimination is maintained by what Kollath (1950) has described as 'the flow equilibrium' (Fig. 4.1). Adequate circulation and drainage depend on the regulation of waste products through the transit mesenchyme, what we would now regard as the connective tissues. Kollath termed 'the slow, imperceptible decline in the health of the cell owing

to poor nutrition' mesotrophy and this is considered to be the basis of many chronic degenerative diseases. Reckeweg (1971) described this as the accumulation of the products of intermediate metabolism at the site of a metabolic block.

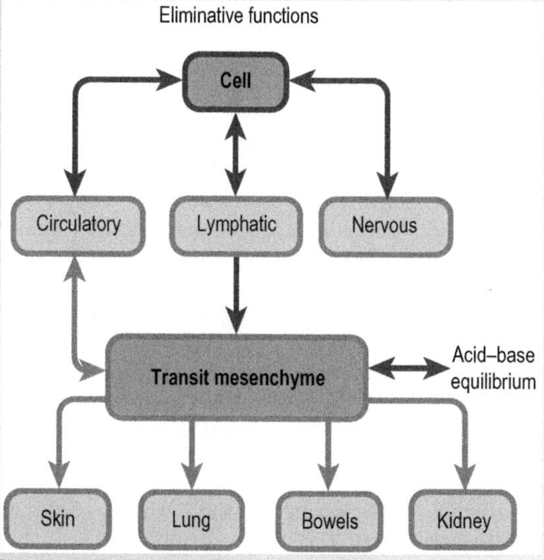

The principal objective of detoxification is, therefore, the removal of obstacles to circulation, innervation, lymphatic drainage and tissue perfusion.

Detoxification physiology

In recent years detoxification physiology has focused on the two-phase biotransformation functions of the liver, but Jefferey (2006) has suggested that a phase III efflux system involves the bowel microflora, the filtering processes of the transit mesenchyme, and lymphatic vessels, and a phase IV which is the distal channels of elimination. Indeed, the intestinal mucosa may account for 25% of biotransformation, even before transport to the liver, and all cells have some detoxification capacity (Liska 2002).

Phase I detoxification involves the mixed function oxidase system catalyzed by a number of enzymes, the most important of which are the cytochrome P450 family (CYP 450). These metabolize a wide range of lipid-soluble substances in the liver, kidneys, lungs and skin. This phase does, however, generate metabolites which are more reactive and therefore more toxic than the parent compounds. Phase II conjugates these reactive substances to more soluble compounds by processes which include glucuronidation, sulfation, methylation and acetylation. Both these phases are highly nutrient dependent.

Toxemia in physical medicine

There is a growing body of evidence to suggest an association between exposure to toxic compounds and the etiology of a number of chronic conditions, in particular chronic fatigue syndrome, fibromyalgia and late-onset Parkinson's disease (Perlmutter 1997, Sherer et al 2002, Steventon et al 1989).

Levine & Reinhardt (1983) suggest that chemical hypersensitivity is a manifestation of free radical peroxidative damage to cellular membranes resulting in the release of inflammatory and immune mediators. Hydroxyl radicals also react readily with sugars which result in the prostaglandin and leukotriene release that promotes joint inflammation via the arachidonic acid cascade. Kjelsden-Kragh et al (1991) were able to demonstrate that patients undertaking a vegetarian diet (low in arachidonic acid) for 1 year following a fasting regime showed objective improvement in the symptoms of rheumatoid arthritis.

Figure 4.1 The flow equilibrium

Continued

Box 4.2 Detoxification continued

Managing detoxification

There are certain signs and symptoms that should alert the practitioner to the need for further action in reducing toxic load, as follows:

- Poor complexion, skin lesions, rashes, greasiness
- Digestive dyscrasias, halitosis, taste disturbances
- Lethargy, cognitive dysfunction
- Muscular aches and pains
- Increasing sensitivity to exogenous exposures, odors, etc.
- Hyper-reactivity to medications or supplements
- History of heavy medical or recreational drug use or exposure to environmental chemicals.

Many chronic physical and systemic disorders may require detoxification measures for their successful management. The following should be considered:

- Reduce toxic load by reduction or exclusion of potential toxicants
- Provide balanced nutritional support for biotransformation and conjugation reactions
- Support healthy digestion and intestinal ecology
- Promote phase IV functions of skin, lungs, bowels and kidneys by hydrotherapy, dry brushing, exercise and breathing rehabilitation.

Naturopaths view the immune system from a holistic perspective and have always considered how other systems affect its functioning. This is particularly true of the effect of the psycho-emotional aspect on immune function, as demonstrated by the field of psychoneuroimmunology (PNI; discussed later in this chapter and in Chapter 1). It is also true of the effect of the physical tissues and their role in both cell-mediated and humoral immunity. Figure 4.2 illustrates the interaction between these systems.

There are a number of osteopathic studies (Radjieski et al 1998) showing effects of physical methods on enhanced immune function, and many of these are described in Chapters 7 and 8, as well as in Chapter 10. The relationship between structure and function appears to play a role in this, where immobilized parts become immunosuppressed, possibly because of the stasis of lymphatic fluid and a resultant congestive state. The normalization of movement, both structural (e.g. range of motion) and functional (e.g. respiratory capacity), is aimed at reducing such stasis, where it exists. A brief review of lymphatic function is required to understand this approach.

Lymphatic function

A primary influence on the immune response is the health of the lymphoid tissue, and optimal lymphatic circulation supports this. Increased lymphatic flow results in increased production and distribution of lymphoid cells (Mesina et al 1998). The volume of fluid exchange between the compartments of the body is determined by Starling's Law. This states (Guyton & Hall 2006) that:

Hydrostatic pressure (capillary – tissue) – Oncotic pressure (capillary – tissue) = net fluid movement out

of capillary into interstitium (Oncotic pressure is osmotic pressure created by plasma protein molecules that are impermeable across the capillary membrane).

The lymphatic capillaries form a network of small vessels that are distributed throughout the subcutaneous layer. These capillaries branch and interconnect freely into all tissues. Lymph capillaries are blind-ended and one cell in thickness. Pressure from the fluid surrounding the capillary forces these cells to separate, allowing fluid to enter the capillary. There are one-way valves within the lymphatic capillaries that ensure the continued one-way flow of the lymph away from the tissues.

This interaction between compartment and vessel pressures is what drives nutrients into, and drainage of wastes out of, tissues, and this is a vital dynamic in maintaining optimal health and healing. The thin-walled lymphatic vessels require compression to empty, and this is accomplished against gravity from the lower limbs by, for example, the rhythmic contraction of the soleus muscles in the calf.

Physical therapies, including massage, have been shown to affect the flow of lymphatic fluid. One example is the effect of decreased upper limb edema post mastectomy surgery (Mesina et al 1998).

Manual therapy techniques that assist in fluid movement have been shown to:

- enhance local circulation and drainage (Foldi & Strossenreuther 2003)
- reduce swelling and improve washout of inflammatory chemicals (Wittlinger & Wittlinger 1982)
- assist post-surgical recovery (Cantieri 1997).

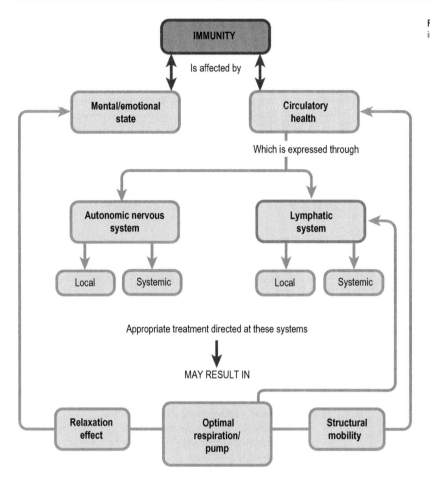

Figure 4.2 Flow chart of systems interaction

Lymphatic drainage is further discussed in Chapter 7, with additional research examples in Chapter 10, including in patients with fibromyalgia and immune function.

There are known to be other beneficial effects of massage, other than from the effects of increased circulation. For instance, the fluctuating levels of circulating immune cells have a direct impact on the speed and efficacy of the immediate immune response, and changes to these levels have been noticed in small trials of lymphatic massage. A significant increase in natural killer cell number, natural killer cell cytotoxicity, soluble CD8 and the cytotoxic subset of CD8 cells was found in a study of 29 gay men (20 HIV positive, 9 HIV negative) who received daily massages for 1 month (Ironson et al 1996). A subgroup of 11 of the HIV-positive subjects served as a within-subject control group (1 month with and without massages).

In another clinical trial (Hernandez-Reif et al 2005), 58 women diagnosed with breast cancer were ran-domized into massage therapy, progressive muscle relaxation or standard treatment groups. The massage therapy was applied in 30-minute sessions, three times a week for 5 weeks, and dopamine levels, natural killer cells and lymphocytes increased from the first to the last day of the study for the massage therapy group. In an uncontrolled multimodality treatment program of 149 females with breast cancer, quality of life, anxiety, depression and the tumor marker CA 15-3 were measured before and after an individualized rehabilitation program incorporating manual lymph drainage, exercise therapy, massages, psychological counseling, relaxation training, carbon dioxide baths and mud packs. Quality of life and mood improved significantly and CA 15-3 declined significantly to follow-up (Strauss-Blasche et al 2005).

The integration of physical medicine with multidisciplinary approaches to immune enhancement shows promise, but requires further research to reveal which modalities produce particular effects (see Chapter 10 for more discussion on the effects of immune enhancement in relation to physical medicine).

Fever

The management of fever is central to the optimization of the immune response in the context of naturopathic medicine (Box 4.3).

Circulatory stimulation

The function of circulation in the body is primarily to transport the nutrients into the cells and then to remove wastes that result from metabolic activities. Massage therapy can increase local capillary flow by a number of mechanisms (Yates 1990):

1. *Physical and mechanical effects*: One effect of massage is emptying venous beds, which has a subsequent effect of lowering the venous pressure and increasing capillary blood flow.
2. *Vasodilator release*: The effect of friction on the skin and subcutaneous tissues creates a disruption of mast cells and a chemically mediated release of the potent vasodilator histamine.

Box 4.3 Fever

Eric Blake ND MSOM Dipl Ac

The elevation of the body temperature 1°F beyond normal indicates a febrile state. The elevation of the body temperature in infectious processes is mediated via the hypothalamus due to pyrogen influence (primarily lipopolysaccharides), either directly or through production of interleukin-1 (IL-1) by macrophages, leukocytes or granular lymphocytes. The elevation of the hypothalamic set point induces heat conservation and increased heat production for a net increase in temperature. Once the initiating factor is withdrawn or resolved, heat dispersion occurs via vasodilation and sweating. This signifies the 'crisis' and predicts the anticipated reduction of oral temperature (Guyton & Hall 2006).

It is understood that when infectious processes produce fever it is an adaptive response by the organism. It is also acknowledged that this leads to beneficial effects such as increased interferon production and enhanced T-cell activity. Mild febrile states are also associated with better prognosis in viral and bacterial infections (Kluger 1986).

Conventional approaches to fever management include antipyretic therapy to reduce the febrile temperature to normal. Internal debate as to the necessity or usefulness of this approach is acknowledged (Beers & Berkow 1999). Underlying the prescription of antipyretics is the assumption that fever is detrimental and that reduction of fever will have benefit; however, neither assumption has been demonstrated (Mackowiak 2000).

Recent research is demonstrating that antipyretic treatment can prolong viral illnesses and enhance and prolong the period of communicability. Additionally, antipyretics do not show any benefit in reducing the length of viral illness (Geisman 2002).

The naturopathic approach to fever management is quite different from conventional approaches. Based on the understanding that the organism contains self-healing means fever is considered a potentially beneficial expression of the *vis medicatrix naturae* (Lindlahr 1918b). The accelerated metabolic rate, increased oxidation and increased tissue perfusion are predictable physiological results of a febrile state. The associated immune benefits previously described, in association with the increased total metabolic rate, are indicators of enhanced vital reactivity (Acharan 1956).

Hallmarks of the general naturopathic approach to acute febrile states were clearly articulated by Lindlahr (1918c):

1. Fresh air
2. Caloric restriction
3. Free water drinking
4. Hydrotherapy.

Access to fresh air is necessary due to the increased oxidation and elimination via the pulmonary system that is associated with increased metabolic states. For every 1°C increase over 37°C, oxygen consumption increases 13% (Beers & Berkow 1999). The restriction of calories is beneficial, presumably due to the decreased peristaltic activity during febrile episodes because of the influence of IL-1 (Bodnar et al 1989). Increased caloric intake during periods of decreased peristalsis will presumably lead to increased toxemic states (Rauch 1993). Free water drinking is encouraged to minimize the risks of dehydration attendant to febrile episodes. Dehydration can worsen febrile states and dehydration has been reported as the most common cause of fever in the first week of life (Tiker et al 2004). Hydrotherapy treatment is instituted to encourage heat radiation and to maintain the fever within beneficial limits in a manner that effectively harnesses this expression of the *vis medicatrix naturae*.

3. *Reflex response*: Massage has been shown to stimulate the autonomic nervous system, in particular to produce a systemic sympathetic reflex (Lederman 2005). This can result in initial tachycardia and elevated blood pressure. Over time, this settles into the relaxation response with a withdrawal of sympathetic stimulation and a decrease in pulse and blood pressure.

Additional discussion of the biomechanical and other influences of massage therapy (including evidence of modification of anxiety levels) is to be found in Chapters 7, 8 and 10.

Massage is likely to be of benefit to patients who have circulatory insufficiency (e.g. those with paralysis) or who demonstrate sustained muscular contraction, or who require enhanced circulation to an area healing from nerve/tissue trauma.

Optimize respiratory function

See Box 4.4.

Box 4.4 Optimizing respiratory function

Leon Chaitow ND DO

Respiration is a vital function in maintaining optimal wellness, and a breathing pattern disorder (the extreme of which is hyperventilation) produces an astonishing array of adaptive imbalances affecting both the biochemical and psychological stability of the body, while also creating a degree of structural change.

Hyperventilation (overbreathing) is a breathing pattern disorder (BPD) that produces a drop in arterial CO_2 (expressed as partial pressure of CO_2 – $PaCO_2$), caused when ventilation patterns exceed metabolic demands for O_2 (Schleifer et al 2002). The incidence of BPD in the general population has been variously estimated to be in a range of anything from 3.5 to 28% (Huey & West 1983).

Symptoms as diverse as neck and head pain, chronic fatigue, anxiety and panic attacks, cardiovascular distress, gastrointestinal dysfunction, lowered pain threshold, spinal instability and hypertension (this is not a comprehensive listing) may result – caused directly, or more commonly aggravated and maintained, by breathing pattern disorders such as hyperventilation (Timmons & Ley 1994).

The adaptational processes involved in this pattern of breathing can include excessive loss of CO_2, due to an increase in the rate of flow of CO_2 from cells to lungs, and a rise in blood pH (normal is ±7.4) during hyperventilation, creating respiratory alkalosis (Pryor & Prasad 2002). With the onset of respiratory alkalosis there is an immediate disruption in the acid–base equilibrium, triggering a chain of systemic physiological changes, many of which have adverse implications for musculoskeletal health. There are, in addition, negative effects on balance (Balaban & Thayer 2001), motor control (Van Dieën et al 2003), pain thresholds (Rhudy & Meagher 2000) and autonomic imbalance characterized by sympathetic arousal (Dempsey et al 2002).

Some of the immediate effects of respiratory alkalosis include altered autonomic control, together with a tendency for smooth muscles to constrict, leading to narrowing of blood vessels, as well as other tubular structures such as the intestines and urethra (Dempsey et al 2002), resulting in reduced delivery of blood to tissues (Ford et al 1995). Hyperventilation is usually characterized by a shift from a diaphragmatic to a thoracic breathing pattern, which imposes biomechanical stress on the neck/shoulder region due to the excessive recruitment of sternocleidomastoid, scalene and trapezius muscles in support of thoracic breathing (Schleifer et al 2002).

There are major implications of breathing pattern disorders for spinal stability. According to Schleifer et al (2002), hyperventilation can compromise spinal stability in a number of ways, including increasing any tendency to greater muscle tension, muscle spasm, amplified response to catecholamines, and muscle ischemia and hypoxia, as well as by interfering with the intra-abdominal pressure stabilization functions of the diaphragm. Motor control is commonly compromised as a result (Chaitow 2004). Recent data confirm that the stabilization activity of the diaphragm is compromised during tasks that challenge both the stability of the spine as well as making respiratory demands – 'shoveling snow' is a reasonable example (Hodges & Gandevia 2002a,b, Hodges et al 1997). When such a challenge occurs, it is the stabilizing potential of the diaphragm that suffers (Hodges et al 2001). Lee (1999) has demonstrated a clear connection between respiratory (diaphragmatic) dysfunction and pelvic floor problems (high tone or low tone), potentially involving associated effects including stress incontinence, prostatic symptoms, interstitial cystitis (see Chapter 7) and chronic pelvic pain.

Strategies that can help to normalize such a cascade of health problems have been shown in many studies to require (for optimum results) a combination of breathing retraining and physical medicine interventions that focus

Continued

Box 4.4 Optimizing respiratory function continued

attention on the thoracic cage, diaphragm and accessory respiratory muscles (Lum 1994).

Reducing levels of apprehension, anxiety and fear may be seen to have the potential for encouraging improvement in breathing patterns and all the negative symptoms that flow from these. There is also good evidence that breathing rehabilitation is a useful method for achieving reduced anxiety/panic levels, and for improving postural control (Aust & Fischer 1997) and somatic complaints such as low back pain (Mehling & Hamel 2005), as well as conditions such as chronic fatigue (Nixon & Andrews 1996).

A combination of breathing rehabilitation and physical therapy has been shown to allow normalization of

habitual breathing pattern disorders in the vast majority of cases (Han et al 1996).

In a study by Lum (1987), more than 1000 anxious and phobic patients were treated using a combination of breathing retraining, physical therapy and relaxation. Symptoms were usually abolished in 1–6 months, with some younger patients requiring only a few weeks. At 12 months, 75% were free of all symptoms, 20% had only mild symptoms and about one patient in 20 had intractable symptoms.

(See Figure 2.7 for a flow chart that outlines the multiple changes that occur as a result of breathing pattern disorders.)

Provide optimal rest/sleep and reduce stress

Therapeutic rest is a high priority intervention in naturopathic medicine; according to Lindlahr (1918d), 'the reserve of vital energy is accumulated by sleep'. The effects of adequate rest are well known, and are mostly modulated through the autonomic nervous system and central nervous system. These include decreased blood pressure and pulse rate, as well as enhanced muscle relaxation.

Sleep is similar to waking rest, in therapeutic effect. The benefits include dilation of skin vessels, improved gastrointestinal function and a reduction in the basal metabolic rate of between 10 and 30%. Sleep disorders are known to be associated with conditions as wide ranging as fibromyalgia and psychosis (Watkins 1997).

Massage therapy has known effects on the psychological state of the recipient. These include:

- reduction in anxiety
- modulation of depression
- relaxation response.

The physiological response to stress can be modulated by NPM, as evidenced by studies showing a short-term relaxation effect from massage, as well as decreases in serum cortisol, the main hormonal expression of chronic stress (Ferrell-Torry & Glick 1993, Field et al 2005, Ironson et al 1996, Labyak & Metzger 1997, Richards 1998).

- In a study of the effects of massage on 50 palliative care patients, self-perceived pain, anxiety, stress and depression all improved significantly after gentle relaxation techniques at the bedside (Barnes & Orrock 2004).

- Chronic fatigue syndrome patients reported reduced depression and somatic symptoms, as well as improved sleep, following massage (Field et al 1997).
- There was immediate decreased anxiety and depressed mood, long-term increased sleep hours and decreased sleep movements in fibromyalgia patients following massage. Substance P levels dropped, as did pain ratings (Field et al 2002).

Normalize vitality/metabolic energy

Vitality is a key component in the NM approach to health. Although difficult to define, it is an expression of what can be described as metabolic energy, and is a useful focus in solving clinical problems with a naturopathic medicine approach (refer to Chapters 1, 2, 7, 8, 9 and 10). The fluctuations in available energy, and the relationship of this to the wellness concept, impact most human functions.

The potential for physical medicine methods to influence the overall vitality of the organism can be understood from a perspective of *optimization of function*. An individual may be free of pathological disease and have reasonable health, but have an inability to adequately adapt to higher levels of functional demand in terms of exercise, occupation or stress. Another individual may be sensitive to the environment to the point of needing to exclude specific foods and substances to avoid becoming ill. There are clearly systemic functions that are less than optimal in such cases, and these are often identified and treated in naturopathic medicine in order to increase overall adaptive capacity, and therefore wellness and vitality. For example, to have high-level wellness, the circulatory system should be functioning efficiently, perfusing all tissues with nutrients, and draining away waste fluids and materials. Many physical medicine modalities – including massage, mobilization, lymphatic drainage, movement therapies and hydrotherapy – have the potential to enhance circulation (see discussion and evidence in Chapter 7) and so will have an effect on the vitality of the whole organism.

In order to be independent, able to adapt to environmental stressors and to express life through the physical body, the expression 'motion is life' may be appropriate. NPM aims to enhance this aspect of health, and links this improved functionality to vitality.

There is well-established and documented evidence of the influence of physical (aerobic) exercise and training on rehabilitation from conditions that feature clinical presentations of extreme pain and fatigue, such as fibromyalgia (Bagge et al 1998, Mannerkorpi & Iversen 2003, Nichols & Glenn 1994, Richards & Scott 2002).

Prevent or retard degeneration

Patients consulting a practitioner of NPM will commonly be prescribed an individualized exercise program along with advice regarding movement and posture, as explained more fully in Chapter 9. Musculoskeletal development depends on normal movements and regular weight-bearing exercise. This is equally true in relation to the prevention of degenerative changes (Malone et al 1997). Carefully designed exercise programs have been shown to help prevent diseases of aging and slow the progression of some degenerative diseases. Examples of degeneration prevention via methods commonly used in naturopathic settings include the following:

- It is estimated that approximately half the decline in function that occurs with aging is the result of a reduction in skeletal muscle (accelerated by physical inactivity and disuse of muscle) rather than illness (Evans & Campbell 1993, Penhall 1994).
- Lean body mass (muscle) declines progressively throughout adult life and is associated with a reduction in performance, loss of strength, decrease in protein reserves, increased disability and increased risk of falls and injury (Bales & Ritchie 2002, Iannuzzi-Sucich et al 2002).
- Gerontological exercise physiology confirms that maintenance of a physically active lifestyle arrests or significantly delays age-related changes in cardiovascular, respiratory and

musculoskeletal function (Eastell & Lambert 2002).
- Arthritis, osteoporosis, accidents and fractures are major causes of injury and suffering in this age group. According to the World Health Organization, the prevalence of musculoskeletal disease has reached epidemic proportions (Kai et al 2003). There is consensus that physical activity can delay the functional decline and reduce the morbidity associated with aging (Delmas 2002, Fiechtner 2003).

Enhance biomechanical functionality

A primary goal of physical medicine in any field is maximizing biomechanical efficiency. The characteristic of NPM is its understanding of how this efficiency affects all aspects of an individual's health, in a vitalistic sense.

According to Yates (1990), the known effects of physical therapy on *skeletal muscle* can be grouped into a number of clinical goals:

- Relaxation and softening through neuromuscular reflex effects
- Relief of spasms and cramps by inhibition of reflex activity and increased local circulation
- Relief of pain of myofascial origin, including release of trigger points
- Treating delayed muscle soreness after vigorous activity
- Enhancing athletic performance.

These known physical therapy effects would be well applied in enhancing performance in sports, and may also be helpful in the management of the following conditions:

- Muscle spasm and hypertonicity
- Myofascial trigger point syndrome
- Spinal curvatures – hypertonic/shortened postural muscles
- Respiratory disorders – hypertonic/shortened postural muscles
- Torticollis
- Whiplash after-effects
- Temporomandibular joint dysfunction
- Overuse injuries
- Thoracic outlet syndrome
- Tension headache.

Re-education of the individual – prevention

In order to ensure long-term recovery, a program based on education and understanding is the greatest preventive.

The long-term success of most health interventions is usually contingent on the extent to which individuals are willing to change behavior. Public health campaigns in particular emphasize the need to adopt healthier lifestyles, exercise more regularly, moderate alcohol intake and cease smoking. If an individual believes that a particular course of action will help to solve a health problem, adherence to the prescribed program is more likely (Conner & Norman 1995). This makes the educational/informational aspect of naturopathic medicine of fundamental importance. As an example, something as simple as learning that 'hurt does not necessarily mean harm', can dramatically change a person's compliance with an exercise program.

According to Prochaska et al (1992), progression towards desirable health behavior can be assisted by using such techniques as:

- consciousness raising
- self-re-evaluation
- self-liberation
- counter-conditioning
- stimulus control
- reinforcement management
- dramatic relief
- environmental re-evaluation and social liberation.

Understanding the condition, its causes and its likely remedies, as well as having appropriate educational tools, is a pivotal role for the practitioner of naturopathic medicine

In naturopathic physical medicine, this becomes central to healing, as lifestyle modification, management of physical and occupational activities, and the need for rehabilitation all require compliance from the individual. Prevention of further injury and physical dysfunction results from skillful and coherent educational processes in the clinical setting. Empowering the individual is a cogent expression of the *vis medicatrix naturae*, or, to use modern terminology, homeostasis, or self-regulation. (These issues are discussed fully in Chapters 1 and 2, while compliance and patient education are explored in Chapter 9.)

Reduce pain and discomfort

Reducing or modulating the level of pain an individual is experiencing can be an appropriate clinical goal in itself, even if the underlying condition is not modified. Pain is a complex symptom of variable acuity and chronicity, and affects the target tissues, the sensory receptor function and the central processing of pain perception (see Chapter 10 for a review of physical medicine therapeutic measures that significantly influence pain).

- Massage and other physical therapy modalities (mobilization, manipulation, specific exercise protocols, etc.) have been shown to decrease pain perception and/or enhance function, as well as having an evidence base of relief of low back and articular pain (Clelland et al 1987, Cochrane Database of Systematic Reviews 2006, Delitto et al 1995, Ernst 1999, Zusman 1988).
- Complex painful conditions (e.g. fibromyalgia) have been shown to benefit from a combination of hydrotherapy and exercise approaches (Buskila et al 2001, Evcik et al 2002, Mannerkorpi et al 2000, Nichols & Glenn 1994).

Numerous additional citations and examples of pain relief via massage (and other manual modalities and hydrotherapy) are to be found in Chapters 7 and 10.

Practicing whole-body physical medicine

Definition

Whole-body physical medicine could be defined as diagnosing and treating disorders of the somatic tissues within a conceptual basis of the interdependency and continuity of all the tissues of the body, including their reciprocal influence on (and by) the state of mind and emotions (Ferrell-Torry & Glick 1993, Shulman & Jones 1996).

NPM modalities, including manipulation, massage, mobilization, exercise, hydrotherapy, etc., are commonly employed in the treatment of patients (and their symptoms) with conditions of a pathological nature – pneumonia (Noll et al 2000), Parkinson's disease (Hernandez-Reif et al 2002), cancer (Field et al 2001, Hernandez-Reif et al 2004), hypertension (Hernandez-Reif et al 2000) and premenstrual syndrome (Walsh & Polus 1998) – unrelated to obvious musculoskeletal dysfunction.

Chapters 7, 8 and 10 provide a wide range of information on this area of NPM usage.

Constitutional types in NPM

Individualization of treatment is a key feature of NPM, and this is often based on the concept of constitutional types. Two perspectives on the use of constitutional types in NPM are outlined in Boxes 4.5 and 4.6.

Box 4.5 Constitutional considerations

Roger Newman Turner ND DO BAc

Constitution in the context of anthropomorphic classification is based on a simple description of body shape and mass, such as thin, fat, athletic or stocky. Sheldon (1940), whose classification is the clearest and most applicable to assessing patients for physical interventions, stated that the constitution 'refers to those aspects of the individual which are relatively more fixed and unchanging – morphology, endocrine function, etc., – and may be contrasted with those aspects which are more labile and susceptible to modification by environmental pressures'. His system was developed from a study of over 4000 students whom he photographed and classified according to three main components based on the predominance of the body layers: the endoderm, mesoderm and ectoderm.

The *endomorphic* constitution has a predominance of soft roundness in which the digestive organs dominate the body economy. *Mesomorphy* refers to a relative predominance of muscles, bone and connective tissue. The physique tends to the heavy and rectangular. *Ectomorphy* is characterized by length and fragility. In proportion to body mass, the ectomorph has a greater surface area and, therefore, greater sensory exposure to the outside world.

Whilst many people have elements of more than one group, Sheldon's system provides broad guidelines to the resilience and likely response of the patient to physical therapy, especially when supported by palpatory findings, use of the cardiovascular index and observation of the iris (see below). Within each broad classification, treatment must be tailored to the individual response and tolerance of the patient.

The endomorphic individual, for example, tends to have a slower metabolism and requires stronger stimuli. The contrasts of hydrotherapy applications can be greater, soft tissue procedures may need to be stronger and deeper, and such patients can generally endure longer treatment sessions. The ectomorphic types, or those of slim build, on the other hand, require lighter, shorter approaches and may need less extremes of hydrotherapy. Mesomorphs are more sturdy and athletic in build and can usually tolerate reasonably strong stimuli.

Somatotype has also been shown to have correlations with aerobic trainability, adaptability and blood pressure. Chaouachi et al (2005) conducted a series of exercise tests and measures of ventilatory capacity on subjects divided into four somatotype groups – endo-mesomorphs, mesomorphs, meso-ectomorphs and ectomorphs – who were then subjected to a 12-week endurance training program for two sessions per week.

At re-evaluation, there were significant differences among the groups, with the meso-ectomorphs and mesomorphs showing the greatest improvement in aerobic capacity.

Salivon & Polina (2005) carried out a comparative analysis of anthropometric indices, matching these to cardiovascular vegetative regulation. The researchers observed typological specificity of organism reactivity to unfavorable geochemical situations in young males and females, in different stages of the adaptation process. They noted variations of adaptability to adverse environmental factors such as nutrient mineral deficiencies in the soil ('vital macro- and micro-elements in soils and drinkable water').

A study of over 700 subjects of each gender carried out by Kalitchman et al (2004) revealed an association between somatotype and blood pressure. Individuals of robust physique (high endomorphic and mesomorphic components) showed higher mean values of systolic and diastolic blood pressure. The researchers note that their findings suggest:

> ... the existence of common physiological paths in the development of body physique and blood pressure regulation and may possibly be indicative of the involvement of pleiotropic genetic and/or epigenetic mechanisms in this regulation.

This study adds weight to the value of the cardiovascular index (CVI – see below) as a tool for gauging vital reserve.

Cardiovascular index

The cardiovascular index (CVI) is the sum of the systolic plus diastolic blood pressures, multiplied by the pulse rate. The normal range is between 12 000 and 24 000. Figures in the lower quintile, or below the range, suggest degrees of hypotonia and weakness (Priest 1959). The author's clinical observations have found a low CVI to be common in ectomorphic individuals tending towards sympathicotonia, as suggested by iridological findings.

Iris diagnosis

A further guide to the vital reserve of the patient is possible using observation of the iris of the eye. The overall color and texture of the irids is considered to be indicative of hereditary traits and inherent constitutional integrity. Observation may be made with a hand lens and penlight although, for more detailed analysis, a desktop ophthalmoscope or camera designed for close imaging of the iris is preferable.

The system is based on what A.W. Priest (Newman Turner 2000) has described as 'symbolic topography'

Continued

Box 4.5 Constitutional considerations continued

because radial and concentric circular zones are said to represent tissues and organs of the whole body, although no definite anatomic basis has been established for this belief. Nevertheless, empirical evidence suggests that the tightness or otherwise of the structure of the iris can give a good indication of the overall tissue tone. A loose radial structure indicates a

greater fragility whereas more compact radii suggest greater resilience (Schimmel 1984).

The degree of autonomic tone is also indicated by the tightness of the autonomic wreath, a radial zone lying outside the pupil, as well as the dilation of the pupil itself (Kriege 1969). A chronically dilated pupil correlates with excessive sympathicotonia (see Table 4.1).

Table 4.1 Some possible constitutional signs and indications

Somatotype (Sheldon)	Physique	CVI*	Iris	Therapeutic considerations
Endomorph	Rotund, fleshy	Tends to be >18 000	Compact structure Narrow pupil	Strong stimuli, strong contrasts Greater tolerance to strength and duration of treatment
Mesomorph	Muscular	Mid-range	Mixed type	Tolerance varies with condition Generally good resilience
Ectomorph	Slim, angular	Tends to be <12 000	Loose structure Dilated pupil	Milder stimuli with less contrast Shorter treatment duration

* Normal range: 12 000–24 000.

Box 4.6 Constitutional diagnosis

Eric Blake ND MSOM Dipl Ac

There exist several approaches to constitutional diagnosis in naturopathic medicine. Facial diagnosis was initially advocated by Kuhne (1902) in his widely influential work. Havard further elaborated on the cranial structures alongside his work at Dr Lindlahr's college and hospital (Lindlahr 1924). While Kuhne's diagnosis focused upon identification of the pattern of accumulation of waste products, whose elimination was the goal of therapeutic intervention, Havard's method identified constitutional types based upon a hierarchy of organ strengths and weaknesses. Rank categorization based upon the relative size of the occipital, parietal or temporal lobes, as evidenced visually in the corresponding cranial structures, allowed a ranking of the digestive, genitourinary or cardiopulmonary systems, respectively. Ranking of the organ systems would then allow prediction of healing crises, in the secondary strength during adulthood, and in the weakest organ system at childhood. Pathological derangement of the strongest organ system was considered a poor prognosis. This method was referred to as 'basic diagnosis' and Lindlahr advocated a combination of this and iris diagnosis.

Another approach to constitutional diagnosis was the chemical typology advocated by Rocine (1925). This method identified chemical elements that predominated in the individual. Based on characteristic physical, mental and emotional patterns, individuals could be categorized and therapeutic interventions designed. Naturopathic physicians such as Shadduck (1930), Verbon (1948), Shanklin (1950) and Jensen (1983) advocated and expanded upon Rocine's approach.

Iris diagnosis, a unique naturopathic diagnostic method (McCain 1936), has also developed a constitutional typology. The earliest model by Madaus (1925) incorporated some facial and fingernail diagnosis as well. The later taxonomy of Deck (1965) has certain similarities; however, the focus is upon the iris. This approach is gaining greater international acceptance and is advocated as a basic identification model by the Felke Institut (Hauser et al 2000). The genetically determined iris color is thought to identify the primary constitution, the overarching structural pattern of the fibers the secondary disposition, and finally tertiary categorization is determined by accumulation patterns. Upon this basic constitutional classification further iris diagnosis is then elaborated.

Box 4.6 Constitutional diagnosis continued

Contemporary research is validating and expanding our understanding of the model of the iridological constitutions. For example, the connective tissue weakness disposition, characterized by a general laxity of the iris fibers, has a statistically significant higher genetic expression of the IL-1 beta genotype, a pro-inflammatory cytokine associated with irritable bowel disease (Um et al 2004). Similarly, the neurogenic disposition, characterized by a relatively tight and taut iris fiber pattern, has increased expression of genotype associated with hypertension (Um et al 2005). The methods of constitutional diagnosis are in accord with the modern understanding of genetic phenotypic expressions.

Interdependency

Anatomic

Fascial mapping

The perspective of interdependency in NPM is well illustrated by a focus on the tissues gathered under the global category of fascia. Fascia is one component of connective tissue in the body, which includes fascia, tendons and ligaments. These tissues have particular characteristics that influence their function – they have parallel collagen fibers, various degrees of undulations and are low in elastin. This category of tissue has many functions (Manheim 2001):

- Supports matrix
- Provides pathways for nerves, blood vessels, lymphatic vessels
- Facilitates movement
- Bursal sacs minimize friction and pressure
- Restraining mechanism of ligament/tendons
- Ensheaths limbs – promotes circulation
- Sites for muscle attachment
- Stores fat – conserves heat
- Fibroblastic activity – scar formation
- Histiocytes act as phagocytes – immune reaction
- Plasma cells – antibody formation
- Tissue fluids – nutrition to cells ... and more.

The principles that guide attention to fascia in physical medicine are based on the knowledge that fascia covers, separates, attaches to and gives cohesion to all organs, muscles and other bodily tissues, so that there is true structural interdependence between all regions – literally from the plantar fascia to the reciprocal tension membranes of the cranium. With the functions of fascia being intimately involved with many of the clinical goals of NPM and the principles illustrating its holistic and interdependent nature, fascial (or myofascial) techniques are particularly suited to naturopathic physical medicine. As noted below – see notes on the work of Langevin (Box 4.7) and Ingber

Box 4.7 Langevin's communication networks

Leon Chaitow ND DO

Langevin & Yandow (2002) have presented evidence that links the network of acupuncture points and meridians to a network formed by interstitial connective tissue, which has major implications for manual/physical therapies. Using a unique dissection and charting method for location of the connective tissue (fascial) planes, acupuncture points and acupuncture meridians of the arm, they note that 'overall, more than 80% of acupuncture points and 50% of meridian intersections of the arm appeared to coincide with intermuscular or intramuscular connective tissue planes'.

Langevin & Yandow's research further shows microscopic evidence that when an acupuncture needle is inserted and rotated (as is classically performed in acupuncture treatment), a 'whorl' of connective tissue forms around the needle, thereby creating a tight mechanical coupling between the tissue and the needle. The tension placed on the connective tissue as a result of further movements of the needle delivers a mechanical stimulus at the cellular level. They note that changes in the extracellular matrix '... may, in turn, influence the various cell populations sharing this connective tissue matrix (e.g. fibroblasts, sensory afferents, immune and vascular cells)'.

In 2005, Langevin et al observed that: 'The dynamic, cytoskeleton-dependent responses of fibroblasts to changes in tissue length have important implications for our understanding of normal movement and posture, as well as therapies using mechanical stimulation of connective tissue, including physical therapy, massage and acupuncture.'

(Box 4.8) – this interconnection involves all tissues, down to cellular cytoskeletal structures.

Langevin's research (see Box 4.7) has shown that the influences of fascia extend beyond the obvious biomechanical functions of tissues, to the strong possibility

Box 4.8 Ingber's research

Leon Chaitow ND DO

Changes in the shape of cells also alter their ability to function normally, even in regard to how they handle nutrients.

Ingber conducted research (1993, 2003), much of it for NASA, into the reasons astronauts lose bone density after a few months in space. He showed that as cells deform when gravity is removed or reduced, the behavior of cells changes to the extent that, irrespective of how good the overall nutritional state, or how much exercise (static cycling in space) is taking place, when they are distorted, individual cells cannot process nutrients normally, and problems such as decalcification emerge.

This research is a confirmation, were any needed, that structure is the governing feature of function, a validation in naturopathic medicine of the essential role of manual and other physical modalities that have the potential to beneficially modify structural components of the body, so enhancing functional features. As noted in Chapter 2, the corollary to this relationship is, of course, that functional factors such as overuse and misuse imposed on tissues will modify their structure (shortening, fibrosis, etc.), making the structure–function equation a two-way process.

that as yet only partially uncharted communication functions are inherent aspects of connective tissue.

Physiological

Neuromuscular system

Neuromuscular activity in human physiology is a major adaptive system that facilitates and controls movement and stability in both skeletal and smooth muscle function. Movement can be disturbed by unexpected events, as well as by the normal activities of life, and the level of stability in the system can be defined as the ability of a system to return to its original state after any adaptive challenge, evident in the process of homeostasis. It can also be considered as the ability to return to a desired movement pattern after such a demand or disturbance.

Sensory systems in the body, such as the proprioceptive, visual and equilibrium systems, monitor structural, postural and other changes, demands and disturbances, and send informational feedback signals to the central control cortex, which in turn adapts its output to the musculoskeletal system to compensate, adapt and correct imbalances. This type of feedback control – which is clearly dependent on accurate infor-

mation gathering and processing – adds to stability (van Leeuwen 1999).

Because of this complex interplay between movement, stability, strength and coordination, many systems can be affected by any dysfunction in neuromuscular control. This system can be put under duress by stressors as simple as gravity, and as complex as multiple trauma and immune system dysfunction. Reflex patterns associated with visceral inflammation also recruit neuromuscular adaptive activity, and naturopathic practitioners – as well as other holistic professions – consider that a detailed analysis of the neuromuscular system is vital in making a coherent and complete diagnosis (Kuchera 1997). Some elements of such assessment are to be found in Chapter 6, which discusses and gives examples of palpation and assessment skills.

Most commonly this aspect of understanding the interdependency in human function is faced with the patient in pain, especially when caused by trauma and/or postural imbalance. An analysis of how neuromuscular adaptation has occurred, in which tissues, and a strategy of assisting in the optimal outcome of balanced movement, stability and muscle function, is one focus of naturopathic physical medicine.

Two examples of neuromuscular adaptive patterns are those based on the work of Janda and Zink, as described in Boxes 4.9 and 4.10. Additional discussion is to be found in Chapter 2, where adaptation processes are dealt with in depth.

Body–mind

The link between the body and the mind has been well established in the literature over the past three decades, and confirms the traditional naturopathic and holistic view that these two realms of the individual cannot be separated in their functions.

There are historical precedents in naturopathic medicine, as early *nature cure* physicians such as Alfred Brauchle instituted what he called 'naturopathic psychotherapy' as early as 1934, and included a chapter titled 'Psychological Nature Cure' in his 1937 book *History of Nature Cure in Biographies* (Kirchfeld & Boyle 2000). The technique was based mostly on suggestion and hypnosis, although he also believed in the clinical effects of group therapy.

European naturopaths have also demonstrated a wide interest in this area of health care, most notably the British naturopathic practitioner Milton Powell who for many years contributed a series of articles on naturopathic psychotherapy to the *British Naturopathic Journal & Osteopathic Review*. In one example, when discussing the topic of phobia, his naturopathic perspective involved, among other aspects of care,

Box 4.9 Janda: Categorization of change

Leon Chaitow ND DO

As adaptive changes take place in the musculoskeletal system, and as decompensation progresses toward more compromised degrees of dysfunction, structural modifications appear and whole-body, regional and local postural changes emerge.

These changes in response to postural and overuse (and disuse) influences have been categorized in different ways. Amongst the simplest and most useful ways of envisioning adaptational changes affecting the muscles of the body is to use the descriptions and descriptors given by Janda (1978) and Lewit (1999).

They have both noted that particular muscles and groups of muscles function primarily as guardians of stability ('postural' muscles), whereas others have a more active role ('phasic' muscles).

In truth all muscles perform both functions; however, some have a predominant role in one direction or the other (as well as having different ratios of Type 1 and

Type 2 fibers). There is evidence that deeper muscles (also described as 'inner unit', or 'stabilizer' or 'local' muscles) contain proportionately greater numbers of slow twitch (postural) fibers, whereas superficial muscles (also described as 'outer unit', or 'mobilizer' or 'global' muscles; Norris 1998) are dominated by faster (Type 2) fibers (Ng et al 1998).

A simplistic summary of the effects of poor posture would be that a combination of this, together with aging, overuse, misuse, abuse (trauma) and disuse, lead inevitably to adaptation exhaustion, decompensation and ultimately symptoms (see Chapters 2 and 9 for more on adaptation).

Tissues gradually change from a state of normotonicity to a palpably dysfunctional state, at times involving hypertonicity, and at others hypotonicity, the presence of myofascial trigger points (Simons et al 1999), along with altered firing sequences, modified motor control, abnormal postural and/or movement patterns, and ultimately dysfunctional chain reactions.

Box 4.10 The common compensatory pattern

Leon Chaitow ND DO

Defeo & Hicks (1993) have noted that:

Osteopathic physicians Zink and Lawson have observed clinically that a significant percentage of the population assumes a consistently predictable postural adaptation, arising from nonspecific mechanical forces such as gravity, gross and micro-trauma, and other physiological stressors. These forces appear to have their greatest impact on the articular facets in the transitional areas of the vertebral column.

It is clearly important for the naturopathic practitioner to have an awareness, as best this can be ascertained, as to the patient's current level of vitality and vulnerability – both of which can be considered as reflections of the degree to which the person (or the local tissues) have adapted. The principle this reflects, in naturopathic terms, would be the desire to avoid interfering with self-regulation ('*vis*') by further overloading adaptation mechanisms.

Zink & Lawson (1979) described methods for testing tissue preference in these transitional areas where fascial and other tensions and restrictions can most easily be noted, i.e. the occipitoatlantal (OA), cervicothoracic (CT), thoracolumbar (TL) and lumbosacral (LS) levels of the spine. These sites are tested for rotation and side-flexion preference.

Zink & Lawson's research showed that most people display (assessing the occipitoatlantal pattern first)

alternating patterns of rotatory preference, with about 80% of people showing a common pattern of left-right-left-right (L-R-L-R) compensation, termed the 'common compensatory pattern' (CCP).

In a hospital-based study involving over 1000 patients they also observed that the approximately 20% of people whose compensatory pattern did not alternate in the CCP manner had poor health histories, low levels of 'wellness' and had poor stress-coping abilities.

More recent clinical evidence has emerged for the value of this attempt at reading the levels of adaptation exhaustion present in the physical structures of the body. The German osteopath Torsten Liem (2004) has suggested that if the rotational preferences alternate (L-R-L-R) when supine, and display a greater tendency to not alternate (i.e. they rotate in the same directions – for example, L-L-L-R or L-L-R-L or R-R-R-R, or some other variation on a non-alternating pattern) when standing, a dysfunctional adaptation pattern that is 'ascending' is more likely, i.e. the major dysfunctional influences lie in the lower body, pelvis or lower extremities.

If the rotational pattern remains the same when supine and standing this suggests that the adaptation pattern is primarily 'descending', i.e. the major dysfunctional influences lie in the upper body, cranium or jaw.

Methods for evaluation of the CCP and the accompanying imbalances are to be found in Chapter 6 on palpation and assessment methods; Chapter 9 (Rehabilitation) contains ways of addressing problems associated with such imbalances and asymmetries.

exploring with the patient any possible 'purpose' for the phobia, as well as predisposing or contributory factors, followed by what today would be termed cognitive-behavioral measures (Powell 1973).

There have been movements in the study of mind–body interactions during the last 80 years, both from a bodyworker's perspective and the point of view of the psychologically oriented practitioner/physician. The 'bodymind' writings refer to the seminal works by Freud's student Wilhelm Reich (1961), and to his student Alexander Lowen's bioenergetic theories (Lowen 1975). Another major contributor to the understanding in this field was Ida Rolf and her consideration of deep connective tissue holding emotional memory and expression (Rolf 1977).

Dychtwald's book *Bodymind* (1977) further explained for practitioners of bodywork a methodology for applying these theories. The formation of the individual *bodymind* is thought to develop from a combination of influences including heredity, physical activity, emotional and psychological activity, nutrition and the environment. The effects of these domains are considered integral to body structure, leading to the evolution of imbalances that are identifiable (such as 'splits' in development of sides or limbs), with treatment being aimed at a deep consideration of the causes and effects of these.

The parallel movement in 'mind body' medicine has resulted in a more pathophysiological consideration of the effects of emotional distress on the human immune and endocrine systems, termed psychoneuroimmunology (Lutgendorf & Costanzo 2003) (see notes on this in Chapter 1). This concept is supported by substantial scientific evidence, emphasizing the need for naturopaths to practice evidence-informed medicine within a holistic framework, including consideration of all elements of an individual's makeup – mental, physical and spiritual.

From a naturopathic perspective, the study of psychoneuroimmunology has put a scientific theoretical underpinning to the traditional notion that the effects of physical medicine extend beyond the musculoskeletal system. There are many studies showing the body–mind effect of physical medicine – particularly massage but also various forms of manipulation and exercise (Pilkington et al 2005, Yates et al 1988) – on anxiety and depression (Field et al 1992, Fraser & Kerr 1993, McKechnie et al 1983, Meek 1993).

Writers such as Louise Hay (1984) and Peter Levine (1997) take this concept further with methods of accessing the body's expression of inner emotional stressors. Hay puts forward a self-healing framework for exploring the emotional states associated with the specific ailment, and then suggests affirmations to resolve the dysfunctional relationship between that state and the body tissue. Levine studied post-traumatic stress disorder and developed a way of the individual reconnecting with their body tissue (somatic experiencing). The insight gained from these and other mind–body techniques is thought to enhance healing when complex psychosomatic dysfunction is present.

In naturopathic physical medicine the interplay between the physical, emotional and mental spheres is central to diagnosis and therapy, and integrating methods such as those outlined is common. Hypnosis, somatic psychotherapies, emotional supportive counseling and trauma healing, as well as the use of manual methods, all lie within the scope of naturopathic physical medicine, commonly within an (hopefully) integrated multimodality and interdisciplinary team.

Technique choice

Choice of therapeutic approaches

In naturopathic thinking the ideal selection of therapeutic methods and modalities, in any given case, can be seen to require a need for choices that match that individual's current levels of decompensation/maladaptation, vitality and vulnerability.

Treatment approaches should have as objectives a necessity to either reduce adaptive load or enhance functionality (or both), thus allowing self-regulation to operate more effectively. The only other therapeutic choice would be to focus attention mainly on symptomatic relief, with little or no immediate attention as to cause.

Indeed, symptom-oriented treatment may at times be the only choice initially available; however, in a naturopathic setting, objectives that incorporate the possibility of assisting self-regulation ('lighten the load/enhance functionality') would usually be the primary choices.

The other principle that comes to the fore when choosing from the wide array of modalities is the 'first do no harm' tenet. This should guide the practitioner to consider rest as a primary healer, and provide a test for the necessity of each level of intervention. Each intervention is considered against this background, and generally pushes the choices towards the most gentle and least provocative.

A schema of interventions could thus be constructed, based on risk of harm. It should be kept in mind that one of the significant risks in medicine is that of omission – not doing enough, or not having enough knowledge to act on the patient's condition. The

---

Box 4.11 A schema for increasing provocation and risk in modality choice

The list below represents a (far from comprehensive) selection of choices/modalities that are increasingly demanding of the body's adaptive capacities. As discussed in this chapter, therapeutic choices should reflect the individual's current levels of vitality or vulnerability. The more robust the person, the greater the therapeutic load that can be safely managed without negative consequences. Conversely, the more frail, and the greater the current adaptive burden, the lighter and less invasive should be any therapeutic input.

Choices include:

- Do nothing – allow self-regulation to operate uninterrupted
- Educational, informational, cognitive provision
- Rest, relaxation, autonomic training, etc.
- Subtle energy approaches (Reiki, Therapeutic Touch, etc.)
- Nutritional, homeopathic, botanical and/or pharmaceutical substances

- Hydrotherapy (see Chapter 11)
- Electrotherapy (ultrasound etc., see Chapter 12)
- Acupuncture
- Gentle passive exercise (see Chapter 9)
- Functional/indirect manual methods (e.g. positional release methods, see Chapter 7)
- General non-specific mobilization (see Chapter 8)
- Soft tissue/myofascial release/muscle energy/proprioceptive neuromuscular facilitation, etc. (see Chapter 7)
- Prolotherapy (see Chapter 7)
- Active exercises appropriate to the situation (see Chapter 9)
- Direct soft tissue/articular techniques (see Chapter 7)
- Direct manipulation (HVLA) (see Chapter 7)
- Joint injection
- Surgery.

---

knowledgeable practitioner, whilst allowing natural healing to occur by minimal intervention, should be constantly vigilant in a diagnostic and review sense.

It should be recalled that all therapeutic interventions, however minimal, represent an adaptational load for the individual's system to respond to (this is discussed more fully in Chapter 10). Current evidence (Dhabhar & Viswanathan 2005) suggests that there is the potential for both positive and negative effects to derive from what can be termed therapeutically focused stress.

This makes therapeutic choices critical: matching clinical judgment of the patient's ability to respond to whatever modality (physical, chemical, psychological, etc.) or combination of modalities may be involved – a key element in decision-making (see Box 4.11).

Conclusion

This chapter has outlined a definition, a scope of practice based on unique principles, and a set of clinical goals in the practice of naturopathic physical medicine.

Placing these concepts in context for students and practitioners is vital for establishing and expanding the understanding of this style of medical practice, and to promote the use of this characteristic practice in mainstream health care provision.

References

Acharan M 1956 Medicina natural alcance de todos. Carlos Cesarman, Santa Cruz, Mexico

Aust G, Fischer K 1997 Changes in body equilibrium response caused by breathing. A posturographic study with visual feedback. Laryngorhinootologie 76(10):577–582

Bagge E, Bengtsson BA, Carlsson L, Carlsson J 1998 Low growth hormone secretion in patients with fibromyalgia. Journal of Rheumatology 25:145–148

Balaban C, Thayer J 2001 Neurological bases for balance–anxiety links. Journal of Anxiety Disorders 15(1–2):53–79

Bales CW, Ritchie CS 2002 Sarcopenia, weight loss, and nutritional frailty in the elderly. Annual Review of Nutrition 22:309–323

Barnes L, Orrock PJ 2004 The self-perceived effects of massage in palliative care patients. Honours thesis, Southern Cross University, Australia

Beers MH, Berkow R 1999 The Merck manual of diagnosis and therapy, 17th edn. Merck Research Laboratory, Whitehouse Station, NJ

Bodnar RJ, Pasternak GW, Mann PE et al 1989 Mediation of anorexia by human recombinant tumor necrosis factor through a peripheral action in the rat. Cancer Research 49(22):6280–6284

Buskila D, Abu-Shakra M, Neumann L et al 2001 Balneotherapy for fibromyalgia at the Dead Sea. Rheumatology International 20(3):105–108

Cantieri MS 1997 Inpatient osteopathic manipulative treatment: impact on length of stay. American Academy of Osteopathy Journal 7(4):25–29

Chaitow L 2004 Breathing pattern disorders, motor control, and low back pain. Journal of Osteopathic Medicine 7(1):34–41

Chaitow L, DeLany J 2000 Clinical applications of neuromuscular techniques, vol 1: upper body. Churchill Livingstone, Edinburgh

Chaouachi M, Chaouachi A, Chamari K et al 2005 Effects of dominant somatotype on aerobic capacity trainability. British Journal of Sports Medicine 39(12):954–959

Clelland J, Savinar E, Shepard K 1987 Role of physical therapist in chronic pain management. In: Burrows G, Elton D, Stanley GV (eds) Handbook of chronic pain management. Elsevier, London, p 243–258

Cochrane Database of Systematic Reviews 2006 Issue 4. The Cochrane Collaboration. Wiley, Chichester

Conner M, Norman P 1995 Predicting health behaviour: research and practice with social cognition models. Open University Press, Buckingham

Cordingley EW 1925 Principles and practice of naturopathy: a compendium of natural healing. O'Fallon, Bazan, CA

Deck J 1965 Principles of iris diagnosis. Josef Deck, Ettlingen, Germany

Defeo G, Hicks L 1993 A description of the common compensatory pattern in relationship to the osteopathic postural examination. Dynamic Chiropractic 24:11

Delitto A, Erhard RE, Bowling RW 1995 A treatment-based classification approach to low back syndrome: identifying and staging patients for conservative management. Physical Therapy 75:470–479

Delmas PD 2002 Treatment of postmenopausal osteoporosis. Lancet 359(9322):2018–2026

Dempsey J, Sheel A, St Croix C 2002 Respiratory influences on sympathetic vasomotor outflow in humans. Respiratory Physiology and Neurobiology 130(1):3–20

Dhabhar F, Viswanathan K 2005 Stress-induced enhancement of leukocyte trafficking to sites of surgery or immune activation. Brain, Behavior and Immunity 19(4 Suppl 1):e15

Draper G 1924 Human constitution: a consideration of its relationship to disease. WB Saunders, Philadelphia

Dychtwald K 1977 Bodymind. Tarcher, New York

Eastell R, Lambert H 2002 Strategies for skeletal health in the elderly. Proceedings of the Nutrition Society 61(2):173–180

Ernst E 1999 Massage therapy for low back pain: a systematic review. Journal of Pain and Symptom Management 17:65–69

Ernst E 2001 Life-threatening complications after spinal manipulation. Stroke 32:809–810

Evans WJ, Campbell WW 1993 Sarcopenia and age-related changes in body composition and functional capacity. Journal of Nutrition 123:465–468

Evcik D, Kizilay B, Gokcen E 2002 The effects of balneotherapy on FMS patients. Rheumatology International 22(2):56–59

Ferrell-Torry AT, Glick OJ 1993 The use of therapeutic massage as a nursing intervention to modify anxiety and the perception of cancer pain. Cancer Nursing 16:93–101

Fiechtner J 2003 Hip fracture prevention. Drug therapies and lifestyle modification that can reduce risk. Postgraduate Medicine 114(3):22–28, 32

Field T, Morrow C, Valdeon C et al 1992 Massage reduces anxiety in child and adolescent psychiatric patients. Journal of the American Academy of Child and Adolescent Psychiatry 31:125–131

Field T, Sunshine W, Hernandez-Reif M 1997 Chronic fatigue syndrome: massage therapy effects on depression and somatic symptoms in chronic fatigue syndrome. Journal of Chronic Fatigue Syndrome 3:43–51

Field T, Cullen C, Diego M et al 2001 Leukemia immune changes following massage therapy. Journal of Bodywork and Movement Therapies 5:271–274

Field T, Diego M, Cullen C et al 2002 Fibromyalgia pain and substance P decrease and sleep improves after massage therapy. Journal of Clinical Rheumatology 8:72–76

Field T, Hernandez-Reif M, Diego M et al 2005 Cortisol decreases and serotonin and dopamine increase following massage therapy. International Journal of Neuroscience 115:1397–1413

Foldi M, Strossenreuther R 2003 Foundations of manual lymph drainage, 3rd edn. Mosby, St Louis

Ford M, Camilleri M, Hanson R 1995 Hyperventilation, central autonomic control, and colonic tone in humans. Gut 37:499–504

Fraser J, Kerr JR 1993 Psychophysiological effects of back massage on elderly institutionalized patients. Journal of Advanced Nursing 18(2):238–245

Geisman LA 2002 Fever: beneficial and detrimental effects of antipyretics. Current Opinion in Infectious Diseases 15(3):241–245

Govan ADT, MacFarlane R 2004 Pathology illustrated. Churchill Livingstone, New York

Greenman PE 1997 Principles of manual medicine. Churchill Livingstone, Philadelphia

Guyton AC, Hall JE 2006 Textbook of medical physiology, 11th edn. WB Saunders, Oxford

Han J, Stegen K, De Valck C et al 1996 Influence of breathing therapy on complaints, anxiety and breathing pattern in patients with hyperventilation syndrome and anxiety disorders. Journal of Psychosomatic Research 41(5):481–493

Hauser H, Karl J, Stolz R 2000 Information from structure and colour. Felke Institut, Heimsheim

Hay L 1984 Heal your body. Hay House, Carlsbad, CA

Hernandez-Reif M, Field T, Krasnegor J et al 2000 High blood pressure an associated symptoms reduced by massage therapy. Journal of Bodywork and Movement Therapies 4:31–38

Hernandez-Reif M, Field T, Largie S et al 2002 Parkinson's disease symptoms reduced by massage therapy. Journal of Bodywork and Movement Therapies 6:177–182

Hernandez-Reif M, Ironson G, Field T et al 2004 Breast cancer patients have improved immune functions following massage therapy. Journal of Psychosomatic Research 57(1):45–52

Hernandez-Reif M, Field T, Ironson G et al 2005 Natural killer cells and lymphocytes are increased in women with breast cancer following massage therapy. International Journal of Neuroscience 115(3):495–510

Hodges P, Gandevia S 2000a Activation of the human diaphragm during a repetitive postural task. Journal of Physiology 522:165–175

Hodges P, Gandevia S 2000b Changes in intra-abdominal pressure during postural and respiratory activation of the human diaphragm. Journal of Applied Physiology 89:967

Hodges P, Butler J, McKenzie D, Gandevia SC 1997 Contraction of the human diaphragm during postural adjustments. Journal of Physiology 505:539–548

Hodges P, Heijnen I, Gandevia S 2001 Postural activity of the diaphragm is reduced in humans when respiratory demand increases. Journal of Physiology 537(3):999–1008

Huey S, West S 1983 Hyperventilation: its relation to symptom experience and anxiety. Journal of Abnormal Psychology 92:422–432

Hunter G 1998 Specific soft tissue mobilization in management of soft tissue dysfunction. Manual Therapy 3(1):2–11

Iannuzzi-Sucich M, Prestwood KM, Kenny AM 2002 Prevalence of sarcopenia and predictors of skeletal muscle mass in healthy, older men and women. Journals of Gerontology Series A: Biological Sciences & Medical Sciences 57(12):M772–777

Ingber DE 1993 Cellular tensegrity: defining new rules of biological design that govern the cytoskeleton. Journal of Cell Science 104:613–627

Ingber DE 2003 Mechanobiology and diseases of mechanotransduction. Annals of Medicine 35(8):564–577

Ironson G, Field T, Scafidi F et al 1996 Massage therapy is associated with enhancement of the immune systems cytotoxic capacity. International Journal of Neuroscience 84(1–4):205–217

Janda V 1978 Muscles, central nervous motor regulation, and back problems. In: Korr IM (ed) Neurobiologic mechanisms in manipulative therapy. Plenum Press, New York

Jefferey E 2006 Detoxification basics. Managing biotransformation: metabolic, genomic, and detoxification balance points. 13th International Symposium on Functional Medicine, Tampa, Florida

Jensen B 1983 The chemistry of man. Bernard Jensen. Escondido, CA

Kai M, Anderson M, Lau E 2003 Exercise intervention: defusing the world's osteoporosis time bomb. Bulletin of the World Health Organization 81(11):827–830

Kalitchman L, Livshits G, Kobyliansky E 2004 Association between somatotypes and blood pressure Annals of Human Biology 31(4):466–476

Kasseroller R 1998 Compendium of Dr Vodder's manual lymph drainage. Haug, Heidelberg, p 190

Kirchfeld F, Boyle W 2000 Nature doctors: pioneers in naturopathic medicine. Medicine Biologica, Portland, OR, p 173

Kjelsden-Kragh J, Haugen M, Borchgrevink CF, Laerum E 1991 Controlled trial of fasting and one-year vegetarian diet in rheumatoid arthritis. Lancet 338(8772):899–902

Kluger MJ 1986 Fever: a hot topic. News in Physiological Sciences 1:25–27

Kollath W 1950 Uber die Mesotrophie, ihre Ursachen und praktische Bedeutung. In: Grote LRR, Kollath W (eds) Ernahrungswirkungen. Schriftenreihe fur Ganzheitsmedizin Band 3. Hippokrates Verlag, Stuttgart

Kretchmer E 1921 Physique and character. Translated by WH Sprott, 1925, Kegan Paul, Trench, Trubner, London (from Körperbau und Charakter, Springer, Berlin)

Kriege T 1969 Fundamental basis of iris diagnosis. Fowler, London

Kuchera M 1997 Treatment of gravitational strain pathophysiology. In: Vleeming A, Mooney V, Dorman T, Snijders C, Stoeckart R (eds) Movement, stability and low back pain. Churchill Livingstone, New York

Kuhne L 1902 Handbook of the science of facial expression. Kuhne, Leipsic; The International News Co., New York

Labyak SE, Metzger BL 1997 The effects of effleurage backrub on the physiological components of relaxation: a meta-analysis. Nursing Research 46(1):59–62

Langevin H, Yandow J 2002 Relationship of acupuncture points and meridians to connective tissue planes. Anatomical Record 269(6):257–265

Langevin H, Bouffard N, Badger G et al 2005 Dynamic fibroblast cytoskeletal response to subcutaneous tissue stretch ex vivo and in vivo. American Journal of Physiology. Cell Physiology 288:C747–756

Lederman E 2005 Science and practice of manual therapy, 2nd edn. Churchill Livingstone, Edinburgh, p 277–293

Lee D 1999 The pelvic girdle. Churchill Livingstone, Edinburgh

Levine P 1997 Waking the tiger: healing trauma. North Atlantic Books, Berkeley

Levine SA, Reinhardt JH 1983 Biochemical pathology initiated by free radicals, oxidant chemicals, and therapeutic drugs in the aetiology of chemical hypersensitivity disease. Journal of Orthomolecular Psychiatry 12:166–183

Lewit K 1999 Manipulative therapy in rehabilitation of the locomotor system, 3rd edn. Butterworths, London

Liem T 2004 Cranial osteopathy: principles and practice. Churchill Livingstone, Edinburgh, p 340–342

Lindlahr H 1918a Natural therapeutics, vol 2: practice. Lindlahr Publishing, Chicago, p 47

Lindlahr H 1918b Philosophy of natural therapeutics: the classic nature cure guide to health and healing. Edited and revised by JCP Proby. Maidstone Osteopathic Clinic, Maidstone, Kent, 1975

Lindlahr H 1918c Acute diseases: their uniform treatment by natural methods. Lindlahr Publishing, Chicago

Lindlahr H 1918d Natural therapeutics, vol 2: practice. Lindlahr Publishing, Chicago, p 16

Lindlahr H 1924 Iridiagnosis and other diagnostic methods, 6th edn. Lindlahr Publishing, Chicago

Liska DJ 2002 The role of detoxification in the prevention of chronic degenerative diseases. Applied Nutritional Science Reports. Advanced Nutrition Publications Inc

Lowen A 1975 Bioenergetics. Coward, McCann & Geoghegan, New York

Lum L 1987 Hyperventilation syndromes in medicine and psychiatry. Journal of the Royal Society of Medicine 80:229–231

Lum L 1994 Hyperventilation syndromes. In: Timmons B, Ley R (eds) Behavioral and psychological approaches to breathing disorders. Plenum Press, New York, p 113–123

Lutgendorf S, Costanzo E 2003 Psychoneuroimmunology and health psychology: an integrative model. Brain, Behavior and Immunity 17:225–232

Mackowiak PA 2000 Physiological rationale for suppression of fever. Clinical Infectious Diseases Supplement 5:S185–189

Madaus M 1925 Lehrbuch uber Irisdiagnose. Rohrmoser, Bonn Am Rhein

Malone TR, McPoil T, Nitz A 1997 Sports and orthopaedic physical therapy. Mosby, St Louis, p 83–110

Manheim CJ 2001 Myofascial release manual. Slack, Thorofare, NJ

Mannerkorpi K, Iversen M 2003 Physical exercise in fibromyalgia and related syndromes. Baillière's Best Practice and Research in Clinical Rheumatology 17(4):629–647

Mannerkorpi K, Nyberg B, Ahlmen M, Ekdahl C 2000 Pool exercise combined with an education program for patients with FMS. A prospective, randomized study. Journal of Rheumatology 10:2473–2481

McCain RM 1936 Iridiagnosis. Naturopath and Herald of Health 41(3):72

McKechnie AA, Wilson F, Watson N, Scott D 1983 Anxiety states: a preliminary report on the value of connective tissue massage. Journal of Psychosomatic Research 27(2):125–129

Meek SS 1993 Effects of slow stroke back massage on relaxation in hospice clients. Journal of Nursing Scholarship 25(1):17–21

Mehling W, Hamel K 2005 Randomized, controlled trial of breath therapy for patients with chronic low-back pain. Alternative Therapies in Health and Medicine 11(4):44–52

Mesina J, Hampton D, Evans R et al 1998 Transient basophilia following the application of lymphatic pump techniques: a pilot study. Journal of the American Osteopathic Association 98:91–99

Newman Turner R 1996 Free radicals and disease: the toxaemia hypothesis. Complementary and Therapeutic Medicine 4:43–47

Newman Turner R 2000 Naturopathic medicine. Heall, Letchworth Garden City

Ng J, Richardson C, Kippers V, Parnianpour M 1998 Relationship between muscle fiber composition and functional capacity of back muscles in healthy subjects and patients with back pain. Journal of Orthopaedic and Sports Physical Therapy 27(6):389–402

Nichols DS, Glenn TM 1994 Effect of aerobic exercise on pain perception, affect, and level of disability in individuals with fibromyalgia. Physical Therapy 74:327–332

Nixon P, Andrews J 1996 A study of anaerobic threshold in chronic fatigue syndrome (CFS). Biological Psychology 43(3):264

Noll D, Shores J, Gamber R et al 2000 Benefits of osteopathic manipulative treatment for hospitalized elderly patients with pneumonia. Journal of the American Osteopathic Association 100(12):776–782

Norris C 1998 Functional load abdominal training: part 1. Journal of Bodywork and Movement Therapies 3(3):150–158

Penhall RK 1994 Wasting away of the old: can it and should it be prevented? Modern Medicine of Australia March:16–26

Perlmutter D 1997 Parkinson's disease – new perspectives. Townsend Letters Jan:48–50

Pilkington K, Kirkwood G, Rampe H 2005 Yoga for depression: the research evidence. Journal of Affective Disorders 89(1–3):13–24

Powell M 1973 The practice of naturopathic psychotherapy (xvi phobias). British Naturopathic Journal and Osteopathic Review 9(2):35–37

Priest AW 1959 The iridological assessment of the patient and its relationship to subsequent therapeutics. Proceedings of the Research Society for Natural Therapeutics, London

Prochaska JO, DiClemente CC, Norcross JC 1992 In search of how people change: applications to addictive behaviors. American Psychologist 47:1102–1114

Pryor J, Prasad S 2002 Physiotherapy for respiratory and cardiac problems, 3rd edn. Churchill Livingstone, Edinburgh, p 81

Radjieski JM, Lumley MA, Cantieri MS 1998 Effect of osteopathic manipulative treatment on length of stay for pancreatitis: a randomized pilot study. Journal of the American Osteopathic Association 98:264–272

Rauch E 1993 Naturopathic treatment of colds and infectious diseases. Haug, Brussels

Reckeweg HH 1971 Die Wissenschaftlichen Grundlagen der biologischen Medizin. Homotoxin-Journal 10:345–359

Reich W 1961 The function of the orgasm. Farrar, Straus & Cudahy, New York

Rhudy J, Meagher M 2000 Fear and anxiety: divergent effects on human pain thresholds. Pain 84.65–75

Richards KC 1998 Effect of a back massage and relaxation intervention on sleep in critically ill patients. American Journal of Critical Care 7:288–299

Richards S, Scott D 2002 Prescribed exercise in people with fibromyalgia: parallel group randomised controlled trial. British Medical Journal 325:185

Rocine V 1925 Chemical diagnosis. Rocine, Chicago

Rolf I 1977 Structural integration: the re-creation of the balanced human body. Viking Press, New York

Salivon I, Polina N 2005 Constitution and reactivity of the organism. Journal of Physiological Anthropology and Applied Human Science 24(4):497–502

Schimmel HW 1984 Constitution and disposition from the eye. Translated by B Kelly. Pascoe, Giessen

Schleifer LM, Ley R, Spalding T 2002 A hyperventilation theory of job stress and musculoskeletal disorders. American Journal of Industrial Medicine 41(5):420–432

Shadduck R 1930 Body chemicals and their relationship to health. Nature Way Institute, Salt Lake City, UT

Shanklin L 1950 The chemical types of people and their foods. Harmony Health Foods, Homestead, FL

Sheldon WH 1940 The varieties of human physique. Harper, New York.

Sherer TB, Betarbet R, Greenamyre JT 2002 Environment, mitochondria, and Parkinson's disease. Neuroscientist 8(3):2315–2321

Shulman K, Jones G 1996 Effectiveness of massage therapy intervention on reducing anxiety in the workplace. Journal of Applied Behavioral Science 32:160–173

Simons D, Travell J, Simons L 1999 Myofascial pain and dysfunction: the trigger point manual, vol 1: upper half of body, 2nd edn. Williams & Wilkins, Baltimore

Southern Cross University, Naturopathic Nutrition panel definition, 2003

Steventon GB, Heafield MT, Waring RH, Williams AC 1989 Xenobiotic metabolisms in Alzheimer's disease. Neurology 39:883–887

Strauss-Blasche G, Gnad E, Ekmekcioglu C et al 2005 Combined inpatient rehabilitation and spa therapy for breast cancer patients: effects on quality of life and CA 15-3. Cancer Nursing 28(5):390–398

Tiker F, Gurakan B, Kilicdag H, Tarcan A 2004 Dehydration: the main cause of fever in the first week of life. Archives of Disease in Childhood Fetal and Neonatal Edition 89:F373

Timmons B, Ley R (eds) 1994 Behavioral and psychological approaches to breathing disorders. Plenum Press, New York

Um JY, Do KR, Hwang WJ et al 2004 Interleukin-1 beta gene polymorphism related with allergic pathogenesis in iris constitution. Immunopharmacology and Immunotoxicology 26(4):653–661

Um JY, An NH, Yang GB et al 2005 A novel approach of molecular genetic understanding of iridology: relationship between iris constitution and angiotensin converting enzyme gene polymorphism. American Journal of Chinese Medicine 33(3):501–505

Van Dieën J, Selen L, Cholewicki J 2003 Trunk muscle activation in low-back pain patients, an analysis of the literature. Journal of Electromyographic Kinesiology 13:333–351

van Leeuwen JL 1999 Neuromuscular control: introduction and overview. Philosophical Transactions of the Royal Society of London, Series B 354(1385):841–847

Verbon L 1948 A transcript of lectures on chemical types of people. Verbon, Portland, OR

Walsh M, Polus B 1998 A randomized placebo controlled clinical trial on the efficacy of chiropractic therapy on premenstrual syndrome. In: Proceedings of International Conference on Spinal Manipulation, Vancouver, BC, July 16–19 1998

Watkins A (ed) 1997 Mind–body medicine: a clinician's guide to psycho-neuroimmunology. Churchill Livingstone, New York

Wittlinger H, Wittlinger G 1982 Textbook of Dr Vodder's manual lymph drainage, vol 1: basic course, 3rd edn. Haug, Heidelberg

Yates J 1990 A physician's guide to therapeutic massage. Massage Therapists Association of British Columbia, Vancouver

Yates RG, Lamping DL, Abram NL, Wright C 1988 Effects of chiropractic treatment on blood pressure and anxiety: a randomized controlled trial. Journal of Manipulative and Physiological Therapeutics 11:484–488

Zink G, Lawson W 1979 An osteopathic structural examination and functional interpretation of the soma. Osteopathic Annals 7(12):433–440

Zusman M 1988 Prolonged relief from articular soft tissue pain with passive joint movement. Journal of Manual Medicine 3:100–102

5

Leon Chaitow ND DO

With contributions from:

Matthew Wallden ND DO

Assessment and Palpation: Accuracy and Reliability Issues

Clinical decision-making needs to be based on accurate information. This is no less the case in naturopathic physical medicine than in professions such as chiropractic, osteopathy, massage and physical therapy, where clinical decisions are frequently based on subjectively gathered information, combined with objective evidence and the individual's history and presenting symptoms.

In manual medicine it is necessary for the practitioner to be able to extract non-verbal information by means of observation, touch and movement. A high degree of palpatory literacy and observational accuracy is necessary for this to be a meaningful process, and the skills required need development and refinement – as do the skills and knowledge required to appropriately interpret the information gathered. Chapter 6 contains numerous examples and exercises for acquisition and/or polishing of just such skills.

Because so much of palpation and observation evidence is subjective ('What does it *feel* (or look) like?'), questions are frequently raised regarding the validity and accuracy of palpation and observation (Meijne et al 1999, Panzer 1992, Van Dillen et al 1998).

Research on intra- and inter-examiner reliability generally, across all manual medicine and physical therapy professions, shows poor results.

Such evaluation can be divided into:

- the individual practitioner's degree of consistency in performing palpation assessment methods (intra-rater reliability) (Love & Brodeur 1987)
- the degree of agreement of findings between different practitioners all performing the same palpation assessment (inter-rater reliability) (Gerwin et al 1997, Strender et al 1997).

Examples of, and many of the issues involved in, inter- and intra-rater (un)reliability, in the field of manual assessment and palpation, are discussed in this chapter.

Questions

Questions that have emerged from the many studies showing poor inter- and intra-examiner reliability relate to whether the problems reside in palpation itself, as a method of assessment, or in the way palpation is taught and practiced.

In an editorial in the *Journal of Bodywork and Movement Therapies*, the following questions were asked of an interdisciplinary group of physical medicine experts (Chaitow 2001):

1. *Does the reported poor inter-observer reliability of palpation methods make you question the validity and usefulness of an examination based upon this skill? If not, why not?*
2. *How do you think palpation and clinical assessment should be taught/studied so that its validity and clinical potential can be best demonstrated?*
3. *Should we depend less on palpation and assessment methods in clinical settings, since their reliability seems to be so poor?*
4. *What other tests do you use so that your clinical examination's reliability can be bolstered?*
5. *If treatment based on possibly unreliable assessment and palpation methods is apparently effective, what does this say about the value of the methods being used? (For example, is apparently successful treatment, based on apparently unreliable assessment methods, valuable mainly for its placebo effects?)*
6. *Should palpatory diagnostic findings be accepted as having a subjective/interpretative value similar to interpretation of radiographic findings or other laboratory data, and therefore be capable of being integrated into a treatment plan by a skilled therapist?*

The main conclusions arrived at by an interdisciplinary group of manual medicine experts (Joanne Bullock-Saxton PhD PT, Leon Chaitow ND DO, Peter Gibbons DO, Shannon Goossen LMT DAc, Diane Lee PT, Karel Lewit MD, Craig Liebenson DC, Don Murphy DC, David Simons MD and Phillip Tehan DO) were (Bullock-Saxton et al 2002):

1. Individual palpation-based assessments and tests have limited value, but *when combined with other indicators and tests*, along with the patient's history and presenting symptoms, are invaluable.
2. The apparent inadequacies in palpation results are similar to results noted with other assessment methods that depend on subjective interpretation of evidence, such as radiographic interpretation (Christensen et al 2001), and *can be remedied by appropriate training and precise application of agreed methodology*.
3. Training in palpation skills demands a sound knowledge of the terrain, as well as *diligent practicing of assessment techniques, in a standardized manner*, until results are routinely reproducible by the individual, and between individual practitioners.

A selection of insightful individual responses from these experts will be found towards the end of this chapter.

Context

The *context* of the setting within which palpation is being utilized has a bearing on its efficacy. Take, for example, a scenario where a patient presents with right-sided sacroiliac joint pain.

Practitioner 1 might assess the left and right sacroiliac joints (and associated tissues, e.g. piriformis, lumbar erectors; see descriptions of assessments in Chapter 6) for tissue texture changes, pain, temperature, edematous features, range of motion, etc., and conclude that the left SIJ is restricted in its range, suggesting that the right SIJ may be overworked in compensation, and may have undergone cumulative myoligamentous adaptive strain. This would certainly be what an osteopathically or chiropractically oriented naturopath might *expect* to find. However, because we do tend to find what we look for, the assessment might at times be self-fulfilling. A question worth considering is whether patterns of dysfunction revealed in the symptomatic patient, which are interpreted as being etiological, may sometimes (often) be identified in symptom-free individuals if they were assessed in the same manner. The individual practitioner/therapist, whose skill relates to an ability to proficiently mobilize/manipulate restricted joints/tissues, will conduct tests designed to assess joint play features.

Practitioner 2 may have a different perspective, and might assess the relative ranges of motion in the ankle, knee, hip and SI joints bilaterally, as well as lower abdominal wall strength/coordination and transversus abdominis activation, and follow on with an active straight leg raise test. This practitioner might also assess the position of the atlas, evaluate digestive function, undertake a gait analysis and perform a box step-up test, a toe touch drill, a lunge, a squat, a multifidus activation test and a gluteus medius strength test. Finally, the SIJ might be assessed using some local motion palpation tests. Most of these tests (barring perhaps digestive function) would have a palpatory or observation element – and all might provide valuable information about how the SIJ and surrounding musculature are functioning. In gathering such a broad spectrum of information, the practitioner is less prone to skewing the outcome due to 'expectations' than the first example above, since the number of possible outcomes increases exponentially with each additional assessment/test. There is therefore arguably less margin for subjective bias. The data would then be assessed for patterns of dysfunction and, if identified, the findings of practitioner 2 may be seen to probably have greater validity than example 1.

This latter set of tests might be chosen by a practitioner with a background in corrective exercise provision. Hence, what that practitioner is looking for is different from the focus of the first example.

The depth of the second set of assessments would fall well outside the confines of a traditional 30-minute consultation, which suggests that palpation may be of differing values in differing clinical contexts. And, if this is true, and if the lengthier evaluation offers greater insight into the breadth of the problem, naturopaths in their physical medicine mode of operation might consider that 'working outside the box', in the manner described for Practitioner 2, offers a fuller assessment protocol for the patient. This search for information, conducted *before* suggesting or applying corrective measures, would seem to offer a more naturopathic approach than that offered by Practitioner 1.

The clinical context, therefore, is critical!

The thesis of this section is that, although subjective by nature, palpation and observation are valid and reliable assessment methods *when performed by practiced examiners, and when used in conjunction with other assessment methods*. It is seldom the case that a single positive test should be relied on as offering conclusive evidence in clinical decision-making.

Interpreting palpation and assessment findings

Gathering information is one thing, interpreting the findings and making clinical decisions as to appropriate treatment quite another.

To some extent this will always remain an individual matter for the naturopathically trained clinician, who – it is to be hoped – will rely on an amalgam of information, gathered in a variety of ways, that will be placed alongside palpation and assessment findings, allowing safe and rational decisions to be made, supported by clinical and research evidence All this should ideally take place in a setting that maintains a primary focus on safely assisting self-regulation, in ways that impose the minimum of secondary adaptive demands.

Naturopathic physical medicine practice requires that palpation and assessment findings should be screened through a filter that asks pertinent questions, such as:

- *Which tissues or areas are dysfunctional, based on these findings, and why are they in this state?*
- *What do these findings mean in terms of this individual's symptoms and his/her place in the spectrum of adaptation?*
- *Do these findings indicate that self-regulation is operating appropriately, and what can I do to assist this without impeding progress?*
- *Are these tissues too loose, too tight, too damaged, too weak (etc.) – and what are the least invasive, and most effective, means of assisting them towards normality?*
- *Based on these findings, and the history and symptoms and signs of the patient, and the state of the tissues involved, is there a reasonable expectation of benefit if appropriate treatment is initiated?*
- *What is the appropriate initial treatment for this situation?*
- *With the complexity of symptoms on display, including pain and dysfunctional tissues, joints, etc., where would it be most appropriate to initiate treatment?*
- *Does the evidence of palpation and assessment support the probability that this is a self-limiting*

condition that will normalize itself via self-regulation with minimal therapeutic input?

- *Does the evidence of palpation and assessment support the probability that this is not a self-limiting condition that will normalize itself, and, if this is the case, what is likely to be the most helpful initial therapeutic approach?*
- *How do these findings equate with the evidence gathered from the Zink and Lawson (common compensatory pattern) assessment (see pages 138/139) regarding where this individual is to be located in the compensation/decompensation spectrum?*
- *What whole body, constitutional methods might be most suitable for this individual, rather than specific interventions?*

The following paradigm may be found to be constructive when making clinical decisions:

- *Identifying the physiological status of the tissues and the context in which these exist +*
- *Understanding the physiological effects of treatment modalities →*
- *Rational, effective, evidence-based treatment choices.*

The first step in this process is identifying the physiological status of the tissues and this step requires answers to three questions:

1. **Which** *tissues are dysfunctional?*
2. **What** *is the physiological status of these tissues?*
3. **Why** *are these tissues in this state?*

Questions 1 and 2 relate to the type, location and condition of the tissues involved, and palpation is central to answering these questions.

Question 3 is about identifying the process that may have led (or contributed) to, or that is maintaining, this state.

Some answers to these questions lie in the patient's history, and some can be found by examining the patient's entire body, especially those areas that directly relate to the area in question. For example, the answer to 'Why is this knee restricted?' might be found in a hypermobile talus or in an irritated hip joint, or possibly an imbalance/restriction in the temporomandibular area (Schamberger 2002).

The practiced examiner will recognize signs of physiological disturbance, or adaptation, in the tissues being palpated. This recognition will assist in making sound therapeutic choices, based on as clear an understanding as possible of the context out of which symptoms have emerged. In this way skilled palpation and observation can contribute to improved clinical choices, and therefore of results.

Palpation accuracy issues

Beal, in his 1989 *Louisa Burns Memorial Lecture*, focused on the issue of palpation which, he suggested, involves three operations:

1. The sensing of stimuli
2. The transmission of these responses to the brain, and
3. The interpretation or analysis or perception of the information.

Clearly, if any aspect of these operations is distorted or inaccurate, the conclusions drawn from them are likely to be suspect.

Numerous examples exist of poor inter-examiner reliability in use of palpation and motion assessment detection of spinal (cervical or elsewhere) dysfunction. There are, however, also examples of excellent assessment outcomes (Christensen et al 2002, Downey et al 2003, Gibbons et al 2002, Mior et al 1985).

The problem of consistency in diagnosis is a fundamental one, common to all medical professionals as well as bodyworkers. Whether interpreting symptoms and signs, radiographic evidence (Aprill & Bogduk 1992) or the degree of restriction in a spinal joint, there is likely to be inconsistency among practitioners.

These issues are important to our credibility and our effectiveness as clinicians.

The problem of poor inter-examiner agreement is most often phrased in terms of reliability, the inference being that if others agree with our findings, the problem must be real, although this is clearly not necessarily true (Comeaux et al 2001).

Posing questions to the body

All motion testing represents the posing by the examiner of questions to the tissues involved, and to the body as a whole.

Comeaux et al (2001) report that functional osteopathic spinal assessment should include comparison of tissue texture cues at rest, as well as during gentle provocative regionally induced passive motions, proceeding ideally from a regional screen to ultimately being able to identify a single spinal segment that is most implicated, compared to the segments immediately above and below it. This is detective work, seeking information from witnesses that can only offer information in a minimalist manner – Yes? No? Perhaps?

The questions asked to a large extent determine whether appropriate answers will emerge, for clearly, assessment of flexion potential in the wrist will tell you very little about pelvic function.

The way the question is phrased, i.e. the position of the patient and the tissues, the manner of execution, the handling of the structures, the degree of apprehension or relaxation of the individual, will all influence the 'answer', the response, and therefore the accuracy of the information gathered.

The mindset of the examiner is another important factor. If the examiner has already decided that he or she knows what and where the problem is, the accuracy and completeness of the examination may be endangered. Palpation and observation is a process of mining for data, not a process of proving one's suspicions correct.

In seeking palpatory efficacy we have something of a paradox. We need to use the unconscious, non-judgmental mind (more right-brain function) to gain unbiased information, and then switch to the conscious, decision-making mind (more left-brain function) to interpret the data. This is a difficult paradoxical skill switch for the clinician; however, if a clinician is skilled in this way, it is likely that there will be greater efficacy and decreased error.

More questions

A full functional joint evaluation could include (depending on the joints involved) a wide range of motion assessments (including flexion, extension, side-flexion right and left, rotation right and left, translation in various directions, compression and distraction) to assess for freedom/restriction (ease/bind). However, it is commonly useful to restrict assessment to just three cardinal axes of movement: rotation, side-bending and flexion/extension.

The questions being asked during any such assessment represent a progression that may include:

- *Is there a problem?*
- *Where is the problem?*
- *What is the precise nature of the problem?*
- *Why has this problem occurred – and what action (if any) is needed to assist it toward recovery?*

Given the traditional time frame for assessment (30–60 minutes maximum), arriving at accurate answers to these questions may be extremely difficult to achieve – particularly if the clinician has a holistic understanding of biomechanics.

However, there are composite tests that could be used to optimize the efficiency of such examination. For example, watching someone do a full squat means that you have multiple joints and body segments coupling in their motion (see 'Archetypal postures' in Chapter 9). This means that a pattern of restriction or dysfunction becomes magnified by the attempted coupling of multiple joints (this is the premise in preparation for the use of a high velocity, low amplitude thrust for 'locking a joint', where the coupling of motions within a given joint limits the range of motion, allowing it to be moved out of its physiological range of motion via a *low amplitude* thrust) (Hartman 1997).

STAR

Authors in the field of manual therapy claim that intervertebral dysfunction – known as somatic dysfunction, segmental dysfunction, chiropractic subluxation, joint blockage or fixation, by various professions (DiGiovanna & Schiowitz 1997, Gatterman 1995, Greenman 1996, Grieve 1981, Kappler 1997, Kuchera et al 1997, Leach 1994) – can be detected by skilled manual palpation (DiGiovanna & Schiowitz 1997, Greenman 1996).

In osteopathy, the diagnostic indicators of segmental dysfunction – previously known as the 'osteopathic lesion' (Still 1902) – are said to be:

- **S**ensitivity/tenderness (Gibbons & Tehan 2000)
- **T**issue texture changes
- **A**symmetry of bony landmarks
- **R**ange of motion abnormality (increased, decreased or a change in quality).

Other manual medicine professions use similar diagnostic criteria to diagnose manipulable dysfunction. For example, physiotherapists (physical therapists in the USA) place emphasis on the altered *quality* of joint motion or 'end-feel' (Corrigan & Maitland 1983, Jull et al 1988, 1994).

Jull and co-workers (1988, 1994) concluded that symptomatic cervical zygapophyseal joints have a number of pathognomonic findings, using manual diagnosis including 'abnormal end-feel, abnormal quality of resistance to motion, and reproduction of pain'.

Jull et al suggest that one reason for the often reported 'fair to poor' reliability of motion palpation in the neck region (DeBoer et al 1985, Mior et al 1985) is that repeated, consecutive palpatory procedures might alter joint play within the cervical spine, and therefore either induce a new biomechanical dysfunction or modify a dysfunction that was previously present. This underlines the need for minimal contact when palpating and as few repetitions of active or passive movements as possible.

The chiropractic profession used to emphasize static asymmetry, sometimes employing radiographic analysis to determine positional asymmetry (Leach 1994).

Palpatory acronyms

The acronyms STAR, TART and ART are commonly referred to in manual therapy literature to define 'somatic dysfunction', biomechanical dysfunction or 'chiropractic subluxation' (DeBoer et al 1985, Greenman 1989, Kappler 1997).

- ART stands for asymmetry, range of motion and tissue texture changes, with some authors suggesting that tenderness (T) should also be included in the diagnostic criteria.
- STAR is a similar acronym that incorporates the same ingredients, labeled in this version as sensitivity, tissue texture change, asymmetry and range of motion change, whereas TART = tenderness, asymmetry, range of motion change and tissue texture modification.

How valid are these components of dysfunction, and how accurately they can be assessed by palpation?

A study by Jull et al (1988) concluded that manual diagnosis, performed by *an experienced manual therapist*, was as accurate at identifying symptomatic cervical zygapophyseal joints as diagnostic nerve blocks, which is the criterion standard for this diagnosis.

Whilst results for determining the inter-examiner reliability in detection of cervical spine dysfunction are promising, there remains a continuing need for studies that investigate the reliability and validity of this diagnostic approach. From the current research literature, it would appear that the TART/ART descriptors are reasonable diagnostic criteria for spinal dysfunctions (Jull et al 1988).

It seems that the value of palpation is established when examinations are well executed, but the question remains, how well are these assessments commonly performed?

Tenderness (or sensitivity)

Tenderness is usually the end result of ART (asymmetry, restriction, texture/tone changes).

Since only *one* of these factors needs to be present for a diagnosis of dysfunction to be made (Jones 1997), dysfunction can be present *before* the advent of pain. This, then, is of greater application in preventive medicine, rather than just reactive work – which, of course, is where most of our time as therapists is spent.

Most studies of athletic/sporting injury rates only reflect the 'tenderness' or pain component of dysfunction, as subjects are generally only considered 'injured' if they miss a competitive match, miss a training session or report to a clinic with pain. In sports analyses it is generally only if someone misses a match that they are considered 'injured' for the purposes of data collection (Wallden & Walters 2005). Hence there are rafts of sports people and members of the general public who manifest 'dysfunction', and unless corrected it is just a matter of time before that dysfunction manifests with 'tenderness' or pain, so that they become one of the statistics. To be truly naturopathic we need to identify systems that can be used to prevent or minimize tissue texture changes, asymmetry and restriction, in order to avoid the end result, which is tissue damage and pain.

Tenderness on its own is seen to have some problems as a diagnostic tool (Jull et al 1994). For example, because of age or infirmity patients cannot always communicate, and what is communicated may be colored by emotion or confusion.

Pain thresholds differ from person to person, and in the same person, depending on, among other things, how worried the person is about the pain, and what meaning they ascribe to the pain (Jensen & Karoly 1991).

A stomach-ache after overeating will be less worrying than a stomach-ache that has no obvious cause, especially if someone you know has recently been diagnosed with abdominal cancer!

While one person may report a muscle or joint as being 'painful', another might report the very same joint as 'uncomfortable'. There are cultural as well physiological, ethnic and gender reasons for this (Hong et al 1996, Melzack & Katz 1999).

Some may find it surprising to learn that women, on average, have a far lower pain threshold than men. Wolfe and colleagues (1995) showed that although approximately 60% of women can tolerate 4 kg (9 lb) of pressure before reporting pain, approximately 90% of men can tolerate that amount of pressure without feeling what they would describe as pain. Less than 5% of women can tolerate 12 kg (27 lb) of pressure, while nearly 50% of men can do so.

Nevertheless, information regarding sensitivity can be valuable, particularly when used in combination with other diagnostic criteria, such as asymmetry, range of motion and tissue texture changes. When other findings are made, a pain report by the patient can positively complement the practitioner's diagnosis.

Tissue texture

Fryer et al (2004a) report that little direct evidence exists for the actual *nature* of abnormal paraspinal tissue texture detected by palpation, and note that palpation for tenderness is more reliable than palpation for tissue texture change.

Indirect evidence from animal studies and experimental muscle inflammation support the plausibility of protective paraspinal muscle contraction, which should be palpable.

Increased paraspinal electromyographic (EMG) activity observed in subjects with low back pain (LBP) appears to be a result of both voluntary and involuntary changes in motor control, modified by psychophysiological responses to perceived stress, rather than a simple protective reflex.

Fryer et al (2004b) have evaluated the relative pain threshold of areas of paraspinal texture change, as compared with adjacent tissues, where no texture changes were perceived:

The study demonstrated that medial, paraspinal sites, identified as having abnormal tissue texture and tenderness during palpation, were significantly more tender than sites immediately above, below, and on the opposite side to the abnormal region.

What texture change is being palpated?

It seems possible that most reports of increased paraspinal EMG activity in LBP patients may be explained as a combination of voluntary guarding behavior (Ahern et al 1990, Nouwen et al 1987) and a change in CNS strategy, producing exaggerated 'pain mode' muscle activity designed to limit excessive or unanticipated movement (Zedka et al 1999).

Emotional and psychological experience of chronic pain may further modify or reinforce this altered CNS strategy to produce stereotypical patterns of guarding activity in response to real or imagined stress (Flor et al 1985).

The relevance of abnormally increased muscle activity to paraspinal regions that are tender, and that feel abnormal to palpation, remains untested, but it is feasible – indeed probable – that increased muscle activity would be detectable with palpation, and possibly that the act of palpation itself might provoke further muscle guarding (Fryer et al 2004a).

Actual structural modifications may be present, as demonstrated by Hides et al (1994), who employed diagnostic ultrasound to study the multifidus lumbar muscles of individuals with first episode unilateral acute or subacute low back pain. They observed marked wasting on the symptomatic side, located at just one vertebral level. Similar observations have been made using magnetic resonance imaging (MRI) and computed tomography (CT) (Danneels et al 2000, Kader et al 2000).

There seems little doubt that such atrophy would be palpable, displaying altered texture compared with normal paraspinal tissues. And there is clearly asymmetry involved, and, as Fryer et al have shown, the tissues are indeed more tender than surrounding tissues – therefore the majority of the criteria for TART evaluation are clearly present.

What is palpable in the paraspinal tissues of people with low back pain?

A variety of studies offer information and most suggest that there are changes that discriminating palpation would be able to identify.

- Decreased paraspinal muscle activity and strength associated with low back pain is well established, and, as observed in the ultrasound, MRI and CT studies reported above, there is evidence of changes in muscle fiber composition and localized selective multifidus atrophy – which may well be palpable as being 'different from more normal tissue' (Mannion et al 2001, Mooney et al 1997).

- There appears to be a complex relationship between deep paraspinal muscle inhibition that occurs during dynamic activity, and involuntary guarding behavior that takes place during static activity, in relation to chronic low back pain (Kaser et al 2001). At least some of these changes should be palpable as differences in tone.

- The effect of spinal manipulation on paraspinal EMG activity is inconclusive but promising (Lehman et al 2001, Schiller 2001). Variations in EMG would translate as heightened or reduced tone that should be palpable as an asymmetrical difference (Fryer et al 2004c).

In 1993, Cassisi et al disagreed, stating that there was little direct evidence to support the existence, or nature, of paraspinal tissue texture change that was claimed to be detected with palpation. The concept of segmental reflex paraspinal muscle contraction had not at that time been supported, they said, at least in association with low back pain.

Ten years later the evidence has changed, and it safe to say that their supposition was incorrect.

Asymmetry and range of motion issues

It seems that tissue texture changes and tenderness can indeed be located by palpation, if they are present, and if the examiner has acquired the skills required to identify such characteristics.

Much of the effort in motion palpation is aimed at establishing asymmetry, and this may emerge as a result of a combination of indicators involving observation and palpation as well as assessment of the range and quality of motion of a joint, as it is moved both actively and passively.

For example, if a joint moves further in right rotation than left, or side-flexion one way rather than another, a degree of asymmetry will have been established. Subsequent palpation of the shortened or lengthened structures associated with such an imbalance might reveal altered tone and/or abnormal texture and/or tenderness. If this were so, then all of the elements of STAR or TART would have been identified.

The importance of asymmetry cannot be overemphasized – in the same way that a muscle imbalance, such as an upper crossed syndrome (see page 184) creates a level of inevitability of tissue damage, albeit microscopic, so does asymmetry.

With the cumulative load of asymmetry and the repetitive microtrauma this entails, the eventual result is macrotrauma. Commonly, the sufferer will make compensatory postural changes to accommodate the pain or dysfunction. This results in a pattern of migrating or 'roving' pain(s) around the body.

Frequently, by the time the patient seeks professional help they have compensated several times from the original 'dysfunction' until, eventually, their body is unable to compensate any more. This is technically termed a state of 'decompensation'. Like that famous analogy of 'peeling an onion', the skilled practitioner must now trace back through the patient's history (their biography) and through their biomechanics (their biology) to locate the root cause of their symptom profile. As Myss (1997) states, 'your biography becomes your biology'.

It is common to hear that a patient's asymmetries have come about as a result of adaptation to their leisure activities or their occupation, and that to work to correct these asymmetries may hamper their performance. This suggestion, however, has no grounding in physiology and more grounding in fear of a change in performance. Physiological principles dictate that relative symmetry is not only a requirement for functional biomechanics (see discussion of 'Laterality' in Chapter 9) but also for attractiveness and reproduction (Enquist & Arak 1994), something noted by Darwin (1882) in the 19th century.

Is quality of movement palpable?

The quality of any movement offers further information, both during the arc of motion and most importantly as the end of range is approached.

A spectrum of possibilities exist – for example, as an arm is moved passively from flexion to extension of the shoulder – ranging from a sense of the structures floating freely and unimpeded, with an end-feel that is gentle and 'soft', to feelings of there being boggy, restricted, hesitant movement, with an end-feel that is harsh, wooden or 'blocked'.

The interpretation of these sensations (and the descriptors you give them), perceived during palpation of active or passive movement, is clearly at least as important as being aware of the variables involved.

1. Does 'floating and free' mean poor muscle tone? neural deficit? – or simply an optimal degree of relaxation and balance?
2. Does the 'restricted, hesitant' movement indicate pathology? apprehension? – or simply an inability to adequately relax – or possibly poor technique on the part of the practitioner?
3. And what do the different end-feel sensations indicate? Is the end-feel:
   • normal but soft?
   • normal but firm?
   • normal but hard?
4. Or is there a pathological end-feel such as reduced elasticity – relating perhaps to scar tissue? Or is it elastic, but not soft – possibly due to increased tonus? Or is there an 'empty' end-feel because the movement has been stopped by the patient, perhaps to avoid pain or because of psychological reasons (Kaltenborn 1985, Mennell 1964)?
5. Do the differences (from perceived normal) suggest structural, neural, psychological, functional abnormalities – or a combination of these?

Repetitive practice, ideally on 'real' patients rather than fellow students, is probably the only way to achieve literacy in this subjective, interpretive skill.

Malalignment implications – including visceral

Schamberger (2002) has condensed much of the discussion of the variables associated with dysfunctional structures into a model that sees *malalignment* as the key issue, with all the different shortenings, weaknesses, restrictions, tissue texture changes and sensitivities being component parts of *malalignment syndromes*.

This is a compelling way of presenting the issues – with malalignment at the center of the picture, and all other features (texture changes, tenderness, altered ranges of motion) flowing inevitably from the deviant structures – the malalignment.

In fact, all these elements represent aspects of adaptive processes that are ongoing in any such area of dysfunction (see Chapter 2 for discussion of adaptation issues).

Tissue overuse, misuse, abuse

Placing malalignment at the center is no more logical than placing soft tissue changes ('texture') at the center. These features coincide, and one is impossible without the other. If, due to overuse or misuse (or disuse), specific muscle groups shorten or lengthen over time they will reciprocally influence their antagonists, raising or reducing tone in those, and there will be an inevitable and automatic change in symmetry – leading to malalignment (Janda 1996).

Sahrmann (2002) describes the malalignment concept of Schamberger using standard biomechanical descriptors. She explains the importance of maintaining the optimal instantaneous axis of rotation of any given joint. If this is not achieved (commonly due to muscle imbalance; Gleeson et al 1998), then the passive subsystem of joint stability becomes cumulatively stressed. The end result is that the cumulative microstress evolves into macro-strain. This natural history of joint dysfunction emphasizes the concept that the joint must remain on its optimal path of rotation at all times during posture and acture – to use Myer's (1997) terminology – or during static and dynamic postures.

Did the chicken cause the egg or vice versa?

Or did these changes emerge out of process of functional imbalance (inappropriate use of the part or the self), involving microtrauma perhaps, that resulted in structural modifications?

Since 85% of patients attending for orthopedic consultation describe having no specific onset of symptoms (Vleeming 2003), experience suggests that these emerge from a process of functional imbalance that, perpetuated over time, emerges as symptoms as adaptation fails. For example, the upper crossed syndrome (see page 183 for description and Fig. 6.33) is also:

- a 'red light posture' (Hanna 1988)
- a flexor response/startle response, and a
- fetal posture (Kolár 1999).

Problems involving cumulative systemic stressors include musculoskeletal pain, temporomandibular joint dysfunction, breathing pattern disorders, dysmenorrhea, irritable bowel syndrome, depression, fibromyalgia and many more, pointing to a naturopathic model of treatment and rehabilitation as offering effective long-term strategies.

Naturopathic assessment calls for consideration of process

From the perspective of evaluation, when trying to make sense of what can be assessed or palpated, it is important for the naturopathically inclined manual practitioner to hold onto a view that it is not only *the features* (what's short? what's weak? etc.) but also *the process* that needs to be evaluated and understood, if the patient is to be helped towards recovery and prevention.

The nuts and bolts – the state of the muscles, joints and other structures – are merely the clues that illuminate the process.

Whether the palpating hands, or observation, deduce changes in tissue texture, increased sensitivity, asymmetry (malalignment) or altered range of motion is less relevant than an understanding, not only of the 'what and where?' but also the 'why?'

More examples of palpation accuracy issues

Most practitioners and therapists do not have easy access to equipment to evaluate tissue change by means of MRI, CT scans or ultrasound, and need to rely on palpation assessments. Palpation may have issues with accuracy, and to a lesser extent with precision, but it *is* real-world. The availability of MRI scanners, real-time ultrasound and Cybex dynamometers to the average clinician, and/or average patient's temporal/financial budget, is very limited.

Palpation is a living, real-time, dynamic process that holds its own unique value. Other more 'high-tech' methods of assessment bring with them their own flaws; as Gracovetsky (2003) delights in pointing out, x-ray and other imaging techniques cannot, for example, distinguish between the spine of a living patient and a cadaver! His point is that they provide information about structure and only loose assumptions about consequent function based on that structure.

Is palpation adequate to the task, and if not what can be done to ensure that it improves?

Downey et al (2003) conducted a study to investigate whether physiotherapists, with postgraduate qualifications in manipulative physiotherapy, could reliably palpate and name the spinal level, in people presenting to clinics with low back pain, using central anteroposterior pressure as the means of assessment.

This is one element of the methodology used in assessment prior to mobilization, based on the Maitland approach, which claims that the palpation methods used are more accurate than others (Maitland et al 2001).

The criteria used to decide relative dysfunction, during anteroposterior pressure on the spinous process, were:

- abnormal end-feel
- abnormal quality of resistance to motion
- reproduction of pain, local or referred.

In this study, each therapist located the level that was considered to be most likely to be contributing to symptoms and then marked the skin overlying the spinous process of the comparable level with an ultraviolet pen, and these marks were transcribed on to transparencies for analysis.

Therapists demonstrated only fair agreement for palpating the location of a comparable spinal level (k = 0.37).

In addition, when asked to name the located level the overall agreement (k = 0.09) was no greater than due to chance alone, suggesting that the therapists were frequently palpating the wrong lumbar spinous processes.

Downey et al (2003) suggest that if therapists cannot agree on which level is the most likely source of the patient's symptoms from the manual assessment, then it follows that treatment decisions based on the palpation findings will also be unreliable between therapists.

It is worth observing that some practitioners do not use palpation in their assessment of patients with vertebral complaints, as they consider these methods unreliable (McKenzie & Taylor 1997). Instead, for example, the McKenzie approach focuses on the *behavior* and location of a patient's pain during repetition of physiological movements, such as lumbar flexion or extension, in order to identify what actions improve, and what actions worsen, symptoms. This information is used as a guide to prescription of exercise methods. (See Chapter 7 for more detail on the McKenzie approach.)

What emerges is that while inter-rater reliability is not particularly good in such settings the patient would not necessarily receive inappropriate or unhelpful treatment. Misnaming the spinal level is relatively unimportant unless the patient is being referred to another therapist, who might depend on the previously recorded spinal level as a starting point for treatment. It is more important to determine that the problem is 'right here', rather than stating that 'right here' is L2, L3 or L4.

This study further confirms that skilled palpation requires application and practice, since – although many were not – some of the therapists were indeed accurate in their judgment of spinal levels.

Since individual tests are frequently unreliable as a basis for a decision regarding manipulation, the use of a cluster of indicators clearly offers more reliable evidence than any single piece of evidence on which to base any clinical decision regarding high velocity thrust manipulation or other specific attention to the implicated segment.

The need for a wider evidence base

In addition to palpation evidence, outcome measures need to inform clinicians when making clinical decisions.

Finch (2006) has pointed out:

In an evidence informed practice model, the clinician bases treatment decisions on a blend of information gleaned from best research evidence, patient values, and clinical expertise, the latter encompassing experience and skills (Sackett et al 2001). In addition to this, it has been shown that patient and practitioner preference, and peer group advice also influence decision making (Gabbay & LeMay 2004).

Fundamental to evidence-informed practice is not only the existence of relevant research evidence but also the ability of practitioners to evaluate the literature in an informed and reasonable fashion. This reflects the notion that one of the early steps in developing an evidence-informed approach to practice, within a professional group, is the creation of a research-literate cadre of practitioners, research literacy being defined as understanding research language and its application to practice (Williams et al 2002).

Finch has proposed a model (Fig. 5.1) that he terms the 'evidence funnel'. This incorporates the 'best' evidence from numerous sources, which are ultimately processed to arrive at a clinical decision:

The structure of the Evidence Funnel is such that the responsibility of the health care professional for decision making based on reasonable assessment of the available best evidence, in addition to clinical expertise and patient values, is emphasized. In this model, as in the clinical reality of the practitioner, evidence gained through different research designs and from many different sources flows to the clinician. The contents of the Funnel reflect these different sources, and although not intended to be an exhaustive listing, does [intend to] reflect the diversity of information sources relevant

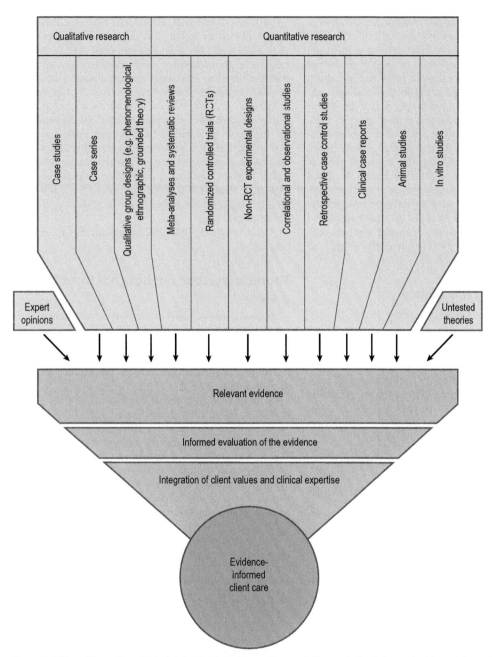

Figure 5.1 The evidence funnel: highlighting the importance of research literacy in the delivery of evidence-informed complementary health care. Reproduced with permission from Finch P. *Journal of Bodywork and Movement Therapies* 2006;11(1):78–81

to patient care. In the Funnel, information from various sources enters the Relevant Evidence section, after which it is only through assessment by the research literate practitioner that the best, most impactful evidence will influence therapeutic decisions.

Other variables

Although it is recognized that palpation is a component of 'the process' of clinical decision-making, the fact is that the physiology of the body is constantly changing under our hands as we observe a dynamic interplay between the practitioner and the patient. Other variables include what the patient is thinking (potentially influenced positively or negatively by the therapist) and how the treatment 'feels' to the patient (pleasant/beneficial, or painful/detrimental, or even a 'good hurt'). Physiology may be affected by attention and intention. For example, if the patient is fully present, and the practitioner is fully present, the outcome is likely to be better than if one or both are thinking about their shopping list, or what they're having for dinner that night (Blackburn & Price 2006).

This highlights exactly why the naturopathic model is so important. It's not just about 'biomechanics' – it is about emotions, biochemistry, belief systems and hard evidence, all interacting concurrently, integrated with the biomechanical picture.

Thoracic palpation accuracy

How accurate are motion palpation assessments applied to the thoracic spine?

In a Danish research study (Christensen et al 2002), two chiropractors examined 29 patients and 27 non-patients in the inter-observer part of the study, while one chiropractor examined 14 patients and 15 non-patients in the intra-observer aspect.

Three types of palpation were performed:

- Seated motion palpation for biomechanical dysfunction
- Prone motion palpation for biomechanical dysfunction
- Paraspinal palpation for tenderness.

Each dimension was rated as 'absent' or 'present' for each segment.

The results showed good hour-to-hour and day-to-day intra-observer reliability with all three palpation procedures, and good inter-observer reliability for paraspinal tenderness.

However, the inter-observer reliability was unacceptably poor when results of prone motion palpation were compared with seated motion palpation.

The authors of the research noted that, with respect to sitting and prone motion palpation, the results suggest that an experienced observer can achieve acceptably low variability (i.e. good results), hour-to-hour and day-to-day, after a training session, as long as exact anatomic localization is less important than the presence or absence of a positive finding in a certain region (i.e. the thoracic spine).

They also report that, after some training, it is possible to obtain acceptably low intra- and inter-observer variability with regard to diagnosing spinal tenderness in the thoracic spine, and to achieve results comparable to those reported from palpation of other spinal regions (Hestboek & Leboeuf 2000, Levoska et al 1993).

This suggests that results of individual assessments of this type, performed in different positions (e.g. prone and seated), should be viewed with caution, but that with adequate training, findings can be reliable.

This further confirms the need for individual findings (e.g. tenderness) to be supported by additional results (e.g. reduced range of motion) during clinical decision-making.

It also confirms that palpation can be accurately employed!

Thoracic percussion: how *not* to conduct a study

Ghoukassian et al (2001) note that while motion palpation is an assessment tool utilized by the majority of manual medicine practitioners, when attempting to diagnose or treat spinal dysfunction, the clinical usefulness of this method of palpation remains questionable.

As this poses a problem for manual therapists as they seek other, more reliable assessment methods, a study (Ghoukassian et al 2001) was designed to examine the inter-examiner reliability of Johnston & Friedman's (Johnston & Friedman 1994, Johnston et al 1983) thoracic spinal percussion scan.

Following two training sessions, 10 examiners performed the percussion scan once on each of 19 asymptomatic male subjects, resulting in 190 assessments in total.

The examination involved the thumb and third finger of the examiner straddling the vertebral spinous processes to percuss the paravertebral muscles that overlie the transverse processes bilaterally (Johnston et al 1983). The examiner then proceeded down the vertebral column of the seated patient, with one percussion strike per segment, comparing the tissue tension of one segment with that of adjacent segments, above and below.

Once the level of most significantly altered tissue tension had been identified, positional and tissue characteristics were palpated, looking for tenderness, asymmetry, motion restriction, changes in texture, etc., in order to gather further clues as to the nature of the dysfunction.

Analysis yielded 'slight' inter-examiner reliability (k = 0.07) significant at the 0.01 level, suggesting that the reliability of this examination procedure used in isolation remains questionable.

Accurate evaluation of the findings of this study is seen to be questionable for various reasons, and – irrespective of the palpation method(s) being used – offers useful guidelines of how *not* to conduct a study:

- This study employed asymptomatic subjects rather than individuals with discomfort, pain or restrictions in the region being evaluated. This common study fault suggests a reluctance (or difficulty) in recruiting symptomatic subjects, and almost guarantees that palpation will not yield much of clinical value, as there may be little in the way of variation between different muscles to identify.
- There were only two training sessions for those conducting the examination, which – based on reports of difficulties during the study – suggests that training failed to meet Bogduk's (1998) logical suggestion that diagnostic procedures employed in musculoskeletal medicine should be standardized, and that examiners should be well trained in the procedures (percussion, or any other palpation method).
- Problems arose during application of the percussion, partly due to the variable height of examiners in relation to the seated subjects being assessed, something that could have been solved by use of adjustable height plinths on which the patient could be seated.

The study therefore failed to demonstrate the value or lack of value of this percussion palpation method, since – for all the reasons outlined above – there was little chance of the result being other than the one that emerged.

Simons' perspective

In a quite different setting, trigger point researcher David Simons MD has described a similar situation:

Reports of the poor inter-observer reliability of palpation methods serves as a warning flag that some examiners use different criteria than others, or have a significant difference in skill level. If no study can demonstrate satisfactory inter-observer reliability by palpation, then that diagnostic method is seriously suspect.

In the case of myofascial trigger points (MTrPs), five well-designed studies used raters that were either experienced or trained – but not both. All five studies reported reliability ratings that were unsatisfactory. One other reliability study by four physicians who were recognized for their expertise in treating MTrPs started out making the same mistake, and assumed that because of their individual expertise, they would have high inter-observer reliability. They did poorly on their first study so, before repeating it, they spent 3 hours comparing their examination techniques on a human subject, and came to agreement regarding details as to what constituted each specific diagnostic finding. This time the study resulted in good to excellent agreement (Gerwin et al 1997). My conclusion is that reliable diagnosis of MTrPs takes more training and skill than most teachers or investigators realize.

Simons highlights the difficulty faced by clinicians employing widely divergent methods and vocabularies (osteopathy, chiropractic, manual medicine, physiatry, physiotherapy, etc.). If inter-examiner reliability of palpation and observation is to be improved and enhanced, then we need to agree on what we are looking for, and what we should call it when we find it.

Moderately successful palpation study of lumbar spine

As we have seen, many studies that have attempted to demonstrate the accuracy of spinal evaluation by physical means have been only moderately accurate in terms of reproducibility – commonly it would seem for reasons other than any fault with the method being used.

One of the more successful such studies was that of Keating et al (1990) who investigated the lumbar spine by studying individual segments from T11/12 to L5/S1.

They used a multidimensional approach that analyzed the reliability of four tests:

1. Palpation for pain over bony structures of each joint
2. Pain on palpation of paravertebral tissues
3. Temperature readings with a dermathermograph
4. Visual inspection for gross asymmetry, hyperemia, edema and skin lesions.

In this study, three chiropractors examined 25 asymptomatic subjects and 21 low back pain patients.

Across the segments, the intraclass correlation coefficient ranged from 0.34 to 0.62 with a mean of 0.46, demonstrating marginal to good reproducibility.

This study demonstrates that with the use of a variety of assessments – some subjective, others objective – involving reported pain, heat variations and observation, it was possible to achieve reasonable levels of accuracy and agreement. This study also emphasizes the value of patient feedback (pain levels) as part of the assessment process.

The need for such multidimensional assessment methods has been underlined by Medicare requirements as explained below.

Medicare requirements

Gemmell & Miller (2005) observe that the need for a multidimensional approach by chiropractors during physical examination that is evaluating for spinal dysfunction has been demonstrated by the requirements of the Health Care Financing Administration (Medicare Carriers Manual).

Initially, between 1974 and 1999, Medicare required x-rays to demonstrate subluxation of the spine. From 2000 Medicare allowed physical examination findings for the demonstration of subluxation, in place of x-rays.

The requirements they laid down state that: 'To demonstrate a subluxation based on physical examination, two of the four criteria listed below are required.'

These include:

- asymmetry/misalignment
- range of motion abnormality
- restricted motion
- excessive motion
- muscle and osseous tenderness
- muscle spasm
- osseous malposition
- trophic changes and edema,

identified by means of visual inspection including postural analysis, motion testing, joint play analysis, manual muscle testing, etc.

All of the criteria listed above depend, to some extent, on palpation and observation by the examiner. Based on the research we have reviewed so far in this chapter, the variability of findings among practitioners is sometimes high. If diagnostic criteria are based on methods with poor reliability, it is difficult to establish a standard of care under Medicare guidelines, and the public may be asked to bear the cost of unnecessary treatment. In a very real way, the variability of findings is a potentially costly affair. Naturopathic physical medicine needs to ensure that its students are trained to be aware of the need for a high standard of palpation, observation and assessment.

The way forward – focus on kinetics and kinematics

Marcotte et al have shown one way forward in achieving standardized assessment protocols. The focus of palpation assessment in the first study on which they reported was rotational dysfunction in the cervical spine.

Reporting in 2002 they noted that:

A review of the chiropractic literature demonstrates the difficulty in standardizing the test of motion palpation; thus it often produces poor to fair reliability. Our study attempts to highlight the advantageous effect of supervised training and standardization of the test.

It was hoped that standardization would avoid situations where, for example, a fixation at C5, identified by an experienced examiner, using standardized methodology, would subsequently be reported by a non-standardized examiner as being at the level of C2, or by another as being at C7.

The inexperienced/non-standardized examiners would not agree with the experienced examiner, nor would they agree between themselves.

To achieve standardization of motion palpation, two technical variables are involved:

1. There is a need for standardization of the force of pressure employed during the test – the kinetics
2. There is seen to be an essential need to standardize the spatial orientation – the kinematics.

The researchers noted that palpation involving movement should ideally be parallel to the plane of pure movement, as accepted by the international system of coordinates, i.e. the horizontal (transverse), frontal (coronal) and sagittal planes.

The researchers ensured that, before the study was carried out, the examiners undertook sessions of practical and theoretical technical training, and that a total of 12 hours of supervised training were completed. This meant that, by the start of the study, the examiners were able to reproduce accurately the kinematics of motion palpation in cervical rotation as described in the experimental protocol.

The results of palpation in the study were excellent, confirming the value of training.

Marcotte et al (2002) make another important point (noted earlier in the percussion discussion) when they suggest that there is little value in attempting to judge the usefulness of palpation skills when testing subjects/patients who are unlikely to have dysfunctional sites worth locating: 'Only patients with a history of mechanical disorders of the area tested should be selected.'

They continue:

In the future all parameters (position of the patient and the examiner, point of contact, forces, pressure of palpation, etc.) must also become the subject of standardization. Moreover, the examined subject-patient must present a strong probability of intervertebral dysfunction (fixation) to be detected at the time of palpation.

In subsequent research, Marcotte et al (2005) demonstrated that, providing the kinematic standards are maintained accurately, the degree of pressure used during assessment of spinal dysfunction is relatively unimportant.

They report:

*The pressure applied during palpation as a parameter of the test of motion palpation does not seem to represent a variable relating to interexaminer reliability. Strong reliability of the test was obtained by using subjects with a history of mechanical neck disorders, and by standardizing the kinematics of the test. The pressure applied during motion palpation for cervical spine rotation is light to moderate but always comfortable for the patient. Applied pressures can vary tenfold (4–41 N/cm^2) and remain reliable **provided the kinematics of the test are standardized**.*

The topic of the degree of pressure used in palpation will be covered in Chapter 6, on skill acquisition.

Leg-length discrepancy measurement by palpation

In order to accurately assess leg-length discrepancy (see Chapter 2 for some of the adaptive implications of such imbalances) a variety of validated methods have been described and assessed for accuracy.

One relatively inaccurate method involved palpation of the iliac crests of the standing subject, in order to estimate the extent of the asymmetry (Clarke 1972). In one study only 32% of therapists who used this technique alone were within 5 mm of the radiographic measurement of leg-length discrepancy (LLD).

A more accurate method also used the levels of the iliac crests (Jonson & Gross 1997), as well as wooden blocks (5 mm thickness) to correct for LLD. This achieved intra- and inter-rater reliability of 0.87 and 0.70, respectively.

In 2001, Hanada et al attempted to improve on the sensitivity of this approach by using an 'iliac crest palpation and book correction' (ICPBC) method.

- The healthy subjects of the study all had leg-length discrepancies induced by standing on various thicknesses (small: 7–17 mm; medium: 18–35 mm; large: 36–53 mm) of paper (pages of a book), masked from the examiner.
- LLD was screened for by palpation of the iliac crests in the standing position
- If the extent of the LLD appeared to be clinically significant, the extent of the difference was measured by correcting the LLD with the pages of a book.
- The book would be opened to the number of pages required and then placed under the foot of the shorter leg until the iliac crests were judged to be level based on palpation.
- In a study of this method the intra- and inter-rater reliabilities were 0.98 and 0.91, respectively.

The researchers suggest that:

The ICPBC technique for measuring LLD is highly reliable and moderately valid. When there is no history of pelvic deformity and the iliac crests can be readily palpated, we recommend using iliac crest palpation to detect LLD, and the book correction to quantify it.

A contrary view

In virtually complete disagreement with Hanada et al were the results of a study by Gibbons et al (2002) who evaluated attempts to assess LLD using heel inserts to create an inequality.

In that study, 27 subjects (mean age = 23) were examined by eight examiners. Assessment of leg length was performed by palpation of iliac crest heights, posterior superior iliac spines, greater trochanters and gluteal folds with the subjects standing. Examiners indicated whether leg length was equal, or if there was a longer leg on the left or right. Subjects were assessed with no heel insert and with heel inserts of 0.5 cm and 1 cm in their shoes. Each insert intervention was examined twice on each subject by each examiner.

The results of this study indicate that examiners were unable to reliably detect simulated leg-length discrepancies of 1 cm or less by standing assessment.

Reasons for different results

It is difficult to reconcile the excellent results of one study with the poor results of the other apart from referral to the insistence of Marcotte et al, and Simons, on the need for training and precise protocols.

One clear difference between the two studies is the magnitude of the simulated leg-length differences. In the study with higher reliability, the simulated leg-length differences were 0.7–5.3 cm. In the study with the poor reliability, the simulated leg-length differences were 0.5–1.0 cm. Future research can explore the threshold for inter-examiner reliability. For example, we might find that at leg-length inequality greater than 1.5 cm there is greater than 0.90 reliability, but below 1.25 cm reliability is less than chance. This might have significant implications for clinical practice, as leg-length inequality is a common cause of pelvic, hip and lumbar pain and dysfunction, and there is disagreement about how to find it and what to do about it once it is discovered.

Aside from the differences already highlighted, this scenario provides good rationale for the use of multiple assessment methodologies in order to provide a comprehensive and accurate picture. The body reflexively makes adjustments to maintain the eyes, ears and jaw on the optic, otic and occlusal planes (Chek 1994), shifting the pelvis in the frontal plane to adjust for simulated leg-length discrepancy or uneven ground. This dampening mechanism provides further explanation as to why Gibbon's study was apparently unfruitful. If Gibbon's team had assessed for both iliac crest heights *and* shifts in the frontal plane, they may have produced a different result.

Are there indicators that can suggest successful palpation outcomes?

Is the focus on inter-examiner reliability the best way to evaluate the usefulness or otherwise of palpation and assessment prior to treatment?

Gemmell & Miller (2005) note that, in recent years, there has been a trend away from inter-examiner reliability studies towards a focus on outcome-based investigations (Borge et al 2001, Flynn et al 2002).

For example, Flynn et al (2002) were able to identify patients with low back pain that was more likely than not to respond to manipulation. They found that the presence of four of five predictor variables suggested a 95% likelihood of success with use of manipulation.

The five variables suggesting a likely *positive* outcome were:

1. Duration of symptoms less than 16 days
2. Fear-Avoidance Beliefs Questionnaire (FABQ) with subscale score less than 19
3. At least one hip with more than 35° of internal rotation
4. Hypomobility on lumbar spinous springing
5. No symptoms below the knee.

It is obvious that only two of these five criteria depend on examination findings, and only one of those on palpation. Although these variables may be useful in predicting the efficacy of manipulation, they do not assist the practitioner in answering the questions 'Where is the problem?' and 'What is the state of these tissues?'

These questions still depend on skilled palpation – among other assessment methods (scan etc.) – for their answers.

Are there indicators that can suggest unsuccessful outcomes?

In contrast, Fritz et al (2004) have identified six variables that predict *non-response* (negative outcome) to manipulation in treatment of patients with low back pain.

These are:

1. Longer than 3 weeks' duration of symptoms
2. Symptoms in the buttock or leg
3. No hypomobility on spinous process springing
4. Reduced hip rotation range
5. Reduced discrepancy in left-to-right hip medial rotation
6. A *negative* Gaenslen sign (pain provocation test with the patient supine, one hip taken into full flexion and the other into hyperextension (leg over edge of table) in order to apply torsion to the pelvis). The test is *positive* if pain is reported in the sacroiliac joint (and/or thigh) on the side of the hyperextended leg.

Using such protocols would seem to offer useful information as to who is more likely and who is less likely to respond to particular forms of treatment. However, as in the case of the positive predictors above, they do not assist the practitioner in making a diagnosis or localizing the problem.

Employment of a broader prediction model such as that of Zink & Lawson (1979), as described in Chapter 2, offers further guidance as to the degree of adaptation exhaustion currently being demonstrated by the patient.

Such predictive methods should not result in the abandonment of palpation and assessment methods, but should be seen to complement such methods.

And – based on the evidence at hand – these should be applied with confidence once skills have been refined and standardized.

The opinions of experts

As mentioned earlier, a team of experts were assembled in 2002 to evaluate the problems highlighted by studies that showed poor palpation outcomes (Bullock-Saxton et al 2002).

A selection of pertinent extracts from their opinions is given below.

Dr Joanne Bullock-Saxton PhD, MAppPhty St (Manips), BPhty (Hons)

When reviewing the literature in this area, it is very important to keep in mind the quality of the research question asked, whether the protocol was sufficiently well designed to answer this question and whether the conclusions drawn by the authors are confined to the limits of the study. Much research has been published that throws a negative light on clinical practice because of poor inception or design. This has resulted in ramifications that go far beyond clinical practice to stakeholders in the health care system whose agenda may be to prove or disprove the efficacy of practice on the basis of any literature (regardless of its quality).

Researchers need to be careful that their design is not doomed to failure before starting due to the potential of incorporating other confounding variables that, if not revealed, will produce results that reflect poorly on the profession as a whole. It takes time to develop manual palpation skills, and novices of palpation should not be included in a research design unless the protocol is specifically interested in a question about skill acquisition. I am not yet convinced that there is sufficient evidence in the current literature to condemn the use of some commonly taught palpation techniques.

Essential elements to develop clinical reasoning skills in students are as follows:

- Knowledge that is discipline-specific, well-understood, easy to recall and commonly applied
- Cognitive skills of analysis, synthesis and data evaluation practiced
- Context specific, i.e. that presenting conditions or events are associated with the development or maintenance of the presenting problem.

Conversely, experts in clinical practice tend to use a pattern recognition/inductive reasoning model that has superseded the hypothetical deductive approach. With the development of expertise, large meaningful patterns of information are interpreted quickly for problem solving. These individuals demonstrate a highly developed short- and long-term memory regarding the above three essential elements, as well as a deeper understanding of the problem that is inclusive of the patient's perspective. While this model of diagnosis is rapid, if employed too early there is a chance that the pattern recognition model may be responsible for the clinician's making assumptions without clarification, failing to collect sufficient information and demonstrating confirmation bias. The final outcome is that all presentations may be placed into a single diagnostic box.

Peter Gibbons MB, BS, DO, DM-SMed and Philip Tehan DipPhysio, DO, MMPAA

There are many components of the clinical examination leading to a final diagnosis. Poor inter-observer reliability of palpatory findings should not be considered as necessarily devaluing the use of palpation as a diagnostic tool. Different practitioners respond in different ways to different palpatory cues, formulating their own manipulative prescription based upon individual experience.

We believe that reliability of palpatory diagnosis could be improved by:

- standardization of palpatory assessment procedures
- utilization of multiple tests
- increased focus upon linking palpation with pain provocation.

Despite extensive research, involving numerous different palpation procedures, the reliability and validity of many of these procedures remain questionable. Poor research design, use of inappropriate statistical methods and unsubstantiated conclusions have prevented musculoskeletal medicine from drawing substantive or definitive conclusions concerning the reliability of palpation as a diagnostic procedure. One might argue that the jury is still out.

Research to date has focused largely on the reliability of palpation in diagnosis but has not adequately explored the relationship between palpatory skills and the delivery and monitoring of manipulative techniques. Even where diagnosis is not predicated upon the use of palpatory cues, palpation is still critical to the safe and effective application of 'hands-on techniques'.

The authors would contend that highly refined palpatory skills are essential for the development of the psychomotor skills necessary to perform manual therapy techniques. It has been our experience, in teaching high velocity, low amplitude (HVLA) thrust techniques for over 20 years, that the development of palpatory proficiency is necessary for both the initial development and the subsequent refinement of the psychomotor skills necessary for the effective delivery of HVLA thrust techniques.

Shannon Goossen AP, BA, LMT, CMTPT

Before the days of MRIs, CAT scans, diagnostic spinal injections, needle EMGs and sEMG, the skilled practitioner relied upon listening to a history, observation skills and the ability to perform an examination with all of their senses. From this, practitioners formed a provisional diagnosis to explain their patient's complaints and/or suffering. New diagnostic tests came to us in the 1980s with big hopes for the definitive answers to pain and suffering. This was followed in 1990 by Boden et al's (1990) landmark study which showed that a portion of the population happily walks about the planet, pain free, even after an MRI has demonstrated that they have a herniated disc in the lumbar spine. Yet would anyone actually question the validity of an MRI demonstrating an L5–S1 disc herniation in a patient suffering desperately from leg pain? Well, they might, if the leg pain is on the right and the MRI report is a herniation on the left. Should we therefore discount the value of MRIs? Obviously not; they are tremendously valuable when combined with a properly focused examination. The appropriately trained manual therapist, skilled in identifying myofascial pain syndromes, should, using palpation skills, be able to differentiate an active myofascial trigger point in the gluteus minimus from a pinched L5 or S1 nerve root, both of which refer pain in similar trajectories, with subtle but clear differences.

Palpation is no more subjective than the motor sensory examination carried out by a neurologist or determining the usefulness of an x-ray or MRI. To be meaningful in developing a treatment plan, these methods all require subjective information from the patient and then subjective interpretation on the part of the examiner. Such interpretation is clearly influenced by the level of experience and training of the particular practitioner. There are not many findings in medicine which are purely objective, where findings are consistently reproducible between different qualified observers, in which cooperation is not required on the part of the patient.

Diane Lee PT, BSR FCAMT

Confidence in these [palpation and assessment] techniques grows as experience is gained; I would not want to be without them in the clinic. Much research quoted pertains to joints with small amplitude of motion (vertebral zygapophyseal and sacroiliac joints) which poses a greater reliability challenge than the larger peripheral joints.

I believe that we have not been able to show inter- or intra-tester reliability when motion (either active or passive) of these [sacroiliac] joints is assessed because we have not paid attention to the dynamic and changing nature of the individual being tested. To investigate, determine and then compare findings such as articular range of motion implies that the tester 'knows' what the range of motion for that joint should be. In addition, we have assumed that the range of motion will be constant from moment to moment for that individual. Recent research (Richardson et al 2000) in the pelvic girdle has shown that the stiffness value, directly related to range of motion (Buyruk et al 1995) of the sacroiliac joint, is related to compression within the pelvis, and compression was increased by activation of transversus abdominis, multifidus, erector spinae, gluteus maximus and/or biceps femoris. Whenever these muscles were activated (in isolation or combination), the stiffness value (measured with oscillations and the echo Doppler) of the SIJ increased (and thus the range of motion decreased). Unless the specific muscle activation pattern is noted during whatever range of motion test (active or passive) is being evaluated for reliability, there is no way of knowing what amount of compression the SIJ is under (at that moment) and therefore what the available range of motion should be.

[There needs to be] a clinical correlation between the subjective examination and objective examination (Lee & Vleeming 1998) which includes tests for:

- form closure (structure and anatomic restraints to motion) – stability and ligamentous stress and motion tests
- force closure (myofascial activation and relaxation tests)
- motor control (sequencing or timing of muscle activation)
- influence of the emotional state on resting muscle tone.

Craig Liebenson DC and Karel Lewit MD

We still lack the ability to identify subgroups of low back pain patients who would respond to specific therapeutic interventions. From this we can only conclude that our science is in its infancy. The question about palpation's reliability should not be turned against palpation but should be turned towards asking how to develop reliable, responsive and valid instruments.

The difficulty of establishing motion palpation's reliability may, in fact, point to the conclusion that our ability to measure the parameters involved in motion palpation is insufficient. The Nobel prize-winning microbiologist Rene Dubos said, 'the measurable drives out the useful'. To abandon a tool because it is hard to measure does not make much sense when we are in a field where over 85% of our patients are labeled as having a 'non-specific disorder' (Bigos et al 1994, Erhard & Delitto 1994). If we were able to identify, specifically, what was wrong with most back pain patients with non-palpation tools and thereby determine the most appropriate treatment, then it would be foolish to hold onto techniques with questionable reliability and validity. However, in our field, we're just beginning to crawl. While we strive to establish proof as our goal for creating a 'best practice' scenario, we are a long way from being able to reasonably justify throwing away such a safe, low-cost, although admittedly difficult to measure technique as palpation of joint, muscle or soft tissue motion and stiffness.

The craft of palpation has the merit that it encourages the development of 'palpatory literacy' (Chaitow 1997) since one at least attempts to feel restricted mobility and end-feel. In fact, although palpation is too complex to measure with a gold standard instrument, like seeing with photography or hearing with tape recorders, this does not make palpation useless.

Since functional disturbances are so variable, our patient populations are likely very heterogeneous. Therefore, it should be expected that no single palpatory test will have high validity. Perhaps, instead of abandoning the palpation of our patients, we should perform a thorough physical examination using a battery of tests so that the heterogeneity of our patient population will not lead us to falsely conclude that there is nothing mechanically wrong.

Erhard & Delitto (1994) concluded that:

- a collection of palpation tests was more valid than any one test by itself
- classification by a combination of palpation findings and other physical examination tests has predictive validity for assigning patients into different meaningful conservative care treatment groups
- non-specific back pain patients represent a heterogeneous group.

Donald R. Murphy DC, DACAN

I think that students should be taught to palpate for both joint restriction and pain provocation when palpating joints (Defranca 2000), as this is the only method that has been shown to be reliable, and should be taught tissue texture changes during joint and myofascial palpation of other tissues. . . . It would be [most] effective to teach the art of palpation and to develop the sensitivity to detect differences in texture, movement and muscle activity, in a stepwise fashion, starting with simple tasks and gradually progressing to more difficult tasks. There is some recent evidence which suggests that starting with non-biological materials may be an effective starting point for students to be able to detect levels of stiffness in isolation from the other nuances of biological tissue (Nicholson et al 1997).

The purpose of the clinical examination is to answer what I call the Three Essential Questions of Diagnosis (Murphy 2000):

- Does this patient have a potentially serious or life-threatening condition?
- What tissue(s) is(are) the primary source(s) of the patient's symptoms?
- What has gone wrong with the patient as a whole that these symptoms would have developed and persisted?

We then set out to answer these questions with the process of examination. . . . The patient examination is a multilevel process that begins when the practitioner first lays eyes on the patient and continues through history taking, neurological and general physical examination, examination for pain provocation, and examination for key dysfunctional chains and localized dysfunction. In this process, there are a variety of individual clinical tests that are available to us, some of which have been demonstrated to be reliable and valid, some of which have been demonstrated to have relatively poor reliability and validity, and most of which have not yet been evaluated for reliability and validity. By being aware of the literature in the area of reliability and validity, we may then apply a 'levels of evidence' approach to the examination. That is, we can go through the examination process and arrive at a working diagnosis, the 'diagnostic hypothesis'. Those aspects of the hypothesis that are based on tests that are known to be reliable and valid will be given greater emphasis and the level of evidence for these will be high. Those aspects that are based on tests of questionable reliability and validity will be given less emphasis. From this we will come up with our greatest suspicion of what is the most likely diagnosis and will test our hypothesis with treatment.

David G. Simons MD

In my experience of teaching physical therapists, the most effective way to teach palpation of MTrPs is one-on-one training. Have the student first study (and learn) that muscle's attachments, structure and function, then understand what they are looking for in their examination and finally realize the pathophysiological basis for the MTrP's clinical characteristics. At that point, I have the student examine one of my muscles (the SCM for pincer palpation and the third finger extensor for flat palpation for starters). First, I check the muscle myself to make sure I know what is there and then see what they can find. If they are having trouble finding it, it is easy for me to see why based on what I see them doing and what their palpation of that muscle feels like, compared to what it felt like when I palpated myself. This process can be applied to most of the muscles in the body.

Another approach that is less demanding of teaching time is to have the students work in teams of three and have them take turns being paired examiners of the subject. Each examiner examines the muscle with the other examiner blinded and fills out a worksheet listing individual examination findings and what MTrPs were found. After the second examiner fills out a similar worksheet, they then compare results and, with the help of an instructor, see how they could have examined the muscle so they would have agreed as to their findings. The person who served as subject then similarly examines one of the previous examiners.

Take a thorough history and consider the circumstances associated with the onset [of symptoms].

- What muscles were likely overloaded or were held in a shortened position for a long time?
- Ask the patient precisely what movements or positions increase their pain or relieve it.
- Sleeping position problems can be very revealing as to which muscles are likely involved.
- Carefully make a drawing of the patient's pain pattern and use that as a guide for further testing.

Examine the suspected muscles for painfully restricted stretch range of motion. Look for skeletal and muscular perpetuating factors such as pronated feet, a short lower extremity, an asymmetrical pelvis, short upper arms, forward head posture, paradoxical breathing, gait or movement patterns that indicate muscle imbalances, mild to moderate muscle weakness (reflex inhibition from TrPs in the same or functionally related muscles), etc.

Now you are ready to start palpating the muscles for the MTrPs that are very likely the cause of the patient's pain. Finding what you expected to find at this point greatly bolsters your confidence in the validity of your palpation findings. Not finding it presents a serious diagnostic challenge.

In the next chapter the focus will be on palpation skill acquisition.

References

Ahern DK, Hannon DJ, Goreczny A 1990 Correlation of chronic low-back pain behaviour and muscle function examination of the flexion–relaxation response. Spine 15:92–95

Aprill C, Bogduk N 1992 High-intensity zone: a diagnostic sign of painful lumbar disc on magnetic resonance imaging. British Journal of Radiology 66:361–369

Beal M 1989 Louisa Burns Memorial Lecture: Perception through palpation. Journal of the American Osteopathic Association 89:1334–1352

Bigos S, Bowyer O, Braen G 1994 Acute low back problems in adults. Clinical practice guideline. US Department of Health and Human Services, Public Health Service, Agency for Health Care Policy and Research, Rockville, MD

Blackburn J, Price C 2006 Further implications of presence in manual therapy. Journal of Bodywork and Movement Therapies 11(1):68–77

Boden S, Davis D, Dina T 1990 Abnormal magnetic resonance scans of the lumbar spine in asymptomatic subjects. Journal of Bone and Joint Surgery 72A(3):403–408

Bogduk N 1998 An interview with Nikolai Bogduk. Musculoskeletal medicine, evidence based medicine and the meaning of life. Newsletter of the Australian Association of Musculoskeletal Medicine, p 1–4

Borge J, Leboeuf Y, Lothe J 2001 Prognostic values of physical examination findings in patients with chronic low back pain treated conservatively: a systematic review. Journal of Manipulative and Physiological Therapeutics 24:292–295

Bullock-Saxton J, Chaitow L, Gibbons P et al 2002 The palpation reliability debate: the experts respond. Journal of Bodywork and Movement Therapies 6(1):18–37

Buyruk HM, Snijders CJ, Vleeming A et al 1995 The measurements of sacroiliac joint stiffness with colour Doppler imaging: a study on healthy subjects. European Journal of Radiology 21:117–121

Cassisi JE, Robinson ME, O'Conner P, MacMillan M 1993 Trunk strength and lumbar paraspinal muscle activity during isometric exercise in chronic low-back pain patients and controls. Spine 18:245–251

Chaitow L 1997 Palpation skills. Churchill Livingstone, Edinburgh

Chaitow L 2001 Palpatory literacy – a time to reflect? Journal of Bodywork and Movement Therapies 5(4):223–226

Chek P 1994 Posture and craniofacial pain. In: Curl D (ed) A chiropractic approach to head pain. Lippincott Williams & Wilkins, Philadelphia

Christensen F, Laursen M, Gelineck J et al 2001 Interobserver and intraobserver agreement of radiograph interpretation with and without pedicle screw implants: the need for a detailed classification system in posterolateral spinal fusion. Spine 26(5):538–543; discussion 543–544

Christensen H, Vach W, Vach K et al 2002 Palpation of the upper thoracic spine: an observer reliability study. Journal of Manipulative Physiology and Therapeutics 25:285–292

Clarke G 1972 Unequal leg length: an accurate method of detection and some clinical results. Rheumatology and Physical Medicine 11:385–390

Comeaux Z, Eland D, Chila A et al 2001 Measurement challenges in physical diagnosis: refining inter-rater palpation, perception and communication. Journal of Bodywork and Movement Therapies 5(4):245–253

Corrigan B, Maitland GD 1983 Practical orthopaedic medicine. Butterworths, Cambridge, p 12–15

Danneels L, Vanderstraeten G, Cambier D et al 2000 CT imaging of trunk muscles in chronic low back pain patients and healthy controls. European Spine Journal 9:266–272

Darwin C 1882 The descent of man and selection in relation to sex, 2nd edn. John Murray, London

DeBoer KF, Harmon R, Tuttle CD, Wallace H 1985 Reliability study of detection of somatic dysfunctions in the cervical spine. Journal of Manipulative and Physiological Therapeutics 8(1):9–16

Defranca G 2000 Evaluation of joint dysfunction in the cervical spine. In: Murphy DR (ed) Conservative management of cervical spine syndromes. McGraw-Hill, New York, p 267–306

DiGiovanna EL, Schiowitz S 1997 An osteopathic approach to diagnosis and treatment, 2nd edn. Lippincott, Philadelphia, p 6–12

Downey B, Taylor N, Niere K 2003 Can manipulative physiotherapists agree on which lumbar level to treat based on palpation? Physiotherapy 89(2):74–81

Enquist M, Arak A 1994 Symmetry, beauty, and evolution. Nature 372:169–172

Erhard RE, Delitto A 1994 Relative effectiveness of an extension program and a combined program of manipulation and flexion and extension exercises in patients with acute low back syndrome. Physical Therapy 74:1093–1100

Finch P 2006 The evidence funnel: highlighting the importance of research literacy in the delivery of evidence informed complementary health care. Journal of Bodywork and Movement Therapies 11(1):78–81

Flor H, Turk DC, Birbaumer N 1985 Assessment of stress-related psychophysiological reactions in chronic low back pain patients. Journal of Consulting and Clinical Psychology 53:354–364

Flynn T, Fritz J, Whitman JA 2002 A clinical prediction rule for classifying patients with low back pain who demonstrate short-term improvement with spinal manipulation. Spine 27:2835–2843

Fritz J, Whitman J, Flynn T et al 2004 Factors related to the inability of individuals with low back pain to improve with a spinal manipulation. Physical Therapeutics 84:173–190

Fryer G, Morris T, Gibbons P 2004a Paraspinal muscles and intervertebral dysfunction: Part 1. Journal of Manipulative and Physiological Therapeutics 27:267–274

Fryer G, Morris T, Gibbons P 2004b The relation between thoracic spinal tissues and pressure sensitivity measured by a digital algometer. Journal of Osteopathic Medicine 7(2):64–69

Fryer G, Morris T, Gibbons P 2004c Paraspinal muscles and intervertebral dysfunction: Part 2. Journal of Manipulative and Physiological Therapeutics 27:348–357

Gabbay J, LeMay A 2004 Evidence based guidelines or collectively constructed mindlines? Ethnographic study of knowledge management in primary care. British Medical Journal 329:1013–1017

Gatterman MI 1995 Foundations of chiropractic: subluxation. Mosby, St Louis, p 176–189

Gemmell H, Miller P 2005 Interexaminer reliability of multidimensional examination regimens used for detecting spinal manipulable lesions: a systematic review. Clinical Chiropractic 8(4):199–204

Gerwin RD, Shannon S, Hong CZ et al 1997 Inter-rater reliability in myofascial trigger point examination. Pain 69(1–2):65–73

Ghoukassian M, Nicholls P, McLaughlin P 2001 Inter-examiner reliability of the Johnson and Friedman percussion scan of the thoracic spine. Journal of Osteopathic Medicine 4(1):15–20

Gibbons P, Tehan P 2000 Manipulation of the spine, thorax and pelvis: an osteopathic perspective. Churchill Livingstone, Edinburgh, p 5–6

Gibbons P, Dumper C, Gosling C 2002 Inter-examiner and intra-examiner agreement for assessing simulated leg length inequality using palpation and observation during a standing assessment. Journal of Osteopathic Medicine 5(2):53–58

Gleeson NP, Reilly T, Mercer TH et al 1998 Influence of acute endurance activity on leg neuromuscular and musculoskeletal performance. Medicine and Science in Sports and Exercise 30(4):596–608

Gracovetsky S 2003 The story of the spine. Royal Geographical Society, London, December 2003. Organizer: www.chekclinic.com

Greenman PE 1989 Principles of manual medicine. Williams & Wilkins, Baltimore, p 13–14

Greenman PE 1996 Principles of manual medicine, 2nd edn. William & Wilkins, Baltimore, p 1–30

Grieve GP 1981 Common vertebral joint problems. Churchill Livingstone, Edinburgh

Hanada E, Kirby R, Lee M 2001 Measuring leg-length discrepancy by the 'iliac crest palpation and book correction' method: reliability and validity. Archives of Physical Medicine and Rehabilitation 82:938–942

Hanna T 1988 Somatics. Addison-Wesley, New York

Hartman L 1997 Handbook of osteopathic techniques, 3rd edn. Chapman & Hall, London

Hestboek L, Leboeuf Y 2000 Are chiropractic tests for the lumbo-pelvic spine reliable and valid? A systematic critical literature review. Journal of Manipulative and Physiological Therapeutics 23(4):258–275

Hides J, Stokes M, Saide M et al 1994 Evidence of lumbar multifidus muscle wasting ipsilateral to symptoms in patients with acute/subacute low back pain. Spine 18:165–172

Hong C-Z, Chen Y-N, Twehouse D, Hong D 1996 Pressure threshold for referred pain by compression on trigger point and adjacent area. Journal of Musculoskeletal Pain 4(3):61–79

Janda V 1996 Evaluation of muscular imbalance. In: Liebenson C (ed) Rehabilitation of the spine. Williams & Wilkins, Baltimore

Jensen M, Karoly P 1991 Control beliefs, coping efforts and adjustments to chronic pain. Journal of Consulting and Clinical Psychology 59:431–438

Johnston W, Friedman H 1994 Functional methods. American Academy of Osteopathy, Indianapolis, IN

Johnston W, Russotto A, Hendra J et al 1983 Interexaminer study of palpation in detecting location of spinal segmental dysfunction. Journal of the American Osteopathic Association 82:839–845

Jones J 1997 Glossary of osteopathic terminology (Educational Council on Osteopathic Principle, 1995, Chairman: Jones). In: Ward RC (ed) Foundations for osteopathic medicine. Williams & Wilkins, Baltimore

Jonson S, Gross M 1997 Intraexaminer reliability, interexaminer reliability, and mean values for nine lower extremity skeletal measures in healthy naval midshipmen. Journal of Orthopaedic and Sports Physical Therapy 25:253–263

Jull G, Bogduk N, Marsland A 1988 The accuracy of manual diagnosis for zygapophysial joint pain syndromes. Medical Journal of Australia 148:233–236

Jull G, Treleaven J, Versace G 1994 Manual examination: is pain provocation a major cue for spinal dysfunction? Australian Journal of Physiotherapy 40(3):159–165

Kader D, Wardlaw D, Smith F 2000 Correlation between MRI changes in the lumbar multifidus muscles and leg pain. Clinical Radiology 55:145–149

Kaltenborn F 1985 Mobilization of the extremity joints. Olaf Norlis Bokhandel, Oslo

Kappler RE 1997 Palpatory skills: an introduction. In: Ward RC (ed) Foundations for osteopathic medicine. Williams & Wilkins, Baltimore, p 473–477

Kaser L, Mannion A, Rhyner A et al 2001 Active therapy for chronic low back pain. Part 2. Effects on paraspinal muscle cross-sectional area, fibre type size, and distribution. Spine 26:909–919

Keating J, Bergmann T, Jacobs G et al 1990 Interexaminer reliability of eight evaluative dimensions of lumbar segmental abnormality. Journal of Manipulative and Physiological Therapeutics 13:463–470

Kolár P 1999 The sensomotor nature of postural functions, its fundamental role in rehabilitation. Journal of Orthopedic Medicine 21(2):40–45

Kuchera M, Jones J, Kappler R, Goodridge J 1997 Musculoskeletal examination for somatic dysfunction. In: Ward RC (ed) Foundations for osteopathic medicine. William & Wilkins, Baltimore, p 486–500

Leach RA 1994 The chiropractic theories: principles and clinical applications, 3rd edn. William & Wilkins, Baltimore, p 23–39

Lee D, Vleeming A 1998 Impaired load transfer through the pelvic girdle – a new model of altered neutral zone function. 3rd Interdisciplinary World Congress on Low Back and Pelvic Pain, November 19–21, Vienna, Austria, p 76

Lehman G, Vernon H, McGill S 2001 Effects of a mechanical pain stimulus on erector spinae activity before and after a spinal manipulation in patients with back pain: a preliminary investigation. Journal of Manipulative and Physiological Therapeutics 4:402–406

Levoska S, Keina nen-Kiukaanniemi S, Bloigu R 1993 Repeatability of measurement of tenderness in the neck-shoulder region by dolorimeter and manual palpation. Clinical Journal of Pain 9:229–235

Love RM, Brodeur R 1987 Inter- and intra-examiner reliability of motion palpation for the thoracolumbar spine. Journal of Manipulative and Physiological Therapeutics 10:1–4

Maitland GP, Hengeveld E, Banks K, English K 2001 Maitland's vertebral manipulation, 6th edn. Butterworth-Heinemann, Oxford, p 157

Mannion A, Taimela S, Muntener M, Dvorak J 2001 Active therapy for chronic low back pain. Part 1. Effects on back muscle activation, fatigability, and strength. Spine 26:897–908

Marcotte J, Normand M, Black P 2002 The kinematics of motion palpation and its effect on the reliability for cervical spine rotation. Journal of Manipulative and Physiological Therapeutics 25(7):E7

Marcotte J, Normand M, Black P 2005 Measurement of the pressure applied during motion palpation and reliability for cervical spine rotation. Journal of Manipulative and Physiological Therapeutics 28:591–596

McKenzie A, Taylor N 1997 Can physiotherapists reliably locate lumbar spinal levels by palpation? Physiotherapy 83(5):235–239

Medicare carriers manual, Rev. 1565, Section 2251.2: coverage of chiropractic services. Centers for Medicare & Medicaid Services, Baltimore, MD

Meijne W, van Neerbos K, Aufdenkampe G et al 1999 Intra-examiner and inter-examiner reliability of the Gillet test. Journal of Manipulative and Physiological Therapeutics 22:4–9

Melzack R, Katz J 1999 Pain measurement in persons with pain. In: Wall P, Melzack R (eds) Textbook of pain, 4th edn. Churchill Livingstone, Edinburgh, p 409–420

Mennell J 1964 Joint pain. Churchill, Boston

Mior SA, King RS, McGregor M, Bernard M 1985 Intra- and interexaminer reliability of motion palpation in the cervical spine. Journal of the Canadian Chiropractic Association 29(4):195–198

Mooney V, Gulick J, Perlman M et al 1997 Relationships between myoelectric activity, strength, and MRI of lumbar extensor muscles in back pain patients and normal subjects. Journal of Spinal Disorders 10:348–356

Murphy DR 2000 History and examination. In: Murphy DR (ed) Conservative management of cervical spine syndromes. McGraw-Hill, New York, p 387–419

Myers T 1997 The 'anatomy trains'. Journal of Bodywork and Movement Therapies 1(2):91–101

Myss C 1997 Anatomy of the spirit: the seven stages of power and healing. Bantam, Toronto

Nicholson L, Adams R, Maher C 1997 The reliability of a discrimination measure for judgments of non-biological stiffness. Manual Therapy 2:150–156

Nouwen A, Van Akkerveeken PF, Versloot JM 1987 Patterns of muscular activity during movement in patients with chronic low back pain. Spine 12:777–782

Panzer DM 1992 The reliability of lumbar motion palpation. Journal of Manipulative and Physiological Therapeutics 15:518–524

Richardson CA, Snijders CJ, Hides J et al 2000 The relationship between the transversely oriented abdominal muscles, sacroiliac joint mechanics and low back pain. Proceedings of the 7th Scientific Conference of IFOMT, Perth, Australia, November 2000

Sackett D, Strauss S, Richardson W et al 2001 Evidence based medicine: how to practice and teach EBM. Churchill Livingstone, Toronto

Sahrmann SA 2002 Diagnosis and treatment of movement impairment syndromes. Mosby, St Louis

Schamberger W 2002 The malalignment syndrome. Churchill Livingstone, Edinburgh

Schiller L 2001 Effectiveness of spinal manipulative therapy in the treatment of mechanical thoracic spinal pain: a pilot randomized clinical trial. Journal of Manipulative and Physiological Therapeutics 24:394–401

Still A 1902 The philosophy and mechanical principles of osteopathy. Hudson-Kimberly, Kirksville, MO

Strender LE, Sjoblom A, Sundell K et al 1997 Inter-examiner reliability in physical examination of patients with low back pain. Spine 22:814–820

Van Dillen LR, Sahrmann SA, Norton BJ et al 1998 Reliability of physical examination items used for classification of patients with low back pain. Journal of Orthopedic and Sports Physical Therapy 78:979–988

Vleeming A 2003 Movement, stability and low back pain – the essential role of the pelvis. 1 day seminar, Birbeck College, London, UK. Organizer: www.physiouk.co.uk

Wallden M, Walters N 2005 Does lumbo-pelvic dysfunction predispose to hamstring strain in professional soccer players? Journal of Bodywork and Movement Therapies 9(2):99–108

Williams J, Mulkins A, Verhoef M et al 2002 Needs assessment: research literacy and capacity amongst complementary and alternative health care providers. Perspectives on Natural Health Products, Natural Health Products Directorate, Health Canada, p 14

Wolfe F, Ross K, Anderson J et al 1995 Aspects of fibromyalgia in the general population. Journal of Rheumatology 22:151–156

Zedka M, Prochazka A, Knight B et al 1999 Voluntary and reflex control of human back muscles during induced pain. Journal of Physiology 520:591–604

Zink G, Lawson W 1979 An osteopathic structural examination and functional interpretation of the soma. Osteopathic Annals 7(12):433–440

6

Leon Chaitow ND DO

With contributions from:
David Russ DC
David J. Shipley ND DC

Assessment/ Palpation Section: Skills

What this chapter is and is not

To apply appropriate naturopathic physical medicine effectively, clinical decision-making has to be based on coherent information, gathered by a variety of means, including palpation and physical/structural assessment.

It is, however, beyond the scope of a single chapter – and probably of a single book – to offer a comprehensive compilation of palpation and assessment protocols and skills. This chapter will therefore focus on palpatory skill enhancement, associated with the processes involved in extracting information during palpation and assessment – the means whereby data are derived non-verbally.

- There has been no attempt to describe all variations of assessment of the length, strength, flexibility and endurance of every major muscle
- Nor are there descriptions of assessment of the ideal/normal range of motion of each and every joint.
- There are, however, descriptions of how these palpation/assessments may optimally be performed, on selected muscles, joints and other tissues (e.g. skin), in order to augment currently employed methods, techniques and skills.
- It should be possible, once the application of particular palpation skills have been acquired for use in one area of the body, to extrapolate and utilize the same methods elsewhere in the body.
- To achieve this effectively, a series of exercises have been described that, it is suggested, should be practiced until information extraction, by these means, becomes easy and comfortable.

The tissues, areas and features that are covered include:

- skin palpation, evaluating hydrosis, elasticity, adherence to underlying tissues, thermal qualities, hyperalgesia (Lewit 1999a)
- scar tissue palpation (Lewit 1999a)
- subdermal palpation assessment (fascia, muscle) evaluating qualities of texture, congestion, inflammation, adhesion and fibrosis, as well as the presence of embryonic, latent or active myofascial trigger points, etc. (Fryer & Hodgeson 2005, Simons et al 1999)
- palpation of periosteal pain points (Lewit 1999a)
- evaluation of functional muscle firing sequences, length, strength, tone (Janda 1986, Janda & Schmid 1980)
- assessment of neural mobility in relation to its mechanical interface (Butler & Gifford 1989, Butler & Moseby 2003)
- hypermobility assessment (Keer & Grahame 2003, Nijs 2005)
- evaluation of joint play (Kaltenborn 1985)
- palpation of mobility, stability and functionality of joints, including form and force

closure assessments of the sacroiliac joints (DonTigny 1995, Lee 1999, Norris 1998)
- sacral assessment (Dalstra 1997)
- palpation of the spine and spinal articulations (Cholewicki & McGill 1996, McGill 1991)
- assessment of spinal segmental facilitation (Beal 1983)
- assessment of balance (Liebenson 1996a)
- craniofacial assessment (including temporomandibular joint) (Chek 1994, Pick 1999a, Rocobado 1985)
- visceral palpation and assessment (Barral 1989, 1996)
- orthopedic assessments/tests (Shipley 2000a).

The major methods that have been discussed and/or recommended as part of this assessment/investigation process will include the following:

- Observation: checking key points and aspects of alignment and balance, with patient static and active, standing, walking, sitting, reclining (Janda 1996, Lewit 1999a)
- Postural evaluation: observation of crossed syndrome patterns, layer syndrome, including functional tests such as scapulohumeral rhythm test, core stability (Liebenson 2005, Norris 1995)
- Breathing pattern evaluation (Chaitow et al 2002)
- Off body scanning (Barral 1996, Lewit 1999a)
- Light touch and deeper palpation (Kuchera & Kuchera 1994, Pick 1999a)
- Neuromuscular technique palpation (DeLany 1996)
- Assessment for tissue texture changes, asymmetry, range of motion changes and tenderness (TART) (McPartland & Goodridge 1997, Ward 1997)
- Mechanical interface assessments for nerves (e.g. upper limb tension tests) (Butler & Gifford 1991)
- Evaluation incorporating awareness of fascial continuities (Myers 1997) and of the possible implications of the presence of contractile smooth muscle cells in connective tissue
- Range of motion and functional assessments of joints, including joint play (Kaltenborn 1985)
- Visceral and cranial palpation methodology (Barral 1989).

Descriptions of the assessment and palpation methods in the different areas and tissues listed above and outlined below will attempt to incorporate the safest and most accurate methods.

Excavating for anatomic and physiological evidence

Naturopathy sees dysfunction and disease as being parts of a process, rather than as entities, as discussed in Chapter 1.

When we are palpating and assessing we are operating in present time. What is being revealed, however, relates to the accumulated effects of past mechanical, chemical and emotional adaptations – stresses, strains, micro- and macrotraumas, toxicities, deficiencies, fears, anxieties, somatizations and more – all overlaid on the unique, inborn idiosyncratic characteristics of the individual. The examiner's task is to identify first the present state of the body, and later the processes that gave rise to the present state.

What is being touched, tested, pressed, stretched and evaluated is as it is because of everything that has ever happened to it. Our task is to make sense of the evidence we can gather in order to build a picture.

The evidence that emerges regarding the relative elasticity of skin and fascia, the degree and nature of shortness, strength, stamina and firing sequences of muscles, the changes in range of motion of joints, the presence of periosteal pain points, mechanical interference with nerves and myofascial trigger points, or the status of the individual's posture, breathing and balance – all offer clues as to the current level of adaptation and compensation. These palpable and assessable changes point us to the processes that have taken and are taking place, as the body adapts to age and the stresses of life.

Just as an archaeologist patiently gathers shards and slivers and learns to interpret these fragments in order to construct a picture of what was, so must we put together a coherent representation of why symptoms are as they are and, potentially, what needs to be done to assist the individual towards recovery.

This involves gathering evidence and then interpreting it in the context of the process of which the individual is currently a part. How tight, loose, weak, bunched, flaccid, symmetrical, balanced, sensitive or painful the tissues are, can tell a potent story without words.

Interpretation of findings emerges from the sensations that we perceive with our hands. From the accumulated evidence, we identify the stressors to which the individual is adapting. Inappropriately focusing on symptoms such as restriction, sensitivity, loss of elasticity, reduced range of motion, rather than on trying to understand the larger contextual picture,

and from this framing strategies that will encourage self-regulation, is likely to retard recovery.

From the evidence gathered we make the therapeutic choices designed to reduce adaptive demands and enhance adaptive capacity, allowing self-regulation to operate more efficiently, while simultaneously preventing exacerbations and recurrences.

Accurate information gathering

The skill acquisition exercises are methods that even experienced practitioners can use to improve proficiency, competence and dexterity. Apart from using palpation in the sort of detective work described above, these skills are relevant to the safe, effective delivery of manual therapy.

A major feature of this is the accurate and consistent identification of resistance barriers, something essential to the successful delivery of treatment (see notes on barriers below).

Considering the evidence offered in Chapter 4, *accuracy of information gathering* is a foundational requirement, and this is the aim of this chapter. For students and those early in their careers, this is an opportunity to refine what has been learned. Wherever possible, recommendations will be given as to the particular texts, DVDs, etc. that could be consulted for a deeper study of particular protocols and regions.

Viola Frymann DO, one of the great teachers of subtle palpation skills, summarized what is needed:

Palpation cannot be learned by reading or listening; it can only be learned by palpation . . . The first step in the process of palpation is detection, the second step is amplification, and the third step must therefore be interpretation. The interpretation of the observations made by palpation is the key that makes the study of the structure and function of tissues meaningful. (Frymann 1963)

The skill acquisition process cannot, however, take place in a vacuum.

Kappler (1997) succinctly and accurately expressed what is required:

The art of palpation requires discipline, time, patience and practice. To be most effective and productive, palpatory findings must be correlated with a knowledge of functional anatomy, physiology and pathophysiology. It is much easier to identify frank pathological states, a tumor for example, than to describe signs, symptoms, and palpatory findings that lead to, or identify, pathological mechanisms . . . Palpation with fingers and hands provides sensory information that the brain interprets as: temperature, texture, surface humidity, elasticity, turgor, tissue tension, thickness, shape, irritability, motion. To accomplish this task, it is necessary to teach the fingers to feel, think, see, and know. One feels through the palpating fingers on the patient; one sees the structures under the palpating fingers through a visual image based on knowledge of anatomy; one thinks what is normal and abnormal, and one knows with confidence acquired with practice that what is felt is real and accurate.

Beware imposter symptoms

Grieve (1994) has described conditions that may 'masquerade' as others:

If we take patients off the street, we need ... to be awake to those conditions which may be other than musculoskeletal; this is not 'diagnosis', only an enlightened awareness of when manual or other physical therapy may be ... unsuitable and perhaps foolish. There is also the factor of perhaps delaying more appropriate treatment.

For example, you might become suspicious that a problem is caused by something other than a simple musculoskeletal dysfunction – and seek a definitive diagnosis – when:

- misleading symptoms are reported
- something does not seem quite right regarding the patient's story describing the pain or other symptoms
- your 'gut feeling', instinct, intuition, internal alarm system, alerts you (if this happens you should always err on the side of caution and be particularly diligent in assessment and testing, and possibly refer onward for another opinion)
- the patient reports patterns of activities that aggravate or ease the symptoms that seem unusual, and cause you to have doubts about the case being straightforward.

Symptoms may arise from sinister causes (e.g. tumors) that closely mimic musculoskeletal symptoms, and/or which may coexist alongside actual musculoskeletal dysfunction. When there is lack of progress in symptom reduction, or if there are unusual responses to treatment, this calls for a review of strategies.

Some important cautions with back pain

Cautionary signs are those that may be present, for example, alongside acute back pain, which suggest that factors other than musculoskeletal dysfunction are operating. In most people there are no obvious pathological features associated with their back pain, but:

- around 4% have compression fractures (probably with osteoporosis as a background to that)
- 1% have tumors as the cause of the problem
- between 1 and 3% of people with acute back pain have prolapsed discs (Deyo et al 1992).

Giles (2003) has demonstrated how a number of very different conditions can produce back pain in precisely the same place:

- Carcinoma of the pancreas
- Inflammatory arthropathy
- Abdominal aneurysm
- Leg-length inequality

and that pain distribution covering the same area may result from any of the following:

- Intervertebral disc protrusion
- Sacroiliac joint dysfunction
- A small aortic aneurysm
- Pain following discectomy
- Spondylolisthesis
- Cauda equina syndrome
- Tethered cord syndrome
- Lumbar neuroma
- Perineural fibrosis.

Red and yellow flags

The red and yellow flag lists, given below, are derived from the document *European Guidelines for the Management of Acute Non-specific Low Back Pain in Primary Care* (RCGP 1999).

Red flags suggest (but do not prove) the possibility of more serious pathology.

Suspicion or recognition of red flags emerges from the person's history and symptoms.

If any of the signs listed below are present, further investigation should be suggested before treatment starts, particularly to exclude infection, inflammatory disease or cancer (RCGP 1999).

- The acute back pain started when the person was less than 20 years or more than 55 years old.
- There is an associated recent history of violent trauma such as a motor vehicle accident or a fall.
- There seems to be a constant progressive, non-mechanical pain that is characterized by no relief being experienced with bed rest.

- There is thoracic pain accompanying the back pain.
- The patient reports a past history of malignancy.
- There is a history of prolonged use of corticosteroids.
- The patient has a history of drug abuse, taking of immunosuppressive medication, or a diagnosis of being HIV positive.
- The back pain is accompanied by systemic 'unwellness' and/or unexplained weight loss.
- There are widespread neurological symptoms. For example, there may have been changes in bladder control, or widespread or progressive limb weakness, or changes in gait.
- There is obvious structural deformity such as scoliosis.
- The back pain is accompanied by fever.

Note: It is probable that one form of physical medicine or another would be useful for back pain relating to all or any of these signs and symptoms, but this should not be offered until the real nature of the problem has been investigated.

Yellow flags suggest psychosocial factors that 'increase the risk of developing, or perpetuating chronic pain and long-term disability' (Van Tulder et al 2004). Examples include (Kendall et al 1997):

- inappropriate attitudes about back pain – such as the belief that back pain is actually harmful and potentially disabling, or that bed rest is all that is needed rather than performing specific beneficial exercises: one of the first and most important lessons people need to learn is that 'hurt does not necessarily mean harm'
- inappropriate pain behavior (e.g. reducing activity levels or 'fear-avoidance')
- compensation (the possibility of financial gain if back pain continues) and/or work-related issues (e.g. poor work satisfaction and the 'benefit' of time away from it)
- background emotional problems (e.g. depression, anxiety, high stress levels).

Principles of palpation (Chaitow 2003a, Frymann 1963, Kuchera & Kuchera 1994)

Intention

The intention within the practitioner's mind–body drives the pressure and the rate of movement of the hand, the texture of their skin, the way it feels to the patient and, ultimately, the healing effect. There needs to be a reflective process in the practitioner to ensure that the intention to touch another body is driven purely by service to that person in their need to be diagnosed and treated by a professional. It is important for the health of the practitioner, and patients, to acknowledge any feelings of attraction, revulsion, anger, or any complicating emotion, before any diagnostic or therapeutic touch is commenced.

Centering

Following on from the need to reflect on the inner state before commencing physical touch, a physical and emotional sense of being 'centered' is best developed along with palpation skills. This concept is best described as being strongly aware of the stability in the mind, emotions and physical posture as the procedures described are carried out – a non-distracted state of observation and sensitivity without the loss of self-consciousness. With this continuously present, fluctuations in the patient's state are felt more clearly as 'outside' events, and are not mixed together as in normal social interactions.

Active and passive hands

It is necessary to develop the ability to have one hand, or one part of the hand, being restful and 'listening' (i.e. passive) whilst the other hand, or part of the hand, is active. The first step of tactile evaluation (after verbal consent is given) is to be passive in general – a gently allowing of the hands to rest on the patient's body, and a centering of the practitioner's body–mind to allow the first meeting and dialogue to start. When the various activities of tactile evaluation proceed, it helps to return frequently to the passive 'palposcope' to assess how the tissue is reacting and responding to the palpation activities. This will increase the information/gathered, and help to guide towards finding the pressure and depth that are appropriate and comfortable for that task.

Notes on applied pressure

What degree of digital pressure should be used when palpating?

This varies with the tissues being evaluated:

- When skin is being palpated (see below), no more than touch ('feather light', 'skin-on-skin') may be needed.
- When assessing tissues below the surface, pressure is increased, and there are a number of ways of conceptualizing what is required at this stage.

Upledger & Vredevoogd (1983) speak of using no more than 5 g of pressure in cranial palpation.

Some clinicians advise discovering the degree of pressure required when pressing onto your own (closed) eyeball before discomfort starts, as a means of learning just how lightly to press. Others advise using the least necessary pressure to make contact with, and evaluate, the tissues in question. Early in the process of learning to palpate deep tissues, the amount of pressure needed to feel engaged with deep structures will be greater. When palpation skills are refined, the least necessary pressure is much less than a beginning student would consider possible.

The term 'pressure threshold' is used to describe the least amount of pressure required to produce a report of pain, and/or referred symptoms, when a trigger point is compressed, and this will vary depending on the depth of the trigger in different tissues, locations and body types (Hong et al 1996).

Finding a 'working level'

How much palpation pressure should be used?

- When working with or on the skin: surface level
- When palpating for trigger points: working level
- When testing for pain responses, and when treating trigger points: rejection level.

Pick (1999b) has usefully described identification of these levels of tissue that you should try to reach by application of pressure, when assessing and/or treating the patient.

Pick described the different levels of tissues to be accessed as:

- *Surface level*: This is the first contact, molding to the contours of the structure, involving no actual pressure. This is just touching, without any pressure at all, and is used to start treatment via the skin – as described below.
- *Working level*: 'The working level . . . is the level at which most manipulative procedures begin. Within this level the practitioner can feel pliable counter-resistance to the applied force. The contact feels non-invasive . . . and is usually well within the comfort zone of the subjects.'
- *Rejection levels*: Pick suggests that these levels are reached when tissue resistance is overcome and discomfort/pain is reported. Rejection will

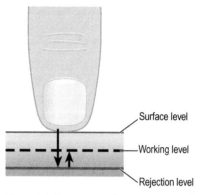

Figure 6.1 The concept of a 'working level'. Surface level involves touch without any pressure at all. Rejection level is where pressure meets a sense of the tissues 'pushing back' defensively. By reducing pressure slightly from the rejection level, the contact arrives at the working level, where perception of tissue change should be keenest, as well as there being an ability to distinguish normal from abnormal tissues (hypertonic, fibrotic, edematous, etc.). Reproduced with permission from Chaitow (2005)

occur at different degrees of pressure, in different areas and in different circumstances.

When you are at the rejection level there is a feeling of the tissues pushing back or resisting, and this has to be overcome to achieve a sustained compression. See Figure 6.1 and Box 6.1.

Sensitivity and filtration of information

The receptors involved in fine touch and pressure are of a rapidly adapting type.

If a constant degree of stimulation of these receptors is being sustained by the palpating hand, sensitivity tends to reduce as the firing rate of the receptors diminishes.

The alteration in sensitivity resulting from rapid adaptation to light touch is something that can be modified by practice. However, because mechanoreceptors serving joint and muscle are slow adapters, as are pain receptors, some experts such as Upledger & Vredevoogd (1983) suggest that use of these proprioceptive receptors should be incorporated into palpation. Their slow adaptation certainly adds weight to this suggestion.

Most of you have been taught to palpate or touch with your fingertips . . . we, however, would urge you to palpate with your whole hand, arm, stomach or whatever part of your body comes into contact with the patient's body. The idea is to 'meld' the palpating part of your body with the body you are examining. As this melding occurs, the palpating part of your body does what the patient's body is doing. It becomes synchronized. Once melding and synchronization have

Box 6.1 Exercise: Variable pressure

- Perform the application of digital pressure to each level (surface, rejection and working) using either a finger or thumb on a variety of tissue areas – for example, on the gluteal region, on the lightly muscled area of a limb, on the cranium, close to the spine, and on the anterior neck muscles.
- Try to locate areas to practice on that are hypertonic and/or flaccid, so that you learn to apply appropriate pressure to a range of tissue types and tones.
- If no palpation partner is available, practice this on yourself.
- Touch the tissues and then slowly apply pressure (sink into the tissues) until you feel a sense of 'rejection' – as though the tissues are pressing back against your digit, or are resisting further pressure.
- Then try to identify a point somewhere between these two levels – between superficial and deep.
- When you do so you will be touching tissues and the pressure you are applying will match the tone of those tissues.
- This will be very similar to what is being achieved during NMT evaluation, only in this instance the pressure is static, rather than on the move (see page 134).
- Practice this approach until you can alight rapidly at the 'working level' of different tissues in all parts of the body.

occurred, use your own proprioceptors to determine what the palpating part of your own body is doing. Your proprioceptors [e.g. mechanoreceptors] are those sensory receptors located in the muscles, tendons, and fascia that tell you where the parts of your body are without using your eyes.

Ford (1989) reminds us that we commonly 'project' our sense of touch, giving the example of writing with a pencil. We feel the texture of the page on which we are writing not at our skin surface, or in our fingertips, but at the end of the pencil, thus demonstrating how our proprioceptive awareness can be projected. Ford suggests you experiment by:

Changing the pressure with which you grasp the pencil – you'll quickly discover that you can't write. The pressure exerted to hold the pencil needs to be constant so you can extend your perception to [the] pencil tip and thereby control the complex task of writing. A good craftsperson knows this instinctively. The woodworker's sense of touch extends to the teeth of the saw, a machinist's to the end of a wrench, a surgeon's to the edge of a scalpel, an artist's to the tip of a brush.

At times during palpation too much information is being received and a degree of discrimination, or filtering, of information is required in order to make sense of it.

Kappler (1997) summarized this as follows.

A more significant component [of palpation skills] is to be able to focus on the mass of information being perceived, paying close attention to those qualities associated with tissue texture abnormality, and bypassing many of the other palpatory clues not relevant at the time. This is a process of developing mental filters . . . The brain cannot process everything at once. By concentrating only on the portion you want, it becomes easy and fast to detect areas of significant tissue texture abnormality.

Kappler et al (1971) found that when student examiners were compared with experienced practitioner examiners, although the students recorded more palpation findings, the practitioners recorded more significant findings. The experienced practitioners were filtering out the unimportant, and focusing on what was meaningful, rather than being 'overwhelmed with the mass of palpatory data'.

Is it possible to learn to apply precise pressure, poundage?

Physical therapy students have been taught to accurately produce specific degrees of pressure on request. They were tested applying posteroanterior pressure force to lumbar tissues, and after training, using bathroom scales to evaluate pressure levels, were able to demonstrate sustained accuracy for up to a month following the initial training (Keating et al 1993).

Meeting barriers

Elasticity is a feature of all tissues – even bone. When pressure is applied to tissues, a very first sense of resistance will be noted. Exercises that incorporate these first sensed barriers are included later in this chapter. See the notes on evaluation of shortness in the medial hamstrings, below.

If greater pressure is slowly applied, more resistance is felt, while further pressure would probably induce pain (see 'rejection level' in notes above).

This first sign of resistance is the point at which the mechanical properties of the tissue reach the end of their easy elasticity. This may be called different things – first endpoint, a first sign of resistance or the first barrier (Lewit 1999a). This can easily be missed if the searching digit moves too rapidly or too heavily.

It is possible to identify this first barrier in all soft tissues, including skin, subdermal tissue, fascia,

Box 6.2 Palpation pressure – and a practical psoas exercise

David Russ DC

Introduction

Examiners should always strive to use the least amount of pressure necessary to palpate a structure of interest. Using light pressure conserves energy, allows for more precise palpation and provides the patient with a more comfortable experience.

It easy to minimize pressure when palpating superficial tissues such as the upper trapezius muscle. When palpating deeper structures, it is more difficult to minimize pressure. This exercise allows the student to experience palpation of a deep structure (the psoas muscle in the abdomen) and pay especially close attention to the amount of pressure applied. If performed repeatedly, the exercise will establish good palpatory skills.

General tips for making palpation easier and minimizing pressure

Room environment

If any factors in the room environment are causing the patient to be tense or guarded, palpation and therapy are impeded. The air should be warm enough for the patient to stay warm with skin exposed. Attention must be paid to noise and light. Blankets and an eye mask are useful.

Patient positioning

- The patient should be well-supported with pillows, bolsters, etc.
- A comfortable, stable treatment table of adequate width is essential.
- The patient should be positioned so that the structure to be palpated is as accessible as possible. The examiner should not be reluctant to ask the patient to change position to access a particular region or structure.
- When palpating deeper structures, position the patient so that more superficial muscles are passively shortened. Inducing slack in superficial muscles will soften them so that palpating through them is easier.
- The height of the table should place the area to be palpated at, or slightly below, the level of the examiner's umbilicus.

Examiner positioning

The examiner should be positioned to easily reach the structures being palpated, to minimize tension in the body. A good rule of thumb is that at all times the examiner's umbilicus should directly face the area being examined.

Examiner's hands

- The examiner's hands should be relaxed but engaged and 'awake'. Tension in the hands will interfere with palpatory sensitivity and may induce use of increased pressure.
- The contact between the examiner's hands and the patient's body should be as broad as possible (i.e. as much of the hand as possible should contact the patient) while still allowing access to the structure being palpated. Experience suggests that broad contacts generally feel more comfortable to the patient than narrow or pointed contacts.
- The hands should increase pressure slowly, move slowly, and transition from one area to another slowly. In learning to trust that the examiner will be gentle and not perform any unexpected movements, the patient will relax and allow for easier access to deeper structures.

Examiner's mind

- Visualizing the structures being palpated can be very helpful.
- If the examiner's mind is anxious, it will be difficult to focus on what the hands are feeling, and there will be tension in the body. Mental tension can be decreased by first noticing its presence, slowly taking the hands off the patient's body, taking two or three deep breaths, shaking and softening the hands, and gently, slowly, replacing the hands on the patient's body.

Practical exercise: palpating the psoas in the abdomen

Note: This exercise should not be performed on anyone with inflammatory bowel disease or a history of arteriosclerosis, or an aneurysm, in case the aorta is contacted.

This exercise should take about 10 minutes for a novice palpation student to complete.

Patient position

Supine with the abdomen exposed, the knees and hips slightly flexed by propping the knees on a bolster or pillows. This position puts slack in the abdominal and psoas muscles.

Examiner position

Standing at the side of the table at the level of the umbilicus or slightly inferior to the umbilicus, facing the patient.

Procedure

The examiner begins by simply placing the hands on the patient's abdomen with the finger pads on the midline just inferior to the umbilicus. The palms and heels of the hands are placed on the abdomen. This makes the contact broad and comfortable for the patient. No pressure should be applied at first.

Box 6.2 Palpation pressure – and a practical psoas exercise continued

The examiner, without moving the hands, pays attention to the texture and tone of the skin and of the tissues directly underlying the skin. With very gentle pressure and small circular movements of the hands, the examiner glides the skin over the underlying tissues.

The examiner gently increases pressure, enough to slightly depress the anterior abdominal wall toward the table, and slides the hands laterally until the lateral border of the rectus abdominis is felt. At the lateral border of the rectus a definite softening of the anterior abdominal wall will be noted. The examiner palpates the lateral edge of the rectus abdominis. Having the patient raise the head and shoulders off the table will increase the tone of the rectus, making it easier to identify. Once it has been identified, the patient should once again rest the head and shoulders on the table.

The examiner begins to increase pressure slowly. The direction of pressure should be medially and posteriorly through the abdomen, toward the anterior surface of the patient's spine.

The examiner will first feel the oblique and transverse abdominal muscles. These will feel elastic and fibrous, and will offer some resistance. This resistance is best overcome by maintaining a slow, steady increase in pressure. The pressure is increased not by increasing tension in the hands, but by transferring weight through the arms and hands.

The examiner slowly increases pressure until a soft, homogeneous sensation just deep to the abdominal muscles is reached. This is the tissue of the abdominal viscera. This tissue will often be quite tender, and the patient is probably not accustomed to deep pressure on the abdomen. Simply maintaining steady pressure, or decreasing pressure slightly before slowly increasing it again, will help the patient to relax into the sensation.

The examiner slowly increases pressure until a firm tissue is reached. This is the anterior surface of the psoas muscle and will most likely be very tender. Maintaining this deep pressure, the examiner moves the fingertips across the fibers of the psoas, slowly, to get a sense of the fibrous nature of this tissue. This fibrous texture, along with the firmness of the muscle, differentiates the psoas from the viscera. Having the patient briefly flex the hip will increase the tone of the psoas, confirming that this is what is being palpated. The examiner should create a visual picture of the muscle's rounded anterior surface, fibrous texture and firm tone.

Note: If the examiner feels a sensation of pulsation deep in the abdomen where the psoas muscle should be, the aorta is probably being contacted. The examiner should gently but immediately release the palpating pressure and the exercise should be stopped.

Once the examiner has identified the psoas and explored its characteristics, pressure should be decreased very slowly and steadily until contact with the psoas is lost. Pressure is then increased slowly until the psoas is securely contacted again, at which time variations in tone may be noted, synchronous with inhalation and exhalation.

Pressure is decreased again and the examiner attends to the transition between definite palpation of the firm, fibrous psoas muscle and palpation of the soft, homogeneous viscera. The examiner can spend a few moments investigating this transition before decreasing the pressure very slightly, just enough to be off of the psoas muscle.

With pressure heavy enough to palpate the viscera but too light to directly contact the psoas, the examiner may still sense the tone and texture of the psoas muscle beneath by moving the fingertips medial and lateral (i.e. perpendicular to the grain of the psoas muscle fibers). Having the patient repeat the brief flexion of the hip will increase the tone of the psoas and make it more readily palpable again.

The examiner decreases the pressure again slightly, and again moves the fingertips across the grain of the psoas. There is still the possibility of sensing the firm tone, rounded shape and fibrous texture of the muscle even though direct contact with the muscle has been definitely lost. Visualization of the muscle is of enormous value during this part of the exercise.

This procedure continues with the examiner slowly and incrementally decreasing pressure, holding onto the mind's visual picture of the muscle, and working to sense the muscle deep to the viscera. This is done until the examiner can no longer sense any trace of the muscle's firmness or texture. The examiner should investigate this transition place – where the muscle is absolutely no longer palpable.

The examiner should then very slowly decrease pressure until the hands are simply resting on the patient's abdomen, and then the hands are removed.

Thank your palpation partner and switch roles.

muscle and joints, and – depending on the quality of the resistance offered – can be judged as normal, flaccid, restricted, dysfunctional or pathological – or other descriptors might be used.

Neuromuscular technique (NMT) palpation, in its assessment mode (as described below), attempts to insinuate finger or thumb movement through the tissues at precisely this 'first resistance' barrier, not introducing any actual lengthening of fibers – at least not until assessment gives way to treatment.

In treatment of muscle shortness, when isometric contractions might be employed (as in MET methodology – see Chapter 7), the very first sign of resistance, the first barrier or just short of this, is identified as the commencement point for a contraction.

To work with tissues that are any more elongated than that might well compromise the success of the treatment because it would be asking for a contraction by tissues already at stretch – a formula for cramp, or pain, or a defensive stretch–reflex response (He 1998).

A host of descriptors exist that reflect the multiple states that tissues and their barriers may represent – from lifeless and flaccid, to boggy and waterlogged, to tense, dense, turgid, indurated, fibrotic, harsh or rigid.

The way the tissues respond when the barrier is released can also offer information. Do the tissues, painlessly and efficiently, spring back to their previous state, as they should? If not, this may offer evidence of dysfunction or pathology.

Discrimination of the relative health, or otherwise, of soft tissues by means of assessment of the barriers, and the springing quality of these, is an important palpation skill that will be further explored in the skin, muscle and joint palpation methods detailed later in this chapter.

Palpation discrimination and cautions

How we make sense of what we feel when palpating has been researched, as have issues of sensitivity and interpretation. Some of these were discussed in Box 6.2.

Note: It is worth keeping in mind that palpation and assessment, when performed improperly (heavy handedly, clumsily, too rapidly, too persistently, etc.), particularly at a time when the body is highly agitated, can worsen an already compromised situation. Such action would not be in line with the tenets of naturopathy – *first do no harm*.

It is also clinically evident that when a particular assessment or palpation is repeated several times, in a short space of time, definite changes occur that may distort the findings – for example, in the firing sequence of muscles or in the degree of sensitivity reported. First impressions are commonly best.

NMT pressure – 'meet and match'

In NMT the required digital (finger or thumb) pressure varies, depending on the tissues being evaluated.

The expression 'meet and match' the tissues, suggests that in assessment mode at least (when NMT moves from assessment to treatment mode greater force is used) there should be no attempt to distract or compress the tissues beyond the 'first barrier' described above. There should merely be a sense of meeting and matching the intrinsic degree of tone or tension of whatever tissues are being palpated.

During layer palpation, pressure would increase incrementally as greater penetration is required, overcoming the resistance of superficial tissue to 'meet and match' deeper fascial or muscular fibers, for example, when seeking to evaluate for areas of dysfunction such as myofascial trigger points (Chaitow & DeLany 2002).

Aspects of the methodology of NMT, in treatment mode, are covered more fully in Chapter 7.

US and UK NMT: similarities and differences

European NMT was developed in the 1930s by British naturopaths Stanley Lief ND DC and Boris Chaitow ND DO DC, who based its methodology on traditional Ayurvedic massage methods (Chaitow 2003b, Varma 1935). American NMT evolved out of the work of chiropractor Raymond Nimmo (Cohen & Gibbons 1998, Nimmo 1957).

Both versions of NMT have evolved over the years since their inception, as explained in later chapters. Both are capable of being employed in therapeutic settings to treat localized dysfunction (such as myofascial trigger points – see Chapter 7) as well as in more general, whole-person applications (see Chapter 8).

Using an algometer

A small spring-loaded, rubber-tipped, pressure threshold meter (algometer) can be used to measure the degree of pressure required to produce symptoms – for example, before and after deactivation of a trigger point. When treatment has been successful, the pressure threshold over the trigger point should increase markedly (Fig. 6.7) (Baldry 1993).

Box 6.3 Exercise: Neuromuscular technique (NMT) evaluation

- Apply a small amount of light creamy lubricant to an area of the back of a prone model/palpation partner (the cream is to ensure that no dragging occurs on the skin, but that there is sufficient traction to avoid slipping).
- The main contact is made with the tip of one thumb, more precisely the medial aspect of the tip (Fig. 6.2).
- In some regions the tip of the index or middle finger can be used instead (Fig. 6.3), as this allows easier access between the ribs for assessment (or treatment) of, for example, intercostal musculature.
- The examination table should be at a height that allows the practitioner to stand erect, legs separated for ease of weight transference, with the assessing arm straight at the elbow, allowing bodyweight to be transferred, so that force can be imparted simply by leaning on the arm (Fig. 6.4).
- The fingers of the assessing/treating hand act as a stationary fulcrum positioned at the front of the contact, allowing the thumb to move across the palm of the hand during each slow assessment stroke.

- This differs from a usual massage stroke, in which the whole hand moves. Here the hand is stationary and only the thumb moves.
- Each stroke, diagnostic or therapeutic, extends for approximately 4–5 cm before the thumb ceases its motion, at which time the fulcrum/fingers are replaced in the direction the thumb needs to travel next.
- The thumb stroke employs a variable pressure that allows it to intelligently 'insinuate' and tease its way through whatever fibrous, indurated or contracted structures it meets.
- The degree of resistance or obstruction presented by the tissues determines the degree of effort required.
- Thus, in very tense tissues, sustained but not invasive pressure may be needed to 'match the tissue tension' during a diagnostic stroke.
- Tense, contracted or fibrous tissues are not overcome by force during treatment, rather the fibers are 'worked through', using substantial pressure at times, but in a

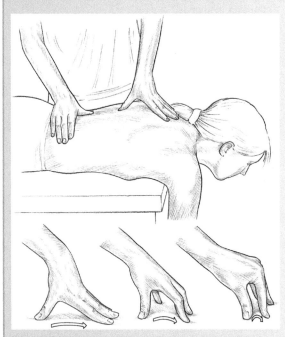

Figure 6.2 NMT thumb technique. Reproduced with permission from Chaitow (2003b)

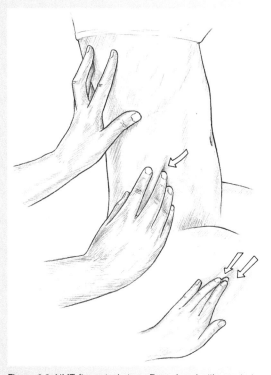

Figure 6.3 NMT finger technique. Reproduced with permission from Chaitow (2003b)

Continued

Box 6.3 Exercise: Neuromuscular technique (NMT) evaluation continued

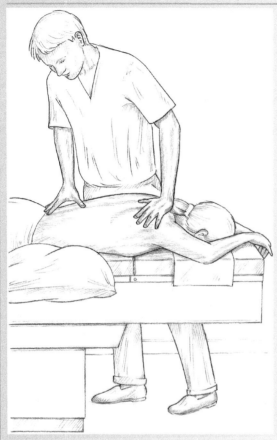

Figure 6.4 NMT – practitioner's posture should ensure a straight treating arm for ease of transmission of body weight, as well as leg positions that allow for the easy transfer of weight and center of gravity. These postures assist in reducing energy expenditure and ease spinal stress. Reproduced with permission from Chaitow (2003b)

constantly varying manner, in which both direction of application of pressure, as well as degree of pressure, are constantly varied as the palpating digit responds to the tissue status.

- The finger fulcrum acts as a stable point of contact for the hand, as the thumb travels towards the fingers.

- Effort, if any is required, is achieved by shifting bodyweight through the almost straight arm, not by using arm or hand strength.
- When a finger contact is used instead of the thumb, the hand is drawn towards the practitioner's body, with the treating finger slightly hooked (usually middle finger supported/braced by one of its neighbors), as in the methods of *bindegewebsmassage*. This allows for optimal control of the palpation effort.
- A major area where finger contact is useful, apart from the intercostal structures, involves the lateral pelvic region and lateral thigh.
- Standing on the side opposite the one being treated, the hooked finger – supported by its adjacent digit – can be inserted into the intercostal space, or the lateral pelvic musculature above the trochanter, and as the practitioner leans back and allows the weight of the patient to apply counterforce, the finger is then slowly drawn through these tissues, assessing the nature of dysfunction or applying cross-fiber or inhibitory contacts, when in therapeutic rather than diagnostic mode.
- Follow the arrows in the NMT sequences from Figures 6.5 and 6.6, as illustrated.
- The objective is to obtain information without causing excessive discomfort to the patient and without stressing the hands.
- NMT in its treatment mode involves greater pressure in order to modify dysfunctional tissues; however, the exercise sequence above is for 'information gathering' only.
- Any findings should be charted – tender areas, stress bands, contracted fibers, edematous areas, nodular structures, hypertonic regions, trigger points and so on.
- If trigger points are located, their target (referral) area should also be noted (trigger point assessment is described below).
- By working methodically, and following the descriptions given, a sense of non-invasive exploration should be experienced.

Once a delicacy of touch has been achieved, by repetition of this exercise, NMT evaluation can be applied anywhere on the body surface – meeting and matching tissue tension to elicit areas that are 'different', and possibly dysfunctional.

Box 6.3 Exercise: Neuromuscular technique (NMT) evaluation continued

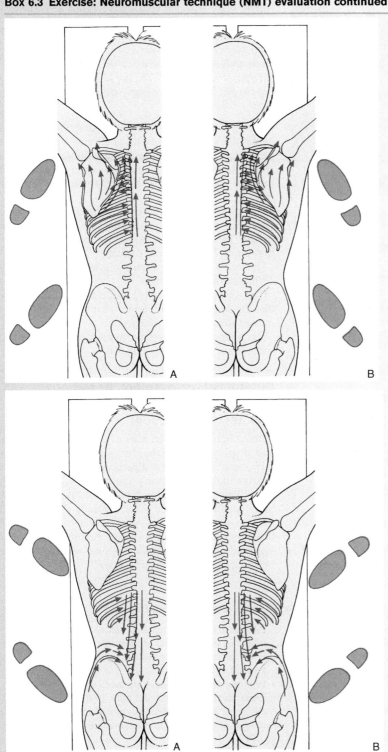

Figure 6.5 **A** Fourth and **B** fifth positions of suggested sequence of applications of NMT. Reproduced with permission from Chaitow (2003b)

Figure 6.6 **A, B** Sixth positions of suggested sequence of applications of NMT. Reproduced with permission from Chaitow (2003b)

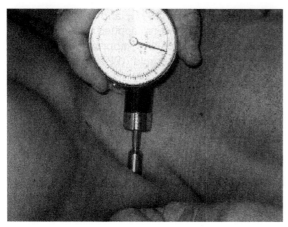

Figure 6.7 Position of the pressure threshold meter over the myofascial trigger point in the upper trapezius muscle. Reproduced with permission from Fernández-de-las-Peñas et al. *Journal of Bodywork and Movement Therapies* 2006;10:3–9

However, as valuable as an algometer may be in research settings, its use is not really practical in everyday clinical work. Newer electronic versions that fit onto a thumb-tip (linked to a computer screen) have made their use both practical and desirable (Fryer et al 2004).

Assessment of the common compensatory pattern (Zink & Lawson 1979)

See page 41 for an introduction to the topic of the common compensatory (adaptation) pattern (CCP).

Defeo & Hicks (1993) have described the observed signs of CCP as follows:

In the common compensatory pattern (CCP), an examiner will note the following observations in the supine patient. The left leg will appear longer than the right. The left iliac crest will appear higher or more

cephalad than the right. The pelvis will roll passively easier to the right than to the left because the lumbar spine is side-flexed left and rotated right. The sternum is displaced to the left as it courses inferiorly. The left infraclavicular parasternal area is more prominent anteriorly, because the thoracic inlet is side-flexed right and rotated right. The upper neck rotates easier to the left. The right arm appears longer than the left when fully extended.

Tissue preference is the sense that the palpating hands derive from the tissues being moved, as to the preferred direction(s) of movement (for example, at its simplest, 'this area turns more easily to the right than the left – and therefore has a "preference" to turn right').

The process of evaluation can be conceived as a series of 'questions' posed by the practitioner, to tissues being moved: 'Are you more comfortable moving in this direction, or that?'

The terms *comfort, position of ease* and *tissue preference* all mean the same thing.

Positions of ease, comfort and tissue preference are directly opposite to directions that *engage barriers*, or move towards *bind* or *restriction*

The methods for assessing tissue preferences in this context are described in Box 6.4.

Differential assessment, based on findings of supine and standing Zink tests (Liem 2004)

If the rotational preferences alternate when supine, and display a greater tendency to not alternate (i.e. they rotate in the same directions) when standing, a dysfunctional adaptation pattern that is 'ascending' is most likely, i.e. the major dysfunctions lie in the lower body, pelvis or lower extremities. If the rotational pattern remains the same when supine and standing this suggests that the adaptation pattern is primarily 'descending', i.e. the major dysfunctional patterns lie in the upper body, cranium or jaw.

Box 6.4 Assessment of tissue preference with patient supine and with patient upright

Note: If a differential assessment is being attempted, the procedures outlined in Box 6.1 should be performed in both supine and standing. Differential assessment is explained below.

Occipitoatlantal (OA) area

- With the patient supine the therapist is seated or standing at the head of the table. Both hands are used to take the neck into *maximal unstressed*

flexion (to lock the segments below C2) and the rotational preference *to an easy end of range – not a forced one,* is assessed. Is rotation more free left or right?

- With the patient standing, the neck is placed in full flexion, and rotation left and right, *of the head on the neck,* is evaluated for the preferred direction (range) of movement. Is rotation more free left or right?

Box 6.4 Assessment of tissue preference with patient supine and with patient upright continued

Cervicothoracic (CT) area

- The patient is supine and the therapist's hands are placed so that they lie, palms upward, beneath the scapulae. The therapist's forearms and elbows should be in touch with the table surface. Leverage can be introduced by one arm at a time as the therapist's weight is introduced toward the floor, through one elbow, and then the other, easing the patient's scapulae anteriorly. This allows a safe and relatively stress-free assessment to be made of the freedom with which one side, and then the other, moves, producing a rotation at the cervicothoracic junction. Rotational preference can easily be ascertained. Is rotation more free left or right?

- The patient is seated or standing in a relaxed posture with the therapist behind, with hands placed to cover the medial aspects of the upper trapezius, so that the fingers rest over the clavicles and thumbs rest on the transverse processes of the T1/T2 area. The hands assess the area being palpated for its 'tightness/looseness' preferences as a slight degree of rotation left and then right is introduced at the level of the cervicothoracic junction. Is rotation more free left or right?

If there was a preference for the OA area to rotate left, then if the CCP applies to this person, there should be a preference for right rotation at the CT junction.

Thoracolumbar (TL) area

- The patient is supine or prone. The therapist stands at waist level facing cephalad and places the hands over the lower thoracic structures, fingers along lower rib (7–10) shafts laterally. Treating the structure being palpated as a cylinder, the hands test the preference for the lower thorax to rotate around its central axis, testing one way and then the other. Is rotation more free left or right?

  The preferred TL rotation direction should be compared with those of OA and CT test results. Alternation in these should be observed if a healthy adaptive process is occurring.

- With the patient standing the therapist stands behind and with hands over the lower thoracic structures, fingers along lower rib shafts laterally, the preference for the lower thorax to rotate around its central axis is tested one way and then the other. Is rotation more free left or right?

  Alternation with previously assessed preferences should be observed if a healthy adaptive process is occurring.

Lumbosacral (LS) area

- The patient is supine. The therapist stands below waist level facing cephalad and places the hands on the anterior pelvic structures, using the contact as a 'steering wheel' to evaluate tissue preference as the pelvis is rotated around its central axis, seeking information as to its 'tightness/looseness' preferences. Is rotation more free left or right?

  Alternation with previously assessed preferences should be observed if a healthy adaptive process is occurring.

- The patient is standing and the therapist, standing behind, places the hands on the pelvic crest, rotating the pelvis around its central axis to identify its rotational preference. Is rotation more free left or right?

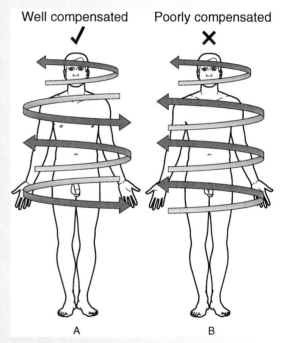

Well compensated   Poorly compensated

A   B

Figure 6.8 Zink's postural (fascial) patterns. Tissue 'preferences' in different areas identify adaptation patterns in clinically useful ways: *ideal* = minimal adaptive load transferred to other regions; *compensated* (**A**) = patterns alternate in direction from area to area; atlanto-occipital, cervicothoracic, thoracolumbar, lumbosacral; *uncompensated* (**B**) = patterns which do not alternate. Therapeutic objectives which encourage better compensation are optimal. Reproduced with permission from Chaitow (2003a)

Questions the therapist should ask him/herself following this assessment

1. *Was there an 'alternating' pattern to the tissue preferences, and was this the same when the patient was supine and when standing?*

2. *Alternatively, was there a tendency for the tissue preference to be in the same direction in all, or most of, the four areas assessed?*

3. *If the latter was the case, was this in an individual whose health is more compromised than average (in line with Zink & Lawson's observations – see Chapter 2).*

4. *What therapeutic methods would help the body to produce a more balanced degree of tissue preference?*

The critically important clinical relevance of the CCP test

If the key spinal transition areas fail to alternate in their rotational preferences, it may be assumed that adaptation potential is close to, or has passed, its ability to compensate any further, without symptoms emerging. The elastic has reached breaking point, metaphorically speaking. Therapeutic focus should shift from specific to constitutional interventions – for example, whole body massage rather than high velocity, low amplitude (HVLA) thrust or a heel lift – as any specific intervention would make demands on tissues that are relatively unable to comply, adapt, compensate.

From a naturopathic perspective this offers an important insight and should help to prevent applications of methods that, under more normal circumstances, would be well tolerated, but which under the circumstances prevailing when a maladapted CCP is evident, would most probably cause exacerbation, rather than assistance, to an already overburdened system.

Assessing the tissues

Much of the remainder of this chapter will be devoted to descriptions and exercises focused on evaluation of the status of skin, subdermal and fascial tissues, muscles, viscera and joints, as well as specific functions such as balance and breathing.

The tests involved are asking key questions as to whether whatever is being assessed is normal, and, if not, what further assessments are required to define the nature of dysfunction or pathology.

Palpation and assessment methods for any structure require an appreciation of its unique properties, so that differentiation and assessment can be accurate.

A reasonable knowledge of basic anatomic and physiological features and characteristics will therefore be assumed.

Thermal assessment

Various forms of thermal assessment are used clinically to identify trigger point activity and other forms of dysfunction, including infrared, electrical and liquid crystal methods (Baldry 1993), as well as manual thermal diagnosis (MTD) (Barral 1996).

Swerdlow & Dieter (1992) examined 365 patients with demonstrable trigger points in the upper back, and noted that: 'Although thermographic "hot-spots" are present in the majority, the sites are not necessarily where the trigger points are located.'

This suggests that:

- 'hot-spots' do not necessarily identify sites of trigger points, and
- trigger points may be located in colder areas, possibly in tissues that are ischemic and/or fibrotic.

Simons (1993a) also suggests that while 'hot-spots' may commonly represent trigger point sites, some triggers may exist in 'normal' temperature regions, and that hot-spots may exist for reasons other than the presence of trigger points.

Thermal examination of the reference zone (target area) to which a trigger point refers or radiates, usually demonstrates that the skin temperature is raised, but not always. Simons attributes this anomaly to the different effects trigger points can have on the autonomic nervous system.

He explains:

Depending upon the degree and manner in which the trigger point is modulating sympathetic control of skin circulation, the reference zone initially may be warmer, isothermic or cooler than unaffected skin. Painful pressure on the trigger point consistently and significantly reduced the temperature in the region of the referred pain and beyond.

Is manual thermal scanning accurate?

Some practitioners who use MTD 'scan' the tissues being investigated, keeping the hand approximately 1 inch (2.5 cm) from the skin surface to try to identify areas that apparently differ from each other in temperature.

Osteopathic pioneer Viola Frymann (1963) observes:

Even passing the hand a quarter of an inch above the skin provides information on the surface temperature. An acute lesion area will be unusually warm, an area of long-standing, chronic dysfunction may be unusually cold, as compared with the skin in other areas.

Are such perceived temperature differences accurate and significant?

Using sophisticated equipment, French osteopath Jean-Pierre Barral (1996) has established that areas that scan (non-touching) as 'hot' are only truly warmer than surrounding areas in 75% of instances.

It seems that scanning for hot and cold areas results in the perception of greater heat whenever *a significant temperature difference* occurs in one area, compared to a neighboring one.

The brain considers any area that is appreciably different from surrounding tissues – in temperature terms – to be 'hot'. This means that scanning over a 'normal' followed by a colder area will often (75% of the time) result in a perception that greater heat is being sensed. However, this misplaced identification of 'heat' does not nullify the usefulness of such approaches in attempting to identify dysfunctional tissues in a non-invasive way. But it does mean that what seems 'hot' may actually be 'cold' (ischemic?).

Manual scanning for heat is therefore an accurate way of assessing 'difference' between tissues, but not for identifying the actual thermal status.

Skin palpation, evaluating hydrosis, elasticity, adherence to underlying tissues, thermal qualities, hyperalgesia

The areas of skin overlying dysfunctional areas have been described by Lewit (1999b) as *hyperalgesic*

Box 6.5 Exercise: Manual thermal assessment

Off-the-body scan

- Stand at waist level, with your palpation partner prone on the treatment table, exposed from the waist up.
- Hold your dominant hand, with palm down, close (1–3 inches/2.5–7.5 cm) to the surface of the back and make steady, deliberate sweeps of the hand to and fro, across the back, until all of it has been scanned. Approximately 4–5 inches (10–12.5 cm) should be scanned per second.
- As you 'scan' for temperature variations 'off the body' in this way, keep the hand moving slowly. If the hand remains still or moves too slowly, you have nothing to compare, and if you move too fast, you will not perceive the slight changes as the hand passes from one area to another.
- Different aspects and areas of the hand may be more sensitive than others, so test whether your sensitivity is greater in the palm, near the wrist or on the dorsum of the hand, as you evaluate areas which feel warmer or cooler than others.
- Does your experience agree with the suggestion by some that the palmar surface is more sensitive than the dorsal surface of the hand?

It is suggested that you make the areas that seem to you to be 'warmest' the focus for subsequent skins tests in this sequence, as these are the areas of greatest difference, and therefore of potential interest. Chart your findings on an outline of the body.

Palpating for temperature differences

- Your palpation partner should be lying prone with the back exposed.
- You should now apply hand or finger contact, without pressure, to the tissues being evaluated, which should involve those that tested as 'warm' in the previous (scan) exercise, as well as those that did not.
- Do not rub or press the tissues, merely mold your hand(s) to the skin surface for a few seconds, before moving to an adjacent area. In this way, slowly and carefully palpate the back for variations of skin temperature, using both hands, one at a time or both at the same time.

To introduce variables you might wish to perform this palpation:

1. when the 'patient' has been lying still for some minutes in a room of normal temperature/humidity
2. when the 'patient' has actively skipped, jogged, danced or performed some other exercise for several minutes
3. when you have performed a similar exercise for some minutes.

Do you note any differences between 1, 2 and 3?

Vary your contact so that you sometimes use the palmar and sometimes the dorsal surface of your palpating hand:

- Is one hand more sensitive than the other?
- Is one palpation contact more accurate than the other?

Do you sense differences in temperature from one area to another of the body surface and, if so, how does this relate to the off-the-body scan in the previous exercise?

How does your, or your partner's, degree of hydrosis/sweating influence what you feel?

Record your findings.

skin zones (HSZ). These dysfunctional areas might involve inflammation, increased tone or even spasm. Alternatively, an HSZ may overlie a trigger point (TrP).

There are a number of palpable characteristics of skin that overlie hyperalgesic zones:

1. The skin adheres to the underlying fascia more tightly, resisting movements such as sliding, lifting or rolling

2. Increased sympathetic activity results in abnormally high sudomotor activity (hydrosis, sweat) in and on the skin, and this is demonstrated by resistance during light finger stroking movements – a quality described as 'skin drag'. (Lightly run your finger across the skin of an area where you have recently been wearing a watch or bracelet, to get an enhanced sense of 'drag'.)

3. The skin appears to have a compacted, inelastic feel, resisting easy separation or stretching.

4. There are usually changes in thermal quality that can commonly be appreciated and discriminated by touch (Adams et al 1982), or by off-the-body scanning, as being warmer or cooler than surrounding skin (Barral 1996) (see discussion above of accuracy of scanning palpation).

Skin palpation test exercises

The information derived from any of the three methods described in Boxes 6.6–6.8 should complement and confirm each other. In clinical practice it is seldom necessary to perform all three assessments (Chaitow 2003a).

Box 6.6 Exercise: Skin on fascia assessment

This approach is based on methods derived from German *bindegewebsmassage* (connective tissue massage) (Bischof & Elmiger 1960).

It will be found that moving skin on fascia is more easily accomplished when assessing slim individuals. There will be greater tissue resistance in patients with a higher subcutaneous fat and water content.

Method

• The patient lies prone with the practitioner standing to one side, at the level of the pelvis.

• The practitioner applies the pads of several fingers of each hand, bilaterally, flat against the skin overlying the sacrum.

• Only light pressure should be used, sufficient to produce adherence between the finger pads and the skin.

• The skin and subcutaneous tissues should be displaced simultaneously, bilaterally, sliding it over the fascia in a cephalad direction, until the 'first sign of resistance' barrier is perceived.

• If the tissues are normal (i.e. no hyperalgesia or underlying dysfunction or pathology) there should be an equal, easy, free range of motion symmetrically.

• Having taken the tissue to the first sign of resistance, it is useful to 'spring' it to its elastic barrier, to assess the quality of response: Does it rapidly return to the starting position, or does it do so only slowly? Do both sides respond similarly? (Any asymmetry suggests a need for further investigation of the tissues below the area of dysfunction.)

• Sequentially the finger pads should then be moved superiorly a few centimeters, and the bilateral skin on fascia test repeated. In this way an assessment can be made of all paraspinal tissues, from the sacrum to the base of the neck.

Pattern of testing/evaluation

Ideally the pattern of testing should be performed from inferior to superior, either moving the skin superiorly as described, or starting the finger contact a little more laterally with movements in an obliquely diagonal direction, toward the spine – provided that the same directions (i.e. toward the spine, or superiorly) are used on each side at the same time.

With each series of skin slides the tissues are being evaluated for symmetry and quality of range of movement of the skin and subcutaneous tissue, to the first resistance and/or to the elastic barriers, where the 'springing' assessment is made. In this way it should be possible to identify local areas where the skin adherence to underlying connective tissue varies from adjacent or surrounding skin. This is likely to be an area housing active myofascial trigger points (TrPs) or tissue that is dysfunctional (possibly inflamed) or hypertonic.

The areas located in this palpation exercise that appear different from surrounding areas should be marked with a skin pencil, and compared with information derived from the next two exercises, both of which involve aspects of skin testing.

Box 6.7 Exercise: Drag palpation assessment

Atrichial sweat glands, controlled by the sympathetic division of the autonomic nervous system, empty directly onto the skin, creating increased hydrosis (sweat) presence, and in the process the mechanical, electrical and heat transfer properties, and characteristics, of the skin are altered (Adams et al 1982).

Lewit (1999b) suggests that clinicians should be able to identify active reflex activities (such as are involved with TrPs) simply by assessing the degree of elasticity in the overlying skin, and comparing this with surrounding tissue. This is one of the mechanical changes resulting from increased sympathetic activity. The simultaneously occurring hydrosis phenomenon explains why, prior to the introduction of methods of electrical detection of acupuncture points, any skilled acupuncturist could quickly locate 'active' points by palpation, and also why measurement of the electrical resistance of the skin can now do this even more rapidly (i.e. when skin is moist it conducts electricity more efficiently than when dry).

Note: There should be no oil or lubricant on the patient's skin or clinician's hands for this method to be efficient.

Method

- Using an extremely light touch ('skin on skin'), without any pressure, the digit (finger, thumb) is stroked across the skin overlying areas suspected of housing dysfunctional changes (e.g. TrPs).
- The areas chosen are commonly those where skin on fascia movement (see previous exercise) was reduced, compared with surrounding skin.
- When the stroking digit passes over areas where a sense of hesitation, or 'drag', is noted, increased hydrosis will have been identified.
- A degree of searching pressure into such tissues, precisely under the area of drag, may locate a taut band of tissue, and when this is compressed a painful response is commonly elicited.
- If pressure is maintained for 2–3 seconds, a report of a radiating or referred sensation may be forthcoming.
- If this sensation replicates symptoms previously noted by the patient, the point located is an active trigger point (Simons et al 1999).

Drag palpation can be used almost anywhere on the body surface and is the least invasive, and for many the most efficient, method for rapidly identifying areas of dysfunction.

Identification of dysfunction via the skin

Modification and often normalization of the reduced elastic status of the skin, as identified by these assessment methods (skin on fascia, skin drag, skin elasticity), is possible by various methods, including sustained light stretching (mini-myofascial releases), by means of positional release techniques, the introduction of isometric contractions into the underlying tissues, via sustained compression, or by acupuncture (Chaitow 2003a).

Scar tissue palpation

Dosch (1984) has described scars as 'interference fields', explaining that such a 'field' is a 'center of irritation' potentially producing strong, persistent interference with the neurovegetative system. It is suggested that scars (and other pathologically damaged tissues) are capable of generating strong, long-standing stimuli that 'mislead the regulating mechanisms'.

These concepts seem very similar to our understanding of sensitization and facilitation, as discussed in Chapter 2.

Scars are also frequently associated with the generation of myofascial trigger points (which are local areas of sensitization) (Defalque 1982).

Lewit & Olanska (2004) have summarized the evolution of treatment strategies involving scar tissue:

As early as in the 1930s, the brothers Huneke (who were not physicians) injected scars with Novocain, obtaining surprising effects mainly in painful conditions of the type now diagnosed as myofascial pain syndromes. They ascribed the therapeutic effect entirely to Novocain. So prompt was the effect that they coined the term 'Sekundenphenoman' (effect within a second). This was the beginning of 'Neuraltherapie', making use of Novocain for painful conditions (mainly in Germany). It was later found that it did not matter what was injected and finally that the same effect could be brought about by just using the needle. It was therefore no coincidence that the same therapists finally adopted acupuncture. In this development, however, the scar was largely forgotten.

They go on to describe how soft tissue methods are equally effective and have described strategies to

Box 6.8 Exercise: Skin stretch method (Lewit 1999b)

Note: At first, it is necessary to practice this method slowly. Eventually, it should be possible to move fairly rapidly over an area that is being searched for evidence of reflex activity (or acupuncture points).

Choose an area to be assessed, where abnormal degrees of skin on fascia adherence, and/or drag sensations, were previously noted.

Method

- The patient should be lying prone.
- Place two index fingers adjacent to each other (touching), on the skin, side by side or pointing toward each other, with no pressure at all onto the skin, just a contact touch.
- Lightly and slowly separate the fingers, feeling the skin stretch to its 'easy' limit, to the point where resistance is first noted.
- When this barrier has been identified it should be possible – in normal tissue – to 'spring' the skin further apart, to its elastic limit.
- Release this stretch and move both fingers between $^1/_4$ and $^1/_2$ inch (0.5 cm) to one side of this first test site, and test again in the same way, and in the same direction of pull, and using the same degree of effort,

separating the fingers, and adding a spring assessment once the first barrier is reached.

- Compare the range and quality of the elasticity and springiness of one test site with the previous one.
- Perform exactly the same sequence over and over again until the entire area of tissue has been searched, ensuring that the rhythm adopted is neither too slow (difficult to remember the kinesthetic feel of the previous stretch if there is too long a delay between test stretches) nor too rapid (difficult to perform the sequence accurately if carried out too rapidly).
- Approximately one stretch per 1–2 seconds should be performed.
- When skin being stretched is not as elastic as it was on the previous stretch a potential HSZ will have been identified.
- This should be marked with a skin pencil for future attention/investigation.
- Light digital pressure to the center of that small zone would commonly locate a sensitive contracture, which on sustained pressure may radiate or refer sensations to a distant site.
- If such sensations are familiar to the patient, the point being pressed is an active trigger point.

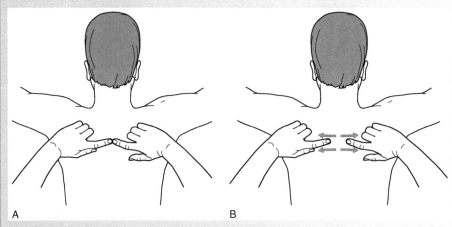

A   B

Figure 6.9 **A** Fingers touch each other directly over skin to be tested – very light skin contact only. **B** Pull apart to assess degree of skin elasticity – compare with neighboring skin area. Reproduced with permission from Chaitow (2003a)

use when palpating for trigger points close to scar tissue.

The characteristic findings on the skin are increased skin drag, owing to increased moisture (sweating); skin stretch will be impaired and the skin fold will be thicker. If the scar covers a wider area, it may adhere

to the underlying tissues, most frequently to bone. In the abdominal cavity, we meet resistance in some direction, which is painful. Just as with other soft tissue, after engaging the barrier and waiting, we obtain release after a short latency, almost without increasing pressure. This can be of great diagnostic value, because if, after engaging the barrier the

Box 6.9 Exercise: Combined scan and skin assessment

It is suggested that you attempt an assessment in which you compare the reliability and accuracy of the scan and of the three skin evaluation methods, with each other, on one individual, at the same time.

Method

- Have someone lie prone.
- Perform an off-the-body scan for temperature variations (remembering that cold may suggest ischemia and hot may indicate irritation/inflammation). Note areas that are 'different'.
- Now palpate directly for thermal (heat) variations by molding your hands lightly to the tissues to assess for temperature differences, avoiding lengthy hand contact so as not to change the status of the tissues you are palpating. A few seconds should be adequate.
- Pay particular attention to those 'different' areas (comparing one area with another, and also comparing the 'touch' palpation with the scan palpation), and then, using those areas where temperature differences are most obvious, assess for dysfunction (HSZ) using the skin adherence to fascia, skin drag and skin elasticity methods.
- In this way identify the most likely target areas for deeper palpation.
- Choose several of these and see if you can identify reflexively active areas (trigger points etc.) by means of single-digit pressure palpation, assessing for: (1) increased sensitivity/pain; (2) pain that radiates or refers; and (3) pain that the patient recognizes as being familiar (i.e. an active trigger point).

Do the scan and palpation findings agree with each other?
Which was the most efficient way of identifying trigger points?

resistance does not change, this is not due to the scar but to some intra-abdominal pathology.

Dosch (1984, p. 143) also points to German research which has demonstrated that scars often display marked differences (up to 10 times greater) in electrical resistance, when compared to surrounding 'normal' skin. This observation correlates with Lewit & Olanska's mention of 'increased moisture' which characterizes areas of greater skin drag.

Lewit (1999a) observes that scars may act as physiological 'saboteurs', demanding special attention. He

suggests deep palpation for painful areas near scars, assessing for increased resistance ('adhesions'), as well as for hyperalgesic skin zones, using skin stretching.

Scar tissue might also block normal lymphatic drainage and may in this way encourage trigger point formation or recurrence (Chikly 1996).

Lewit & Olanska (2004) go on remind us of the use of barrier assessment (as discussed above in relation to skin elasticity) in palpation and assessment of scar tissue:

> *For both diagnosis and treatment, the barrier phenomenon is essential. As in joints, there is always a range of movement in which there is next to no resistance to stretch or shift. The moment the first resistance is met, the barrier is reached. Under normal conditions, this barrier is soft and can easily be sprung or shifted. Under pathological conditions, however, the barrier is abrupt, does not spring ('end feel'), and restricts movement. For treatment, we engage the barrier, and after a short latency, release is obtained.*

They also point out that not all layers of a scar may be 'active', and that it is important to examine all layers as part of the assessment.

After locating an active scar (characterized by pain being produced during stretching of the tissues around the scar), the question needs to be asked whether the scar relates to the patient's condition – whether or not it is 'active', and whether or not the patient recognizes the painful palpation symptoms as being familiar.

Upledger & Vredevoogd (1983) discuss scar tissue, illustrating its importance with the example of a patient with chronic migraine headaches which resulted from chronic fascial drag produced by an appendectomy scar. Deep pressure medially on the scar produced the headache; deep pressure laterally caused relief of the headache. Mobilization of the scar was performed by sustained and deep but gentle pressure. This resulted in freedom from headaches, according to these respected authors, who add: 'Spontaneous relief of low back pain, menstrual disorders and chronic and recurrent cervical somatic dysfunction also occurred following cicatrix [scar] mobilisation.'

Subdermal palpation assessment (fascia, muscle)

This involves evaluating qualities of texture, congestion, inflammation, adhesion and fibrosis, as well as the presence of embryonic, latent or active myofascial trigger points.

Box 6.10 Exercise: Scar palpation

- Palpate a scar, feeling the scar tissue itself and judge how the surrounding tissues – skin and deeper tissues – associate with it.
- Is there a sense of tethering, or does the scar 'float' in reasonable supple, elastic, local tissues?
- Can the scar be moved easily in all directions equally, or are there directions of movement for all, or part, of the scar that are limited, compared with others?
- If possible, palpate a recent and also a very old scar, and compare the characteristics.
- See if local tenderness or actual pain exists around the scar on pressure or distraction of attached structures.
- Evaluate whether the skin elasticity alongside the scar varies.
- Can you release undue tension of the skin attaching to the scar by sustained painless stretching – holding it at its elastic barrier?
- This can be achieved in various ways – as in skin stretching, i.e. holding the skin at stretch for 15–90 seconds while stabilizing the scar with the other hand, or by means of pinching, compressing and/or rolling the scar tissue between the thumb and finger.
- Record your findings, relating what you feel when evaluating as many scars as possible, of different types, of recent and of long standing

Background to soft tissue changes

What happens to soft tissues to make them adapt and alter in texture and function has been discussed in Chapter 2. Tissues modify in response to musculoskeletal overuse, misuse, disuse and abuse (trauma) – involving factors such as age, genetic features, occupational and leisure activities, and posture.

When adaptive changes occur in response to a single, or short-term, unaccustomed demand (e.g. playing tennis for the first time, or digging the garden, or any other unexpected or unaccustomed effort), self-regulatory mechanisms ensure that the stiffness and soreness fade away after a few days. However, if the adaptive demands are repeated, or are constant, different effects are likely.

1. The first phase may be equated with the alarm stage in Selye's (1984) general adaptation syndrome (GAS; see Chapter 2). Indeed, all elements of the GAS can be scaled down to a local level (a single muscle or joint, for example) in which the same stages are passed through (alarm, adaptation, exhaustion). This is then referred to as the local adaptation syndrome (LAS).

2. As would be expected according to both the GAS and LAS, after the acute phase would come the phase of adaptation. In the muscular sense this means that if increased tone is maintained for longer than a few weeks, a chronic stage evolves. This is characterized by indications of structural changes in the supporting tissues with the development of 'contraction knots' (Mense & Simons 2001) and fibrous modification.

3. Simons & Mense (1997) have examined the increased levels of tone associated with clinical muscle pain. They define 'tone' in two ways:
   - Resting muscle tone (in the specific sense) represents the elastic and/or viscoelastic stiffness in the absence of contractile activity (motor unit activity and/or contracture)
   - Muscle tone (in the general sense) represents elastic or viscoelastic stiffness including any involuntary contractile activity.

4. McMakin (2004) has described some of the mechanisms involved in muscles and connective tissue that develop trigger points:

   Local ischemia in muscles that contain myofascial trigger points causes a decrease in ATP production (Cheng et al 1982), disrupts the sodium pump and normal membrane conductance, and increases the presence of metabolic wastes, creating a self-sustaining cycle of dysfunction that encourages trigger point formation (Alvarez & Rockwell 2002). Both spasm and contracture cause a reduction in local blood supply, decreasing oxygen transport and waste removal, leading to a further tightening of the myofascia. Dysfunction in the delicate fascial membrane encasing each myofibril disrupts the flow of neurotransmitters. Ground substance [connective tissue/fascia] within the myofascia undergoes transformation from a solute, to a gel, to a solid state, further stiffening the myofascial tissues.

5. Bauer & Heine (1998) conducted a clinical study to observe fascial perforations in patients suffering from chronic shoulder/neck or shoulder/arm pain. Such perforations had previously been identified in superficial fascial layers (Heine 1995, Staubesand & Li 1997) and are characterized by penetration by venous, arterial and neural structures. The perforations correlate 'identically' with traditional Chinese acupuncture point

locations, which Wall & Melzack noted also correlate – in approximately 80% of cases – with common trigger point sites (Melzack 1977, Wall & Melzack 1989).

6. Bauer & Heine (1998) also found that the perforating vessels were frequently 'strangled' together by a thick ring of collagen fibers, lying just above the perforation aperture.

   These alterations might be considered as part of an 'organizing' (or adaptive) response, in which sustained tone is replaced by concrete, supportive bands. The body may be adapting to the seemingly permanent demand for increased tone in these tissues (Lewit 1999a).

7. Staubesand & Li (1996) have studied human fascia using electron photomicroscopy and have found smooth muscle cells (SMC) widely embedded within the collagen fibers. They describe a rich intrafascial supply of capillaries, autonomic and sensory nerve endings, and concluded that these intrafascial smooth muscle cells enable the autonomic nervous system to regulate a fascial pre-tension, independently of (but probably influencing) muscular tonus.

8. Subsequent research has led to increasing interest in the possible effects that active SMC contractility may have in the many fascial/connective tissue sites in which their presence has now been identified, including ligaments (Meiss 1983), menisci (Ahluwalia 2001), spinal discs (Hastreiter et al 2001) and, as suggested by the research of Yahia et al (1993), the lumbodorsal fascia, which has been shown by Barker & Briggs (1999) to extend from the pelvis to the cervical area.

9. Respiratory alkalosis (Foster et al 2001, Pryor & Prasad 2002) resulting from breathing pattern disorders (BPD) such as hyperventilation causes SMC to adapt by constricting, potentially modifying fascial tone. This may have as yet unspecified influences on general muscular tone and conditions such as low back pain. See notes in this chapter, and in Chapters 7 and 10, on the importance of assessment and rehabilitation of breathing pattern disorders – even in conditions such as low back pain.

   The sequence of adaptive changes listed above, that evolve from a variety of backgrounds, but which influence the functionality of tissues and contribute towards symptom evolution, highlight the need for naturopaths to have a constant awareness of contextual factors, and not just the obvious.

10. For example, in his book *Anatomy Trains*, Myers (2001) has described a number of clinically useful sets of myofascial chains – the connections between different structures ('long functional continuities') that he terms 'anatomy trains'. These involve specific linkages that can help to explain why certain symptoms emerge some distance from an identified area of dysfunction.

    An example of one of the continuities described by Myers (1997) is the so-called 'superficial back line' (Fig. 6.10):
    • This starts with the plantar fascia, linking the plantar surface of the toes to the calcaneus –
    • gastrocnemius, then links the calcaneus to the femoral condyles –
    • the hamstrings, link the femoral condyles to the ischial tuberosities –
    • the sacrotuberous ligament, links the ischial tuberosities to the sacrum –
    • the lumbosacral fascia, erector spinae and nuchal ligament, link the sacrum to the occiput –
    • and the scalp fascia, links the occiput to the brow ridge.

11. The degree of relative ischemia, hypoxia and retention of toxic debris evident, as the various stages of adaptation progress, is likely to vary from person to person (and region to region) in relation to features such as age, exercise, nutritional status, lifestyle, etc.

    It is during these adaptation stages that signs might be noted of myofascial trigger point development, in which discrete areas of the affected soft tissues would evolve into localized areas of facilitation as trigger points appear (Kuchera et al 1990, Norris 1998). These sensitive, discrete and palpable tissue changes are themselves capable of sending noxious impulses to distant target areas where pain and new 'crops' of embryonic trigger points develop (Simons et al 1999).

    Any pain noted would probably have a deep, aching quality and in time palpation may reveal trigger points, as well as a fibrous, stringy muscular texture along with other palpable changes, possibly involving edema (Larsson et al 1990).

12. Bands of stress fibers tend to develop in the hypertonic tissues and the muscles affected in

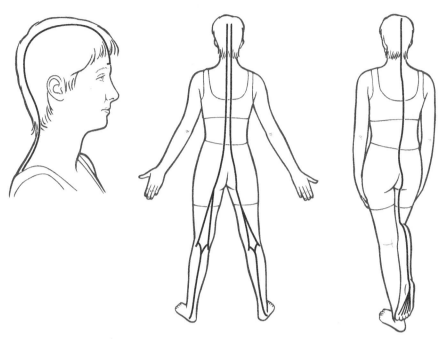

Figure 6.10 The superficial back line. Reproduced with permission from Chaitow (2002)

this way begin to place increasing degrees of tension on their tendons and osseous insertions (Mense & Simons 2001). As these processes evolve, tendon changes begin, at first producing an acute, and later a more chronic adaptation response, which may progress on to degenerative changes (see Chapter 2 discussion on the effects of a short-leg problem).

13. As the load of sustained increased muscular tone affects the tendons and their periosteal insertions it may be possible to palpate very tender periosteal pain points (PPPs), or to note early signs of joint dysfunction if such a muscle crosses a joint (e.g. knee, elbow) (Lewit 1999a). Mense & Simons (2001) report that: 'The muscles crossing involved [blocked] joints are . . . likely to develop trigger points producing secondary muscle-induced pain because of the joint problem.'

14. The inhibitory effect of hypertonic muscles on their antagonists (Janda 1986) produces inappropriate firing sequences (discussed in more detail later in this chapter), leading to a range of functional changes, as demonstrated by crossed syndrome patterns. Functional tests for these patterns are described later in this chapter (Janda 1988, Janda & Schmid 1980).

15. The natural sequence described by Selye (1976), in which tissues progress from an acute phase to an adaptation phase (which can last many years) and ultimately (when adaptive potentials are exhausted) to the final phase of degeneration and disease, is the normal consequence of any unrelieved chronic hypertonicity. The end result could take the form of arthritic joint changes, or chronic muscular or other soft tissue dysfunction, almost always also involving myofascial trigger points (Lewit 1999c, Murphy 2000).

Don't forget TART

In all soft tissue palpation it is useful to recall the earlier discussion (see Chapter 4) of the characteristics of dysfunction:

- Tenderness
- Asymmetry
- Range of motion changes
- Tissue texture modification.

Whether a joint is being evaluated for its behavior, or a muscle is being tested for its length/strength or presence of trigger points, or the periosteum is being palpated for changes relating to excessive tension on tendons, or changes in skin behavior are being evaluated – some or all of these TART characteristics will be present and can aid the decision-making process when your palpating fingers are asking questions such as:

1. *Is this normal?*
2. *In what way is this different from the norm?*
3. *What do these changes signify?*
4. *Do these findings relate to the patient's symptoms?*

Box 6.11 Exercise: Trigger point palpation (Travell & Simons 1983a, Simons et al 1999)

- Areas to target for deeper palpation can be identified using any of the skin palpation methods outlined above, or use of NMT in palpation mode.
- To identify a trigger point may require a systematic palpation of muscles, across the direction of the fibers.
- There may be a palpable ropiness, or nodularity, in muscles containing trigger points, and the muscle will have an altered range of motion (usually shorter than usual).
- By palpating perpendicularly to the fiber direction (using 'flat' or 'pincer' palpation – see next bullet point) it should be possible to locate a taut band.
- *Flat palpation* into the tissues, using the thumb for example, should be slowly achieved, teasing and searching with the thumb-tip, as tissues are slowly compressed toward underlying structures
- Focused compression of individual fibers is possible by using either *pincer compression*, using the tips of the digits, or *flat palpation* against underlying structures. Both methods entrap specific bands of tissue.
- Compression between fingers and thumb has the advantage of offering information from two or more of the examiner's digits simultaneously, whereas flat palpation against underlying tissues offers a more solid and stable background against which to assess the tissue.
- Central trigger points lie close to the motor endpoint.
- Attachment trigger points lie close to the attachments of the muscle (trigger points in these different locations call for contrasting treatment strategies outlined in Chapter 7).
- Sustained digital pressure onto, or stretching of, an active or latent trigger point (or insertion into it of a needle) usually reproduces a referred or radiating pain pattern.
- A trigger point that is active radiates or refers pain to a predictable site, producing symptoms recognizable to the patient.
- A latent trigger point produces symptoms (usually pain) that are not recognized as 'familiar' by the patient.
- Central trigger points are usually palpable either with flat palpation (digital pressure against underlying structures using a thumb or finger) or with pincer compression (tissue held more precisely between thumb and fingers like a C-clamp, or held more broadly, with fingers extended like a clothes pin).
- Trigger points are seldom located where the patient complains of pain.
- The taut band feels like a bundle of contracted, string-like fibers.
- Careful palpation along a taut band may reveal an exquisitely tender nodular area where the tissue can be rolled between fingers and thumb to assess quality, density, fluidity and other characteristics that may offer information.
- When the taut band is 'rolled' briskly by fingers or thumb ('snapping palpation'), this may produce a 'twitch' response (Dexter & Simons 1981).
- Apart from pain, autonomic phenomena may also be evoked. Simons (1993b, 1996) maintains that the high intensity of nerve impulses from an active trigger point can, by reflex, produce vasoconstriction, a reduction of the blood supply to specific areas of the brain, spinal cord and nervous system, provoking a wide range of symptoms capable of affecting almost any part of the body.

In this exercise it is suggested that you:

- identify sites using skin palpation methods and NMT evaluation to assess preferences – which approach offers you the best information?
- locate trigger points using flat and compression palpation
- identify trigger points in different muscles – for example, upper trapezius (patient supine, you seated at the head of the table) and quadratus lumborum (patient prone, you standing at waist level ipsilateral to the palpated area)
- identify both central and attachment trigger points – for example, central in sternocleidomastoid on anterior neck, and attachment in piriformis, posterior to greater trochanter
- identify both active (patient recognizes symptoms as 'familiar') and latent (not familiar to patient) points.

Wider significance of trigger points

Trigger points when active are a source of pain; however, symptoms may also involve functional changes. For example, as far back as the early 1950s there were reports that pelvic pain and bladder symptoms, such as cystitis, could be created by trigger points lying in the abdominal muscles (Kelsey 1951).

Travell & Simons (1983b), the leading researchers into trigger points, have reported that:

Urinary frequency, urinary urgency and 'kidney' pain may be referred from trigger points in the skin of the lower abdominal muscles. Injection of an old appendectomy scar . . . has relieved frequency and urgency, and increased the bladder capacity significantly.

More recent research confirms this, and has shown that symptoms such as chronic pelvic pain and interstitial cystitis can often be relieved by manual deactivation of trigger points, as well as by injection of these, or by acupuncture (Oyama et al 2004, Weiss 2001).

Periosteal pain points (PPPs)
(Lewit 1999a)

As muscle tonus increases and becomes chronic, stresses build up on the tendons and their osseous insertions into the periosteum. The localized pain and resulting palpable changes on the periosteum make them useful as diagnostic aids.

A frequently palpated feature is of a sensitive 'soft bump' at the point of attachment of tendons and ligaments. This can sometimes be noted on spinous processes where one side is tender, relating to sustained heightened tension in the muscles on that side. Rotational restrictions may be identified associated with the involved spinal segments where muscle attachments on one side are 'tighter' than the other.

The cervical joints are most easily accessible for palpation of such attachment sites when the patient is supine, and greater palpation pressure is required through paraspinal tissues with the patient prone, in order to access thoracic or lumbar spinal periosteal sites in those regions.

Many extremity joints are available for direct palpation of the periosteum – for example, the hip attachments can be reached via the groin, if care is taken.

Acromioclavicular and sternoclavicular joints are easily accessed, as is the temporomandibular joint (TMJ) anterior to the tragus.

Brugger (1960) has described a number of syndromes in which altered arthromuscular components produce reflexogenic pain. Ligaments and fascia can therefore be considered as sources of referred pain. Painfully stimulated tissues (such as the origins of tendons or joint capsules) can produce pain in associated muscles, tendons and overlying skin. As an example, irritation and increased sensitivity in the region of the sternum, clavicles and rib attachments to the sternum, through occupational or postural patterns, may influence or cause painful intercostal muscles, scalenes, sternomastoid, pectoralis major and cervical muscles.

The increased tone in these muscles and the resultant stresses which they produce may in turn lead to spondylogenic problems in the cervical region, with further spread of symptoms. Overall, Lewit (1999a) suggests, this syndrome can produce chronic pain in the neck, head, chest wall, arm and hand (even mimicking heart disease).

Some of the major PPPs are listed in Table 6.1.

Evaluation of muscle firing sequences, length, strength, tone (Janda 1983, 1996)

Three 'functional assessments' will be outlined, which examine the way in which muscles are firing when particular actions are performed by the patient/model.

Muscle-firing sequences offer evidence of normality or dysfunction (Janda 1982) and, depending on the muscles involved, can point to the likelihood of particular muscles being either:

- shortened (postural/predominantly Type 1 fibers/deep/inner unit/stabilizer/local muscles) or
- inhibited (phasic/superficial/outer unit/mobilizer/global muscles).

Janda (1988) has shown that postural muscles have a tendency to shorten, not only under pathological conditions, but often under normal circumstances.

Box 6.12 Exercise: Periosteal pain points

- Palpate the PPPs described in Table 6.1 and see how many are present as sensitive, palpable structures.
- Try to assess which soft tissues may be associated with the PPP tenderness.
- Try to establish the connection between a PPP and the soft tissue dysfunction associated with it, by evaluating the tone and general 'feel' of attaching muscles.
- Incorporate tests for shortness of those muscles specifically linked to PPPs (shortness assessments are discussed later in this chapter).
- Chart your findings.

Table 6.1 Some PPPs and their significance according to Lewit (1999a)

PPP	Significance
Head of metatarsals	Metatarsalgia (flat foot)
Calcaneal spur (a classic PPP)	Tension in plantar aponeurosis
Tubercle of tibia	Tension long adductors; hip dysfunction
Attachments of collateral knee ligaments	Dysfunction corresponding meniscus
Fibula head	Tension biceps femoris or restriction fibula head
Posterior superior iliac spines	Common, but no specific indication
Lateral aspect of symphysis pubis	Adductor tension, SIJ or a hip dysfunction
Coccyx	Gluteus maximus, levator ani, piriformis dysfunction
Iliac crest	Gluteus medius, quadratus lumborum or thoracolumbar dysfunction
Greater trochanter	Tension in abductors or a hip dysfunction
T5–T6 spinous process	Dysfunction lower cervical spine
Spinous process of C2	Dysfunction C1–2/C2–3 or levator scapulae tension
Xiphoid process	Tension rectus abdominis or 6th, 7th or 8th rib dysfunction
Ribs, mammary or axillary line	Tension pectoral attachments/visceral problem
Sternocostal junction of upper ribs	Tension in scalene muscles
Sternum, close to the clavicle	Tension in sternomastoid muscle
Transverse process of atlas	A/O problem/SCM or rectus capitis lateralis
Styloid process of the radius	Elbow dysfunction
Epicondyles	Elbow or epicondyle attachment dysfunction
Attachment of deltoid	Scapulohumeral joint lesion
Condyle of the mandible	TMJ or masticatory muscle dysfunction

A/O, atlanto-occipital; SCM, small muscle cells; SIJ, sacroiliac joint; TMJ, temporomandibular joint.

Most problems of the musculoskeletal system involve, as part of their etiology, dysfunction related to aspects of muscle shortening (Janda 1978, Liebenson 1996b).

Where weakness (lack of tone) is apparently a major feature of dysfunction, it will often be found that antagonists are shortened and are reciprocally inhibiting the tone of the weakened muscles.

In most instances it is thought that, before there is any effort to strengthen weakened muscles, hypertonic antagonists should be dealt with by appropriate means, after which spontaneous toning should be anticipated in the previously relatively weak muscles (Lewit 1999a).

If tone remains reduced then, and only then, should exercise and/or isotonic muscle energy technique procedures be brought in (Chaitow 2001).

The following simple observation and/or palpation tests allow for a rapid gathering of information with a minimum of effort. They are based on the work of Janda (1983) and Liebenson (1996b).

Further assessment requirements

If any of the following tests is positive, this requires the additional assessments outlined, all of which are described later in this chapter.

1. Prone hip extension test (Box 6.13):
   - Test for weakness of gluteus maximus
   - Test for shortness if hamstrings are overactive
   - Test for shortness if erector spinae are overactive
   - Search for trigger points in all these muscles.
2. Side-lying hip abduction test (Box 6.14):
   - Test for weakness of gluteus medius
   - Test for shortness if quadratus lumborum was overactive
   - Test for shortness if tensor fascia lata was overactive
   - Search for trigger points in all these muscles.
3. Scapulohumeral rhythm test (Box 6.15):
   - Test for weakness of lower fixators of the shoulder (serratus anterior, lower and middle trapezius)
   - Test for shortness if upper trapezius was overactive
   - Test for shortness if levator scapula was overactive
   - Search for trigger points in all these muscles.

McKenzie classifications (McKenzie 1981)

Perhaps the most defining element of the McKenzie diagnostic approach is the central role it gives to patient response. As the patient is put through a series

---

Box 6.13 Exercise: Prone hip extension test

- The patient lies prone and you stand at waist level facing the patient.
- The cephalad hand spans the lower erector spinae, so that the pads of your fingers touch one side of the erector spinae and the heel of your hand touches the other, while the caudad hand rests with the thenar eminence on gluteus maximus and the fingertips on the hamstrings.
- The patient is asked to raise the leg into extension of the hip.

- The normal activation sequence is gluteus maximus and hamstrings (which of these fires first seems inconsequential; however, they should be the first two to fire), followed by erector spinae (contralateral then ipsilateral).
- If either the contra- or ipsilateral erector spinae adopt the role of gluteus maximus, as indicated by firing first, they are working inappropriately, and are therefore 'stressed' and will – by implication – have shortened.

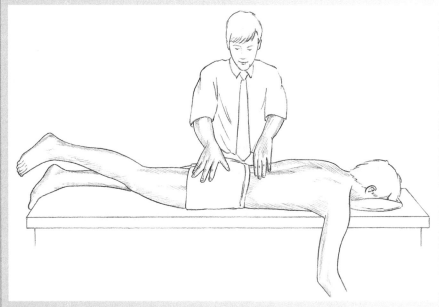

Figure 6.11 Hip extension test: the normal activation sequence is gluteus maximus, hamstrings, contralateral erector spinae, ipsilateral erector spinae. Reproduced with permission from Chaitow (2003a)

Box 6.14 Exercise: Side-lying hip abduction test

Observation

- The patient lies on the side with the lower leg flexed to provide support and the upper leg straight, in line with the trunk.
- The practitioner stands in front of the patient at the level of the feet and observes (no hands on yet) as the patient is asked to abduct the leg slowly.
- Normal = hip abduction to 45°.
- Abnormal = (1) hip flexion occurs during abduction, indicating tensor fascia lata (TFL) shortness; (2) the leg externally rotates (indicating piriformis shortening); and (3) 'hiking' of the hip occurs at the outset of the movement (indicating quadratus overactivity, and therefore, by implication, shortness).
- Individual muscles – as indicated by the test – should then be evaluated for shortness and weakness.

Functional palpation 1

- The test should be repeated with the practitioner standing behind the patient at waist level, with a finger pad on the lateral margin of quadratus lumborum. The other hand palpates simultaneously gluteus medius and TFL (Fig. 6.12).
- As the leg is abducted, if quadratus fires strongly and first (before gluteus medius), a twitch or push will be felt by the palpating finger, indicating overactivity and probable shortness of quadratus lumborum (this would show visually as a 'hip-hike', as mentioned in the observation segment of the test).

- Normal firing sequence is gluteus medius or TFL first and second, followed by quadratus lumborum at about 20–25° of leg abduction.
- If TFL is short, the leg will drift into flexion on abduction.
- If piriformis is short, the leg and foot will externally rotate during abduction.

Functional palpation 2

- The patient is side-lying and the practitioner stands facing the patient's front, at hip level.
- The patient's non-tested leg is slightly flexed to provide stability, and there should be a vertical line to the table between one anterior superior iliac spine (ASIS) and the other (i.e. no forwards or backwards 'roll' of the pelvis).
- The practitioner's cephalad hand rests over the ASIS so that it can also palpate over the trochanter, with the fingers resting on the TFL and the thumb on gluteus medius.
- The caudad hand rests on the mid-thigh to apply slight resistance to the patient's effort to abduct the leg.
- The patient abducts the upper leg (which should be extended at the knee and slightly hyperextended at the hip) and the practitioner should feel the trochanter 'slip away' as this is done.
- If, however, the whole pelvis is felt to move rather than just the trochanter, there is inappropriate muscular imbalance.

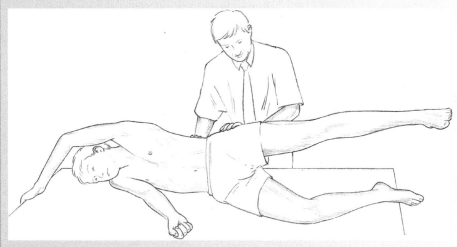

Figure 6.12 Palpation assessment for quadratus lumborum overactivity. The muscle is palpated, as is the gluteus medius and tensor fascia lata (TFL), during abduction of the leg. The correct firing sequence should be gluteus and TFL, followed at around 25° elevation by quadratus. If there is an immediate grabbing action by quadratus it indicates overactivity, and therefore stress, so shortness can be assumed. Reproduced with permission from Chaitow (2003a)

Continued

Box 6.14 Exercise: Side-lying hip abduction test continued

- In balanced abduction, gluteus medius comes into action at the beginning of the movement, with TFL operating later in the pure abduction of the leg.
- If there is overactivity (and therefore shortness) of TFL, then there will be pelvic movement on the abduction, and TFL will be felt to come into play before gluteus medius.
- The abduction of the thigh movement will have been modified to include external rotation and flexion of the thigh (Janda 1996).
- This indicates a stressed postural muscle (TFL), which implies shortness.

It may be possible (depending on the practitioner's hand size and patient anatomic size) to increase the number of palpation elements involved by having the cephalad hand also palpate (with an extended small finger) quadratus lumborum (QL) during leg abduction.

In a balanced muscular effort to lift the leg sideways, QL should not become active until the leg has been abducted to around 25–30°.

When QL is overactive it will often initiate the abduction together with TFL, thus producing a pelvic tilt.

A lateral 'corset' of muscles exists to stabilize the pelvic and low back structures, and if TFL and quadratus (and/or psoas) shorten and tighten, the gluteal muscles will be inhibited. This test strongly suggests existence of such imbalance.

Box 6.15 Exercise: Scapulohumeral rhythm test

This assessment gives information as to the status of some of the most important upper fixators of the shoulder.

This is a purely observational assessment, without touching.

- The patient is seated with the arm at the side, elbow flexed to 90° and facing forwards.
- The practitioner stands behind and observes as the patient is asked to raise the elbow towards the horizontal.
- Normal = elevation of shoulder only after 60° of shoulder abduction.
- Abnormal = elevation of the shoulder, obvious 'bunching' between the shoulder and neck (upper trapezius), or winging of the scapulae, within the first 60° of shoulder abduction.
- Any of these indicators suggests levator scapulae and upper trapezius overactivity and therefore probable shortness, associated with lower and middle trapezius, and serratus anterior inhibition (Fig. 6.13).
- This pattern, of weak lower fixators and overworked and probably shortened upper fixators, is common in postural patterns such as the crossed syndromes, involving a forward head carriage with round-shouldered stance.
- Individual muscles – as indicated by the test – should then be evaluated for shortness and weakness.

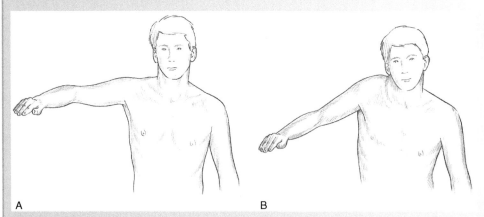

Figure 6.13 Scapulohumeral rhythm test. **A** Normal: elevation of the shoulder after 60° of abduction. **B** Abnormal: elevation of the shoulder before 60° of abduction. Reproduced with permission from Chaitow (2003a)

Box 6.16 Exercise: Greenman's functional assessment of shoulder fixator imbalance

Greenman (1996) describes a functional 'firing sequence' assessment which identifies general imbalance and dysfunction involving the upper and lower fixators of the shoulder.

- The patient is seated and the practitioner stands behind.
- The practitioner rests the right hand over the right shoulder area to assess the firing sequence of muscles during shoulder abduction.
- The other hand can be placed either on the mid-thoracic region, mainly on the side being assessed, or spanning the lower back to palpate quadratus firing.
- The assessment should be performed several times so that various hand contacts are used to evaluate the behavior of different muscles during abduction.

The 'correct' sequence for shoulder abduction (Janda 1983), when seated, involves:

1. supraspinatus
2. deltoid
3. infraspinatus
4. middle and lower trapezius
5. contralateral quadratus.

In dysfunctional states the most common substitutions are said to involve:

- shoulder elevation by levator scapulae and upper trapezius, as well as
- early firing by quadratus lumborum, ipsilateral and contralateral.

Abduction of the arm, in this position during the first 20 degrees or so, should not employ upper trapezius as a prime mover, although it does increase in tone during the procedure.

Inappropriate activity of any of the upper fixators results in shortness.

When overactivity involves the lower fixators, weakness and possible lengthening results (Norris 1999).

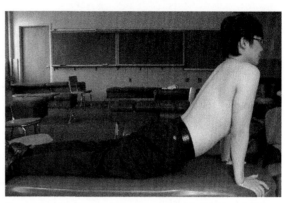

Figure 6.14 McKenzie extension position in prone. Reproduced with permission from Chaitow (2007)

Initially the patient is asked to assume a series of *static sustained* postures at end range. Each position attempts to produce a change in symptomatology by varying the spinal configuration incorporating a range from flexion to extension. This includes sitting slouched, sitting erect, standing slouched and standing erect. After this, the patient lies supine and then prone, introducing relative flexion and extension (Fig. 6.14).

To increase the degree of flexion the patient draws the knees to the chest and to increase extension the patient is supported on the forearms.

If a response is demonstrated during any of these positions no increase in that direction of flexion or extension is added – for example, if symptoms modify when lying supine, the knee-to-chest position would not be necessary.

This sequence is followed by examination of the effects of repetitive end-range movements involving both active and passive motions including standing flexion and standing extension (Table 6.2).

The patient is instructed to perform each of these movements up to 10 times in sequence, with the response assessed after each series of repetitions.

Translation and list

Lisi (2007) points out that:

*In the McKenzie system, a patient who initially presents with an antalgic list is also assessed for the response to side gliding, both standing and prone, active and passive. This assessment is typically reserved only for those patients with an initial list, with the transition movement performed **in the direction that would neutralize the list.***

Centralization

Assessment of this phenomenon is carried out as follows:

of positions and repetitive movements, the response in terms of changes in pain and other symptoms is assessed.

- Does the range of motion increase or decrease in one position or another?
- And/or does pain intensity rise or fall?
- And/or does the location of the pain change – does it become more central or more peripheral? (Aina et al 2004).

Table 6.2 The mechanical examination

Examination	Position
Static (sustained posture at end range)	• Sitting slouched, sitting erect • Standing slouched, standing erect • Lying prone in extension, lying supine in flexion
Dynamic (repetitive end-range movements)	*Active* • Flexion standing, extension standing • Flexion supine (knee to chest); extension prone (prone press up) • Side-gliding, right or left, standing or prone *Passive* • Mobilization (grades III–IV) in flexion, extension, right or left rotation

Adapted from Chaitow (2007).

• When the most distal (peripheral) symptoms (whether pain or paresthesia) are eliminated or substantially decreased during the positioning or repetitive end-range exercise.
• If the patient whose presenting symptoms are local low back pain only, that pain is eliminated.
• When the change in distal pain is the defining element, and is often independent of proximal pain. For example, if a patient with low back pain and leg pain experiences relief of leg pain even though there is an increase of low back pain, that patient has centralized.
• The converse of this is also true: the patient with relief of low back pain and an increase in leg pain has peripheralized.
• The reduction in symptoms must have some duration – seconds to minutes, perhaps hours in excellent responders.
• If, on the other hand, a patient peripheralizes, the distal pain lingers after the posture or repeated movements have stopped.

McKenzie has classified mechanical low back pain into three syndromes, each of which is defined by a theoretical model of the underlying pathology, plus patient history, postural assessment and mechanical examination findings (Razmjou et al 2000):

1. **Postural**: *Examination* findings include full and pain-free active ranges of motion, with repetitive motions also pain-free. Sustained posture at normal end of range causes pain. In such cases normal tissue is probably being strained by prolonged inappropriate posture. *Treatment* involves primarily avoiding painful positions and maintaining correct posture. (Refer to Chapter 2 – this is an example of 'reducing the adaptive load'.)

2. **Dysfunction**: Active ranges of motion are restricted in one or more directions with local pain at end range. Repetitive motions tend to be painful at end range, but such movements may increase the range of motion. The problem probably relates to chronic soft tissue contracture or fibrosis (e.g. facet capsular fibrosis, nerve root adhesions). *Treatment* may involve repetitive motions that increase pain in order to break adhesions and increase elasticity. This might include exercises and/or manual treatment, as well as application of appropriate ergonomics.

3. **Derangement**: Active ranges of motion are restricted in one or more directions as well as being painful at end range. If the cause is discogenic pain with competent annulus, then repetitive motion should reveal centralization. If, on the other hand, the cause is discogenic pain with incompetent annulus (non-contained annular tear, internal disc disruption or herniated disc), then repetitive motion will probably reveal peripheralization. *Treatment* demands that motions which centralize are performed and that motions which peripheralize are not. This might include appropriate exercises (that centralize) and/or manual treatment, as well as application of appropriate ergonomics Patients whose symptoms peripheralize during assessment using positions and movements have a poor prognosis, and usually respond poorly to conservative treatment.

Testing muscles for length (range of motion)

A comprehensive palpation protocol requires assessment for inappropriate shortness of muscles in a standardized manner. Janda (1983) suggests that to obtain a reliable evaluation of muscle shortness, the following criteria be observed during passive testing:

- The starting position, method of fixation and direction of movement must be observed carefully.
- The prime mover muscle must not be exposed to external pressure.
- If possible, the force exerted on the tested muscle must not work over two joints.
- The examiner should perform a slow movement at an even speed that brakes slowly at the end of the range.
- The examiner should keep the stretch and the muscle irritability about equal and the movement must not be jerky.
- Pressure or pull must always act in the required direction of movement.
- Muscle shortening can only be correctly evaluated if the joint range is not decreased, as might be the case should an osseous limitation or joint blockage exist.

It is in shortened muscle fibers, as a rule, that reflex activity is noted. This takes the form of local dysfunction variously called trigger points (Simons et al 1999), hyperalgesic skin zones (Lewit 1999a), tender points (Wolfe et al 1992), zones of irritability, neurovascular and neurolymphatic reflexes (Ward 1997), etc.

Localizing these areas is possible via normal palpatory methods ('drag' palpation, skin elasticity, etc.) or as part of NMT diagnostic treatment.

Identification of tight muscles may also be systematically carried out as described in the example exercises below.

Note that the assessment methods presented are not themselves diagnostic but provide strong indications of probable shortness of the muscles being tested.

Why do we need to identify muscle shortness?

Two opinions are offered in answer to this question, one from osteopathy and one from physiotherapy (physical therapy).

Greenman (1996) offers a summary of his clinical approach that demands knowledge of shortness:

After short tight muscles are stretched, muscles that are inhibited can undergo retraining . . . as in all manual medicine procedures, after assessment, stretching, and strengthening, reevaluation of faulty movement patterns . . . is done.

Dommerholt (2000), discussing enhancement of posture and function in musicians, has summarized an important concept:

In general, assessment and treatment of individual muscles must precede restoration of normal posture and normal patterns of movement. Claims that muscle imbalances would dissolve following lessons in Alexander technique are not substantiated in the scientific literature (Rosenthal 1987). Instead, muscle imbalances must be corrected through very specific strengthening and flexibility exercises . . . myofascial trigger points must be inactivated . . . [and] . . . associated joint dysfunction . . . must be corrected with joint mobilization. Once the musculoskeletal conditions of 'good posture' have been met, postural retraining can proceed.

The functional tests described above offer evidence of overactivity. If they are overactive, postural (Type 1) muscles will shorten.

The assessments below offer methods for identifying the degree of shortness in such stressed muscles.

Understanding 'ease' and 'bind'

The concept and reality of tissues providing the palpating hands or fingers with a sense of their relative 'bind', as opposed to their state of 'ease', is one which needs to be literally felt to be appreciated.

Hoover (1969) describes 'ease' as a state of equilibrium or 'neutral' which the practitioner senses by having at least one completely passive, 'listening' contact, either of the whole hand or a single or several fingers or thumb, in touch with the tissues being assessed.

Bind is, of course, the opposite of ease, and can most easily be noted by lightly palpating the tissues surrounding, or associated with, a joint as this is taken towards its end of range of movement, its resistance barrier.

The examples of assessment of shortness in muscles, given here as exercises, are meant to encourage acquisition and/or refinement of the skills required for postural muscle-length assessment, and are a representative sample only. See also the text earlier in this chapter by David Russ DC, describing abdominal/psoas palpation.

Hamstring notes: Should obviously tight hamstrings always be treated?

Van Wingerden (1997), reporting on the earlier work of Vleeming et al (1989), states that both intrinsic and extrinsic support for the sacroiliac joint derives in part from hamstring (biceps femoris) status.

Box 6.17 Exercise: Evaluation of shortness of medial hamstrings (semi-membranosus, semi-tendinosus as well as gracilis) and short adductors (pectineus, adductors brevis, magnus and longus)

First stage

Is there shortness?

1. The patient lies with the non-tested leg abducted slightly, heel over the end of the examination table.
2. The leg to be tested should be close to the edge of the table, and you should ensure that it is in its anatomically correct position: knee in full extension, and with no external rotation of the hip, which would nullify the test.
3. Stand between the patient's leg and the table, so that control of the tested leg is achieved with your lateral (non-tableside) arm/hand, while the tableside hand can rest on, and palpate, the inner thigh muscles for sensations of 'bind' as the leg is taken slowly into abduction.
4. Abduction of the tested leg is introduced passively until the first sign of resistance (first barrier) is noted (Fig. 6.15). There are three indicators of this resistance:

- A sense of increased effort will be noted by the hand carrying the leg at the moment that the first resistance barrier has been passed.
- A sense of bind should be noted by the palpating hand at this same moment.
- An observation sign can confirm this barrier. After it has been passed there will be movement of the pelvis as a whole, laterally towards the tested side.

5. If a sense of 'bind' is not palpated, and the barrier is passed (pelvis moves), repeat the process over and over until you learn to recognize the subtle 'tightening' under your palpating hand on the inner thigh.
6. If abduction produces an angle with the midline of 45° or more, before a first resistance barrier is reached, then no further testing of these muscles is required, as the degree of abduction is normal and there is probably no shortness in the short or long adductors.

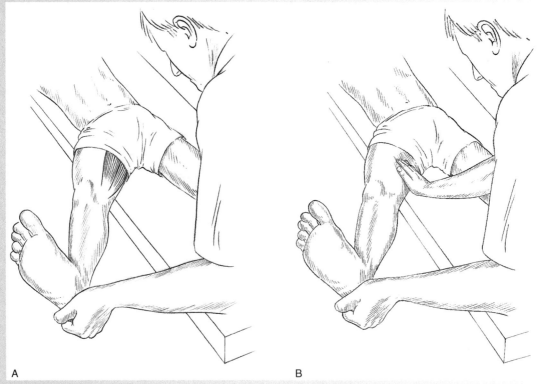

A   B

Figure 6.15 Assessment of 'bind'/restriction barrier with the first sign of resistance in the adductors (medial hamstrings) of the right leg. **A** The practitioner's perception of the transition point, where easy movement alters to demand some degree of effort, is regarded as the barrier. **B** The barrier is identified when the palpating hand notes a sense of bind in tissues which were relaxed (at ease) up to that point. Reproduced with permission from Chaitow (2001)

Box 6.17 Exercise: Evaluation of shortness of medial hamstrings (semi-membranosus, semi-tendinosus as well as gracilis) and short adductors (pectineus, adductors brevis, magnus and longus) continued

7. If, however, the barrier is sensed, or observed, before a 45° angle is achieved (without effort, or a sense of bind in the tissues), then a shortness restriction exists in either the medial hamstrings or the short adductors of the thigh.

8. A screening assessment is required to evaluate which of these has shortened.

Second stage

If there is shortness, does this exist in the short adductors (one-joint muscles) or in the long adductors (two-joint muscles)?

1. Precisely the same test is carried out; however, when the first resistance barrier is reached, flexion of the knee is introduced, so that the lower leg hangs down freely.

2. If, after knee flexion has been introduced, further abduction is now easily achieved to 45° when previously it was restricted, this indicates that any previous limitation into abduction was the result of medial hamstring (long adductor) shortness.

3. If, however, restriction remains once knee flexion has been introduced to the abducted leg, as evidenced by continued restriction in movement towards a 45° excursion, then the short adductors are at fault and are restraining movement towards the barrier.

4. After the short adductors have been appropriately treated/released it will still be necessary to retest abduction with the leg straight, as the fact that the short adductors are short does not remove the possibility that the medial hamstrings (two-joint adductors) may also be short.

Intrinsically, the influence is via the close anatomic and physiological relationship between biceps femoris and the sacrotuberous ligament (they frequently attach via a strong tendinous link):

> Force from the biceps femoris muscle can lead to increased tension of the sacrotuberous ligament in various ways. Since increased tension of the sacrotuberous ligament diminishes the range of sacroiliac joint motion, the biceps femoris can play a role in stabilisation of the SIJ.

Van Wingerden also notes that in low back patients forward flexion is often painful as the load on the spine increases. This happens whether flexion occurs in the spine or via the hip joints (tilting of the pelvis). If the hamstrings are tight and short they effectively prevent pelvic tilting: 'In this respect, an increase in hamstring tension might well be part of a defensive arthrokinematic reflex mechanism of the body to diminish spinal load.' Under such circumstances the hamstrings (biceps femoris) would shorten, possibly influencing sacroiliac and lumbar spine dysfunction.

The decision to treat tight ('tethered') hamstrings should therefore take account of *why there is excessive tightness*, noting that, in some circumstances, this might be offering beneficial support to the sacroiliac joint, or reducing low back stress.

Quadratus lumborum notes

Norris (2002a) describes the divided roles in which quadratus is involved:

- The quadratus lumborum stabilizes lumbar spinal movements (McGill et al 1996), while tightening has also been described.

- The muscle may act functionally differently in its medial and lateral portions, with the medial portion being more active as a stabilizer of the lumbar spine, and the lateral more active as a mobilizer (Janda 1983).

- Quadratus fibers merge with the diaphragm (as do those of psoas), which makes involvement in respiratory dysfunction a possibility since it plays a role in exhalation, both via this merging and by its attachment to the 12th rib.

- Shortness of quadratus, or the presence of trigger points, can result in pain in the lower ribs and along the iliac crest if the lateral fibers are affected.

- Shortness of the medial fibers, or the presence of trigger points, can produce pain in the sacroiliac joint and the buttock.

- Bilateral contraction produces extension and unilateral contraction produces extension and side-flexion to the same side.

- The important transition region, the lumbodorsal junction (LDJ), is the only one in the spine in which two mobile structures meet, and dysfunction results in alteration of the quality of motion between these structures (upper and lower trunk/dorsal and lumbar spines).

Box 6.18 Exercise: Evaluation of shortness of hamstrings

Method A

If the hip flexors (psoas etc.) are short, then the test position for the hamstrings needs to commence with the non-tested leg flexed at both knee and hip, and the foot resting flat on the treatment surface to ensure full pelvic rotation into neutral. If there is no hip flexor shortness, the non-tested leg should lie flat on the surface of the table.

- The patient lies supine with non-tested leg either flexed or straight, depending on hip flexor status.
- The tested leg is taken into a straight leg raised (SLR) position, no flexion of the knee being allowed, with minimal force.
- The first sign of resistance (or palpated bind) is assessed as the barrier of restriction.
- It is useful at this point to gently 'spring' the tissues to obtain a sense of the end-feel (see notes on palpation barrier earlier in this chapter).
- If straight leg raising to 80° is not easily possible, then there is some shortening of the hamstrings and the muscles can be treated in this straight leg position.

Method B

Whether or not an 80° elevation is easily achieved with the leg straight, a variation in testing is needed to evaluate the lower hamstring fibers.

- To achieve this assessment the tested leg is taken into full hip flexion (helped by the patient holding the upper thigh with both hands) (Fig. 6.16).
- The knee is then slowly straightened until resistance is felt, or bind is noted by palpation of the lower hamstrings.

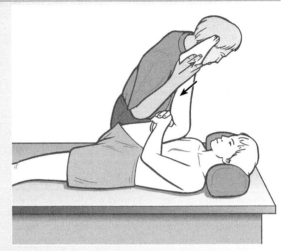

Figure 6.16 Assessment and treatment position for lower hamstring fibers. Reproduced with permission from Chaitow (2001)

- If the knee cannot straighten with the hip flexed, this indicates shortness in the lower hamstring fibers, and the patient will report a degree of pull behind the knee and lower thigh.
- It is useful at this point to gently 'spring' the tissues to obtain a sense of the end-feel (see notes on palpation barrier earlier in this chapter).
- If the knee is capable of being straightened, with the hip flexed, having previously not been capable of achieving an 80° straight leg raise, then the lower fibers are not responsible for the restriction, and it is the upper fibers of hamstrings that require attention.

- In dysfunction there is often a degree of spasm or tightness in the muscles which stabilize the region, notably psoas and erector spinae of the thoracolumbar region, as well as quadratus lumborum and rectus abdominis:

Symptomatic differential diagnosis of muscle involvement at the LDJ is possible as follows:

- Psoas involvement usually triggers abdominal pain if severe and produces flexion of the hip and the typical antalgesic posture of lumbago.
- Erector spinae involvement produces low back pain at its caudad end of attachment and interscapular pain at its thoracic attachment (as far up as the mid-thoracic level).

- Quadratus lumborum involvement causes lumbar pain and pain at the attachment of the iliac crest and lower ribs.
- Rectus abdominis contraction may mimic abdominal pain and result in pain at the attachments at the pubic symphysis and the xiphoid process, as well as forward flexion of the trunk and restricted ability to extend the spine.

Lewit (1999a) points out that even if a number of these muscles are implicated, it is seldom necessary to treat them all since, as the muscles most involved (discovered by tests for shortness, overactivity, sensitivity and direct palpation) are stretched and normalized, so others will begin automatically to normalize.

Box 6.19 Exercise: Evaluation of shortness of paravertebral muscles (e.g. erector spinae)

Assessment for paravertebral muscle shortness

- The patient is seated on a treatment table, legs extended if the hamstrings tested as normal, and with knees slightly flexed if the hamstrings were short.
- The pelvis should be vertical, not tilted backwards or forwards.
- Spinal flexion is introduced in order to approximate the forehead to the knees.
- An even, 'C'-shaped curve should be observed and a distance of about 4 inches (10 cm) from the knees achieved by the forehead.
- The movement should be a spinal one, not involving pelvic tilting.

Interpretation

- Areas of shortening in the paraspinal muscles may be observed as 'flatness', or even, in the lumbar area, as a reversed curve.
- For example, on forward flexion a lordosis may be maintained in the lumbar spine, or flexion may be very limited even without such lordosis.
- There may be evidence of obvious overstretching of the upper back and relative tightness of the lower back.
- All areas of 'flatness' are charted since these represent an inability of those segments to flex, which involves the erector spinae muscles as either a primary or a secondary feature (if the failure to flex lies in the articulation itself).
- Even if the flexion restriction relates to articular factors, the erector group may be shortened.

Note: Lewit (1999a) points out that patients with a long trunk and short thighs may perform the flexion movement without apparent difficulty, even if the paraspinal muscles are short, whereas if the trunk is short and the thighs long, even if the erectors are supple, flexion will not allow the head to approximate the knees.

Box 6.20 Exercise: Evaluation of shortness of quadratus lumborum

Evaluation of quadratus lumborum (QL) overactivity (and by implication shortness) was described in the hip abduction test.
The degree of shortness can be confirmed as follows:

- The patient stands, back towards the crouching practitioner.
- Any leg-length disparity (based on pelvic crest height) is equalized by placing a book or pad under the heel of the short leg.
- With the patient's feet shoulder width apart, a pure side-flexion is requested, so that the patient runs a hand down the lateral thigh/calf. (Normal level of side-flexion excursion allows the fingertips to reach to just below the knee.)
- If side-flexion to one side is limited, then QL on the opposite side is probably short.
- Combined evidence from the functional test (see Fig. 6.12) and this side-flexion test indicates whether or not it is necessary to treat QL for shortness.

monly a posteriority of the ilium associated with short tensor fascia lata (TFL).

In addition:

- Mennell (1964) and Liebenson (2005) maintain that TFL shortness can produce all the symptoms of acute and chronic sacroiliac problems.
- Pain from TFL shortness can be localized to the posterior superior iliac spine (PSIS), radiating to the groin or down any aspect of the thigh to the knee.
- TFL can be 'riddled' with sensitive fibrotic deposits and trigger point activity.
- If TFL and psoas are short, they may, according to Janda (1996), 'dominate' the gluteals on abduction of the thigh, so that a degree of lateral rotation and flexion of the hip will be produced, rotating the pelvis backwards.

Tensor fascia lata notes

Rolf (1977) points out that persistent exercise such as cycling will shorten and toughen the fascial iliotibial band 'until it becomes reminiscent of a steel cable'. This band crosses both hip and knee, and spatial compression allows it to squeeze and compress cartilaginous elements such as the menisci. Ultimately, it will no longer be able to compress, and rotational displacement at knee and hip will take place. There is com-

Upper trapezius notes

Lewit (1999a) simplifies the need to assess for shortness of this muscle, by stating: 'The upper trapezius should be treated if tender and taut.'

Since this is an almost universal state in modern life, it seems that everyone requires MET (muscle energy technique, see Chapter 7) application to this muscle. Lewit also notes that a characteristic mounding of the muscle can often be observed when it is very short,

Box 6.21 Exercise: Evaluation of shortness of tensor fascia lata

- The test recommended is a modified form of Ober's test.
- The patient is side-lying with the back close to the edge of the table.
- The practitioner stands behind the patient, whose lower leg is flexed at hip and knee and held in this position, by the patient, for stability.
- The tested leg is supported by the practitioner, who must ensure that there is no hip flexion, which would nullify the test.
- The leg is extended to the position where the iliotibial band lies over the greater trochanter.
- The tested leg is held by the practitioner at both ankle and knee, with the whole leg in its anatomic position, neither abducted nor adducted, and not forward or backward of the trunk.
- The practitioner carefully introduces flexion at the knee to 90°, without allowing the hip to flex, and then, while supporting the limb at the ankle, allows the knee to fall towards the table.
- If the TFL is normal, the thigh and knee will fall easily, with the knee usually contacting the table surface (unless unusual hip width or a short thigh length prevents this).
- If the tested side leg remains aloft, with little sign of 'falling' towards the table, then either the patient is not letting go, or TFL is short and does not allow it to fall.
- As a rule the band will palpate as tender under such conditions.

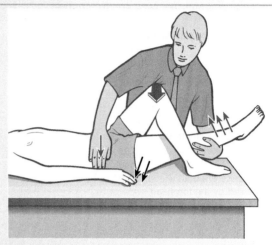

Figure 6.17 MET treatment of tensor fascia lata. If a standard MET method is being used, the stretch will follow the isometric contraction in which the patient will attempt to move the right leg to the right against sustained resistance. It is important for the practitioner to maintain stability of the pelvis during the procedure. Reproduced with permission from Chaitow (2001)

producing the effect of 'Gothic shoulders', similar to the architectural supports of a Gothic church tower.

If the scapulohumeral rhythm test is positive, then, by implication, upper trapezius (and levator scapulae) will be overactive and so will have shortened, and will probably house trigger points (see discussions of postural and phasic muscles earlier in this chapter).

If Greenman's functional assessment of firing sequence is positive, the same implications exist: overactivity leads to shortening of the postural muscles involved (such as upper trapezius and levator scapulae) and inhibition of the antagonists (serratus anterior and lower trapezii) with implications for shoulder dysfunction amongst others.

Assessing and grading muscle weakness and endurance

The functional tests described earlier, in which hip abduction, hip extension and the scapulohumeral rhythm were evaluated, may have offered evidence of imbalances between opposing muscles (e.g. upper trapezius–lower trapezius).

In these functional tests firing sequences may at times have differed from the proposed norm (Janda 1983, Liebenson 2005), with implications for overactivity, and therefore shortness, in specific muscles (postural/Type 1), or inhibition/weakness in others (phasic/Type 2), as discussed earlier.

Further assessment may now have demonstrated actual shortness in muscles implicated in the functional testing sequences.

Inhibition of the phasic muscles involved in those functional tests is probable – but to what degree?

Strength tests of these muscles allow them to be graded from virtually 'no strength/no contraction' to 'movement possible against resistance'.

In order to test a muscle for strength a standard procedure is carried out as follows:

- The area should be relaxed and not influenced by gravity.

Box 6.22 Exercise: Evaluation of shortness of upper trapezius

- The patient is supine with the neck fully (but not forcefully) side-bent contralaterally (away from the side being assessed).
- The practitioner is standing at the head of the table and uses a cupped hand contact on the ipsilateral shoulder (i.e. on the side being tested) to assess the ease with which it can be depressed (moved caudally) (Fig. 6.18).
- There should be an easy 'springing' sensation as the practitioner eases the shoulder towards the feet, with a soft end-feel to the movement.

- If depression of the shoulder is difficult, or if there is a harsh, sudden endpoint, upper trapezius shortness is confirmed.
- This same assessment (always with full lateral flexion) should be performed with the head fully rotated away from the side being tested, half turned away from the side being tested, and slightly turned towards the side being tested, in order to assess the relative shortness and functional efficiency respectively of posterior, middle and anterior subdivisions of the upper portion of trapezius.

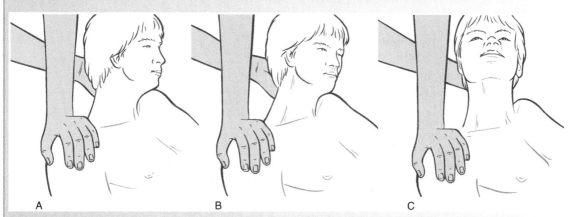

A   B   C

Figure 6.18 MET treatment of right side upper trapezius muscle. **A** Posterior fibers, **B** middle fibers, **C** anterior fibers. Note that stretching in this (or any of the alternative positions which access the middle and posterior fibers) is achieved following the isometric contraction by means of an easing of the shoulder away from the stabilized head, with no force being applied to the neck and head itself. Reproduced with permission from Chaitow (2001)

Box 6.23 Exercise: Evaluation of shortness of levator scapula

- The patient lies supine with the arm of the side to be tested lying flat against the examination table, with the supinated hand and lower arm tucked under the buttocks, to help restrain movement of the shoulder/ scapula.
- The practitioner's contralateral arm is passed across and under the neck to cup the shoulder of the side to be tested, with the forearm supporting the neck.
- The practitioner's other hand supports and guides the head.
- The forearm is used to lift the neck into *full pain-free flexion* (aided by the hand on the head).
- Once fully flexed, the neck/head is placed fully towards side-flexion and rotation, *away* from the side being treated.

- With the shoulder held caudally and the neck/head in the position described (at the resistance barrier), stretch is being placed on levator from both ends.
- If dysfunction exists and/or levator scapula is short, there will be discomfort reported at the attachment on the upper medial border of the scapula, and/or pain reported near the levator attachment on the spinous process of C2.
- The hand on the shoulder should then gently 'spring' it caudally.
- If levator scapula is short there will be a *harsh*, wooden, 'blocked' feel to this action; if it is normal there will be a soft springing response.

- The area/muscle/joint should be positioned so that whatever movement is to be used can be comfortably performed.
- The patient should be asked to perform a concentric contraction that is evaluated against a scale, as outlined below.
- The degree of resistance required to prevent movement is a subjective judgment, unless mechanical resistance and/or electronic measurement is available.

For more detailed understanding of muscle strength evaluation, Janda's *Muscle Function Testing* (1983) is recommended. For an understanding of endurance features, Norris's *Back Stability* (2000b) is recommended.

Scale for evaluation of concentric contractions (Janda 1983)

Grade 0 = no contraction/paralysis

Grade 1 = no motion noted but contraction felt by palpating hand

Grade 2 = some movement possible on contraction, if gravity influence eliminated ('poor')

Grade 3 = motion possible against gravity's influence ('fair')

Grade 4 = movement possible during contraction against resistance ('good')

In the tests described below it is not only strength that is being evaluated, but also endurance. There is little value in strength if it cannot be maintained for more than a few seconds.

In these strength and endurance tests (for gluteus maximus, gluteus medius and psoas) a protocol is suggested by Norris (1999), as follows:

'Inner holding isometric endurance' tests can be performed for muscles which have a tendency to lengthen, in order to assess their ability to maintain joint alignment in a neutral zone. Usually a lengthened muscle will demonstrate a loss of endurance when tested in a shortened position. This can be tested by the practitioner passively pre-positioning the muscle in a shortened position and assessing the duration of time that the patient can hold the muscle in the shortened position. There are various methods used, including:

- *Ten repetitions of the holding position for 10 seconds at a time*
- *Alternatively, a single 30-second hold can be requested.*

If the patient cannot hold the position actively from the moment of passive pre-positioning, this is a sign of inappropriate antagonist muscle shortening.

Box 6.24 Exercise: Evaluation of weakness/endurance of gluteus maximus

- Patient is prone.
- Practitioner lifts one leg into extension at the hip (knee flexed to 90°) by approximately 5 cm (Fig. 6.19).
- Patient is asked to hold the leg in this position.
- Assess results based on criteria outlined above.

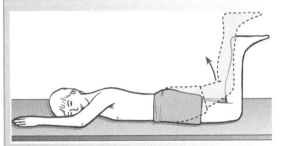

Figure 6.19 Gluteus maximus strength and stamina test. Reproduced with permission from Chaitow (2001)

Box 6.25 Exercise: Evaluation of weakness/endurance of gluteus medius

- Patient is side-lying with uppermost leg flexed at hip and knee so that both the knee and foot are resting on the floor/surface.
- Practitioner places the flexed leg into a position of maximal unforced external rotation at the hip, foot still resting on the floor (Fig. 6.20).
- Patient is asked to maintain this position.
- Assess results based on criteria outlined above.

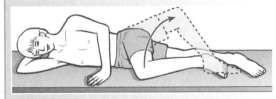

Figure 6.20 Posterior fibers gluteus medius strength and stamina test. Reproduced with permission from Chaitow (2001)

Optimal endurance is indicated when the full inner range position can be held for 10 to 20 seconds.

Muscle lengthening is present if the limb falls away from the inner range position immediately.

Box 6.26 Exercise: Evaluation of weakness/ endurance of psoas

- Patient is seated.
- Practitioner lifts one leg into greater hip flexion so that foot is well clear of the floor.
- Patient is asked to hold this position.
- Assess results based on criteria outlined above.

These testing procedures can become treatment. The patient can be asked to repeat the simple positioning described above, regularly at home, until there is an ability to maintain the test position for 30 seconds without difficulty, or there is an ability to repeat 10 repetitions of 10 seconds.

Assessment of neural mobility in relation to its mechanical interface

The tissues that surround neural structures have been called the mechanical interface (MI). Any pathology in the MI can produce abnormalities in nerve movement, resulting in tension on neural structures with unpredictable ramifications.

Good examples of MI pathology are nerve impingement by disc protrusion or osteophyte contact and carpal tunnel constriction. These problems can be regarded as mechanical in origin as far as the nerve restriction is concerned.

Chemical or inflammatory causes of neural tension can result in 'interneural fibrosis' leading to reduced elasticity and increased 'tension', which would become obvious during tension testing (see below).

Provocation tests that involve movement rather than pure (passive) tension are most effective.

Maitland (1986) suggests that this form of assessment and treatment should be considered as 'mobilization' of the neural structures, rather than simply stretching them, and that these methods be reserved for conditions that fail to respond adequately to normal mobilization of soft and osseous structures (muscles, joints and so on).

Butler & Gifford (1991) described assessment and treatment protocols for those mechanical restrictions that impinge on neural structures in the vertebral canals and elsewhere.

A positive tension test is one in which the patient's symptoms are reproduced by the test procedure and where these symptoms can be altered by variations in what are termed 'sensitising manoeuvres', which are used to 'add weight to', and confirm, the initial diagnosis of AMT [adverse mechanical tension] – for

example, adding dorsiflexion during the straight leg raising test is an example of a sensitising manoeuvre.

Precise symptom reproduction may not be possible, but the test is still relevant if other abnormal symptoms are produced during the test, or its accompanying sensitising procedures.

Comparison with the test findings on an opposite limb, for example, may indicate an abnormality worth exploring.

Altered range of movement is another indicator of abnormality, whether this is noted during the initial test position or during sensitising additions.

When a tension test is positive (i.e. pain or other sensations result from one or another element of the test – for example, initial position alone, or with 'sensitizing' additions) it indicates only that there exists abnormal mechanical tension (AMT) somewhere in the nervous system, and not that this is necessarily at the site of reported pain.

For more detail of this assessment and treatment approach, the book by Butler & Gifford (1991) is recommended.

Two examples of AMT testing are given below: the straight leg raising (SLR) test and two upper limb tension tests (ULTT 1 and 2).

Notes on the straight leg raising (SLR) test

On SLR there is caudad movement of the lumbosacral nerve roots in relation to interfacing tissue (Butler & Gifford 1991), which is why there is a 'positive' indication – pain and limitation of leg-raising potential – from SLR if a prolapsed intervertebral disc exists.

Less well known is the fact that the tibial nerve, proximal to the knee, moves caudad (in relation to the mechanical interface) during SLR, whereas distal to the knee it moves cranially. There is no movement of the tibial nerve behind the knee itself, which is therefore known as a 'tension point'.

Additionally, the common peroneal nerve is attached firmly to the head of the fibula (another 'tension point').

Notes on upper limb tension tests (ULTT) 1 and 2

Butler & Gifford (1991) have demonstrated that a great deal of nerve movement occurs during this test.

- In cadavers, up to 2 cm movement of the median nerve has been observed during neck and wrist movement, in relation to its mechanical interface.

Box 6.27 Exercise: Straight leg raising (SLR) test

It is suggested that this test should be used in all vertebral disorders, all lower limb disorders and some upper limb disorders to establish the possibility of AMT in the nervous system in the lower back or lower limb.

The leg of the supine patient is raised in the sagittal plane, with the knee extended, until a barrier of resistance is noted, or symptoms are reported. Sensitizing additions might include:

- ankle dorsiflexion (this stresses the tibial component of the sciatic nerve)
- ankle plantarflexion, plus inversion (this stresses the common peroneal nerve, which may be useful with anterior shin and dorsal foot symptoms)
- passive neck flexion
- increased medial hip rotation
- increased hip adduction
- altered spinal position (e.g. during left SLR lateral flexion to the right of the spine may produce or modify symptoms).

Perform the SLR test and incorporate each sensitizing addition, in order to assess changes in symptoms, new symptoms, restrictions, etc.

Can the leg be raised as far as it should normally go (approximately 80°), and as easily, without force and without symptoms (new or old) appearing when the sensitizing additions are incorporated?

- 'Tension points' in the upper limb, where nerve is tethered to bone, are found at the shoulder and elbow.
- During ULTTs cervical lateral flexion away from the tested side causes increased arm symptoms in 93% of people, while cervical lateral flexion towards the tested side increases symptoms in 70% of cases.

Additional neurological assessments

This chapter is not designed to provide a comprehensive 'how to' series of evaluation and assessment tools. Rather it offers samples and examples with deeper understanding of the methods involved and the principles behind their use being the role of textbooks, teachers and researchers. Some further reading suggestions are made later in this chapter.

David Shipley DC ND has provided a summary of some of the key issues relating to neurological assessment in Box 6.29. It is suggested that student naturopaths practice such tests on as wide a range of individuals as possible, ideally involving those with, and those without, symptoms, so that 'norms' become familiar.

Notes on hypermobility assessment

Hypermobile ligaments and muscles do not adequately protect joints and therefore fail to prevent excessive ranges of motion from being explored.

Without this stability, overuse and injury stresses evolve and muscular overuse is inevitable, and indeed hypermobility has been shown to be a major risk factor in the evolution of low back pain. Muller et al (2003) studied over 300 patients with back pain, using among other methods Janda's functional tests, and found that approximately one-third (112 patients, predominantly female) demonstrated constitutional hypermobility compared with 13% of normal controls. They conclude: 'Hypermobility proved to be an independent factor in the genesis of chronic back pain. Therefore hypermobility should be considered in the clinical examination of each back pain patient.'

There also appears to be a link between hypermobility and increased risk of musculoskeletal pain in general (Karaaslan et al 2000, Russek 1999).

Janda (1986) observes that, in his experience: 'In races in which hypermobility is common there is a prevalence of muscular and tendon pain, whereas typical back pain or sciatica is rare.'

Significant ethnic differences in the presence of hypermobility have been noted. Al-Rawi et al (1985), supported by subsequent research by Hudson et al (1995), showed that prevalence rates of hypermobility vary markedly, depending upon the population being examined, and range between 5% in Caucasian adults to rates as high as 38% in younger Middle Eastern women.

Logically, the excessive work rate of muscles that are adopting the role of 'pseudoligaments' leads to tendon stress and muscle dysfunction, increasing tone in the antagonists of whatever is already weakened and complicating an already complex set of imbalances, including altered patterns of movement (Beighton 1983).

Notes on evaluation of joint play

Joint play refers to the particular movements between bones associated with either separation of the surfaces (as in traction) or parallel movement of joint surfaces (also known as translation or translatoric gliding). Some degree of such movement is possible between most joints.

Any change in length of a joint's associated soft tissues automatically alters the range of joint mobility – also known as the degree of 'slack' – which is available.

Box 6.28 Exercise: Upper limb tension test (ULTT)

ULTT 1

- Your patient/palpation partner should be supine with the side to be tested close to the edge of the table.
- You stand on that side, at chest level, facing cephalad.
- Your tableside hand should stabilize the shoulder and depresses it slightly, caudally.
- With the non-tableside hand holding the patient's wrist, sequentially place the tested arm into approximately 110° abduction, full extension and lateral rotation of the glenohumeral joint.
- Once these positions are established, supination of the forearm should be introduced, together with elbow extension.
- This is followed by the addition of passive wrist and finger extension.

If pain is experienced at any stage during placement of the person into the test position, or during addition of sensitization maneuvers (below), particularly reproduction of neck, shoulder or arm symptoms that have previously been reported, the test is positive and confirms a degree of mechanical interference affecting neural structures.

Additional sensitization includes:

- adding cervical lateral flexion, away from the side being tested

- introduction of ULTT 1 on the other arm, simultaneously
- the simultaneous use of straight leg raising, bi- or unilaterally
- introduction of pronation rather than supination of the wrist.

ULTT 2

In using ULTT 2, comparison is always made with the other arm.

- For a right side test the patient lies close to the right side of the table, so that the scapula is free of the surface.
- The trunk and legs are angled towards the left foot of the bed so that the patient feels secure.
- The practitioner stands to the side of the patient's head, facing the feet with the practitioner's left thigh depressing the shoulder girdle.
- The patient's fully flexed right arm is supported at both elbow and wrist by the practitioner's hands.
- Slight variations in the degree and angle of shoulder depression ('lifted' towards ceiling, held towards floor) may be used, by alteration of the thigh contact.
- Holding the shoulder depressed, the practitioner's right hand grasps the patient's right wrist while the upper arm is held by the practitioner's left hand (Fig. 6.21).

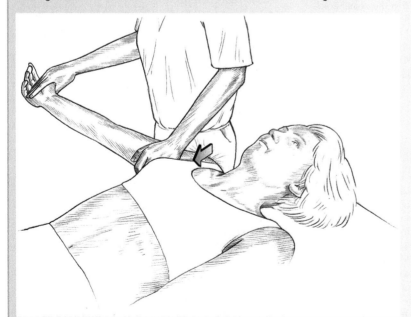

Figure 6.21 Upper limb tension test. Note the practitioner's thigh depresses the shoulder as sensitizing maneuvers are carried out. Reproduced with permission from Chaitow (2003a)

Continued

Box 6.28 Exercise: Upper limb tension test (ULTT) continued

With these contacts, the following sensitization maneuvers can be introduced to the tested arm:

- shoulder internal or external rotation
- elbow flexion or extension
- forearm supination or pronation.

The practitioner then slides the right hand down onto the open hand and introduces supination or pronation or stretching of fingers/thumb or radial and ulnar deviations.

Further sensitization may involve:

- neck movement (side-bend away from tested side, for example), or
- altered shoulder position, such as increased abduction or extension.

A combination of shoulder internal rotation, elbow extension and forearm pronation (with the shoulder constantly depressed) is considered to offer the most sensitive test position.

Box 6.29 Neurological examination

David J. Shipley DC ND

A thorough neurological evaluation ordinarily tests cranial nerves, cognition, muscle strength, reflexes, percussion, vibration and dermatomal sensitivity. While some guidelines are offered below, these are not comprehensive. It is advisable that ND students review the methods of complete neurological testing as presented in the medical literature.

Physiological reflexes

Lower motor neuron reflexes are also known as 'deep tendon reflexes' (DTR). The neuroreflex signal is transmitted to the anterior horn cell in the spinal cord, and immediately returns through the peripheral nerve to the corresponding muscle, without seeking input from the higher centers in the brain. (The information relay takes place at that level of the spinal cord.)

Deep tendon reflexes can be graded as follows:

0	Absent
+1	Diminished
+2	Normal
+3	Increased
+4	Exaggerated (or hyperactive)

- *C5 – Biceps reflex* (*DTR*): With the patient's flexed forearm resting on your non-dominant forearm, place your same side thumb over the biceps tendon. Briskly tap the nail of your thumb with a neurological hammer. There should be an observable rebound, causing the patient's forearm to flex.
- *C6 – Brachioradialis reflex* (*DTR*): Tap the brachioradialis tendon at the distal end of the radius. The patient's hand should rebound to the radial side of their forearm.
- *C7 – Triceps reflex* (*DTR*): Tap the triceps tendon where it crosses the olecranon fossa. There should be a rebound, causing the patient's forearm to extend.

- *L4 – Patellar reflex* (*DTR*): The patient sits with feet hanging freely. Locate and briskly tap their infrapatellar tendon with the narrow end of a reflex hammer. You should observe a notable rebound, i.e. quick extension of the leg. If this reflex is difficult to obtain, Jendrassik's maneuver may be added. Ask the patient to hook the flexed fingers together and pull apart as hard as possible, while you repeat the test.
- *S1 – Achilles reflex* (*DTR*): Bring the Achilles tendon into slight tension by dorsiflexing the patient's foot. With the flat end of the reflex hammer, tap this tendon just superior to the calcaneus bone. Involuntary plantar flexion should occur.
- Achilles reflexes which are sluggish bilaterally, with a slow return to normal position, may be due to insufficient function of the thyroid.

Pathological reflex (Babinski's reflex)

This is tested by rapidly passing a blunt instrument across the plantar surface of the foot, from the heel to the lateral border. In a negative (normal) reaction, either the toes do not move at all, or they all bunch up in plantar flexion.

A positive reaction causes the great toe to extend, while the others plantarflex and splay. This indicates the presence of an upper motor neuron lesion, usually from brain damage brought on by trauma or an expanding tumor. In a newborn baby, however, a positive Babinski's is normal.

Nerve sensitivity tests

Hypoesthesia and hyperesthesia are identified clinically by lightly passing a Wartenberg pinwheel over a patient's neck, arms, forearms, thorax, thighs and legs, and asking for feedback: Does it feel sharp or dull? This test evaluates the dorsal columns of the spinal cord, which are responsible for light touch and joint sensation.

Box 6.29 Neurological examination continued

- *Two-point discrimination and vibratory sense tests* demonstrate the function of receptors in the cerebral cortex.
- *Temperature and nociceptive stimuli* (pain and crude touch) are relayed in the ventrolateral cord.

Percussion testing

Tapping the spinous processes with a neurological hammer helps to identify the level of a spinal lesion. Sharp (acute) pain that dissipates quickly may indicate joint pathology. Dull pain that disappears slowly suggests a fracture, neoplasm, or other bone disease.

Vibration testing

This is performed by striking a C-128 tuning fork and placing its handle on the various bony surfaces, including the spinous and transverse processes. Tenderness over an articulation indicates possible inflammation. Increased pain over an area of direct trauma suggests possible fracture of bone. (It is wise to never rely on this screening test in lieu of x-ray or scan evidence, since false negatives can and do occur.)

Grip strength test

A reliable instrument for determining grip strength is the Jamar hand dynamometer. The patient holds this in one hand, with the elbow flexed to 90° and supported by the side of the thorax. During the grip test, palpate your patient's forearm to determine the level of effort. This reduces the chances of being fooled by malingering. (Petty & Moore (2001a) report that it is advisable (Pryce 1980) for the wrist to be between 0 and 15° of extension during the test.)

Three readings should be taken in succession, and then averaged. As an example, these are recorded as follows: (R) 80/80/80 and (L) 70/70/70. Be sure to note if your patient is right- or left-hand dominant. The testing procedure using a hand dynamometer consists of all the following steps:

1. Opening the hand, which requires simultaneous action of intrinsic muscles and the long extensor muscles of the hand.
2. Closing the fingers to grasp the object and adapt to its shape.
3. Exerted force to perform the test.
4. Release, in which the hand opens to let go of the object.

See orthopedic assessment in Box 6.46, later in this chapter, for additional test descriptions.

Kuchera & Kuchera (1994), discussing the subtalar joint, note:

This is a 'shock-absorber', a designation earned, they say, because, in coordination with the intertarsal joints, it determines the distribution of forces upon the skeleton and soft tissues of the foot.

Mennell (1964) graphically describes this shock-absorbing potential:

Its most important movement is a rocking movement of the talus upon the calcaneus, which is entirely independent of voluntary muscle action. It is this movement which takes up all the stresses and strains of stubbing the toes, and that spares the ankle from gross trauma, both on toe-off and at heel-strike, in the normal function of walking, and when abnormal stresses . . . are inflicted on the ankle joint. If it were not for the involuntary rocking motion at the subtalar joint, fracture dislocations would be more commonplace.

Similar shock-absorbing potential exists at the sacroiliac joint, and when this is lost as in cases where the joint has fused, this can result in fractures of the sacrum (Greenman 1996).

Barriers and end-feel

All joints have 'normal' ranges of motion. The end of a joint's range of motion may be described as having a certain 'end-feel'.

If a joint is taken actively or passively to its maximum range of normal motion it reaches its physiological barrier. This has a firm but not harsh end-feel.

If movement is taken to its absolute limit, the anatomic barrier is engaged and this has a hard end-feel, beyond which any movement would produce damage.

Kaltenborn (1985) has summarized normal end-feel variations: 'The ability to see and feel the quality of movement is of special significance in manual therapy, as slight alterations from the normal may often be the only clue to a correct diagnosis.'

1. *Normal soft* end-feel is due to soft tissue approximation (such as in knee flexion) or soft tissue stretching (as in ankle dorsiflexion).
2. *Normal firm* end-feel results from capsular or ligamentous stretching (internal rotation of the femur, for example).
3. *Normal hard* end-feel occurs when bone meets bone, as in elbow extension.

Box 6.30 Exercise: Hypermobility assessment

Assessment of true hypermobility requires a comprehensive observation and assessment process. This is well described in Chapter 9, *Physiotherapy Assessment of the Hypermobile Adult*, in Keer & Grahame (2003).

Lewit (1992) offers clear clinical guidelines for examination of hypermobility. He suggests ranges of movement that are: (1) hypomobile to normal; (2) slightly hypermobile; or (3) markedly hypermobile.

Lewit (1992, p. 116) makes an important observation: 'There is great variability not only between individuals but also according to age and sex. What may be considered hypermobile in an adult male may be perfectly normal in a female or an adolescent or child.'

Based on the work of Beighton et al (1973), Nijs (2005) offers five specific assessments that abbreviate the comprehensive assessments called for by Lewit and Keer & Grahame, and which offer an accurate indication of hypermobility.

Patients are given a score ranging from 0 to 9, based on 1 point being allocated for the ability to perform each of the following tests unilaterally, and 2 points if they perform them bilaterally.

Can the patient:

- passively dorsiflex the 5th metacarpophalangeal joint to more than 90° (1 point each side)
- oppose the thumb to the volar aspect of the ipsilateral forearm (1 point each side)
- hyperextend the elbow by more than 10° (1 point each side) (Fig. 6.24)
- hyperextend the knee by more than 10° (1 point each side)
- bend forward with knees straight and easily place palms flat on the floor (1 point).

A score of 4 or more defines hypermobility in this assessment (Barrow et al 2002).

Using these illustrations and examples, practice assessing potentially hypermobile individuals.

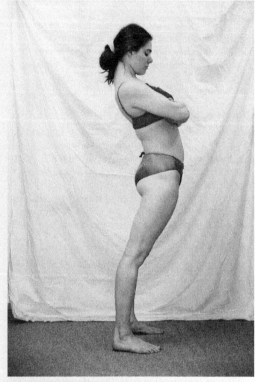

Figure 6.23 Sway-back posture in a hypermobile patient. Reproduced with permission from Keer & Grahame (2003)

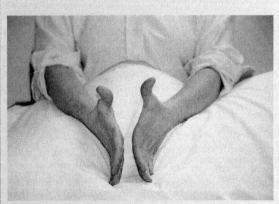

Figure 6.22 Hypermobility in the hands. Reproduced with permission from Keer & Grahame (2003)

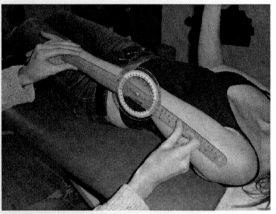

Figure 6.24 The ability to hyperextend the elbow to ≥10°. Reproduced with permission from Nijs J. *Journal of Bodywork and Movement Therapies* 2005;9:310–317

4. *Pathological* end-feel, however, can involve a number of variations such as:
   - a *firmer, less elastic* end-feel when scar tissue restricts movement or when shortened connective tissue exists
   - an *elastic, less soft* end-feel when increased muscle tonus restricts movement.
5. An *empty* end-feel is one in which the patient stops the movement (or asks for it to be stopped) before a true end-feel is reached, as a result of extreme pain (fracture or active inflammation) or psychogenic factors.

Practicing assessment of such variations on normal tissues and joints makes recognition of dysfunctional ones simpler.

Box 6.31 Exercise: Palpating joint play at the proximal tibiofibular joint

- Your palpation partner should be supine with hip and knee flexed so that the sole of the foot is flat on the table.
- You sit so that your buttock rests on the patient's toes, stabilizing the foot to the table. The head of the fibula is grasped between thumb and index finger of one hand, as the other hand holds the tibia firmly, inferior to the patella.
- Care should be taken to avoid excessive pressure on the posterior aspect of the fibular head, as the peroneal nerve lies close by (Kuchera & Goodridge 1997). The thumb resting on the anterior surface of the fibula should be reinforced by placing the thumb of the other hand over it.

A movement that takes the fibular head firmly posteriorly and anteriorly, in a slightly curved manner (i.e. not quite a straight backward and forward movement, but more back and slightly curving inferiorly, followed by forward and slightly curving superiorly, at an angle of approximately 30°), determines whether there is freedom of joint glide in each direction.

If restriction is noted in either direction, repetitive rhythmical but gentle springing of the fibula, at the end of its range, should restore normal joint play.

It is worth noting that when the fibular head glides anteriorly there is automatic reciprocal movement posteriorly at the distal fibula (lateral malleolus), while posterior glide of the fibular head results in anterior movement of the distal fibula. Restrictions at the distal fibula are, therefore, likely to influence behavior proximally and vice versa.

Clinical use of joint play

Mulligan's (1995) remarkably useful 'mobilization with movement' (MWM) method, described in Chapter 7, utilizes joint play as a major feature of its treatment methodology

Wilson (2002) notes:

That a normal joint will follow a normal 'track' or 'path' through any particular normal movement is axiomatic (Kapanji 1987). This articular track – incorporating spin, slide, glide, rotation, etc. – is a genetic inheritance and is dependent upon the shape of joint surfaces and articular cartilage, and upon the orientation and attachments of capsule, ligaments, muscles and tendons. To facilitate controlled, free movement while minimising compressive forces is the overall aim of such a design. Any anomalies in the recruitment or coordination of the sequential elements of the movement pattern will be signalled to the central nervous system (CNS), which may well seek to inhibit that inappropriate movement by pain, stiffness or weakness.

Gently introduced joint play, using 'glide' or translation movements, is a key element of MWM procedures. These are employed in all joints, including the facet (apophyseal) joints, while the patient slowly, repetitively and painlessly introduces previously restricted movements.

The use of these techniques depends on the various articular structure differences being recognized. For example:

- With *hinge joints* such as the elbow and knee, the bones lie end to end and articulate in the sagittal plane. With hinge joints, joint play/translation is applied at right angles to the movement that is introduced (Fig. 6.25). With

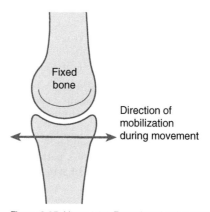

Figure 6.25 Hinge joint. Reproduced with permission from Chaitow (2002)

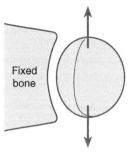

Figure 6.26 Parallel joints. Reproduced with permission from Chaitow (2002)

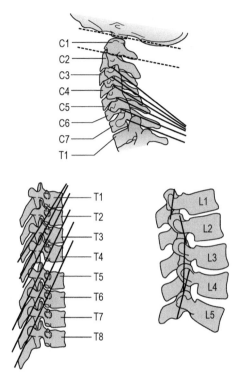

Figure 6.27 Orientation of zygapophyseal joints. Reproduced with permission from Exelby (2002)

the elbow, for example, a lateral glide of the forearm would be introduced on a fixed humerus.

- In *parallel joints* the bones lie alongside each other with their articulation being characterized by variations in that parallel relationship. Examples include the radius and ulna. In treatment settings, one of the pair would be stabilized and the other would be repositioned while the patient performed active movements (Fig. 6.26).

- Spinal *facet joints* have a variety of different planes in different regions of the spine. Gliding of a facet joint requires that the movement takes account of the orientation of the particular facet planes (Fig. 6.27).

Palpation of mobility, stability and functionality of joints

Exercise sequences covering palpation of mobility, stability and functionality of joints, including form and force closure assessments of the sacroiliac joints, are described in Boxes 6.33–6.35.

Sacral assessment

Palpation of the spine and spinal articulations

Normal physiology dictates that side-flexion and rotation in the cervical area (C3–C7) is usually 'Type 2', i.e. segments that are side-flexed will automatically rotate towards the same side.

Most cervical restrictions are compensations – adaptations to ascending or descending stress patterns – and will involve several segments, all of which will adopt this Type 2 pattern.

Exceptions occur if a cervical spinal segment is traumatically induced into a different format of dysfunction, in which case there could be side-flexion to one side combined with rotation to the opposite (Ward 1997).

The concept that general spinal coupling takes place in a predictable manner (apart from in the cervical region) has been challenged (Gibbons & Tehan 1998).

The exercise sequence outlined in Box 6.36 is suggested as an excellent way of becoming familiar with the mechanics of the cervical joints, while simultaneously identifying segmental restriction patterns (Greenman 1996). Palpation assessment of the lumbar spine is outlined in Box 6.37.

Assessment of spinal segmental facilitation (involving viscerosomatic reflexes)

In a study (Rosero et al 1987) of palpatory reliability, relating to thoracic paraspinal tissues in patients with myocardial infarction (MI), the terms most commonly used were selected from 16 descriptive terms provided.

Only five descriptors were consistently used to indicate what was being felt on palpation. The four listed below were significantly more frequently identified

Text continued on p. 178.

Box 6.32 Exercise: Palpation using the joint play of a cervical apophyseal joint

- Identify a person with some degree of restriction in cervical rotation.
- Identify the most restricted segments.
- The translation (gliding/joint play) force (see below) will be applied to the *upper* of the two vertebrae implicated in the movement dysfunction.
- The patient should be seated and the (right-handed) practitioner stands behind.
- The medial border of the distal phalanx of the right thumb is placed on the spinous process (or articular pillar) of the superior of the two vertebrae that have been identified as having less than free movement between them.
- The contact thumb does not apply pressure, but acts as a cushion, onto which the other thumb is placed for the application of pressure (Fig. 6.28). In the cervical area this will be directed to a point between the eyes.
- If the vertebrae in question are in the upper cervical region the practitioner should stabilize the head, with the lateral border of each index finger resting on the zygomatic arches.
- In a lower cervical area an index finger can rest along the jaw line while the other fingers drop onto the clavicle to restrain movement, as the treatment pressure is applied to the spine.
- Light pressure is applied (in this case) by the left thumb, and the patient is asked to slowly rotate the head/neck in the direction of restriction, to the end of a comfortable range, and to then slowly return to the starting position. This may be repeated several times.

- As you are performing this sequence try to become aware of very slight gliding movement of the facet joint during the procedure.
- The patient should have an increased range of rotation, which should persist after the three repetitions of this SNAG (sustained neutral apophyseal glide).

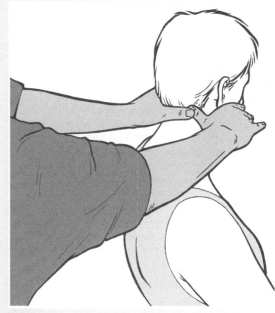

Figure 6.28 Unilateral right C1 SNAG. Reproduced with permission from Chaitow (2002)

Box 6.33 Exercise: Springing the sacroiliac (SI) joint

In practice the SI joint can be separated into a superior and an inferior portion for assessment purposes.

Superior SI assessment

- The patient should be side-lying with the hips flexed at 45° and knees flexed at 90°.
- For patients with a broad pelvis and narrow legs, a pillow placed between the knees will increase stability.
- You sit on the table, facing cephalad, with the patient's knees behind you.
- One of your hands (hypothenar eminence) contacts the lateral and superior aspects of the sacral base, just medial to the PSIS and the SI joint, with fingers palpating for motion.
- The palm of the other hand contacts the patient's ipsilateral ASIS.

- Your forearms should be horizontally positioned in opposition to each other.
- By lightly compressing the hands together, in a scissor-like motion, the first barrier of resistance should be felt.
- The hands then spring the joint to assess relative freedom or restriction.
- A small degree of springing, with no harsh end-feel, should be anticipated in a normal joint.

Inferior SI assessment

- The position of the patient and the practitioner is the same as in the superior SI assessment, described above.
- One of your hands (hypothenar eminence) contacts the lateral sacrum just medial to the inferior aspect of the SI joint, with fingers palpating for motion.

Continued

Box 6.33 Exercise: Springing the sacroiliac (SI) joint continued

- The palm of the other hand contacts the patient's ipsilateral anterior superior iliac spine (ASIS).
- Your forearms should be horizontally positioned in opposition to each other.
- By lightly compressing the hands together, in a scissor-like motion, loading the inferior aspect of

the joint, the first barrier of resistance should be felt.
- The hands then spring the joint to assess relative freedom or restriction.
- A small degree of springing, with no harsh end-feel, should be anticipated in a normal joint.

Box 6.34 Exercise: Functional form and force sacroiliac assessments (Lee 1997, 2000)

Supine form closure assessment

- The supine patient is asked to raise one leg.
- If during the leg raise there is evidence of compensatory rotation of the pelvis toward the side of the raised leg, SI joint instability is suggested.
- You should then apply compressive medially directed force across the pelvis with a hand on the lateral aspect of each innominate, at the level of the ASIS (encouraging *form closure* of the SI joint).
- The same leg should then be raised again.
- If this form closure strategy enhances the ability to easily raise the leg, this suggests that structural factors within the joint may require externally enhanced support, e.g. a trochanter belt.

Supine force closure assessment

- The supine patient is asked to raise one leg.
- If during the leg raise there is evidence of compensatory rotation of the pelvis toward the side of the raised leg, SI joint dysfunction is suggested.
- Before raising the leg again you should apply restraining pressure to the contralateral shoulder, and the patient should be asked to simultaneously slightly flex and rotate the trunk toward the side being tested (against your resistance) while raising the leg.
- This resisted effort increases oblique abdominal muscular activity and force closes the ipsilateral SI joint.
- If the initial leg raising suggests SI dysfunction, and this is markedly reduced or absent during force closure, the prognosis is good.
- The patient should be instructed in appropriate rehabilitation exercises (core stability).

Prone functional form and force SI joint assessment

- The prone patient is asked to extend the leg at the hip by approximately 10°. Hinging should occur at the hip joint and the pelvis should remain in contact with the table throughout.

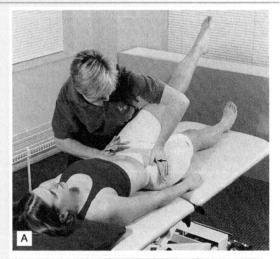

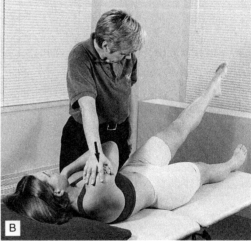

Figure 6.29 Functional test of supine-active straight leg raise: **A** with form closure augmented; **B** with force closure augmented. Reproduced with permission from Chaitow (2006)

Box 6.34 Exercise: Functional form and force sacroiliac assessments (Lee 1997, 2000) **continued**

- Excessive degrees of pelvic rotation in the transverse plane (anterior pelvic rotation) suggest SI joint instability.
- If form features (structural) of the SI joint are at fault, the prone straight leg extension movement will be more normal when medial compression of the joint is introduced by application of firm bilateral medial pressure toward the SI joints, with hands on the innominates.
- Force closure may be enhanced during the assessment if latissimus dorsi can be recruited to increase tension on the thoracolumbar fascia.

- This is achieved by the practitioner resisting extension of the medially rotated contralateral arm prior to, and during, the extension of the leg.
- If force closure enhances more normal SI joint function, the prognosis for improvement is good, via rehabilitation exercises and reformed use patterns.
- If only compressive force across the joint assists the ease of leg extension, then a form (structural) problem exists and a supporting belt may be required.

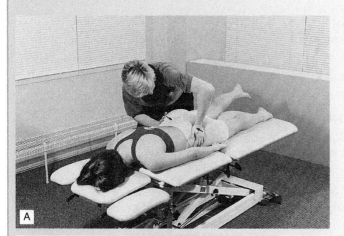

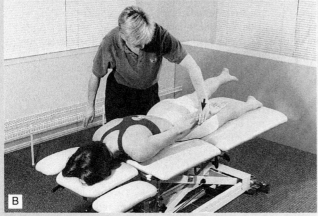

Figure 6.30 Functional test of prone-active straight leg raise: **A** with form closure augmented; **B** with force closure augmented. Reproduced with permission from Chaitow (2006)

Box 6.35 Exercise: Assessment of the hip joint

- The patient should lie supine, close to the edge of the examination table.
- The hip and knee should both be flexed, with the practitioner seated or standing on the same side, facing cephalad.
- The patient's leg should be lifted and the calf rested on the practitioner's shoulder.
- Both hands should then wrap around the proximal thigh, fingers interlaced.
- The hip should be flexed to approximately 90° of flexion.
- The hip joint should then be distracted caudally with the practitioner using bodyweight to achieve this.
- With the hip in this relaxed, distracted position it is possible to spring the joint in an anteroposterior direction, or to introduce medial to lateral motion, or to evaluate motion during circumduction, in varying degrees of hip abduction or adduction.
- Combinations of such movement potentials can be introduced as can circumduction with crowding of the joint, achieved by releasing the distraction, removing the supported calf from the shoulder, and then moving one hand to the fully flexed knee in order to allow long-axis compression.
- The objective of all these movements, and springing assessments, is to assess whether any particular movements are restricted, and also to judge the end-feel in the various directions of motion.

Box 6.36 Exercise: Assessment of cervical joint functionality

To easily palpate for side-flexion and rotation, a side-to-side *translation* ('shunt') movement is used, with the neck in neutral, moderate flexion or moderate extension.

When the neck is in absolute neutral (no flexion or extension – which is an unusual state in the neck), true translation, side-to-side, is possible.

As a cervical segment is translated to one side it automatically creates a side-flexion effect and, because of the anatomic and physiological rules governing it, rotation to the same side occurs (Fryette 1954, Mimura et al 1989).

In order to evaluate cervical function using this knowledge, it is suggested that you are seated at the head of the supine patient and that you place your hands, as follows, on each side of the supine patient's neck:

- The index finger pads rest on the articular pillars of C6, just above the transverse processes of C7
- The middle finger pads will be on C5, the ring finger pads on C4 and the little finger pads on C3, stabilizing these segments.

With these contacts it is possible to examine for sensitivity, fibrosis and hypertonicity, as well as being able to apply lateral translation (side-to-side shunting) to cervical segments while the head is in neutral, flexion or extension.

- In order to do this effectively, it is necessary to stabilize the superior segment to the one being examined.
- The heel of the hand helps to control movement of the head.
- With the head/neck in relative neutral (no flexion and no extension), translation to the right and then left is introduced (any segment) to assess freedom of movement (and, by implication, side-flexion and rotation) in each direction.
- Say C6 is being stabilized with the finger pads; as translation of C6 is introduced, to the left, the ability to freely side-flex and rotate to the right on C7 is being evaluated.
- If the joint (and/or associated soft tissues) is normal, this translation will cause a gapping of the left facet, and a 'closing' of the right facet, as left translation is performed, and vice versa.
- There will be a soft end-feel to the movement, without harsh or sudden braking.
- If, however, translation of the segment towards the right from the left produces a sense of resistance/bind, then the segment is restricted in its ability to side-bend left and (by implication) to rotate left.
- If such a restriction is noted, the translation should be repeated, but this time with the head in extension instead of neutral.
- This is achieved by lifting the contact fingers on C6 (in this example) slightly towards the ceiling before reassessing the side-to-side translation.

Box 6.36 Exercise: Assessment of cervical joint functionality continued

- Once translation to each side has been assessed in extension, the head and neck should be taken into flexion, and the left-to-right translation again assessed.

The objective is to ascertain which position (neutral, flexion, extension) creates the greatest degree of restriction as the translation barrier is engaged.

Is movement more restricted in neutral, extension or flexion – in side-flexion to one side or the other?

In the example given (C6 on C7 translation left to right), if this restriction is greater with the head extended, the diagnosis is of a joint restricted or locked in flexion, side-bent right and rotated right (meaning that there is difficulty in the joint extending and also side-flexing and rotating to the left).

If this restriction is greater when the head is flexed, then the joint is said to be restricted or locked in extension, side-flexed right and rotated right (meaning there is

difficulty in the joint flexing and also side-flexing and rotating to the left).

Once one segment has been assessed you should move to another, and sequentially evaluate the relative freedom of movement into side-flexion and rotation of all levels, from C6 to C2.

Note: As the atlanto-occipital coupling mechanism is not the same as that of the lower cervical segments, it is suggested that you restrict application of this assessment to the segments listed in the exercise.

Treatment options range from HVLA to mobilization – including the use of positional release (PRT) and/or muscle energy (MET) procedures – depending on a host of factors including etiology and the degree of acuteness/chronicity, as well as on the age and status of the patient, and on the training and skill of the practitioner.

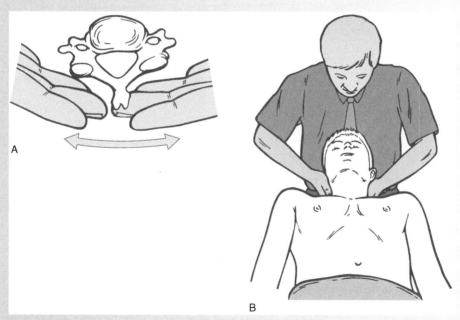

Figure 6.31 **A** The finger pads rest as close to the articular pillars as possible, in order to be able to palpate and guide vertebral motion in a translatory manner. **B** With the head/neck in a neutral position, the practitioner sequentially guides individual segments into translation in both directions in order to sense indications of restriction and tissue modification. If a restriction is sensed, its increase or decrease is evaluated for retesting with the segment held in greater flexion and then extension. MET would be applied from the position of greatest unforced bind/restriction, using muscles which would either take away the area through (antagonists to shortened muscles) or away from (shortened muscles themselves – the agonists) the barrier. Reproduced with permission from Chaitow (2006)

Box 6.37 Exercise: Palpation assessment of the lumbar spine

Rotation

- The patient should lie prone while you stand at waist level.
- By reaching across the patient's trunk your caudal hand can grasp the contralateral pelvic crest.
- This allows you to ease the lumbar spine into rotation by transfer of bodyweight backwards.
- The thumb of your cephalad hand should make contact with the lateral aspect of the ipsilateral spinous process of L5.
- The assessment is performed by you rotating the pelvis posteriorly while firmly palpating the spinous process, so resisting its ability to rotate.
- Note the first resistance barrier as the pelvis rotates and the spinous process of L5 engages your thumb.
- You should then spring the joint to evaluate the quality of end-feel. Is there a springing sensation, or a harsh end-feel?
- The assessment procedure is then sequentially repeated with your thumb contact on L4, L3, L2 and L1.

Once the lumbar joints have been assessed on one side the process is repeated on the other.

Anteroposterior movement

- The patient should be side-lying with knees and hips flexed, and with both knees just off the edge of the table.

- The lumbar spine should be in a relaxed neutral position (but should not be in flexion).
- You should stand facing the table at the level of the patient's knees, which should be level with your abdomen (an adjustable table – hydraulic if possible – is ideal).
- The patient's knees should be in touch with your lower abdomen as you reach across the table to make contact with the L5 spinous process with one middle finger pad. The other hand should be placed on top of the contact hand.

Assessment is made by a combination of: (1) a movement against the flexed knees, with the long-axis compressive force of these driving the pelvis posteriorly, while at precisely the same time, (2) the spinous process of L5 is drawn anteriorly.

In this way you can assess both the quality and quantity of available movement of that segment: Is it free? Is there a harsh end-feel? Is there reported pain? Does the segment 'spring' appropriately?

Precisely the same procedure is applied to all five lumbar vertebrae.

(p <0.001) in patients with MI compared with non-MI (control) patients, mainly relating to the area of T1–T4 (left side):

- 'Resistant' (firm, tense): 10.3% of controls and 34.4% of MI patients
- 'Temperature/warm': 6.5% of controls and 32% of MI patients
- 'Ropiness' (cord-like): 3.6% of controls and 13% of MI patients
- 'Heavy musculature' (increased density): 3% of controls and 13.6% of MI patients.

As can be seen, the terms 'resistant' and 'temperature/warm' were the descriptions most commonly used.

In a randomized study, Nicholas et al (1987) observed that: 'Myocardial infarction is accompanied by characteristic paravertebral soft tissue changes which are readily detected by palpation.'

These researchers hypothesize:

The sympathetic nervous system [acts] as a mediator in such phenomena. This hypothesis is based on the similar embryological origin of the innervation of somatic and visceral tissue. In the case of the heart the cardiac plexus is composed of branches from the cervical sympathetic ganglia and the upper seven thoracic ganglia. About twice as many fibres enter the cardiac plexus from the thoracic nerves as enter from the cervical cardiac nerves (Cathie 1965). Changes in soft tissue in patients with cardiac disturbances were found most often on the thoracic dorsum. It is plausible to attribute their aetiology to efferent and afferent reflex activity during the evolution of myocardial infarction.

According to Lewit (1999a), the first signs of viscerosomatic reflexive influences are vasomotor (increased skin temperature) and sudomotor (increased moisture of the skin) reactions, skin textural changes (e.g. thickening), increased subcutaneous fluid and increased contraction of muscle.

Korr (1976) has compared any facilitated area of the spine to a 'neurological lens', in which stress factors which impinge upon any aspect of the body or mind are automatically targeted through the facilitated segment, further focusing and intensifying activity through its neurological structures.

A simple diagnostic palpation method for 'compressing' or 'springing' the paraspinal tissues is outlined below.

McFarlane Tilley (1961) listed the possible implications of segmental facilitation, in various spinal regions, based on osteopathic clinical observations:

- Myocardial ischemia: rigid musculature in any two adjacent segments between T1 and T4 (usually left, but not essentially so).
- Cardiopulmonary pathology: any two adjacent segments of muscular paraspinal rigidity in the upper thoracic spine, either side or bilaterally.
- Duodenal pathology: any two adjacent segments of muscular paraspinal rigidity and tenderness, right side thoracic spine, levels 6, 7 and 8.
- Pancreatic dysfunction: any two adjacent segments of muscular paraspinal rigidity and tenderness, bilaterally, thoracics 6, 7, 8 and 9.
- Liver and gall bladder: any two adjacent segments of muscular paraspinal rigidity and tenderness, right side thoracics 8, 9 and 10.
- Chronic fatigue related to 'adrenal exhaustion' or stress: any two adjacent segments of muscular paraspinal rigidity and tenderness in thoracics 9, 10, 11 and 12.
- Renal disease: tenderness and painful on pressure, aggravated by percussion, thoracics 11 and 12, and lumbars 1 and 2.
- Female and male reproductive organ problems: lumbosacral area tenderness or rigidity.

Johnston's recommendations regarding somatic findings of visceral origin

Johnston, over many years of clinical research, has identified a number of predictable segmental (spinal) locations and motion characteristics that relate to viscerosomatic reflex activity. He terms these 'linkages' (Johnston 1988). These have all been demonstrated to have a high inter-rater reliability when tested by other clinicians.

Hypertension linkages

- T2 central and 2nd rib (left) resistance to gross passive axial rotation to the right, side-bending right; extension and translation anteriorly and left.

- T6 central and right 6th rib, resistant to passive axial rotation to the left, side-bending right, flexion; translation anterior and left.

Bronchial asthma linkages

- T4 and right 4th rib, resistant to passive axial rotation left and side-bending right.

Cholelithiasis linkages

- 'At 10th (and sometimes 11th) thoracic level the paraspinal tissues will usually display responses to facilitation' (Larson 1977), resulting in immediate increased tissue resistance to passive axial rotation to the left, side-bending left, and extension.

Upper gastrointestinal complaint linkages

- T5 and left 5th rib, palpable tissue resistance to passive axial rotation to the left, side-bending right, and flexion.
- Magoun (1962) has described treatment of this restriction pattern in a child with 'stomach symptoms of a dyspeptic nature' as follows: 'With the patient in left side-lying position, a final slight direct thrusting force was applied [HVLA] to address primarily the local restriction to sidebending right and translation left.'

Beal (1983) has noted that the major palpatory finding associated with segmental facilitation was of: 'hypertonicity of the superficial and deep paraspinal muscles, with fibrotic thickening'.

Beal reports that superficial hypertonicity lessened when the patient was supine, making assessment of deeper tissue states easier in that position. An exercise derived from Beal's work is illustrated in Box 6.38.

These observations from premier osteopathic researchers should inform naturopathic practitioners and physicians of the potential for influencing somatic structures in order to encourage resolution of dysfunctional segmental patterns and indirectly (reflexively) the somatic sources of these patterns. It is clear from a naturopathic perspective that this would not be the end of the story, but in conjunction with appropriate focus on digestive status and function, and on any associated psychosocial factors, would ensure that the full spectrum of influences would have been addressed – truly whole-person medicine.

Note: It is important to differentiate between segmental facilitation, as discussed above, and spinal 'splinting' that occurs as a result of underlying pathology such as TB spine, vertebral metastasis (primary or secondary) and osteoporosis.

Box 6.38 Exercise: Segmental palpation for facilitated areas

- The patient is supine.
- The practitioner is seated at the head of the table.
- One hand is inserted under the patient so that the thoracic spine can be palpated.
- Middle and index fingers lie each side of the segment to be assessed, with one of these fingers directly beneath the transverse processes.
- An anteriorly directed (toward the ceiling), compressive force is applied, assessing the status of the superficial and deep paraspinal tissues, as well as the response of the transverse process to this springing force.
- This compression is performed, one segment at a time, progressively down the spine, until control becomes difficult or tissues inaccessible.
- It is also possible to perform the test with the patient seated or side-lying, though neither is as effective as the supine position.

Box 6.39 Exercise: Assessment of balance

- The patient stands on one leg with eyes open.
- The non-standing leg is flexed to 45° at the hip and 90° at the knee, so that the flexed knee is in front and the foot behind the other leg (Liebenson & Oslance 1996).
- The non-supporting leg should at no time touch the supporting leg.
- The hands are at the side (and should not be used to touch anything for balance).
- Having flexed the hip and knee, the patient is asked to close the eyes and remain balanced on one leg without the standing foot shifting or the eyes opening.
- The length of time during which single leg balance can be maintained (without balance being lost, the hands being used to reassert balance, or the supporting foot shifting to assist in restoration of balance) is measured.
- If balance is lost, several more attempts should be made to evaluate the greatest length of time balance can be held. The test becomes part of self-treatment when the patient is asked to perform the test regularly at home to encourage enhanced balance.

Splinting will usually be more widespread than the two adjacent segments commonly associated with segmental facilitation, and no attempt should be made to reduce such splinting, which is protective.

Assessing balance

The next three exercises (Boxes 6.39–6.41) relate to observation and not palpation.

Balance represents an accurate snapshot of the current functional efficiency of the individual's neuromusculoskeletal integration.

Bohannon et al (1984) have identified widely accepted (Liebenson 2005) 'normal balance times' – single leg stance, eyes closed – in relation to age:

- Between the ages of 20 and 49 a maintained balance time of between approximately 25 and 29 seconds is normal
- Between ages 49 and 59, 21 seconds is normal
- Between 60 and 69, just over 10 seconds is acceptable
- After 70 years of age, 4 seconds is normal.

In order to evaluate the patient's balance status, the single leg stance test is performed (Box 6.39).

Cervical involvement with balance problems

Lewit (1999a) has shown the importance of Hautant's test (Box 6.40) as a screening tool for identifying cervical dysfunction as a factor in balance problems. He has presented evidence showing that correcting cervical dysfunction can improve standing posture if disequilibrium problems can be shown to be associated with cervical dysfunction.

The test is suggested – according to Lewit (1999a, p. 250) – if: 'the patient complains of disturbed balance and if a test standing on 2 scales shows a difference greater than 4 kg'.

Lewit describes a 'characteristic pattern' in which deviation of the outstretched arms occurs in the opposite direction to the rotation of the head/neck, and also at retroflexion of the neck, when disturbed balance relates to a cervical dysfunction. Cervical association (most commonly involving C1, C2 and C3) may be present in all forms of vertigo and dizziness, although the form of vertigo that seems least responsive to cervical manipulative treatment appears to be positional vertigo.

Liebenson (2001) explains the need for precision in assessment when faced with patients with balance and gait disturbances: 'Differentiating between primary feet, lumbar and cervical disorders is crucial.'

Box 6.40 Exercise: Hautant's test

- The patient is seated with arms extended in the 'sleepwalking' position.
- The practitioner stands in front and observes changes in position of the extended arms as the patient, eyes closed, on instruction, moves the head in various directions (side, flexion, rotation, flexion, extension, etc.) to evaluate the effect.
- Movements are performed slowly, on instruction, before a slow return to neutral ('Turn your head as far as you comfortably can to the left' etc.).
- The test is positive if the arms deviate with specific directions of neck movement.

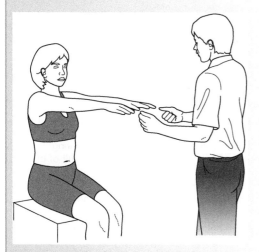

Figure 6.32 Hautant's test

Box 6.41 Exercise: The Fukuda-Unterberger test

During performance of the test there should be no sound or light source present which could suggest a direction.

- A normal individual's body, while stepping in place with eyes closed or blindfold, rotates between 20° and 30° after taking 50 steps in place (i.e. 'marching on the spot') (Fukuda 1984).
- When stepping in place the individual should not raise the thighs by more than approximately 45°.
- The pace of stepping in place should not be excessively rapid.
- A blindfold (better than just 'close your eyes') should be placed over the eyes with the head facing forward, without rotation or tilting.
- The arms should be placed in 'sleepwalking' mode, stretched forward, horizontal and parallel.
- Stepping in place should commence.
- If the degree of rotation, after 50 steps, is in excess of 30° deviation from the start position, then a degree of pathological asymmetry may be assumed, and a further assessment is required, ideally by a skilled neuro-optometrist.

It is possible for a skilled practitioner to use this type of refinement to calculate the degree of abnormal asymmetry, and to then use tactics that encourage more normal spinal, oculomotor and/or plantar input to modify this imbalance.

If the test results in an abnormal degree of rotation then it should be repeated periodically during and after the use of therapeutic tactics directed at normalizing dysfunctional patterns revealed during normal assessment, possibly involving the feet, spine, pelvis, neck or the eyes.

In addition, Gagey & Gentaz suggest other possible causes of, and treatment options for, disturbed balance, including:

- oculomotor, in which there may be a need for use of prisms to influence oculomotor muscles, using 'the law of semicircular canals'
- plantar input, where mechanoreceptors in the soles can be manipulated by means of the precise attachment/placement of extremely thin microwedges
- mandibular interference with postural balance.

Notes on other balance influences

Gagey & Gentaz (1996) note:

When a normal subject keeps his or her head turned to the right, the tone of the extensor muscles of the right leg increases, and vice versa for the left side. When a normal subject performs the . . . [Fukuda-Unterberger] . . . test [see Box 6.41] with the head turned to the right, he or she rotates farther leftward than if the test is performed with the head facing forward. The difference between these two angles of rotation [i.e. the difference in degree of body rotation after 50 steps, with head in neutral, and with head rotated] is a measure of the gain of the right neck reflex.

Box 6.42 Exercise: Kinetic coronal (or other) suture palpation

- The patient should be side-lying on the right, or supine, with the head on a cushion, and head turned to the right to allow examination of the left side.
- You are on the patient's right, at head level.
- Your cephalad (left) hand holds the head to support and stabilize it, with the finger pads (usually index and/or middle) placed strategically to palpate whichever suture is being examined.
- For the coronal suture, the left (palpation) hand rests so that the index and/or middle fingers lie on the left side of the coronal suture, the thumb rests on the frontal bone.
- Your gloved right hand is placed so that the index and middle fingers (spread apart) are in contact with the crown surfaces of the posterior molars, allowing these contacts to be used to introduce light rocking movements, from side to side, or forward and backward, as motion at the suture is evaluated.
- This is then compared with findings noted on the right side coronal suture, which should be palpated with all hand and patient positions reversed.
- This same basic position can be used to palpate motion at the sphenofrontal, sphenoparietal, sphenosquamous, squamoparietal and even the parietomastoid sutures, by altering the palpating left hand contacts to rest on the appropriate suture, as the same rocking motion is introduced via the action of the right hand contacts on the maxillae.

Is a gentle springing motion palpable? Are there any areas where this is diminished? And, if so, what might the significance of this be?

Box 6.43 Exercise: Observation and palpation of the temporomandibular joint

- The patient should be lying supine with you seated at the head.
- Your palpating fingers should be placed over the bilateral temporomandibular joints to assess local tenderness in response to mild or moderate pressure on the joint capsule.
- The angle of the mandible may be pressed gently toward the top of the head to assess for intra-joint tenderness (a form of joint play involving translation that allows for assessment of end-feel as well as feedback on sensitivity).
- The condylar heads should be externally palpated during active translation of the jaw, and compared for symmetry of movement.
- Are there the same degrees of motion bilaterally?
- The adult incisal opening should measure 50–60 mm (*Gray's Anatomy* 1999), with minimal normal opening being 36–44 mm (Simons et al 1999) and with 5–10 mm of range allowed in protrusion and lateral displacement in each direction, with much individual variation.
- As the mandible is depressed during opening of the mouth, observe the lower central incisor pathway to note deviations or unusual movements during tracking. Such deviations may be the result of trigger points or shortened fibers within the musculature (deviation will usually be towards the side of shortening), internal derangement of the disc or other internal pathologies.
- A hard end-feel to opening, especially when the range is significantly reduced, may indicate anterior displacement without reduction, or onset, or presence of, degenerative arthritis.

Cranial assessment, including temporomandibular joint

Coronal suture palpation, and observation and palpation of the temporomandibular joint, are outlined in Boxes 6.42 and 6.43, respectively.

Notes on visceral palpation

Accurate visceral palpation requires a high degree of palpatory literacy that can only be accomplished by practice.

Barral & Mercier (1988) outline what it is necessary to know regarding visceral motility and mobility:

There is an inherent axis of rotation in each of these motions (mobility and motility). In healthy organs, the axes of mobility and motility are generally the same. With disease, they are often at variance with one another, as certain restrictions affect one motion more

than another. What a surprise it was for us to discover that the axes of motion reproduce exactly those of embryological development! Neither preconceived ideas nor hypotheses directed this research. The discovery of this phenomenon was purely empirical, and tends to confirm the idea that 'cells do not forget'.

Additionally, visceral motion is influenced by:

- the somatic nervous system (body movement, muscular tone and activity, posture)
- autonomic nervous system.

Stone (1999) has described the movement of organs:

Visceral biomechanics relate to the movements that the organs make against each other, and against the walls

Box 6.44 Exercise: Palpating the motility of an organ

Barral & Mercier (1988) advise using the following approach:

Place your hand over the organ to be tested, with a pressure of 20–100 g, depending on the depth of the organ. In some cases the hand can adapt itself to the form of the organ. The hand is totally passive, but there is an extension of the sense of touch used during this examination. Let the hand passively follow what it feels – a slow movement of feeble amplitude which will show itself, stop and then begin again (7–8 per minute in health).

This is visceral motility.

It is then desirable, after a few cycles, to estimate elements such as frequency, amplitude and direction of the motility, and to not have preconceived ideas as to what will be felt. Trust what you feel. Empty the mind and let the hand listen. (Both organs of a pair should be assessed and compared.)

One visceral palpation exercise for motility – of the liver – is described in Chapter 7 under the subheading 'Visceral manipulation' (see page 273).

of the body cavities that contain them. The viscera 'articulate' by utilizing sliding surfaces formed by the peritoneal (and pleural or pericardial) membranes that surround the organs and line the body cavities. [Due to normal body movement, including bending and locomotion, as well as body process such as micturition] . . . as the body cavities distort and change their shape, so the individual organs must adapt to those changes, and they do so by slightly sliding over each other, given the constraints of their attachments and surrounds.

See also visceral manipulation notes in Chapter 7.

Visceral palpation and assessment are described in Box 6.44.

General assessments: posture and respiration

The adaptational influence on the body's constant battle with gravity, which is slowly lost over a lifetime, and which can be observed in the crossed syndrome patterns, has been described by Vleeming et al (1997) as 'postural decay'.

Crossed syndrome patterns (see also discussion of crossed and layered syndromes in Chapter 9)

As compensation occurs due to overuse, misuse and disuse of muscles of the spine and pelvis, some muscles become overworked, shortened and restricted, with others becoming inhibited and weak, and body-wide postural changes take place that have been characterized as 'crossed syndromes' (Lewit 1999c) (Fig. 6.33). These crossed patterns demonstrate the imbalances that occur as antagonists become inhibited due to the overactivity of specific postural muscles.

The effect on spinal and pelvic mechanics of these imbalances would be to create an environment in which pain and dysfunction would become more likely to occur.

One of the main tasks in rehabilitation of such pain and dysfunction is to normalize these imbalances, to release and stretch whatever is over-short and tight, and to encourage tone in those muscles that have become inhibited and weakened (Liebenson 2005).

In his classic text on body mechanics, Goldthwait (1945) described the changes that are commonly found in association with a 'slumped posture' (an example of 'postural decay'), leading to loss of diaphragmatic efficiency and abdominal ptosis.

- Breathing dysfunction and restrictions develop.
- There is drag on the fascia supporting the heart, displacing this organ and resulting in traction on the aorta.
- Nerve structures supplying the heart are similarly stressed mechanically.
- The cervical fascia is stretched.
- Venous stasis develops below the diaphragm as its pumping action is inhibited and diminished, leading to development of varicose veins and hemorrhoids.
- The stomach becomes crowded and tilted, affecting its efficiency mechanically.
- The esophagus becomes stretched, as does the coeliac artery.
- Symptoms ranging from hiatal hernia to dyspepsia and constipation become more likely.
- The pancreas is mechanically affected, interfering with its circulation.
- The liver is tilted backwards, there is inversion of the bladder, the support of the kidneys is altered while the colon and intestines generally become mechanically crowded and depressed (as does the bladder). None of these can therefore function optimally.

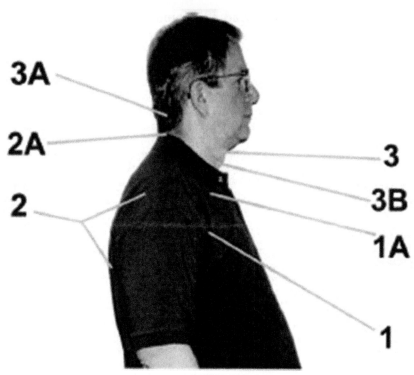

Figure 6.33 Upper crossed syndrome. Weak muscles: (**1**) serratus anterior; (**2**) lower and middle trapezius; (**3**) deep neck flexors. Shortened muscles: (**1A**) pectoralis major; (**2A**) upper trapezius and levator scapulae; (**3A**) suboccipitals; (**3B**) sternocleidomastoid. Reproduced with permission from Moore (2004)

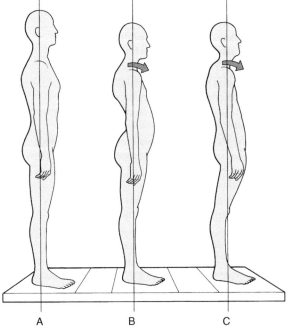

Figure 6.34 Balanced posture **A** compared with two patterns of musculoskeletal imbalance that involve fascial, and general, tissue and joint adaptations; **B** represents a crossed pattern with posterior pelvic shift, while **C** represents an anterior pelvic shift (Key et al 2008). Reproduced with permission from Chaitow (2003b)

- The prostate becomes affected due to circulatory dysfunction and increased pressure, making hypertrophy more likely.
- Similarly, menstrual irregularities become more likely.
- Increased muscular tension becomes a drain on energy, leading to fatigue which is aggravated by inefficient oxygen intake and poor elimination of wastes.
- Spinal and rib restrictions become chronic, making this problem worse.
- Postural joints become stressed, leading to spinal, hip, knee and foot dysfunction, increasing wear and tear.

Kuchera (1997) discusses gravitational influences on posture:

Gravitational force is constant and a greatly underestimated systemic stressor. Of the many signature manifestations of gravitational strain pathophysiology (GSP), the most prominent are altered postural alignment and recurrent somatic dysfunction . . . Recognizing gravitational strain pathophysiology facilitates the selection of new and different therapeutic approaches for familiar problems. The precise approach selected for each patient and its predicted outcome are strongly influenced by the ratio of functional disturbance to structural change.

Kuchera & Kuchera (1997) add a perspective that makes clear how varied are other contextual influences on 'postural decay':

Posture is distribution of body mass in relation to gravity over a base of support. The efficiency with which weight is distributed over the base of support depends on the levels of energy needed to maintain equilibrium (homeostasis), as well as on the status of the musculo-ligamentous structures of the body. These factors – weight distribution, energy availability and musculo-ligamentous condition – interact with the (usually) multiple adaptations and compensations which take place below the base of the skull, all of which can influence the visual and balance functions of the body.

In order to evaluate posture, observation, palpation and specific assessments are needed. The basic requirements include:

- Observation – checking key points and aspects of alignment and balance, with patient static and active, standing, walking, sitting, reclining (Janda 1996, Lewit 1999a)
- Postural evaluation – observation of crossed syndrome patterns, layer syndrome, including functional tests such as scapulohumeral rhythm test, core stability (Liebenson 2005, Norris 1995)
- Gait analysis is described in Chapter 9. This is a skill that requires diligent supervision and explanation.

Further reading

The scope of this chapter does not allow a detailed summary of these topics, and the following texts are recommended:

- Chaitow L 2003 Palpation and assessment skills, 2nd edn. Churchill Livingstone, Edinburgh
- Lewit K 1999 Manipulation in rehabilitation of the motor system, 3rd edn. Butterworth-Heinemann, London
- Liebenson C 2005 Rehabilitation of the spine, 2nd edn. Lippincott Williams & Wilkins, Philadelphia
- Perry J 1992 Gait analysis: normal and pathological function. Slack, Thorofare, NJ
- Petty N, Moore A 1998 Neuromuscular examination and assessment. Churchill Livingstone, Edinburgh
- Valmassy RL 1996 Clinical biomechanics of the lower extremities. Mosby, St Louis

Breathing pattern evaluation

Garland (1994) has summarized the structural modifications that are likely to inhibit successful breathing retraining, as well as psychological intervention, until they are, at least in part, normalized.

He describes a series of changes including:

. . . visceral stasis/pelvic floor weakness, abdominal and erector spinae muscle imbalance, fascial restrictions from the central tendon via the pericardial fascia to the basi-occiput, upper rib elevation with increased costal cartilage tension, thoracic spine dysfunction and possible sympathetic disturbance, accessory breathing muscle hypertonia and fibrosis, promotion of rigidity in the cervical spine with promotion of fixed lordosis, reduction in mobility of 2nd cervical segment and disturbance of vagal outflow . . . and more.

These changes, he states:

. . . run physically and physiologically against biologically sustainable patterns, and in a vicious circle, promote abnormal function which alters structure which then disallows a return to normal function.

The most obvious evidence of poor respiratory function is the raising of the upper chest structures by means of contraction of the upper fixators of the shoulder and the auxiliary cervical muscles (upper trapezius, levator scapulae, scalenes, sternomastoid).

This is both inefficient as a means of breathing and the cause of stress and overuse to the cervical structures. It is clearly evident when severe but may require a deep inhalation to show itself if only slight (Chaitow et al 2002).

In many ways the breathing pattern assessment described in Box 6.45 offers an opportunity to combine many of the skills that have been touched on through-out this chapter, since evidence of dysfunction is almost always accompanied by structural modification of muscles and other soft tissues, as well as joints.

Orthopedic testing and assessment

A selection of standard tests/assessment methods are described in Box 6.46. The descriptions provided are not intended to offer a fully comprehensive series of orthopedic assessment methods; rather, these represent examples of methods that can be used to help to

---

Box 6.45 Exercise: Palpating and assessing respiratory function

- The person to be evaluated should be seated.
- You stand behind and place your hands, fingers facing forwards, resting on the lower ribs, thumbs touching on the midline posteriorly.
- The person exhales to a comfortable limit (i.e. not a forced exhalation) and then inhales slowly and fully.
- Is there a lateral widening and, if so, to what degree?
- Or do your hands seem to be raised upwards?

Your hands should not move superiorly at all, but ideally should move apart slightly. Pryor & Prasad (2002) report that normal total excursion is between 1.5 and 2 inches (3 and 5 cm).

The hands should move apart but they will rise if inappropriate breathing is being performed, involving the accessory breathing muscles and upper fixators of the shoulders.

These muscles should be assessed for shortness and other dysfunctional features:

- Does one side seem to move more than the other?
- If so, local restrictions (ribs? thoracic spine?) or muscle tensions are probably involved.
- Is there evidence of paradoxical breathing?

Pryor & Prasad (2002) report: 'Paradoxical breathing is where some or all of the chest wall moves inward on inspiration and outward on expiration . . . localized paradox occurs when the integrity of the chest wall is disrupted.' Causes can range from rib fracture to diaphragmatic paralysis and cases involving chronic airflow limitation.

While the person being evaluated continues to breathe slowly and deeply you should try to assess 'continuity of motion' in the inhalation/exhalation phases.

Observe any starting and stopping, asymmetry or apparent mal-coordination and any unexpected departures from smooth mobility.

Scalene evaluation

- Rest your hands over the upper shoulder area, finger pads resting on the superior aspect of the clavicles.
- On inhalation, do the hands rise? Does either clavicle rise on inhalation? (Neither the clavicles nor your hands should rise, except on maximal inhalation. If they do, scalene overactivity is implicated and these require further assessment for shortness and presence of trigger points.)
- While in this position, assess whether one side moves more than the other. If so, local restrictions (clavicles, upper ribs) or muscle tensions may be implicated. These muscles should be assessed for shortness and other dysfunctional features.

Upper trapezius evaluation

Observe the upper trapezius muscles as they curve towards the neck:

- Are they convex (bowing outwards)?
- If so, these so-called 'gothic' shoulders are very taut and probably accompany inappropriate breathing, lifting the upper ribs (along with scalenes, sternomastoid and levator scapulae) (Janda 1983, Lewit 1999a).
- Palpate these muscles and test them for shortness.

Upright paradoxical breathing assessment

- With the person still seated, and inhaling deeply, palpate the abdomen.
- Does the abdomen (slightly) bulge on inhalation? (This is normal.)
- In some instances, breathing is so faulty that the abdomen is drawn in on inhalation, and pushed outwards on exhalation – further evidence of a paradoxical pattern.

Box 6.45 Exercise: Palpating and assessing respiratory function continued

Inhalation and exhalation

Evaluation of aspects of inhalation and exhalation demonstrates the functionality of the individual's breathing pattern:

- Return to the first position, with your hands on the sides of the lower ribs.
- Feel the degree of contraction on exhalation: Does this seem to be a complete exhalation?
- Alternatively, does the person not quite get the end of the breath exhaled before commencing the next inhalation? If so, this leads to retention of excessive levels of tidal air, preventing a full inhalation.
- Inhalation efficiency can be said to depend on the completeness of the exhalation.
- Now ask the person to take as long as possible to breathe in completely.
- How long did it take? If less than 5 seconds, there is probably dysfunction.
- Next, after a complete inhalation, ask the person to take as long as possible to exhale, breathing out slowly all the time.
- This should also take not less than 5 seconds, although people with dysfunctional breathing status or who hyperventilate, and those in states of anxiety, often fail to take even as long as 3 seconds to inhale or exhale.
- Time the complete cycle of breathing (inhalation plus exhalation). This should take not less than 10 seconds in good function.

Supine palpation

- The person should now lie supine, knees flexed.
- Rest a hand, lightly, just above the umbilicus and have the patient inhale deeply. Does your hand move towards the ceiling (ideally 'yes')?
- Are the abdominal muscles relaxed (ideally 'yes')?
- Or did your hand actually move toward the floor on inhalation (ideally 'no')?
- If the abdomen rose, was this the first part of the respiratory mechanism to move or did it inappropriately follow an initial movement of the upper or lower chest?
- Paradoxical breathing such as this involves the mechanism being used in just such an uncoordinated manner.

Breathing wave assessment

- Next ask your palpation partner to lie prone.
- Observe the wave as inhalation occurs, moving upwards in a fan-like manner from the lumbars to the base of the neck (Fig. 6.35).

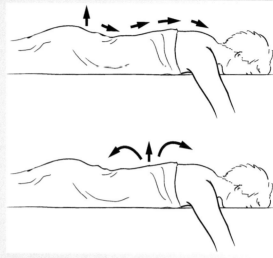

Figure 6.35 Functional (top) and dysfunctional breathing wave movement patterns. Reproduced with permission from Chaitow et al (2002)

- This wave can be observed by watching the spinous processes or the paraspinal musculature, or the 'wave' can be palpated by a feather-light touch on the spine or paraspinal structures during respiration.
- Areas of the thoracic or lumbar spine that are restricted in their ability to flex will probably rise *en bloc* (see Box 6.19).
- A full breath, where the diaphragm is functioning normally and where the spine is flexible, will be demonstrated by a wave-like movement, starting close to the sacrum and ceasing in the upper thoracic region (Lewit 1999a).
- The joints (spinal and rib) and muscles of the region should be assessed for restriction, shortness and other evidence of dysfunction.

Breathing function evaluation

The following features should be observed when breathing function is being evaluated, whether in the presence of pathology or a habitual breathing pattern disorder (Chaitow et al 2002).

1. What is the resting respiratory rate? Normal adult range is 10–14 per minute (West 2000).
2. Is the patient a nose or a mouth breather?
3. Resting breathing pattern. Is there:
   - effortless upper chest breathing or hyperinflation?
   - accessory muscle overactivity (i.e. shoulders rise on inhalation)?
   - frequent sighs/yawns?

Continued

Box 6.45 Exercise: Palpating and assessing respiratory function continued

- breath-holding ('statue breathing')?
- abdominal splinting?
- air hunger (where an attempt to inhale seems almost strangled as there has not been a full exhalation, limiting capacity for inhalation)?
- combinations of the above?
- repeated throat clearing/air gulping?

Possible features associated with upper chest breathing patterns

1. Jaw, facial and general postural tension, tremor, tics, twitches, bitten nails.

2. Adaptive upper thoracic and shoulder girdle muscle changes, e.g. raised shoulders, protracted scapulae.
3. Kyphosis.
4. Scoliosis.
5. Kyphoscoliosis: chest wall abnormalities – for example:
   - pectus carinatum (anterior sternal protrusion)
   - pectus excavatum (depression or hollowing of the sternum).

See also 'Breathing rehabilitation methods' in Chapter 9.

Box 6.46 Orthopedic assessment examples

Note: Many of the orthopedic tests described in this section are taken or modified, with permission, from *Manipulation Therapy for the Naturopathic Physician* (2nd edn) by David Shipley DC ND (publication details in Further reading list below).

Cervical region

Standard vertebral artery test (Grant 1994)

In order to be cautious regarding cervical manipulation it is necessary to evaluate the effects of various cervical positions with the patient seated or supine: (1) extension; (2) rotation left and right; (3) rotation/extension left and right; and (4) position assessed as being required for manipulation.

- Each position is achieved actively by the patient and should be maintained (possibly with slight overpressure) by the practitioner for not less than 10 seconds.
- A return to neutral is then actively produced by the patient and maintained for 10 seconds, before the next position is adopted.

If any of these positions produces symptoms of vertigo, nausea, nystagmus or other sensations associated with vertebrobasilar insufficiency, manipulation is strongly contraindicated.

Differential assessment

Petty & Moore (2001b) suggest that in order to differentiate dizziness resulting from a compromised vertebral artery from dizziness caused by the vestibular apparatus, the following test should also be conducted:

- The patient should be standing and the practitioner maintains the head position facing forward.
- The patient moves the trunk to produce cervical rotation to the end of range.

- This is held for 10 seconds before the patient returns the trunk to a neutral position.
- The patient then introduces trunk rotation in the opposite direction in the same way.
- A positive test is noted if symptoms are produced in either position, indicating that the cause does not lie in the vestibular apparatus, and confirming that cervical manipulation is contraindicated.

Valsalva maneuver

In order to assess for a space-occupying lesion in the spinal canal the patient is requested to breathe in fully; to hold the nose with one hand, compressing both nostrils; and to attempt while doing so to blow out through the nose. The pressure created will increase pressure on neural structures caused by a herniated disc, a tumor and/or other space-occupying structures, increasing pain and associated symptoms.

Note: There are variations in the way this test is performed, as well as cautions that the maneuver itself may aggravate or cause cardiovascular, venous, neurological or cord-related problems (Han et al 2004, Uber-Zak & Venkateshme 2002). This test should not be employed if the patient suffers from glaucoma or severe hypertension.

Distraction tests

- With the patient seated, place one hand under the chin and the other under the occiput. Gently apply distraction, lifting the head towards the ceiling. Symptomatic relief (such as a decrease in pain or paresthesia) is considered positive as it indicates easing of pressure on *nerve roots*. This version of the assessment is also known as Spurling's test.
- Pain noted or increased during this test suggests *muscular involvement* in the patient's symptoms.
- A variation evaluates joint integrity following whiplash or other cervical trauma of the effect of gentle

Box 6.46 Orthopedic assessment examples continued

distraction. If when the distraction test is applied as described above there are no increased symptoms, it is repeated with the head flexed on the neck. Symptoms occurring in that position, on distraction, implicate the *tectorial membrane*, which connects the occiput to the axis, lying posterior to the transverse ligament – a continuation of the posterior longitudinal ligament (Pettman 1994).

Nerve root compression tests

• Foraminal compression: the patient is seated or supine and side-flexed to one side or the other (say to the right in this example). Compression is applied to the vertex of the skull directed towards the contralateral shoulder (left). If *nerve root compression* is present, pain will radiate into the right arm (i.e. on the side to which the neck is flexed).

• A variation has the patient's head rotated to one side (right in this example). Pressure is applied to the vertex of the skull towards the side being turned towards. Radiating pain noted in the arm indicates *nerve root compression.*

• The seated patient side-flexes and rotates the head to one side (right in this example), and then extends the neck, crowding the intervertebral foramina. If pain radiates into the arm the test is positive for *nerve root compression*. The distribution of the pain identifies the cervical level(s) involved.

Brachial plexus dysfunction and Tinel's sign
(Devor & Rapport 1990)

The spinal cord, nerve roots, plexi and peripheral nerves move with different body postures. These neural structures can be trapped at the level of the foraminal exit canals (nerve roots), in the thoracic inlet or outlet (brachial plexus), or in tendinous canals or tunnels (peripheral nerve). These anatomic entrapments form the basis of positions of comfort assumed by patients in pain, as well as the various maneuvers and stretch tests that irritate sensitized nerves.

The nerve roots, plexi and peripheral nerves have their own nerve and blood supply. Irritation by mechanical stimuli, inflammatory mediators, cytokines, prostanoids and kinins sensitizes these roots, nerves and plexi and usually causes mechano-allodynia and hyperalgesia when they are compressed.

A Tinel's sign can be elicited over any nerve root, trunk or cord of the brachial plexus or peripheral nerve where they can be palpated. For example, Tinel's sign may be evoked by the practitioner tapping the skin overlying the brachial plexus. If distal pain or paresthesia is reproduced, this suggests regeneration of previously damaged sensory nerves.

Various standard tests

• *Phalen's test* (wrist flexion test): Have the patient flex the wrists maximally by pushing the backs of the hands together, with forearms parallel to the floor. This position needs to be held for 1 minute. Tingling in the thumb, index finger, middle finger and radial half of ring finger is positive for carpal tunnel syndrome.

• *Froment's test*: With the patient pressing the tip of the thumb to the tip of the little finger on the same hand, have him 'resist' as you attempt to separate the two digits. Inability to resist separation is positive for loss of motor function of the ulnar nerve.

• *Patrick's test*: Another name for this test is the acronym 'FABERE', which indicates the motions used to perform it: *f*lexion, *ab*duction, *e*xternal *r*otation and *e*xtension.
With the patient supine, place the ankle of one limb over the opposite knee (note that the opposite limb remains stationary throughout this procedure). Stabilize the pelvis by anchoring the ASIS on the stationary side with one of your hands. Now carefully push the knee of the test leg towards the examination table with your other hand. If the patient's knee touches the table, or is able to go parallel to it, the test is negative for hip dysfunction.
If, however, the hip socket cannot fully comply, or the patient reports pain with this maneuver, Patrick's test is positive. This could indicate hip joint pathology, iliopsoas spasm or sacroiliac joint fixation.

• *Trendelenburg's test*: With the erect patient facing away from you, place your hands below the waist on either side and with your thumbs on the posterior superior iliac spine (PSIS), ask the patient to raise one leg at a time as if stepping onto a low bench.
If the patient's ipsilateral PSIS dips inferiorly when the limb on that side is flexed, this indicates mechanical, neurological or functional pelvic dysfunction requiring further investigation.

• *Valgus (abduction) knee stress test*: With the patient supine and legs straight, stabilize the ankle with your caudal hand, then push the lateral aspect of the knee toward the midline. If the tibia gives way from the femur excessively, the test is positive for weakness or tearing of the medial collateral ligament.

• *Varus (adduction) knee stress test*: Position the patient as above, with one hand stabilizing the ankle. Now push the medial aspect of the knee away from the midline. If the tibia moves away from the femur excessively, the test is positive for weakness or tearing of the lateral collateral ligament.

identify particular dysfunctional features as part of a comprehensive assessment of the individual.

Most of these tests have been established by long usage in physical therapy, osteopathy, chiropractic and/or orthopedics. Some, but not all, have also been subjected to close evaluation and scrutiny in research studies.

It is always worth remembering that the results of a single assessment method or test should not be taken as an absolute indication for a course of action, but should ideally be supported by additional information, other tests and different sources of data before clinical decisions are made. As Shipley (2000b) observes: 'It is generally good practice to confirm a positive finding with one or two other tests before concluding that a pathology/dysfunction exists.'

See the discussions in Chapter 5 on 'Palpation accuracy issues' for more on this topic.

Further reading

For further information on orthopedic testing methods, the following books are recommended:

- Boyling J, Jull G 2004 Grieve's modern manual therapy, 3rd edn. Churchill Livingstone, Edinburgh
- Petty N, Moore A 2001 Neuromuscular examination and assessment. Churchill Livingstone, Edinburgh
- Shipley D 2000 Manipulation therapy for the naturopathic physician, 2nd edn. Asclepias Publishing, Beaverton, OR

Radiographic examination

It is not within the scope of this text to discuss diagnostic imaging and the reader is referred to many excellent sources of information on this topic. Shipley (2000a) notes that:

In general practice, the most useful spinal views are generally the anteroposterior, lateral, and oblique projections. Care should be taken to review films for visible masses and questionable shadows, as well as musculoskeletal anomalies. X-rays should be used as clinical correlation to confirm a diagnosis, not to make one. Computerized tomography (CT) or magnetic resonance imaging (MRI) may be indicated after a standard radiographic examination.

The numerous exercises and examples covered in this chapter offer the opportunity to refine skills required to assess and evaluate somatic dysfunction involving skin, fascia, muscle, joints and various functions.

These skills, it is strongly suggested, are prerequisites for safe and effective application of the multiple manual modalities that make up naturopathic physical medicine. Many of these modalities are described in the next chapter.

References

Adams T, Steinmetz M, Heisey S, Holmes K, Greenman P 1982 Physiologic basis for skin properties in palpatory physical diagnosis. Journal of the American Osteopathic Association 81(6):366–377

Ahluwalia S 2001 Distribution of smooth muscle actin-containing cells in the human meniscus. Journal of Orthopaedic Research 19(4):659–664

Aina A, May S, Clare H 2004 The centralization phenomenon of spinal symptoms – a systematic review. Manual Therapy 9(3):134–143

Al-Rawi ZS, Adnan J, Al-Aszawi A et al 1985 Joint mobility among university students in Iraq. British Journal of Rheumatology 24:326–331

Alvarez DJ, Rockwell PG 2002 Trigger points – diagnosis and management. American Family Physician 65:653–660

Baldry P 1993 Acupuncture trigger points and musculoskeletal pain. Churchill Livingstone, Edinburgh

Barker P, Briggs C 1999 Attachments of the posterior layer of lumbar fascia. Spine 24(17):1757–1764

Barral J-P 1989 Visceral manipulation II. Eastland Press, Seattle

Barral J-P 1996 Manual thermal diagnosis. Eastland Press, Seattle

Barral J-P, Mercier P 1988 Visceral manipulation. Eastland Press, Seattle

Barrow DF, Cohen BA, Geraghty M et al 2002 Joint hypermobility is more common in children with chronic fatigue syndrome than in healthy controls. Journal of Pediatrics 141:421–425

Bauer J, Heine H 1998 Akupunkturpunkte und Fibromyalgie – M'glichkeiten chirurgischer Intervention. Biologische Medizin 6(12):257–261

Beal M 1983 Palpatory testing of somatic dysfunction in patients with cardiovascular disease. Journal of the American Osteopathic Association 82(11):73–82

Beighton P 1983 Hypermobility of joints. Springer, Berlin

Beighton PH, Solomon L, Soskolne CL 1973 Articular mobility in an African population. Annals of the Rheumatic Diseases 32:413–417

Bischof I, Elmiger G 1960 Connective tissue massage. In: Licht S (ed) Massage, manipulation and traction. Licht, New Haven, CT

Bohannon R, Larkin P, Cook A 1984 Decrease in timed balance test scores with aging. Physical Therapy 64:1067–1070

Brugger A 1960 Pseudoradikulara syndrome. Acta Rheumatologica 18:1

Butler D, Gifford L 1989 Adverse mechanical tensions in the nervous system. Physiotherapy 75:622–629

Butler D, Gifford L 1991 Mobilisation of the nervous system. Churchill Livingstone, Edinburgh

Butler D, Moseby L 2003 Explain pain. Noigroup Publications, Adelaide

Cathie A 1965 Some anatomicophysiologic aspects of vascular and visceral disturbances. Yearbook of the Academy of Applied Osteopathy, p 92–97

Chaitow L 2001 Muscle energy techniques, 2nd edn. Churchill Livingstone, Edinburgh

Chaitow L 2002 Positional release techniques, 2nd edn. Churchill Livingstone, Edinburgh

Chaitow L 2003a Palpation and assessment skills: assessment and diagnosis through touch, 2nd edn. Churchill Livingstone, Edinburgh

Chaitow L 2003b Modern neuromuscular techniques, 2nd edn. Churchill Livingstone, Edinburgh

Chaitow L 2005 Cranial manipulation theory and practice: osseous and soft tissue approaches, 2nd edn. Churchill Livingstone, Edinburgh

Chaitow L 2006 Muscle energy techniques, 3rd edn. Churchill Livingstone, Edinburgh

Chaitow L 2007 Positional release techniques, 3rd edn. Churchill Livingstone, Edinburgh

Chaitow L, DeLany J 2002 Clinical application of neuromuscular techniques, vol 2: the lower body. Churchill Livingstone, Edinburgh

Chaitow L, Bradley D, Gilbert C 2002 Multidisciplinary approaches to breathing pattern disorders. Churchill Livingstone, Edinburgh

Chek P 1994 Posture and craniofacial pain. In: Curl D (ed) A chiropractic approach to head pain. Lippincott Williams & Wilkins, Philadelphia

Cheng N, Van Hoof H, Bockx E et al 1982 The effects of electric currents on ATP generation, protein synthesis and membrane transport in rat skin. Clinical Orthopedics 171:264–272

Chikly B 1996 Lymph drainage therapy: study guide level I. UI Publishing, Palm Beach Gardens, FL

Cholewicki J, McGill S 1996 Mechanical stability of the in vivo lumbar spine. Clinical Biomechanics 11:1–15

Cohen J, Gibbons R 1998 Raymond Nimmo and the evolution of trigger point therapy. Journal of Manipulation and Physiological Therapeutics 21(3):167–172

Dalstra M 1997 Biomechanics of the human pelvic bone. In: Vleeming A, Mooney V, Dorman T, Snijders C, Stoeckart R (eds) Movement, stability and low back pain. Churchill Livingstone, Edinburgh

Defalque R 1982 Painful trigger points in surgical scars. Anesthesia and Analgesia 61(6):518–520

Defeo G, Hicks L 1993 Description of the common compensatory pattern in relationship to the osteopathic postural examination. Dynamic Chiropractic 24:11

DeLany J 1996 American neuromuscular therapy. In: Chaitow L (ed) Modern neuromuscular techniques. Churchill Livingstone, Edinburgh

Devor M, Rapport Z 1990 Pain and the pathophysiology of damaged nerve. In: Fields HL (ed) Pain syndromes in neurology. Butterworths, London, p 51

Dexter J, Simons D 1981 Local twitch response in human muscle evoked by palpation and needle penetration of a trigger point. Archives of Physical Medicine and Rehabilitation 62:521–522

Deyo R, Rainville J, Kent D 1992 What can the history and physical examination tell us about low back pain? Journal of the American Medical Association 268:760–765

Dommerholt J 2000 Posture. In: Tubiana R, Amadio P (eds) Medical problems of the instrumentalist musician. Martin Dunitz, London, p 405–406

DonTigny R 1995 Function of the lumbosacroiliac complex as a self compensating force couple. In: Vleeming A, Mooney V, Dorman T, Snijders C (eds) 2nd Interdisciplinary World Congress on Low Back Pain. San Diego, California, 9–11 November

Dosch P 1984 Manual of neural therapy, 11th edn. Haug, Heidelberg, p 112–166

Exelby L 2002 The Mulligan concept: its application in the management of spinal conditions. Manual Therapy 7(2):64–70

Fernández-de-las-Peñas C, Alonso-Blanco C, Fernández-Carnero J, Miangolarra-Page J 2006 The immediate effect of ischemic compression technique and transverse friction massage on tenderness of active and latent myofascial trigger points: a pilot study. Journal of Bodywork and Movement Therapies 10:3–9

Ford C 1989 Where healing waters meet. Station Hill Press, New York

Foster G, Vaziri N, Sassoon C 2001 Respiratory alkalosis. Respiratory Care 46(4):384–391

Fryer G, Hodgeson L 2005 The effect of manual pressure release on myofascial trigger points in the upper trapezius muscle. Journal of Bodywork and Movement Therapies 9(4):248–255

Fryer G, Morris T, Gibbons P 2004 The relation between thoracic spinal tissues and pressure sensitivity measured by a digital algometer. Journal of Osteopathic Medicine 7(2):64–69

Fryette H 1954 Principles of osteopathic technique. American Academy of Osteopathy, Newark, OH

Frymann V 1963 Palpation – its study in the workshop. Academy of Applied Osteopathy Yearbook, Newark, OH, p 16–30

Fukuda T 1984 Statokinetic reflexes in equilibrium and movement. University of Tokyo Press, Tokyo, p 5

Gagey P, Gentaz R 1996 Postural disorders of the body axis. In: Liebenson C (ed) Rehabilitation of the spine. Williams & Wilkins, Baltimore

Garland W 1994 Somatic changes in the hyperventilating subject. Presentation at Respiratory Function Congress, Paris

Gibbons P, Tehan P 1998 Muscle energy concepts and coupled motion of the spine. Manual Therapy 3(2):95–101

Giles L 2003 50 Challenging spinal pain syndrome cases. Butterworth-Heinemann, Edinburgh

Goldthwait JE 1945 Essentials of body mechanics in health and disease, 4th edn. Lippincott, Philadelphia

Grant R 1994 Vertebral artery concerns. In: Grant R (ed) Physical therapy of the cervical and thoracic spine, 2nd edn. Churchill Livingstone, New York, p 145

Gray's anatomy 1999 (Williams P, ed) 38th edn. Churchill Livingstone, Edinburgh

Greenman P 1996 Principles of manual medicine, 2nd edn. Williams & Wilkins, Baltimore

Grieve G 1994 The masqueraders. In: Boyling JD, Palastanga N (eds) Grieve's modern manual therapy of the vertebral column, 2nd edn. Churchill Livingstone, Edinburgh

Han JJ, Massagli TL, Jaffe KM 2004 Fibrocartilaginous embolism – an uncommon cause of spinal cord infarction: a case report and review of the literature. Archives of Physical Medicine and Rehabilitation 85(1):153–157

Hastreiter D, Ozuna RM, Spector M 2001 Regional variations in certain cellular characteristics in human lumbar intervertebral discs, including the presence of smooth muscle actin. Journal of Orthopaedic Research 19(4):597–604

He J 1998 Stretch reflex sensitivity: effects of postural and muscle length changes. IEEE Transactions on Rehabilitation Engineering 6(2):182–189

Heine H 1995 Functional anatomy of traditional Chinese acupuncture points. Acta Anatomica 152:293

Hong C-Z, Chen Y-N, Twehouse D, Hong D 1996 Pressure threshold for referred pain by compression on trigger point and adjacent area. Journal of Musculoskeletal Pain 4(3):61–79

Hoover H 1969 Method for teaching functional technique. Yearbook of the Academy of Applied Osteopathy, Newark, OH

Hudson N, Starr MR, Esdaile JM, Fitzcharles MA 1995 Diagnostic associations with hypermobility in new rheumatology referrals. British Journal of Rheumatology 34:1157–1161

Janda V 1978 Muscles, central nervous motor regulation, and back problems. In: Korr IM (ed) Neurobiologic mechanisms in manipulative therapy. Plenum, New York

Janda V 1982 Introduction to functional pathology of the motor system. Proceedings of the VII Commonwealth and International Conference on Sport. Physiotherapy in Sport 3:39

Janda V 1983 Muscle function testing. Butterworths, London

Janda V 1986 Muscle weakness and inhibition (pseudoparesis) in back pain syndromes. In: Grieve G (ed) Modern manual therapy of the vertebral column. Churchill Livingstone, Edinburgh, p 197–201

Janda V 1988 Postural and phasic muscles in the pathogenesis of low back pain. In: Proceedings of the XIth Congress of the International Society of Rehabilitation and Disability, Dublin, Ireland, p 553–554

Janda V 1996 Evaluation of muscular imbalance. In: Liebenson C (ed) Rehabilitation of the spine. Williams & Wilkins, Baltimore

Janda V, Schmid HJA 1980 Muscles as a pathogenic factor in back pain. Proceedings of the International Federation of Orthopaedic Manipulative Therapists 4th Conference, New Zealand, p 17–18

Johnston W 1988 Segmental definitions III. Journal of the American Osteopathic Association 8:347–353

Kaltenborn F 1985 Mobilization of the extremity joints. Olaf Norlis Bokhandel, Oslo

Kapanji IA 1987 The physiology of the joints, vols 1, 2 and 3. Churchill Livingstone, Edinburgh

Kappler R 1997 Palpatory skills. In: Ward R (ed) Foundations for osteopathic medicine. Williams & Wilkins, Baltimore, p 473–479

Kappler R, Larson N, Kelso A 1971 A comparison of osteopathic findings on hospitalized patients obtained by trained student examiners and experienced physicians. Journal of the American Osteopathic Association 70(10):1091–1092

Karaaslan Y, Haznedaroglu S, Ozturk M 2000 Joint hypermobility and primary fibromyalgia. Journal of Rheumatology 27:1774–1776

Keating J, Matuyas T, Bach T 1993 The effect of training on physical therapist's ability to apply specified forces of palpation. Physical Therapy 73(1):38–46

Kecr R, Grahame R 2003 Hypermobility syndrome: recognition and management for physiotherapists. Butterworth-Heinemann, Edinburgh, p 80

Kelsey M 1951 Diagnosis of upper abdominal pain. Texas State Journal of Medicine 47:82–86

Kendall N, Linton S, Main C 1997 Guide to assessing psychosocial yellow flags in acute low back pain. Accident Rehabilitation & Compensation Insurance Corporation of New Zealand, Wellington, NZ

Key J, Clift A, Condie F 2008 A model of movement dysfunction Part 2. Journal of Bodywork and Movement Therapies 12(2):135.

Korr I 1976 Proprioceptors and somatic dysfunction. Yearbook of the Academy of Applied Osteopathy, Newark, OH

Kuchera M 1997 Treatment of gravitational strain. In: Vleeming A, Mooney V, Dorman T, Snijders C, Stoeckart R (eds) Movement, stability, and low back pain. Churchill Livingstone, New York

Kuchera M, Goodridge J 1997 Lower extremity. In: Ward R (ed) Foundations for osteopathic medicine. Williams & Wilkins, Baltimore

Kuchera W, Kuchera M 1994 Osteopathic principles in practice. Greyden Press, Columbus, OH

Kuchera M, Kuchera W 1997 General postural considerations. In: Ward R (ed) Foundations for osteopathic medicine. Williams & Wilkins, Baltimore

Kuchera M et al 1990 Athletic functional demand and posture. Journal of the American Osteopathic Association 90(9):843–844

Larson N 1977 Manipulative care before and after surgery. Osteopathic Medicine 2:41–49

Larsson SE, Bodegard L, Henriksson KG et al 1990 Chronic trapezius myalgia. Morphology and blood flow studied in 17 patients. Acta Orthopaedica Scandinavica 61:394–398

Lee D 1997 Treatment of pelvic instability. In: Vleeming A, Mooney V, Dorman T, Snijders C, Stoeckart R (eds) Movement, stability and low back pain. Churchill Livingstone, New York

Lee D 1999 The pelvic girdle. Churchill Livingstone, Edinburgh

Lee D 2000 The pelvic girdle: an approach to the examination and treatment of the lumbo-pelvic-hip region, 2nd edn. Churchill Livingstone, Edinburgh

Lewit K 1992 Manipulative therapy in rehabilitation of the locomotor system, 2nd edn. Churchill Livingstone, Edinburgh, p 116–121

Lewit K 1999a Manipulative therapy in rehabilitation of the locomotor system, 3rd edn. Butterworth-Heinemann, Oxford

Lewit K 1999b Manipulative therapy in rehabilitation of the locomotor system, 3rd edn. Butterworth-Heinemann, Oxford, p 81

Lewit K 1999c Chain reactions in the locomotor system. Journal of Orthopaedic Medicine 21:52–58

Lewit K, Olanska S 2004 Clinical importance of active scars: abnormal scars as a cause of myofascial pain. Journal of Manipulative and Physiological Therapeutics 27(6):399–402

Liebenson C 1996a Integrating rehabilitation into chiropractic practice. In: Liebenson C (ed) Rehabilitation of the spine. Williams & Wilkins, Baltimore

Liebenson C (ed) 1996b Rehabilitation of the spine: a practitioner's manual. Williams & Wilkins, Baltimore

Liebenson C 2001 Sensory motor training. Journal of Bodywork and Movement Therapies 5(1):21–27

Liebenson C (ed) 2005 Rehabilitation of the spine: a practitioner's manual, 2nd edn. Lippincott Williams & Wilkins, Philadelphia

Liebenson C, Oslance J 1996 Outcome assessment in the small private practice. In: Liebenson C (ed) Rehabilitation of the spine. Williams & Wilkins, Baltimore

Liem T 2004 Cranial osteopathy: principles and practice. Churchill Livingstone, Edinburgh, p 340–342

Lisi A 2007 Overview of the McKenzie method. In: Chaitow L (ed) Positional release techniques, 3rd edn. Churchill Livingstone, Edinburgh

Magoun H 1962 Gastroduodenal ulcers from the osteopathic viewpoint. American Academy of Osteopathy Yearbook, Indianapolis, IN, p 117–120

Maitland G 1986 Vertebral manipulation, 5th edn. Butterworths, London

McFarlane Tilley R 1961 Spinal stress palpation. Yearbook of the Academy of Applied Osteopathy, Newark, OH

McGill S 1991 Electromyographic activity of the abdominal and low back musculature during generation of isometric and dynamic axial trunk torque. Journal of Orthopedic Research 9:91–103

McGill SM, Juker D, Kropf P 1996 Quantitative intramuscular myoelectric activity of quadratus lumborum during a wide variety of tasks. Clinical Biomechanics 11:170–172

McKenzie R 1981 The lumbar spine: mechanical diagnosis and therapy. Spinal Publications, Waikanae, NZ

McMakin C 2004 Microcurrent therapy: a novel treatment method for chronic low back myofascial pain. Journal of Bodywork and Movement Therapies 8(2):143–153

McPartland J, Goodridge J 1997 Osteopathic examination of the cervical spine. Journal of Bodywork and Movement Therapies 1(3):173–178

Meiss RA 1993 Persistent mechanical effects of decreasing length during isometric contraction of ovarian ligament smooth muscle. Journal of Muscle Research and Cell Motility 14(2):205–218

Melzack R 1977 Trigger points and acupuncture points of pain. Pain 3:3–23

Mennell J 1964 Back pain. Churchill, Boston

Mense S, Simons D 2001 Muscle pain. Lippincott Williams & Wilkins, Philadelphia

Mimura M, Moriya H, Watanabe T et al 1989 Three-dimensional motion analysis of the cervical spine with special reference to the axial rotation. Spine 14(11):1135–1139

Moore M 2004 Upper crossed syndrome and its relationship to cervicogenic headache. Journal of Manipulative Physiology and Therapeutics 27:414–420

Muller K, Kreutzfeldt A, Schwesig R et al 2003 Hypermobility and chronic back pain. Manuelle Medizin 41:105–109

Mulligan BR 1995 Spinal mobilisations with leg movement (further mobilisations with movement). Journal of Manual and Manipulative Therapy 3(1):25–27

Murphy D 2000 Conservative management of cervical spine syndromes. McGraw-Hill, New York

Myers T 1997 Anatomy trains. Journal of Bodywork and Movement Therapies 1(2):91–101 and 1(3):134–145

Myers T 2001 Anatomy trains: myofascial meridians for manual and movement therapists. Churchill Livingstone, Edinburgh

Nicholas A, DeBias D, Ehrenfeuchter W et al 1987 A somatic component to myocardial infarction. Journal of the American Osteopathic Association 87(2):123–133

Nijs J 2005 Generalized joint hypermobility: an issue in fibromyalgia and chronic fatigue syndrome? Journal of Bodywork and Movement Therapies 9(4):310–317

Nimmo R 1957 Receptors, effectors and tonus. Journal of the National Chiropractic Association 27(11):21

Norris C 1995 Spinal stabilisation. 4. Muscle imbalance and the low back. Physiotherapy 81(3):127–138

Norris C 1998 Sports injuries, diagnosis and management, 2nd edn. Butterworths, London

Norris C 1999 Functional load abdominal training (part 1). Journal of Bodywork and Movement Therapies 3(3):150–158

Norris C 2000a The muscle designation debate. Journal of Bodywork and Movement Therapies 4(4):225–241

Norris C 2000b Back stability. Human Kinetics, Champaign, IL

Oyama I, Rejba A, Lukban J et al 2004 Modified Thiele massage as therapeutic intervention for female patients with interstitial cystitis and high-tone pelvic floor dysfunction. Urology 64(5):862–886

Pettman E 1994 Stress tests of the craniovertebral joints. In: Boyling J, Palastanga N (eds) Grieve's modern manual therapy, 2nd edn. Churchill Livingstone, Edinburgh, p 529

Petty N, Moore A 2001a Neuromuscular examination and assessment, 2nd edn. Churchill Livingstone, Edinburgh, p 242

Petty N, Moore A 2001b Neuromuscular examination and assessment, 2nd edn. Churchill Livingstone, Edinburgh, p 162

Pick M 1999a Cranial sutures: analysis, morphology and manipulative strategies. Eastland Press, Seattle

Pick M 1999b Cranial sutures: analysis, morphology and manipulative strategies. Eastland Press, Seattle, p xx–xxi

Pryce J 1980 Wrist position between neutral and ulnar deviation that facilitates maximum power grip strength. Journal of Biomechanics 13:505–511

Pryor J, Prasad S 2002 Physiotherapy for respiratory and cardiac problems, 3rd edn. Churchill Livingstone, Edinburgh

Razmjou H, Kramer JF, Yamada R 2000 Intertester reliability of the McKenzie evaluation in assessing patients with mechanical low-back pain. Journal of Orthopaedic and Sports Physical Therapy 30(7): 368–389

RCGP 1999 Clinical guidelines for management of acute low back pain. Royal College of General Practitioners, London

Rocobado M 1985 Arthrokinematics of the temporomandibular joint. In: Gelb H (ed) Clinical management of head, neck and TMJ pain and dysfunction. WB Saunders, Philadelphia

Rolf I 1977 Rolfing – integration of human structures. Harper & Row, New York

Rosenthal E 1987 Alexander technique and how it works. Medical Problems in the Performing Arts 2:53–57

Rosero H, Greene C, DeBias D 1987 Correlation of palpatory observations with anatomic locus of acute myocardial infarction. Journal of the American Osteopathic Association 87(2):118–122

Russek LN 1999 Hypermobility syndrome. Physical Therapy 79(6):591–599

Selye H 1976 Stress in health and disease. Butterworths, Reading, MA

Selye H 1984 The stress of life. McGraw-Hill, New York

Shipley D 2000a Manipulation therapy for the naturopathic physician, 2nd edn. Asclepias Publishing, Beaverton, OR

Shipley D 2000b Manipulation therapy for the naturopathic physician, 2nd edn. Asclepias Publishing, Beaverton, OR, p 36

Simons D 1993a Myofascial pain and dysfunction review. Journal of Musculoskeletal Pain 1(2):131

Simons D 1993b Referred phenomena of myofascial trigger points. In: Vecchiet L, Albe-Fessard D, Lindbolm U (eds) New trends in referred pain and hyperalgesia. Elsevier, Amsterdam

Simons D 1996 Clinical and etiological update of myofascial pain from trigger points. Journal of Musculoskeletal Pain 4:93–121

Simons D, Mense S 1997 Understanding and measurement of muscle tone as related to clinical muscle pain. Pain 75(1):1–17

Simons D, Travell J, Simons L 1999 Myofascial pain and dysfunction: the trigger point manual, vol. 1: upper half of body, 2nd edn. Williams & Wilkins, Baltimore

Staubesand J, Li Y 1996 Zum Feinbau der Fascia cruris mit besonderer Berücksichtigung epi- und intrafaszialer Nerven. Manuelle Medizin 34:196–200

Staubesand J, Li Y 1997 Begriff und Substrat der Faziensklerose bei chronisch-venöser Insuffizienz. Phlebologie 26:72–79

Stone C 1999 The science and art of osteopathy. Stanley Thornes, Cheltenham

Swerdlow B, Dieter N 1992 Evaluation of thermography. Pain 48:205–213

Travell J, Simons D 1983a Myofascial pain and dysfunction: the trigger point manual, vol. 1: the upper body. Williams & Wilkins, Baltimore

Travell J, Simons D 1983b Myofascial pain and dysfunction, vol 1: the upper body. Williams & Wilkins, Baltimore, p 671

Uber-Zak L, Venkateshme Y 2002 Neurologic complications of sit-ups associated with the valsalva maneuver: 2 case reports. Archives of Physical Medicine and Rehabilitation 83(2):278–282

Upledger J, Vredevoogd J 1983 Craniosacral therapy. Eastland Press, Seattle

Van Tulder M, Becker A, Nekkering T et al 2004 European guidelines for the management of acute nonspecific low back pain in primary care. Proceedings of 5th Interdisciplinary World Congress on Low Back and Pelvic Pain, Melbourne, Australia, p 56–79

van Wingerden J-P 1997 The role of the hamstrings in pelvic and spinal function. In: Vleeming A (ed) Movement, stability and low back pain. Churchill Livingstone, New York

Varma D 1935 The human machine and its forces. Health For All Publishing, London

Vleeming A, Mooney A, Dorman T et al 1989 Load application to the sacrotuberous ligament: influences on sacroiliac joint mechanics. Clinical Biomechanics 4:204–209

Vleeming A, Mooney V, Dorman T, Snijders C, Stoeckart R (eds) 1997 Movement, stability and low back pain. Churchill Livingstone, New York

Wall P, Melzack R 1989 Textbook of pain, 2nd edn. Churchill Livingstone, London

Ward R (ed) 1997 Foundations of osteopathic medicine. Williams & Wilkins, Baltimore

Weiss J 2001 Pelvic floor myofascial trigger points: manual therapy for interstitial cystitis and the urgency–frequency syndrome. Journal of Urology 166:2226–2231

West J 2000 Respiratory physiology. Williams & Wilkins, Philadelphia

Wilson E 2002 The Mulligan concept: NAGs, SNAGs and MWMs etc. In: Chaitow L (ed) Positional release techniques, 2nd edn. Churchill Livingstone, Edinburgh, p 172

Wolfe F, Simons DG, Fricton J et al 1992 The fibromyalgia and myofascial pain syndromes: a preliminary study of tender points and trigger points in persons with fibromyalgia, myofascial pain syndrome and no disease. Journal of Rheumatology 19(6):944–951

Yahia L, Pigeon P, DesRosiers E 1993 Viscoelastic properties of the human lumbodorsal fascia. Journal of Biomedical Engineering 15:425–429

Zink G, Lawson W 1979 An osteopathic structural examination and functional interpretation of the soma. Osteopathic Annals 7(12):433–440

7

Leon Chaitow ND DO

With contributions from:
Hal Brown ND DC
Douglas C. Lewis ND
Dean E. Neary Jr ND
Roger Newman Turner ND DO
Lisa Maeckel MA CHT
Brian K. Youngs ND DO
Nick Buratovich ND

Modalities, Methods and Techniques

Chapter objectives

The focus of this chapter is to present information regarding a wide range of modalities, methods and techniques that comprise some of the most useful physical medicine approaches employed in naturopathic medicine. These modalities are commonly used to address local dysfunction, or they may be utilized as part of a comprehensive, whole-body, constitutional approach to the patient, individually or in combination with each other.

Constitutional approaches

In Chapter 8 various distinctively naturopathic, constitutional (whole-body) means of evaluating and treating general health, as well as locally dysfunctional conditions, are described and explored in the context of the use of neuromuscular technique, or of a general mobilization approach known as general naturopathic tonic technique (GNTT). There is inevitably an overlap between some of the material covered in this chapter and that outlined in Chapter 8, specifically in relation to neuromuscular technique (NMT), mobilization methods, and in the discussion of what can be termed 'wellness massage'.

As mentioned above, in Chapter 8 details are presented of general (or universal) naturopathic tonic technique (GNTT or UNTT), a universally applicable method developed in the 1920s by Frederick Collins MD ND, and described by Cordingly (1925).

Individual modalities may be interchangeable

In numerous instances, many of the modalities discussed and outlined in this chapter may be seen to be virtually interchangeable. For example, where an area of soft tissue dysfunction is characterized by excessive tone and shortness in muscle, the choice between employing muscle energy technique methods or myofascial release technique methods may simply represent a personal preference on the part of the practitioner, rather than any intrinsic difference in the potential outcome, or the choice of modality may represent an intuitive 'feel' as to which treatment a patient with a particular presentation would best respond.

The selection of modalities outlined in this chapter is not meant to simply provide a cookbook collection in which 'this technique for that condition' is suggested. Instead, it approaches the discussion by outlining the methods, their suggested physiological effects, and how these methods are best applied in the context of musculoskeletal distress in particular, and wider health problems in general.

Methods and modalities are discussed in relation to their general applicability to a wide range of conditions or situations, as well as to specific clinical circumstances where evidence exists for the value of one approach rather than another. Examples of such 'specific' indicators are to be found later in this chapter where methods of categorization of low back pain (used as an example) are discussed.

In that section of this chapter it will become clear that some classes of back problem respond well to manipulation – such as high velocity, low amplitude (HVLA) thrust methods – while others benefit mainly from identifiable patterns of exercise. Evidence shows that manipulation of the 'exercise sensitive' class of back pain would offer little benefit and, likewise, specific exercises are unlikely to help 'manipulation sensitive' back problems (Flynn et al 2002). Of course there are also back problems that are unlikely to respond to either manipulation or exercise, and some that may respond to both.

The key to successful outcomes in rehabilitating dysfunction – whether involving back pain or anything else – lies in identification of the processes that are operating, and, as best possible, recognizing underlying causative and maintaining features. Recovery can then be encouraged as 'load' is reduced and function enhanced – allowing self-regulating, homeostatic systems and mechanisms to operate as nature intended. As was expressed in Chapter 1, this reliance on self-regulation lies at the heart of naturopathic physical medicine.

Efficacy and safety

In this chapter evidence of efficacy of individual methods, techniques and modalities will be graded in a spectrum ranging from 'very good' (systematic review evidence) to 'poor' (rumor, tradition). That said, it is worth reminding ourselves that *lack of proof of efficacy does not represent proof of a lack of efficacy*.

Safety, on the other hand, is non-negotiable, and issues relating to evidence of risk will also be highlighted in presentation of the various methods, techniques and modalities that make up the bulk of this chapter. (See Box 7.5 for a deeper discussion of HVLA safety issues.)

The constituent characteristics that make up a technique are also described – for example, myofascial release (MFR) technique incorporates a combination of compression and distraction (lengthening) features that are common to many other techniques (proprioceptive neuromuscular facilitation, muscle energy, etc.), but which are used in particular ways in MFR. The relative advantages of incorporating different features in various clinical settings are explained wherever evidence exists for such discussion.

Low back pain as an example

Taking low back pain (LBP) disorders as a common and easily comprehended example, a review of the literature demonstrates that there is no universally applicable technique, method, approach or modality that will always be helpful in restoring pain-free functionality, since the causes and features of the condition (LBP) are anything but uniform.

An individualized approach is demanded, since two seemingly identical sets of symptoms might have completely different etiological and aggravating features. These would benefit from quite different therapeutic and rehabilitation strategies – one possibly requiring deactivation of myofascial trigger points followed by postural re-education, the other calling for joint mobilization achieved by high velocity thrust methodology, supported by appropriate soft tissue normalization possibly involving stretching and/or core stability training.

On the other hand, it is possible to generalize and say that, since by definition pain is always a feature of LBP, in many instances accompanied by hypomobility, it may be possible to identify methods and techniques that are likely to modulate both features (pain and hypomobility) in most cases – for example, massage therapy (Ernst 1999, Furlan et al 2002). Massage therapy – as with all modalities, methods and techniques – is itself made up of a series of generic 'building-blocks' or different means of application of load (see discussion below regarding the therapeutic application of load).

Massage is capable of being deep or shallow, rapid and stimulating or slow and relaxing, incorporating specific attention to dysfunctional features, or of being completely non-invasive in order to offer a period of calm. These variables make use of the word 'massage' potentially uninformative, since that word covers everything from deep tissue work to superficial stroking. The descriptions later in this chapter take account of the need for greater specificity.

There has been some success in attempts to categorize 'low back pain', and examples are outlined later in this chapter as to how this has led to the possibility of making evidence-based clinical choices – for example, in regard to the use of manipulation, or exercise, or other modality.

Caution over evidence

In a comprehensive review evaluating the evidence base for use of a variety of approaches in treatment of 'musculoskeletal conditions', Ernst (2004) highlights the usefulness of massage, but questions spinal manipulation's value in treatment of back pain (Assendelft et al 2003) (see also Ernst & Canter 2006):

For acute back pain, spinal manipulation [high velocity, low amplitude thrust – HVLA] was superior to sham therapy and to treatments known to have detrimental effects on back pain. Spinal manipulation generated no advantage over general practitioner care, analgesics, physical therapy, exercise or back school. For chronic back pain, the results proved to be similar.

Unpicking this quoted statement brings sharply into focus the danger of relying on such evidence.

- 'Acute back pain' may have a wide variety of causes, ranging from biomechanical to pathological, psychological and functional features, possibly involving intervertebral disc problems, facet joint dysfunction, hypermobility, muscular and/or ligamentous imbalances, sacroiliac restrictions, trigger points and disturbed emotion/somatization (among others), making it a virtual certainty that 'acute back pain' will not respond to a single intervention, whether HVLA manipulation or anything else.

- The term 'spinal manipulation' may mean HVLA, or it might refer to employment of mobilizing articulation, or soft tissue methods such as muscle energy technique, or combinations of these, or use of chiropractic 'activator' adjustments. And even where HVLA is the specified intervention, there are a wide range of possibilities as to how, and where, this was applied, making evaluation of 'manipulation' for 'acute back pain' a virtually meaningless exercise, or at best a questionable one – unless each patient (irrespective of etiology) received precisely the same manipulative attention, at precisely the same spinal region.

- Similar variables exist in other words in the quoted text above. What, for example, can it be assumed that 'general practitioner care', 'physical therapy' and 'exercise' actually mean, emerging as they do from a systematic review of numerous research papers in which untold variations of each of these areas of care might have been included?

- Rosner (2003) has summarized the relative futility of randomized controlled trials (RCTs) in the study of problems such as low back pain, with all its variables, as well as the validity of conclusions of systematic reviews based on summaries of such trials.

- As an example of the denseness of the fog surrounding much research it is useful to consider that some osteopathic medicine studies describe manual interventions as 'OMT' (osteopathic manipulative treatment). When the content of OMT is broken down, it is sometimes stated to include – amongst others – HVLA, myofascial release, ligamentous balancing, muscle energy and strain/counterstrain techniques (Yates et al 2002). As will become clearer to those unfamiliar with these methods (see the descriptions later in this chapter), there can hardly be more diverse methods for modifying tissue status, or mobilizing joints, than those listed. There is frequently therefore no uniformity in application of OMT, apart from the fact that one or other, or a combination of these methods may be employed. This is not a criticism of the use of OMT, since a selection of diverse methods is essential if patients are to receive individualized attention. However, it is a criticism of reviewers who attempt to homogenize outcomes where actual treatment – uniformly listed as OMT – might have involved all or any of the methods mentioned.
- This is why it has long been recognized that the only true way to evaluate the efficacy of a given discipline – such as chiropractic, osteopathic or for that matter naturopathic care – is to conduct outcome studies. In these, the elements of treatment used to help the patient are not tested – only the intervention of the discipline. This allows a greater opportunity for a non-linear dynamic interplay between patient and practitioner – which characterizes these manual therapies – to play out, rather than a linearized, artificial, dose–response assessment of individual techniques.
- In some studies, precise descriptions are offered of which elements of OMT were utilized. For example, in a study of the use of OMT in treatment of chronic asthma (Bockenhauer et al 2002), it is clearly stated that four methods (balancing ligamentous tension in the upper cervical and upper thoracic junctions; normalization of elevated first rib; mobilization of lower rib exhalation restrictions; diaphragmatic release) were employed sequentially in each patient, compared with sham treatment, making the positive outcomes (increased upper thoracic and lower thoracic forced respiratory excursion) credible, useful and potentially reproducible.
- The OMT issue is, however, no more confusing than the use of terms such as 'physical therapy'. Mehling et al (2005) compared 'gold standard physical therapy' with breathing rehabilitation (also not clearly defined) in treatment of chronic low back pain. Both approaches produced good to excellent results; however, since the reader is left with the mystery as to what 'gold standard physical therapy' is, and just how breathing rehabilitation is achieved, the chances of reproducing the results remains questionable.

For these reasons Ernst's controversial assertion that osteopathic and chiropractic manipulation has little value, is itself of little value, flying as it does in the face of the clinical experience of the chiropractic and osteopathic professions, where manipulation, *when appropriately applied, to match the specific needs of the individual*, appears to offer clear benefit in a range of back and other problems.

This highlights the need in our descriptions of naturopathic physical medicine methodology to describe both generic and specific use of modalities, methods and techniques – not least massage and manipulation (HVLA).

It behoves us to be as precise as possible in our descriptions of methods, modalities and techniques, as well as in the evidence for the use of these in general and in specific settings.

It is also important that we regularly refer to the underlying principles – as outlined in Chapter 1 – that inform clinical decision-making in naturopathic medicine in general and naturopathic physical medicine in particular.

Principles consistent with all techniques of manual medicine

Objectives determine choice of therapeutic load application

Therapeutic objectives derive from evidence that emerges from the individual's history, as well as from observation, assessment, palpation, etc. These elements inform the practitioner as to what needs to be achieved in order to enhance endogenous self-regulatory processes, whether this involves reduction of pain, increased range of motion (ROM), greater stability or a modification of some other feature of the patient's condition.

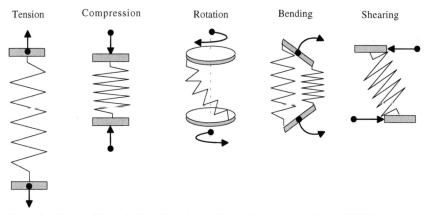

Tension   Compression   Rotation   Bending   Shearing

Figure 7.1 Modes of tissue loading. Reproduced with permission from Lederman (1997a)

Although there exist a wide range of variations of manual techniques, each of these is made up of a number of basic generic elements and carries inherent potentials for physiological change.

Lederman (1997a) has summarized these as incorporating various 'modes of loading' (Fig. 7.1):

- *Tension loading*: may involve traction, extension, elongation or other longitudinal lengthening procedures affecting fiber length
- *Compression loading*: involves crowding, increased pressure, encouraging movement of fluids out of tissues, with little change in actual fiber length resulting
- *Rotation loading*: produces some lengthening effects in soft tissues, along with a great deal of compression; this form of loading is used more in mobilization and articulation of joints
- *Bending loading*: in soft tissues this produces lengthening on the convex side of the tissues, along with compression on the concave side; in joints this produces extension, flexion and side-flexion movements
- *Shearing loading*: translation (shear) movements have some effect on soft tissues (a combination of compression and lengthening); shear forces are used more significantly in attempts to induce joint play and articulation
- *Combined loading*: incorporation of combinations of other loading variables creates progressive degrees of tension and compression.

Combinations of modes of loading – varied by the degree of force employed, directions of force (direct towards the restriction barrier, or indirect involving disengagement from the barrier, or alternating combinations of these), the amount of time involved (continuous, rhythmic, brief, lengthy, etc.), the rate at which loads are applied (rapidly, slowly, variably), whether the method is passive or active, or involves a combination of patient and practitioner effort, as well as which tissues are involved (muscle, fascia, scar tissue, joint, etc.) and their properties, along with practitioner intent – create a huge range of variables that make up the orchestral variety of therapeutic options open to the practitioner.

Consider just a few of these loads as they might combine in the context of therapeutic massage or soft tissue manipulation (see Box 7.1).

A musculoskeletal model of care

Liebenson (1996a) has summarized the ways in which dysfunction in the musculoskeletal system can usually be improved or corrected.

1. Identify local and general imbalances (posture, patterns of use, local dysfunction).
2. Identify, relax and stretch overactive, tight muscles.
3. Mobilize and/or manipulate restricted joints.
4. Facilitate and strengthen weak muscles.
5. Re-educate movement patterns (including postural imbalances) on a reflex, subcortical basis.

This sequence is based on sound biomechanical principles (Jull & Janda 1987, Lewit 1999) and serves as a useful basis for care and rehabilitation of the patient with musculoskeletal problems, although it fails to embrace the psychological and biochemical features of such problems. A variety of soft tissue normalization methods are incorporated into this

Box 7.1 Shear and other forces

Massage and soft tissue manipulation methods that involve kneading, introduce torsional load forces. As tissues are kneaded, soft tissues are lifted, rolled and squeezed, involving compressive, bending, shearing and torsion loads. This may have as an objective the stretching of tissues or encouragement of fluid movement within the tissues.

During massage or soft tissue manipulation shear loading may move soft tissues in a translatory manner – for example, back and forth involving sliding forces that compress and elongate tissues. Friction occurs between the sliding structures, potentially generating physiological change by increasing connective tissue pliability (hysteresis; Norkin & Levangie 1992), as well as possibly inducing a mild therapeutic inflammatory response (Mock 1997).

Cross-fiber friction involves a series of localized shear forces, consisting of small, deep movements, performed on a local area, usually across the line of fiber direction. Friction will increase blood flow to the area (and may induce edema if appropriate measures are not taken to obviate this). Cross-fiber friction has been used effectively in deactivation of trigger points. In a study by Fernández-de-las-Peñas et al (2006) comparing a commonly employed element of massage – compression with friction – an equal degree of improvement in pain threshold and reduction of painful symptoms was achieved (Hou et al 2002).

Note: Whether friction or compression is employed in attempting to deactivate myofascial trigger points, a rapid inflow of oxygenated blood to the tissues occurs (Simons et al 1999). The therapeutic benefits that follow may variously involve reduction of ischemia, as well as release of local endorphins, and possibly enkephalins (Baldry 1993, Kiser et al 1983), and also a degree of mechanoreceptor stimulation affecting pain transmission (Melzack & Wall 1994). A combination of circulatory, endocrine and neurological changes therefore follows in response to simple applications of focused compression or repetitive shear loading.

model in most schools of manual medicine (DiGiovanna & Schiowitz 1991, Greenman 1989).

A broader model of care

The biomechanical model described by Liebenson (above) is one of many variants. Other proposed models for effective management of musculoskeletal dysfunction incorporate somatic as well as behavioral features. Langevin & Sherman (2006) have described a pathophysiological model in which a broader – and therefore possibly more naturopathic – therapeutic approach to low back problems in particular, and

musculoskeletal dysfunction in general, can be understood. This 'integrative mechanistic' model that addresses behavioral and structural aspects of dysfunction, as well as pain psychology, postural control and neuroplasticity, strengthens the rationale for multidisciplinary treatment protocols. These might include direct biomechanical tissue approaches, movement re-education, psychosocial interventions and, where necessary, pharmacological and/or nutritional treatment methods and modalities that meet the needs of the individual (Fig. 7.2A,B).

General health applications of naturopathic physical medicine methods

A defining feature of osteopathic and chiropractic methodology for well over 100 years has been that patients with a wide range of general health problems have been treated, in part at least, by use of manipulation and mobilization methods. This is equally true of naturopathic medicine, which has, in regard to manual methods, been greatly influenced by both osteopathic and chiropractic concepts and methods.

The perspective of the naturopathic profession to manipulative modalities is outlined in the extract from Buratovich et al's 2006 *Position Paper on Naturopathic Manipulative Therapy*, by the American Association of Naturopathic Physicians (AANP), found in Chapter 1 (Box 1.5).

In this Position Paper the following key points are made:

1. Naturopathic physicians use the diverse methods and therapies described as naturopathic physical medicine in a safe, healthful and clinically integrated manner consistent with naturopathic principles and philosophy
2. Naturopathic manipulative treatment as a traditional, integral and essential part of naturopathic medical practice, is a distinct and unique manipulative technique
3. Naturopathic medical educational programs educate and train naturopathic physicians to safely and effectively perform naturopathic physical medicine and naturopathic manipulative treatment
4. Naturopathic medical education programs educate and train naturopathic physicians to safely and effectively utilize physiotherapeutic medical devices, modalities, procedures and injection therapies
5. Naturopathic medical education programs educate and train naturopathic physicians to safely and effectively prescribe movement

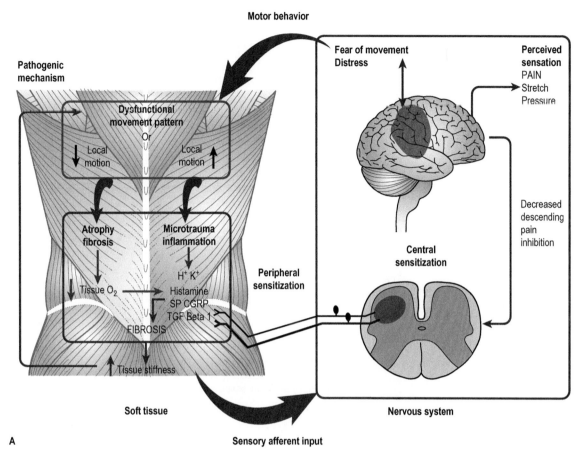

Figure 7.2 **A** Pathophysiological model for chronic low back pain linking somatic and behavioral components. CGRP, calcitonin gene-related peptide; SP, substance P, TGF Beta 1, transforming growth factor-β1. Reproduced with permission from Langevin & Sherman (2006)

integration, functional training and therapeutic exercise programs

6. Naturopathic physical medicine continues to evolve and integrate new therapeutic methods consistent with naturopathic principles and philosophy.

Examples of manipulative treatment where benefit has resulted in treatment of pathological conditions (see separate list of beneficial massage influences later in this chapter) are listed in Box 7.2.

In Chapter 10 a number of the conditions listed in Box 7.2 (and others) will be discussed in terms of appropriate naturopathic physical medicine approaches that may support self-regulating systems and mechanisms.

Therapy as a form of stress

The use of the word 'load' has been prominent in these descriptions of manual methods of treatment.

Whether applying pressure to help deactivate a trigger point, or to take out slack prior to application of a high velocity thrust technique, or in mobilizing and articulating joints, or in use of basic massage methods, load is a feature – indeed, these treatment methods are virtually unimaginable without some force/load involvement.

Load is also a key word (see Chapter 2) used to describe stressors (of all sorts, not just biomechanical ones).

All forms of load create adaptive demands, and when prolonged or repetitive this becomes a feature of the progression towards adaptive overload, decompensation, symptoms and ill-health (see notes on the general and local adaptation syndromes (GAS and LAS) in Chapter 2).

These thoughts highlight the observation that all forms of therapy, manual or otherwise – involving anything from the insertion of an acupuncture needle, to modification of lifestyle or diet, to the taking of

Therapeutic interventions

B

Figure 7.2, cont'd **B** Relationship of proposed chronic low back pain pathogenic mechanism to precipitating factors and non-pharmacological therapeutic interventions. Reproduced with permission from Langevin & Sherman (2006)

Box 7.2 Conditions where manipulation has been reported to offer benefit

- ADHD (Giesen et al 1989, Upledger 1978)
- Asthma (pediatric) (Bachman & Lantz 1991, Guiney et al 2005)
- Asthma (adult) (Rowane & Rowane 1999)
- Cardiac arrhythmia (Jarmel et al 1995)
- Duodenal ulceration (Pikalov & Kharin 1994)
- Dysmenorrhea (Boesler et al 1993, Hondras et al 1999)
- Enuresis (Gemmell & Jacobson 1989)
- Fibromyalgia (Gamber et al 2002)
- Headache (Mootz et al 1994)
- Hypertension (Johnston & Kelso 1995, Yates et al 1988)
- Infantile colic (Klougart & Nilsson 1989, Tanaka et al 1998)

- Multiple sclerosis (enhancing exercise effects) (Yates et al 2002)
- Otitis media (Fallon 1997, Vallone & Fallon 1997)
- Parkinson's disease (enhanced gait) (Wells et al 1999)
- Pneumonia (decreased antibiotic usage, shorter hospital stay) (Noll et al 2000)
- Premenstrual syndrome (Walsh & Polus 1998)
- Prenatal care (improved outcomes for labor and delivery) (King et al 2003)
- Pyloric stenosis (Fallon & Lok 1994)
- Visual acuity enhancement (Kessinger & Boneva 1998)

nutrients or botanical substances, or application of manual pressure – demand a response from the tissues or the body, and are therefore forms of stress.

Appropriate treatment – of all sorts – may therefore accurately be described as 'therapeutic stress' (Selye 1978).

In naturopathic medicine the objective should always be to use the least invasive, most appropriate form of *therapeutic stress* to achieve a positive homeostatic response, ideally involving the least possible demand for additional adaptation, i.e. side-effects.

Categories and classification models: low back pain as an example (McKenzie 1981, McKenzie & May 2003)

Because a pathoanatomic diagnosis is only available in approximately 20% of all LBP cases, the identification of subgroups of patients with low back pain who respond favorably to particular therapeutic interventions has been (and continues to be) an important objective of clinical research (Borkan et al 1998).

A randomized clinical trial (Brennan et al 2006) has put this concept to the test. Of the many classification approaches that have been developed, those reported below are among the most useful.

Staging

The model reported by Delitto et al (1995) has been shown to be a clinically useful tool. This uses staging in an attempt to classify patients into one of several categories. Staging classifies patients based on their symptoms and degree of functional disability, utilizing disability indices such as the *Oswestry Disability Index* (ODI) and the *Fear Avoidance Belief Questionnaire* (FABQ).

This classification system divides patients into three distinct stages, with different treatment objectives emerging for each classification subgroup.

- **Stage 1** patients are unable to perform basic functions, such as walking for more than 1 mile, standing for more than 15 minutes or sitting for more than 30 minutes, and typically have an ODI score of between 40 and 60%. The primary goal of treatment during this stage is suggested to be *pain modulation*.
- **Stage 2** patients can accomplish basic functions, but are limited in their activities of daily living. Their ODI scores typically fall to between 20 and 40%. The objective of treatment at this stage is considered to be to *modulate pain and to begin addressing impairments*.

- **Stage 3** involves the patient's *inability to return to high demand activity* such as manual labor or athletic competition. The ODI scores for patients in this stage are typically below 20%. The aim of treatment at this stage focuses on facilitation of a return to previous levels of activity.

The value of using staging as part of a classification model has been confirmed by studies such as that by Fritz et al (2003) who compared patients who had been classified into 'stages' with the value of using the *Agency for Health Care Policy and Research* (AHCPR) guidelines:

Seventy-six patients with work-related low back pain of less than 3 weeks' duration were randomized into either the AHCPR group or the Classification group (as described above).

1. Based on physical examination criteria in the peer-reviewed literature, patients in the Classification group were placed into one of four categories requiring:
   - mobilization (see Table 7.1)
   - specific exercise
   - stabilization
   - traction.
2. Patients in the AHCPR group were advised to stay active, and were offered reassurance as well as being prescribed low stress aerobic exercises and general muscle conditioning.

ODI measures taken at intake and at 4 weeks demonstrated a statistically significant difference ($p = 0.031$) in favor of the Classification group.

Table 7.1 Classification criteria for mobilization category

Mobilization category	Examination findings
Sacroiliac joint pattern	Unilateral symptoms without signs of nerve root compression
	Positive findings for SI joint dysfunction using pelvic symmetry and standing and seated flexion tests
Lumbar pattern	Unilateral symptoms without signs of nerve root compression; lumbar side-bending asymmetry; lumbar hypomobility

Adapted from Fritz et al (2003).

Return to work status was also measured at the 4-week mark, demonstrating a statistically significant difference ($p = 0.017$) in favor of the Classification group.

Clinical prediction

Taking the classification model a stage further, and in order to evaluate those features that might predict benefit from manipulation, Flynn et al (2002) developed what they termed the *clinical prediction rule* (CPR) based upon five factors:

- Duration of symptoms less than 16 days
- FABQ work subscale less than 19 points
- Symptoms not distal to the knee
- At least one hip with internal rotation greater than 35°
- Hypomobility and pain at one or more lumbar levels when tested using posteroanterior springing testing.

It is suggested that the more of these feature that are present, the greater the chance of success with manipulation (Box 7.3).

Flynn et al suggest that, of these features, the most significant is 'duration of symptoms less than 16 days'.

The development of this clinical prediction rule can be seen to be an important step in establishing reproducible examination findings in order to classify patients for whom manipulation is the manual treatment option most likely to offer benefit.

As noted in Chapter 5, Fritz et al (2004) identified six variables that predict a *negative* response to manipulation (HVLA) in treatment of patients with low back pain. These are:

1. Longer than 3 weeks' duration of symptoms
2. Symptoms in the buttock or leg
3. No hypomobility on spinous process springing
4. Reduced hip rotation range
5. Reduced discrepancy in left-to-right hip medial rotation

Box 7.3 Clinical predictors for success with SI joint manipulation (Flynn et al 2002)

- Duration of symptoms <16 days
- FABQ work subscale <19 points
- No symptoms distal to the knee
- At least one hip with >35° internal rotation
- At least one lumbar segment with positive posteroanterior spring test (hypomobility + pain)

---

6. A *negative* Gaenslen sign (pain provocation test with the patient supine, one hip taken into full flexion and the other hyperextension (leg over edge of table) in order to apply torsion to the pelvis). The test is *positive* if pain is reported in the sacroiliac joint (and/or thigh) on the side of the hyperextended leg.

Using such protocols would seem to offer useful information as to who is more likely and who is less likely to respond to particular forms of treatment such as HVLA.

What choices are there for those for whom manipulation is not indicated (or is contraindicated) based on classification? For many of these the answer may lie in a quite different form of categorization, based on the answer to a simple question: Do the symptoms change for the better based on positioning?

This approach to back pain has been discussed more fully in Chapter 6. A brief summary is given below.

Centralization/peripheralization categorization

McKenzie (1981) has identified three major groups of back pain patients. To understand the differences we need to look at the processes of centralization and peripheralization (McKenzie & May 2003), discussed more fully in Chapter 6.

- When someone with backache (or neck pain) has symptoms that extend into the leg (or the arm), this is a *peripheralization* of the pain (whatever the cause).
- If that person has treatment, performs exercises or adopts particular positions (such as extending the low back, or flexing it) that result in distal symptoms reducing in that limb, i.e. becoming more proximal, even temporarily, this is an example of *centralization*.

The importance clinically is that anything that increases *peripheralization* – whether this involves exercise, change of position or manual treatment – is contraindicated as it will slow down recovery, and may significantly increase symptoms.

The three syndrome models identified by McKenzie are 'postural', 'dysfunction' and 'derangement' (or pathology). The characteristics of these are as follows.

1. *Postural*: Both active ROM and repetitive movements are full and pain free, but static postures at the normal end of range cause pain. In such individuals it is considered that normal tissue is being strained by prolonged inappropriate posture. Treatment and advice

focus on encouraging better posture and good ergonomics, and the avoidance of pain-inducing positions.

2. *Dysfunction*: Active ROM is commonly restricted in one or more directions, with local pain being felt at the end of range. Repetitive motions are also painful at the end of range (bending for example), although such movements may increase the range of motion. Causes may include chronic soft tissue contracture or fibrosis and/or nerve root impingement/restrictions. The recommendation is that exercise, repetitive movement (even if briefly uncomfortable) and manual treatment should aim to reduce fibrosis and increase elasticity.

3. *Derangement* (*pathology*): Active ROM is commonly restricted in one or more directions, with local pain being felt at the end of range. Repetitive motions produce either centralization (likely causes include discogenic changes such as herniation that are 'contained', i.e. the annulus has preserved the material of the disc internally; Laslett et al 2005) or peripheralization (likely causes include non-contained discogenic changes). Exercise, repetitive movement and treatment should aim to avoid anything that increases peripheralization of symptoms. In this last category, *if there are no positions, movements or treatments that encourage centralization, the prognosis is poor, with poor responses likely to almost all therapeutic interventions* (Aina et al 2004).

Using directional preference in rehabilitation

Precisely this McKenzie-informed thinking, regarding the choice of exercise prescription, is evidenced in studies where patients with chronic low back pain are encouraged to exercise using what is termed 'directional preference'.

In one study (Long et al 2004) directional preference (DP) was identified when posture or repeated end-range movements in a single direction (flexion, extension or side-glide/rotation) were shown to decrease or abolish lumbar midline pain, or cause referred pain to progressively retreat toward the lumbar midline (i.e. centralization).

DP was identified in 230 (74%) of 312 patients with acute, subacute or chronic LBP with or without sciatica. Those with DP showed lasting improvement in pain from performing repeated lumbar flexion, extension or side-glide/rotation, and were randomized to receive directional exercises that 'matched' their DP, were directionally 'opposite' to their DP or were 'non-directional'.

One-third of both the 'opposite' and 'non-directionally' exercised patients withdrew within 2 weeks because of no improvement or worsening; however, no patient assigned to 'matched DP' withdrew. The 'matched DP' group had greater improvements in every outcome (p <0.001), including a threefold decrease in medication use.

Biopsychosocial factors: a broader classification approach

O'Sullivan (2005) has produced a much wider model for classification of chronic low back problems, within a biopsychosocial framework. This helps to illustrate why taking a generic rather than a cookbook approach to the selection of therapeutic interventions is likely to produce the most useful filter for such decision-making.

Among the elements that make up this framework O'Sullivan includes genetic, social, pathoanatomic, physical (including trauma and microtrauma), psychological and neurophysiological factors, with each factor containing a number of elements and variables, all of which interact (Fig. 7.3).

Tight/loose indicators

When evaluating the status of joints and soft tissues there should be a sense of the degrees of tension and relaxation (the shorthand words for these two states are 'ease' and 'bind'). The tissues provide the palpating hands or fingers with a sense of these states which can be interpreted to reflect the tissue's current degree of activity, comfort or distress.

Ward (1997) states that: 'Tightness suggests tethering, while looseness suggests joint and/or soft tissue laxity, with or without neural inhibition.'

Many leading clinicians and researchers maintain that most problems of the musculoskeletal system involve, as part of their etiology, dysfunction related to muscle shortening (Janda 1978, Liebenson 1996a).

Where weakness (lack of tone) is apparently a major element, it will often be found that antagonists are shortened, reciprocally inhibiting their tone, and that prior to any effort to strengthen weak muscles, hypertonic antagonists should be dealt with by appropriate means (e.g. use of muscle energy technique; see later in this chapter), after which spontaneous toning occurs in the previously hypotonic or relatively weak muscles.

If tone remains reduced, then there should be specific focus on toning weak or inhibited antagonists to these muscles (Lewit 1999).

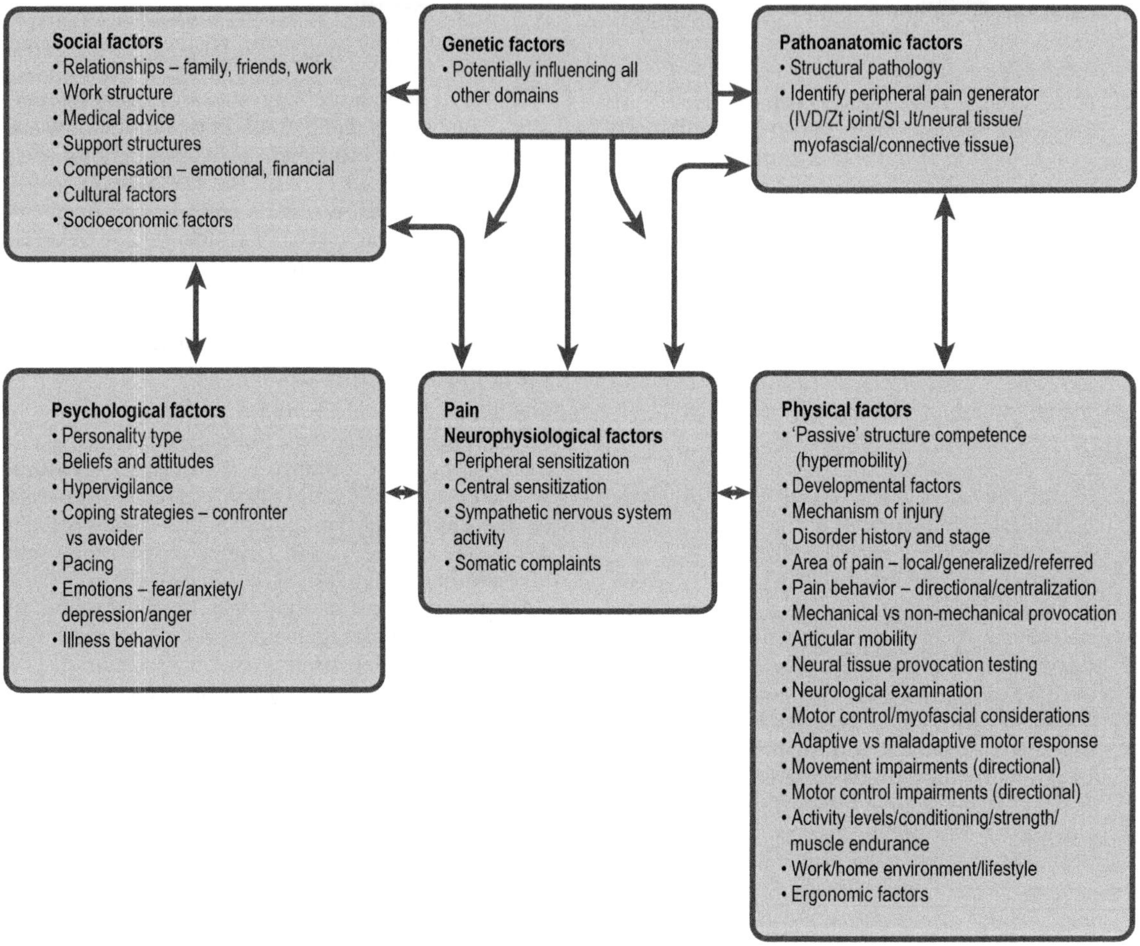

Social factors
- Relationships – family, friends, work
- Work structure
- Medical advice
- Support structures
- Compensation – emotional, financial
- Cultural factors
- Socioeconomic factors

Genetic factors
- Potentially influencing all other domains

Pathoanatomic factors
- Structural pathology
- Identify peripheral pain generator (IVD/Zt joint/SI Jt/neural tissue/ myofascial/connective tissue)

Psychological factors
- Personality type
- Beliefs and attitudes
- Hypervigilance
- Coping strategies – confronter vs avoider
- Pacing
- Emotions – fear/anxiety/ depression/anger
- Illness behavior

Pain Neurophysiological factors
- Peripheral sensitization
- Central sensitization
- Sympathetic nervous system activity
- Somatic complaints

Physical factors
- 'Passive' structure competence (hypermobility)
- Developmental factors
- Mechanism of injury
- Disorder history and stage
- Area of pain – local/generalized/referred
- Pain behavior – directional/centralization
- Mechanical vs non-mechanical provocation
- Articular mobility
- Neural tissue provocation testing
- Neurological examination
- Motor control/myofascial considerations
- Adaptive vs maladaptive motor response
- Movement impairments (directional)
- Motor control impairments (directional)
- Activity levels/conditioning/strength/ muscle endurance
- Work/home environment/lifestyle
- Ergonomic factors

Figure 7.3 Factors that need consideration within a biopsychosocial framework, for the diagnosis and classification of chronic low back pain disorders. IVD, intervertebral joint; SI Jt, sacroiliac joint; Zt joint, zygapophyseal joint. Reproduced with permission from O'Sullivan (2005)

SI joint and tight/loose features

A useful example of 'tight/loose' features can be observed in sacroiliac dysfunction. (*Note*: These assessments are described in Chapter 6.)

To confirm whether sacroiliac (SI) joint problems involve a lack of soft tissue support, the SI joint force closure tests (supine and prone) are performed. To evaluate whether there is a deeper lack of stability, possibly due to structural damage, SI joint form closure tests should be conducted (supine and prone) in which these features are evaluated (Lee 1997).

If *force closure* instability is confirmed, then core stability-type exercises are likely to lead to a restoration of normal function (Fig. 7.4). If problems involving *form closure* are confirmed as a major feature, then an

SI support belt, prolotherapy or surgery may be indicated. If form closure is a feature, there should also be every effort to restore normal balance to the soft tissues of the region; however, without additional support for the joint, muscle toning alone is unlikely to allow restoration of normal function.

It is worth observing, in relation to SI joint problems, that the ipsilateral and/or contralateral hamstring muscles are likely to demonstrate extreme hypertonicity, and possibly trigger point activity. These factors might actually be offering the body an effective means of inducing greater force (via the sacrotuberous ligament for example) across the unstable joint (van Wingerden et al 1997).

Treatment of these features (tight hamstrings housing active trigger points) would be unlikely to

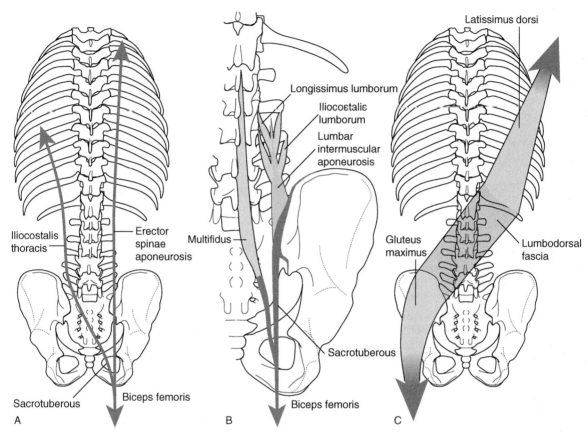

Figure 7.4 **A** The biceps femoris is directly connected to the upper trunk via the sacrotuberous ligament, the erector spinae aponeurosis and iliocostalis thoracis. **B** Enlarged view of the lumbar spine area showing the link between biceps femoris, the lumbar intermuscular aponeurosis, longissimus lumborum, iliocostalis lumborum and multifidus. **C** Relations between gluteus maximus, lumbodorsal fascia and latissimus dorsi. Reproduced with permission from Vleeming et al (1997)

have a beneficial effect until the actual stability issues of the joint are addressed – and indeed stretching the hamstrings, or deactivating trigger points in them that might be helping them to maintain increased tone, could destabilize the SI joint even more (see Hamstring discussion in Chapter 6).

Making choices

Depending on which elements from this selection of staging, categorizations, identified imbalances (tight/loose) and biopsychosocial factors are operating, as well as the degree of chronicity and other features, therapeutic choices might include application to local structures of muscle energy, positional release and/or myofascial release techniques, massage, articulation, oscillatory and/or exercise methods, joint articulation, high velocity thrust methods, and quite possibly

variations of hydrotherapeutic and/or electrotherapeutic attention.

A step back from these immediate, focused, localized approaches lies the strong likelihood that long-term influences are at work, imposing adaptive demands, such as congenital/structural features (anatomic short leg for example), and/or functional influences such as poor posture, overuse, disuse or misuse factors.

And apart from possible pathological changes (disc herniation, arthritis, inflammation as examples), there may also be hyper- and hypomobility conditions, fibrotic changes, active myofascial trigger points, (core) muscular weakness, modified motor control, altered muscular recruitment patterns, breathing pattern and postural disorders.

It is also possible that musculoskeletal problems may be associated with biochemical features (endocrine imbalance, nutritional deficiencies, toxicity, etc.) as at least a part of the etiology.

Similarly, psychosocial issues might play a part, encouraging sympathetic arousal, modified neural function, altered pain threshold, etc.

Along with the classification models outlined above, each of these variables can offer clues as to which of the range of potential treatment and/or rehabilitation approaches might be the most likely to enhance functionality, without undue side-effects.

Faced with this degree of complexity it is all too easy to become confused as to which methods, modalities and techniques to employ.

Remember adaptation

To simplify decision-making it is useful to be reminded of the message (see Chapter 1) from which clinical decision-making in care of all health problems can benefit – *reduce the adaptive load*, and/or *enhance functionality* – so that self-regulating systems and mechanisms can operate more effectively.

Examples include the following:

- As we have seen in the discussion above, using the concepts of categorization it is possible, in some cases, to predict that manipulation (HVLA) is likely to offer the best initial choice.
- Similarly, the McKenzie protocol can offer clear guidelines to suggest where graded specific movements and exercises that encourage centralization might be the best choice.

Pointers to clinical choices are not always as clear as these two examples, in which circumstances the gathering of evidence from palpation and assessment and history should be used to build as clear a picture of the etiology of the current dysfunction as possible. Since naturopathic medicine embraces self-regulation as the key element in recovery or health improvement, it should be a prime aim of the practitioner to remove or modulate obstacles to those endogenous processes – without imposing additional demands on what is, all too often, an already extended, overloaded system.

In short, *appropriate* mobilization or manipulation (joint or soft tissue) is designed to enhance the adaptive potential of the individual, or the area, allowing self-regulatory processes to operate more efficiently. This is therefore a fundamentally naturopathic means of treatment.

What is possible therapeutically?

Selye's general adaptation syndrome (see Chapters 1 and 2) describes a process, following the initial alarm stage of adaptation, that continues until adaptation potential is exhausted. One of the limiting factors in

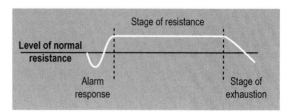

Figure 7.5 Levels of resistance

any area of therapeutics is the stage of exhaustion that the patient may have reached in the spectrum of self-regulation. This defines what Selye termed the stage of exhaustion, or collapse, where frank disease and death follow in an inexorable progression as self-regulating mechanisms fail (see Fig. 7.5 and also Fig. 2.1).

Clearly there is a far greater likelihood of recovery when the person is robust, and the condition is either self-limiting or capable of recovery. However, where degenerative processes have advanced to a certain stage, recovery may be impossible, although stabilization and modulation of symptoms may remain a possibility.

A triage approach can be used to place patients into three broad categories, where objectives would be different, and therapeutic choices probably different.

- *Fix*: Self-regulation is operating, and the condition is likely to improve or normalize. Treatment should offer support to the processes involved, although recovery without any therapeutic input is probable.
- *Maintain*: The potential remains for improvement, or even recovery, if optimal treatment and rehabilitation choices are made. Self-regulation needs help to remove obstacles to recovery and to enhance functionality.
- *Contain*: The likelihood of recovery is minimal; however, there remains the possibility of modulation of symptoms and retardation of what appears to be an inevitable decline. Treatment might be symptom oriented (e.g. pain relief).

To some extent such categorization takes place automatically in most health care settings. There may be value in a more deliberate consideration of such features.

Evaluation of the various modalities

The naturopathic dimension

For clarity in making therapeutic choices we should refer back to the summary towards the end of Chapter

Box 7.4 Key objectives of the application of naturopathic physical medicine approaches

1. To reduce the adaptive load.
2. To enhance functionality (better posture, enhanced breathing function, greater mobility, etc.).
3. To ease symptoms without adding to the patient's adaptive burden (how sensitive and vulnerable, and how far along the road to decompensation, is this individual?).
4. To support self-repair, self-regeneration, self-healing processes (see items 1, 2 and 3 above).
5. To take account of the whole person, the context, and not just the symptoms (see item 6 below).
6. To identify where the individual is in the spectrum of adaptation – judging as best possible the current degree of exhaustion and susceptibility with a rule-of-thumb guideline that the more complex the condition, and/or the more vulnerable the individual, the less that should be done therapeutically at any given time.
7. To focus on causes where possible.
8. To do no harm.

1 in order to evaluate how and where modalities, techniques and methods relate to the principles enshrined in that summary (see Box 7.4).

Questions

The modalities, techniques and methods described later in this chapter therefore need to be evaluated from the perspective of their place within this framework of naturopathic objectives.

- Is the method/technique/modality safe?
- Is there evidence of efficacy?
- Does the method/technique/modality significantly add to the individual's adaptive load, and, if so, is there a less invasive means of achieving similar benefit?
- What are the physiological means of influence of this approach, and in what way, in any given clinical setting, might it assist self-regulation (reducing load and/or assisting functionality)?
- In which situations might it be contraindicated or are cautions suggested?
- If symptom relief is the objective, is this likely to be achieved at the cost of self-regulation? In other words, is the method suppressing or retarding the normal healing processes?

Safety issues

Wherever possible, i.e. where the information is available, an indication is given as to the safety of specific methods/techniques described in this chapter. Where there is evidence of risk, this is highlighted – and the very real risks relative to HVLA when applied to the cervical area (Haldeman et al 2002a, Hurwitz et al 2005) are discussed in detail in Box 7.5.

Validation of efficacy

Living as we do in an age of evidence-based medicine, every effort has been made to give examples of studies that show efficacy (or lack of it) for the methods and techniques under discussion.

Strong et al (2002) discuss the importance of this:

Evidence based practice incorporates evidence of the effectiveness of interventions from research (quantitative and qualitative) with information about the client's needs and goals, and the therapist's clinical experience . . . Many interventions have been examined in research but the quality of the research may be variable.

They list five key steps required by clinicians:

1. Develop a focused question based on the client context, the specific intervention and the expected outcome of the intervention.
2. Collect evidence from the literature that is relevant to the question(s).
3. Critically analyze the validity, reliability and generalizability of the research.
4. Integrate the evidence with clinical experience and client needs, to develop an intervention program.
5. Evaluate the program.

A naturopathic filter needs to be incorporated into this process in order to ensure that 'results' do not conflict with basic principles.

The code used in this chapter in relation to evidence is summarized in Table 7.2.

Alternatives?

Where comparison of methods/techniques is possible, based on either research evidence or the personal clinical experience of the authors, discussion of these issues has been included. There are, for example, a wide range of different methods of stretching soft tissues, and these are compared in relation to their known and purported value in different therapeutic settings.

Table 7.2 Validation of efficacy

Code	Rating	Explanation
5	Good	Evidence of value based on systematic reviews
4	Probably useful	Based on evidence from one or more randomized and/or controlled trials (RCTs)
3	Possibly useful	Based on some evidence from RCTs, with inconclusive or contradictory outcomes, or with methods open to question
2	Opinion	Practitioner conviction, expert view, clinical experience but without reliable research evidence
1	Poor	Rumor, traditional use, with effectiveness doubted, or research evidence suggesting ineffective
0	Anti	Research-derived evidence suggests that this therapy is not useful in the condition or is risky

It is worth reflecting that a great deal of the methodology employed in manual therapy is relatively unresearched. This means that a ranking of '2' should not be seen as a suggestion that the method should not be utilized, only that further study is called for.

How does it work?

If there is evidence as to the physiological effects of particular methods, these have been elaborated on; if not, the conceptual basis on which the method's use is predicated is outlined.

Cautions

Where evidence of potential harm exists, or where there are contraindications, these are listed.

A naturopathic perspective

How particular methods fit with naturopathic concepts is the overarching (or foundational) subtext of each description and discussion relating to techniques and methods of manual treatment.

Manual treatment, enhanced homeostasis and adaptation potential

Evidence of a variety of general health benefits can be shown to result from manual methods of treatment.

Fluid movement

Manual therapy techniques that assist in fluid movement (see manual pump techniques, and manual lymphatic drainage notes, later in this chapter) have been shown to:

- enhance local circulation and drainage (Foldi & Strossenreuther 2003)
- reduce swelling and improve washout of inflammatory chemicals (Wittlinger & Wittlinger 1982)
- assist in normalization of trigger point myalgia (Larsson et al 1990)
- modify neural irritation caused by local edema (Hoyland et al 1989, Rozmaryn et al 1998)
- assist postsurgical recovery (Cantieri 1997).

The types of condition in which these effects are most likely to be a requirement include inflammation, ischemia and wherever there is an impediment to normal blood or lymph flow.

The specific methods that encourage these changes are discussed in the relevant modality sections later in this chapter; for example, manual pump techniques (Ganong 1981) and manual lymphatic drainage. Fluid movement will also be encouraged by aspects of mobilization, massage (Hovind & Nielsen 1974) (including compressive forces; Tamir et al 1999) and muscle energy techniques ('rhythmic muscle contractions'; Sejersted et al 1984), stretching methods (Shustova et al 1985) and oscillatory methodology, all of which are individually described below.

Adaptation enhancement

The aspects of adaptation that are most obviously influenced by manual treatment methods are those resulting from trauma (macro or repetitive micro) as well as the changes that result from long-term overuse, misuse, disuse and abuse of the body (as discussed in Chapter 2), in which tissues modify, shorten or lengthen adaptively over many years.

- Manual modalities appear to be able to encourage optimal regeneration and repair, particularly during the remodeling phase of tissue recovery (Williams 1988, Williams et al 1988).
- Mechanical elongation of chronically shortened, stiff or fibrotically infiltrated soft tissues can be modified, and sometimes normalized, by means of a variety of manual modalities, including massage, mobilization, muscle energy techniques, oscillatory/ vibrational methods and neuromuscular techniques, even though the precise

mechanisms involved remain open to debate (Magnusson S et al 1996, Taylor et al 1990). These approaches, together with validating citation, are outlined later in this chapter.

We should recall that enhanced adaptation arises from two distinct approaches – one that reduces adaptive load (improved posture, ergonomics, breathing function, etc.) and one from methods that encourage tissues to have a greater ability to adapt, by improving flexibility, stability, stamina and function.

In addition to the listed manual methods (and possibly others not listed) this demands consideration of the variety of rehabilitation strategies discussed in Chapter 9, as well as methods such as Pilates and Alexander technique (see below).

The neurological and psychophysiological dimensions

It is beyond the scope of this text to delve, other than superficially, into the neurological influences and consequences of biomechanical dysfunction in particular, and ill-health in general, and of the potential influence on these aspects of ill-health offered by manual modalities.

For an excellent review the reader is referred to Section 2 of Lederman's text *Science and Practice of Manual Therapy* (2nd edition, 2005a), entitled 'The effect of manual therapy techniques in the neurological dimension'.

Whether the therapeutic focus involves pain relief, motor system rehabilitation, enhanced proprioception or other neurologically mediated processes, manual modalities inevitably rely on, or influence, the nervous system – generally, locally, significantly or peripherally (Lederman 2005b).

There is also, of course, the undoubted impact of manual modalities on what can be termed the psychophysiological aspect of the body. This might involve modulating autonomic function, reducing arousal, stimulating parasympathetic functions or assisting in reintegration of the mind–body complex (as in psychodynamic bodywork or somatic experiencing work) (Levine & Frederick 1997).

Manual methods, modalities and techniques used in naturopathic physical medicine

Each of the modalities listed below contains variations and subdivisions.

1. Manipulation: high velocity, low amplitude thrust (HVLA)
2. Manual lymphatic drainage (MLD)
3. Massage
4. Mobilization approaches
5. Muscle energy techniques (MET)/ proprioceptive neuromuscular facilitation (PNF) and variations, and pulsed MET
6. Muscle energy (pulsed) technique
7. Myofascial release methods (MFR)
8. Mobilization with movement (MWM)
9. Neural mobilization of adverse mechanical or neural tension
10. Neuromuscular techniques (NMT)
11. Integrated neuromuscular inhibition technique (INIT)
12. Spray and stretch methods
13. Nasal specific (craniofacial) technique
14. Occupational and ergonomic therapies
15. Oscillatory/vibrational rhythmic methods (including Trager exercise)
16. Pilates methods – see also Chapter 9
17. Positional release techniques (PRT)
18. Postural re-education (e.g. Alexander technique) – see also Chapter 9
19. Prolotherapy: by Hal Brown ND DC RAc
20. Manual pump techniques
21. Rehabilitation methods, including notes on breathing rehabilitation – see also Chapter 9
22. Shiatsu, acupressure, etc.
23. Somatic psychotherapy (a.k.a. body-centered psychotherapy, e.g. Hakomi): by Lisa Maeckel MA CHT
24. Spondylotherapy
25. Thiele massage for pelvic floor dysfunction
26. Visceral manipulation – see also Chapter 3
27. Yoga – see also Chapter 9
28. Zero balancing: by Roger Newman Turner ND DO BAc

In discussing the majority of the modalities and systems listed above, and whenever information is available from responsible sources, this is offered as to:

- indications/description
- methodology
- safety
- validation of efficacy (research evidence if available)
- alternatives
- physiological effects
- cautions

- naturopathic perspectives
- further reading.

Some of the methods and modalities listed (such as Pilates and Alexander technique) are also discussed in Chapter 9 (Rehabilitation) and in those instances only a brief comment will be found in this chapter.

In the description offered of body-centered psychotherapy (under the heading 'Somatic psychotherapy') a broad description is offered, rather than the format used in most of the other modality descriptions.

In some descriptions – where appropriate – exercises in the use of the method have been described. As in Chapter 6 (Palpation and assessment skills) the exercises that are described are designed to allow the reader an opportunity to experience an aspect of the method.

These descriptions and exercises are not meant to provide 'training', but rather to offer a flavor, a sample, that might encourage further study of, or training in, use of the particular approach.

Manipulation: high velocity, low amplitude thrust (HVLA)

Indications/description

Relief/normalization of joint dysfunction and pain are the main objectives of HVLA manipulation.

Changes which indicate that the use of HVLA may be helpful include a selection from the following:

- Local pain or hypersensitivity involving associated tissues, possibly modified by activity
- Altered alignment
- Modified mobility (increased, decreased, aberrant)
- Reduced joint play (movement outside of voluntary control)
- Abnormal end-feel of joint movement
- Abnormal associated muscular features (fibrosis, rigidity, etc.).

Specific indications are listed by Gibbons & Tehan (2000a) as including joint hypomobility (Kenna & Murtagh 1989), motion restriction (Lewit 1999), joint fixation, acute joint locking, motion loss with somatic dysfunction, meniscoid entrapment (Bogduk & Twomey 1991), misalignment, adhesions, disc fragment displacement, a need for reflex relaxation of muscles and release of endorphins (Vernon et al 1986).

Lederman (1997b) has proposed a physiological model of manipulation (Fig. 7.6) that offers three categories in which HVLA may be usefully applied:

1. Biomechanical – in which the effects relate to enhanced elasticity and plasticity as well as improved fluid dynamics
2. Neurological – where tone reduction and pain modulation are the desired effects
3. Psychological/psychophysiological – where the objectives include improved visceral function, reduced pain perception and general relaxation of muscles.

Methodology

There are various definitions of manipulation:

Osteopathic definition (Glossary Review Committee 2005): Therapeutic application of manual force, including all techniques (e.g. muscle energy technique, myofascial release, etc.), as well as thrust (HVLA).

Chiropractic definition (Hurwitz & Haldeman 2004): 'Controlled, judiciously applied dynamic thrust of high or low velocity and low amplitude force directed toward one or more spinal joint segments within patient tolerance that puts the joint within paraphysiological space.' The reference to 'low velocity' methods in this definition incorporates mobilization methods (see Mobilization, later in this chapter).

Other definitions exist for this apparently simple, yet at times confusing word:

- Sandoz (1976), for example, delineated manipulation as 'moving the joint into its paraphysiological space', while he defined mobilization (see Mobilization, later in this chapter) as moving the joint to its endpoint.
- Shipley (D Shipley, personal communication) raises the reasonable question: 'If these definitions are accepted, how is one able to distinguish HVLA, low velocity low amplitude thrust, and/or other manual soft tissue treatment, which also appear to come under the general heading "Manipulation"?' The answer would seem to not be all that easy to establish.

For the purposes of this chapter, the method under consideration as the modality 'Manipulation' is high velocity, low amplitude thrust (a.k.a. 'adjustment' in chiropractic texts).

HVLA involves what can be described as a long-lever procedure in which forces are localized in order to achieve cavitation at a predetermined, specific, vertebral segment (or other joint).

In order to achieve this, focused force-locking is required, achieved by use of facet-locking or ligamen-

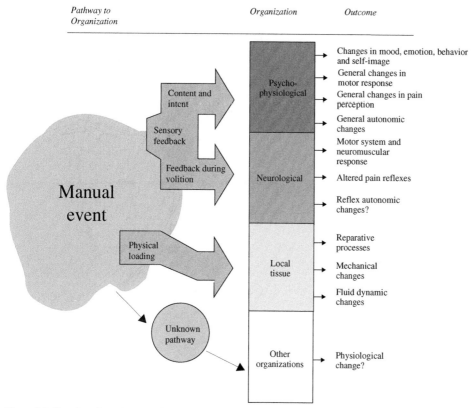

Figure 7.6 The physiological model of manipulation. Reproduced with permission from Lederman (1997b)

tous tension, or a combination of these forces (Gibbons & Tehan 2000b, Greenman 1996).

Achieving facet-locking requires an understanding of spinal coupling whereby side-flexion is automatically accompanied by contralateral rotation (known as Type 1 movement) or by ipsilateral rotation (Type 2 movement) (Fig. 7.7).

Locking is achieved by placing the area of the spine (above or below depending on the location and the levers employed), *but not the joint to be manipulated*, into a position opposite that of normal coupling, so that movement can be forced at the unlocked segment, using HVLA (see Figs 7.7 and 7.8).

There is no universal agreement as to which segments are, and which are not, Type 1 or Type 2, apart from in the cervical region where C1 is Type 1, and C2 to T4 almost universally demonstrate Type 2 behavior – and which therefore require Type 1 positioning to create facet-locking (Penning & Wilmink 1987). Other areas of the spine are less predictable, with coupling being dependent on posture and positioning (i.e. whether the area is flexed, neutral or extended). Some evidence suggests (but there is no consensus) that when the area is flexed, Type 2 mechanics apply, and when neutral or extended, Type 1 mechanics apply (Gibbons & Tehan 1998, Panjabi et al 1989).

Safety

Most issues of safety in relation to use of HVLA involve the cervical spine.

While practitioners using HVLA report that minor side-effects (local discomfort, headache, tiredness, radiating discomfort) occur after approximately 33% of visits, these are usually no longer present after 24 hours (Malone et al 2002a).

Major complications from cervical manipulation are rare (between 1 in 400 000 and 1 in 10 million; Shekelle et al 1992) but serious (Coulter et al 1996). It is worth acknowledging that complications resulting from most other forms of treatment of neck pain, for which data are available, are estimated to be higher than those for manipulation. Haldeman et al (2002b) note that in reviewing nearly 400 cases of vertebrobasilar artery dissection, it was not possible to identify a specific neck movement, type of manipulation or trauma

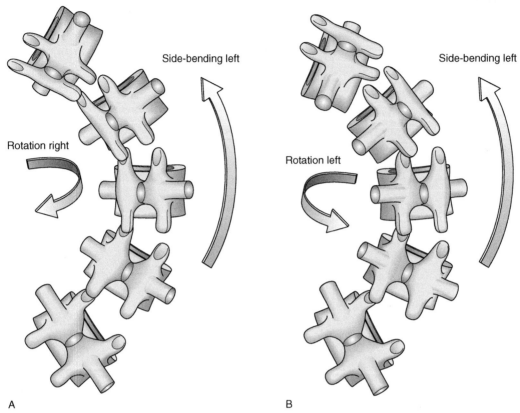

Figure 7.7 A Type 1 movement: side-bending and rotation occur to opposite sides. **B** Type 2 movement: side-bending and rotation occur to the same side. Reproduced with permission from Gibbons & Tehan (2000b)

that would be considered the offending activity in the majority of cases. See Box 7.5 for a deeper discussion of HVLA safety issues.

Validation of efficacy = 5 (see Table 7.2)

Many of the conditions listed in Box 7.2 were treated using HVLA methodology (as well as mobilization).

The value of HVLA in biomechanical conditions has been demonstrated in various studies:

1. For patients with chronic neck pain there is moderate evidence (Bronfort et al 2001) that:
   - manipulation and mobilization are superior to general practitioner management in the short term
   - high-technology exercise results in more pain improvement than manipulation in the long term for a mix of patients with acute and chronic pain
   - mobilization is superior to physical therapy and general medical care and similar to manipulation in both the short and long term.

2. A number of studies that compared use of manipulation with standard medical therapies in treatment of low back pain have shown either greater benefit and cost effectiveness deriving from manipulation, or equal benefit from manipulation when compared with standard medical care (commonly with greater cost effectiveness amongst those receiving manipulation) (Andersson et al 1999, Meade et al 1990, UK BEAM Trial Team 2004).

Alternatives

Exercise and McKenzie methods (see below), as well as mobilization and soft tissue methodology, all offer alternatives to HVLA alone, and in many studies (particularly those where OMT is used – see discussion earlier in this chapter) it is difficult to separate benefits deriving from one or other of the modalities employed. It appears that there is an increasing trend in chiropractic care for combinations of manipulation and other modalities to be offered, as has been standard practice in osteopathic medicine for many years.

Best practice suggests that naturopathic manual therapy should employ treatment strategies that offer the patient treatment approaches which match needs, as indicated by assessment and categorization where this has established clear guidelines (see discussion and examples earlier in this chapter on this topic).

Physiological effects

What actually happens when an HVLA thrust is used?

The audible sound that frequently accompanies HVLA is known as cavitation. This has variously been ascribed to release of dissolved gases in the synovial fluid (Plaugher 1993a), by elastic recoil of the synovial capsule (Bergman 1993) or separation of articular surfaces (Evans 2002).

HVLA-induced cavitation involves intra-articular mechanical changes and neurophysiological changes (Protopapas & Cymet 2002). The neurological repercussions seem to involve both local and central responses, inhibiting pain and spasm, and facilitating motor control (Dishman et al 2002, Sung et al 2005).

In addition to the physiological effects of HVLA thrust, there may well be placebo effects at play.

Cautions

Peterson & Bergmann (2002) suggest that the following contraindications exist for use of HVLA manipulation (*or that they require modified use of manipulation*):

- Atherosclerosis because of risk of vessel rupture or dislodgement of thrombi; soft tissue or mobilizing alternatives suggested
- Vertebrobasilar insufficiency because of risk of stroke; cervical thrust methods to be avoided
- Aneurysm because of risk of rupture or hemorrhage
- Tumors because of risk of disease progression or fracture
- Fractures because of delay to healing and risk of increased instability of tissues
- Severe sprains (and dislocations) due to risk of increasing instability
- Osteoarthritis (late stage) because of potential to increase pain and compromise neural structures

- Clotting disorders because of risk of spinal hematoma
- Osteoporosis because of risk of pathological fracture
- Space-occupying lesions because of permanent neurological deficits
- Diabetic neuropathy because of potential for non-response to pain leading to joint injury
- Malingering, hysteria, hypochondriasis because of treatment dependency risk
- Alzheimer's disease because of inability to respond or comply appropriately.

Senstad et al (1996) also suggest the following absolute contraindications:

- Unstable odontoid peg (os odontoideum)
- Ankylosis
- Acute inflammatory arthritis
- Bone infection.

Also: avoid HVLA in cauda equina syndrome (Haldeman et al 1993a).

Naturopathic perspectives

There is much to consider in relation to use of HVLA in naturopathic practice.

As noted above, much of the benefit deriving from this form of manipulation seems to be capable of being duplicated by more conservative mobilization, and/or soft tissue treatment, and/or exercise methods.

The serious risk implications for some forms of HVLA application – particularly involving the cervical region – demand that care and caution, as well as particular attention, be paid to contraindications (see above).

There are undoubtedly situations where HVLA may be a first choice (where it is essential to improve joint play for example), but where there are potentially equally beneficial and less invasive alternative options for achieving this (Mulligan's mobilization with movement for example, see below), these should be chosen in preference to HVLA.

Murphy (2000) notes the one essential difference between manipulation (HVLA) and mobilization: 'It [HVLA] provides rapid end range loading to dysfunctional joints . . . resulting in increased joint range of motion.'

Further reading

1. Gibbons P, Tehan P 2000 Manipulation of the spine, thorax and pelvis: an osteopathic perspective. Churchill Livingstone, Edinburgh

2. Greenman PE 1996 Principles of manual medicine, 2nd edn. Williams & Wilkins, Baltimore

3. Liebenson C 2006 Rehabilitation of the spine, 2nd edn. Lippincott Williams & Wilkins, Philadelphia

4. Morris C (ed) 2006 Low back syndromes: integrated clinical management. McGraw-Hill, New York

5. Murphy D 2000 Conservative management of cervical spine syndromes. McGraw-Hill, New York

6. Peterson D, Bergmann T 2002 Chiropractic technique: principles and procedures, 2nd edn. Mosby, St Louis

7. Ward R 1997 Foundations for osteopathic medicine. Williams & Wilkins, Baltimore

---

Box 7.5 Safety issues in high velocity manipulation

Hal Brown ND DC RAc

Primum non nocere (first do no harm). Hippocrates (Ligeros 1937)

- About half of all patients will experience adverse events after chiropractic manipulation (HVLA)
- These events, although frequent, are usually mild and transient (Ernst 2001, Senstad et al 1997)
- Local discomfort may occur in 53% of cases
- Headache may occur in 12% of cases
- Tiredness may occur in 11% of cases
- Radiating discomfort may occur in 10% of cases
- 64% of reactions appeared within 4 hours of treatment
- 74% had disappeared within 24 hours (Senstad et al 1997)
- 'Sympathetic storm', fainting, syncope, palpitation, nausea and perspiration occur in 1–2 cases per 1000, lasting 1–2 days (Maigne 1972)
- Perspiration over trunk and axilla is common and of brief duration (Maigne 1972)
- Epigastric, abdominal or pelvic pain is common and of brief duration (Maigne 1972)
- Diffuse pain lasting less than 2 days occurs in 33% (Malone et al 2002a) to 40% of patients (Maigne 1972)
- Muscular aches and pains may occur for 6–14 hours (Haldeman 1980)

A 2001 independent literature review of the most valid studies to identify the safety of spinal manipulation (SM) suggests that about half of all patients will experience adverse events after chiropractic SM. These events, although frequent, are usually mild and transient (Ernst 2001).

Serious effects resulting from spinal manipulation

Manipulation of the cervical spine appears to be associated with the possibility of cervical radiculopathy, myelopathy and disc herniation (Malone et al 2002b). Manipulation of the lumbar spine is associated with a risk of cauda equina syndrome and disc herniation (Stevinson & Ernst 2002).

The possibility of further nerve root damage from mechanical pressure of the herniated disc during the act of manipulation was demonstrated in a study of 400 cases of herniated intervertebral discs verified by surgery (Poppen 1945). It has been also demonstrated that the same manipulations may reduce the size of the disc herniation (Mathew & Yates 1988).

Serious complications of death or paralysis following cervical manipulation

Negative media stories (Abbate 2004, Dynamic Chiropractic 2002) and unsubstantiated medical reports (Norris et al 2000) have put the spotlight on the risk of cervical manipulation. A report from the Canadian Stroke Consortium quoted Dr J.W. Norris, a neurologist, as saying his research indicated a risk of 1 stroke in 5000 manipulations (Norris et al 2000). Dr Norris under oath at an Ontario inquest into the death of a young woman following cervical manipulation stated the numbers he has quoted are 'sheer guesswork' and 'way off'. He was forced to recant his position during the inquest (Sackett 2002).

A literature review at the University of Exeter found that although most adverse events were mild and transient, no reliable data exist about the incidence of serious adverse events (Ernst 2001).

The most serious complication is that of a vascular injury following manipulation which leads to stroke. Such injuries may take the form of:

- intimal laceration
- subintimal hemorrhages
- carotid and vertebral artery dissections
- aneurysms
- thrombus and embolus formation
- trauma to the vertebral artery.

All of these conditions may produce central nervous system infarction, resulting in residual neurological deficit, tetraplegia or death (Terrett 1996a).

Box 7.5 Safety issues in high velocity manipulation continued

Plausible mechanisms of injury leading to serious complications

Stretching, shearing, kinking or crushing forces on the vertebral artery from cervical extension and rotation are often considered as possible mechanisms of injury (Gatterman 1990a, Plaugher 1993b, Terrett 1996b). Cadaver studies of vertebral artery patency during cervical rotation and extension indicate compromise (Brown & Tissington-Tatlow 1963, Tissington-Tatlow & Bammer 1957, Toole & Tucker 1960) in some studies and none (Herzog W 2002) in others. Two in-vivo studies of the vertebral arteries, using Doppler ultrasonography, found that there was no disturbance of blood flow when the head was rotated even in the presence of degenerative changes (Haynes et al 2002, Thiel et al 1994).

A cadaver research study, looking at the biomechanical strain from cervical manipulation, concluded:

- the forces during manipulation were less than those recorded during range of motion and diagnostic testing
- the strains on the vertebral artery during manipulation were less than one-ninth of that required to achieve arterial failure
- the movement of joints during cervical adjustment is done well within the normal range of motion and that cervical adjustment is 'very unlikely to mechanically disrupt the vertebral artery' (Herzog S 2002).

Risk of stroke following cervical manipulation

Although serious complications from manipulation are known to occur, there is an inconsistent and broad range of estimates as to what those risks might be.

- **1 per 5.85 million** cervical manipulations. In 2001 the *Canadian Medical Association Journal* published a study based on Canadian chiropractic malpractice statistics (Haldeman et al 2001).
- **1.3 per 100 000** manipulations 1 week after a manipulation. A study in *Stroke*, based on the case history of stroke patients (Rothwell et al 2001).
- **1 per 500 000** manipulations. A survey of California neurologists (Lee et al 1995).
- **0.65 per million** manipulations. A 1996 literature review reported in *Spine* (Hurwitz et al 1996).
- **1 per 3 million** manipulations. A 1993 study in the *Journal of the Canadian Chiropractic Association* (Carey 1993).
- **0 per 5 million** manipulations. A 1980 review of the clinical files of the National College of Chiropractic performed between 1965 and 1980 (Jaskoviak 1980).

- **0 per 5 million** manipulations. A similar 1988 study of the Canadian Memorial Chiropractic College clinic files for a 9-year period (Henderson & Cassidy 1988).
- **1 per 2 million** manipulations. An extensive 1993 literature review found risk of serious neurological complications (Haldeman et al 1993b).
- **1 per 1.32 million** cervical manipulations and **1 per 414 000** upper cervical manipulations with rotation. A Danish study reviewing insurance claims, complaints and published data of CVA occurrences between 1978 and 1988 (Klougart et al 1996).
- In risk management practices, **1 : 1 000 000** risks are considered acceptable, whereas **1 : 100 000** risks are generally considered unacceptably high (K Green, Risk Assessment Advisor for the Fraser Institute, Vancouver, BC, email communication).

A sample of incidence of stroke in the world male population:

- Finland: 310 per 100 000 persons per year (Sarti et al 1994)
- Eastern Europe and former Soviet Union: 309–156 per 100 000 persons per year
- Western Europe: 100 per 100 000 persons per year
- Trinidad and Tobago: 185 per 100 000 persons per year (Cinzia et al 2000).

Interestingly, the rate of *spontaneous* vertebral artery dissection *without* manipulation is estimated to be about 1–3 per 100 000 persons (Giroud et al 1994, Shievink et al 1993, 1994), about the same rate as the *Stroke* study (Rothwell et al 2001) attributed to spinal manipulation. The authors acknowledge the inherent bias in their study regarding the cause and effect nature of their analysis. They also state that 'the rarity of VBAs makes this association difficult to study despite high volumes of chiropractic treatment'.

It is also important to consider that many persons suffer spontaneous stroke from everyday activities such as turning the head, looking at the sky, shoulder checking while driving, holding a telephone against the shoulder, getting a shampoo at the beauty parlor, doing yoga and many more common activities (Rome 1999, Terrett 1996c).

The wide difference in the statistics of risk of stroke from manipulation and the incidence of stroke and spontaneous arterial dissection in the general population raises questions as to the relationship between the two. Many observers erroneously make a connection between the cause and the effect. If a stroke occurred after a manipulation, then according to Keating (1992), the manipulation must be the cause of the stroke: 'To mistake temporal contiguity of two phenomena for

Continued

Box 7.5 Safety issues in high velocity manipulation continued

causation is a classic fallacy of reasoning known as "post hoc, ergo proctor hoc", from the Latin meaning "after this, therefore caused by this".' It is likely that many vascular accidents that occurred after a manipulation may very well have occurred under other circumstances, and the manipulation may have only been the aggravating factor in an already compromised arterial condition.

This theme is echoed repeatedly in studies evaluating risk of manipulation. As an example, an editorial (Hill 2003) in the *Canadian Journal of Neurological Sciences* stated:

Despite strong circumstantial reports and opinions, the quality of evidence that minor neck trauma including chiropractic neck manipulation causes vertebral or carotid artery dissection remains weak. A majority of papers are case reports or series only representing the weakest tier of clinical evidence.

The editorial also makes the point that is frequently commented on:

Some patients suffer the hallmark neck pain of dissection prior to neck adjustment and seek chiropractic assistance for relief of their neck pain. Neck manipulation may then dislodge a preexisting thrombus.

Identifying at-risk patients for stroke or vertebral dissection

There is no valid screening test for risk of stroke (Cote et al 1996, Terrett 1996d). To date, no particular factor that is useful for physical screening has been identified (Haldeman et al 2002a, McGregor et al 1995). False-negative findings have been reported and the reliability and validity of provocation tests have been unproven (Bolton et al 1989, Ferezy 1988).

The most significant predictor of risk for stroke has been determined to be a transient ischemic attack (TIA). The 90-day risk of stroke in this population is 10%.

Patients with high homocysteine levels are twice as likely to experience spontaneous arterial dissection as those with normal levels (Gallai et al 2001, Graham et al 1997, Pezzini et al 2002).

Hypertension is a well-known risk factor for stroke, as is cigarette smoking, diabetes, heart disease, prior history of stroke, genetics, high RBC count and vascular disease (American Stroke Association 2007).

Reducing the risk of stroke following manipulation

It is usually contraindicated to perform a high velocity manipulation on a patient who:

- has recently suffered a TIA
- has had a history of stroke
- has a known vascular disease
- has an existing neurological deficit
- has displayed any adverse signs or symptoms during treatment. Do not continue to adjust a patient if any possibility of vascular trauma has occurred.

It is a relative contraindication to manipulate a patient who:

- has a history of hypertension or other known risk factor for stroke or vascular disease
- has an elevated homocysteine level
- presents with a bruit
- has a migraine
- is experiencing dizziness, unsteadiness, vertigo or giddiness.

Terrett (1996e) found that 94.6% of the cases of CVA he studied involved rotational manipulation. Other authors have also identified manipulation with rotation (Haldeman et al 2001, Michaud 2002) and extension (Plaugher 1993b) to increase risk of stroke. Cervical techniques that minimize rotation and extension and utilize lateral flexion are associated with lower risk (Plaugher 1993b).

Summary

- About half of all patients will experience mild and transient adverse events after spinal manipulation.
- Manipulation of the cervical spine appears to be associated with the possibility of cervical radiculopathy, myelopathy and disc herniation.
- Manipulation of the lumbar spine is associated with a risk of cauda equina syndrome, disc herniation and increased nerve root damage.
- The most serious complication from manipulation is that of a vascular injury which leads to central nervous system infarction, resulting in residual neurological deficit, tetraplegia or death.
- The risk of stroke with possible permanent neurological damage or death has been estimated to be between 1 per 100 000 and 1 per 5.85 million manipulations.
- The risk assessment tends to be based on a temporal relationship between manipulation and stroke, with no conclusive evidence to date. The evidence is considered to be of a 'post hoc, ergo proctor hoc' nature.
- The risk of spontaneous arterial dissection is 1–3 per 100 000 persons without manipulation.

Box 7.5 Safety issues in high velocity manipulation continued

- The incidence of stroke in the world population is between 70 and 310 per 100 000 persons.
- There is no valid screening test for risk of stroke.
- The most significant predictor of risk for stroke has been determined to be a transient ischemic attack (TIA).
- High homocysteine levels, previous history of stroke, hypertension and vascular disease are also indicators of risk of stroke.

- Most strokes following manipulation are associated with rotational manipulation and extension of the neck.
- Avoiding rotational manipulation and using a more lateral technique is considered to be of less risk.
- If a patient displays any adverse signs or symptoms related to stroke during treatment, stop immediately. Do not continue to manipulate a patient if any possibility of vascular trauma has occurred.

It is more important to know when not to adjust than when to adjust. B.J. Palmer (1934)

Manual lymphatic drainage (MLD)

Indications/description

Numerous conditions, ranging from postoperative or post-traumatic edema to premenstrual fluid retention, may benefit from lymphatic drainage, which enhances lymphatic flow (Foldi & Strossenreuther 2003).

It is worth noting that in areas where MLD is most useful there exists the possibility that deep massage methods might inhibit normal lymph flow (Eliska & Eliskova 1995).

See also (below in this chapter) notes on osteopathic lymphatic pump methods that complement MLD.

Methodology

The manual techniques used in MLD involve extremely light pressure, which significantly increases lymph movement by crosswise and lengthwise stretching of the anchoring filaments that open the lymph capillaries, thus allowing the interstitial fluid to enter the lymphatic system (Braem 1994, Kurz 1987).

Specific protocols have been devised for the most efficient treatment of lymphatic stasis. For example, movements are usually applied proximally first and gradually moved to distal (retrograde) in order to drain and prepare (empty) the lymphatic pathway before congested regions are 'evacuated' of lymph through that same path. After the distal portion is treated, the practitioner proceeds back through the pathway proximally to encourage further (and more complete) drainage of the lymph (Chikly 1997).

Lymph movement is also augmented by respiration as movements of the diaphragm 'pump' the lymphatic fluids through the thoracic duct.

With sound anatomic knowledge, specific directions of drainage can be plotted, usually toward the node group responsible for evacuation of a particular area (lymphotome). Chikly (1999) emphasizes that hand pressure used in lymph drainage should be very light indeed, less than 1 oz (28 g) per cm^2 (under 8 oz per $inch^2$), in order to encourage lymph flow without increasing blood filtration.

Harris & Piller (2004) have summarized the characteristics of MLD when applying one of the five basic techniques (stationary circles, thumb circles, pump technique, scoop technique, rotary technique):

1. Light rhythmic alternating pressure with each stroke
2. Skin stretching and torqued both lengthwise and diagonally
3. Pressure and stretch applied in direction of desired fluid flow (not always in direction of lymph flow)
4. Light pressure over spongy edematous areas and slightly firmer over fibrotic tissue
5. Pressure not to exceed 32 mmHg.

In many instances, in order to maintain the benefits of MLD, additional compression therapy is required (supportive strapping, bandaging, pneumatic, etc.) (Foldi & Strossenreuther 2003).

Safety

Since the degree of pressure used in MLD is so light that tissue damage is virtually impossible, the most likely harm that might derive relates to incorrect usage, or the encouragement (via increased flow) of the spread of infection or malignancy. The cautions set out below offer other areas where problems might arise due to MLD (Kurz 1986).

Validation of efficacy = 5 (see Table 7.2)

MLD is extremely richly validated as being useful in treating the effects of post-traumatic or surgical edema (Fiaschi et al 1998).

Improvements in lymph flow lasting many hours have been shown to result from MLD applied for as little as 15 minutes (Ikimi et al 1996).

Alternatives

Forms of compression and active exercise that encourage circulatory function offer alternatives (Johansseon et al 1998).

Respiratory function is a natural ally of MLD and lymph movement in general.

Osteopathic pump techniques that provide intermittent compression (lymphatic pump, liver pump, etc.) described later in this chapter can support and/or replace MLD in some cases (Szuba & Achalu 2002).

Physiological effects

- Reduction of edema (Ko et al 1998).
- Blood and tissue fluid interchange – for example, enhanced interstitial fluid plasma protein, colloid, and leukocyte uptake into the lymphatic system (Ikimi et al 1996).
- Encouragement of development of secondary/accessory drainage routes (Ferrandez et al 1996).

Cautions (Wittlinger & Wittlinger 1982)

- Acute infections and acute inflammation (generalized and local)
- Thrombosis
- Circulatory problems
- Cardiac conditions
- Hemorrhage
- Malignant cancers
- Thyroid problems
- Acute phlebitis

Conditions that might benefit from lymphatic drainage but for which precautions are indicated, include:

- certain edemas, depending upon their cause, such as cardiac insufficiency
- carotid stenosis
- bronchial asthma
- burns, scars, bruises, moles
- abdominal surgery, radiation or undetermined bleeding or pain
- removed spleen
- major kidney problems or insufficiency
- menstruation (drain prior to menses)
- gynecological infections, fibromas or cysts
- some pregnancies (especially in the first 3 months)
- chronic infections or inflammation
- low blood pressure.

Naturopathic perspectives

It is difficult to imagine a gentler, more supportive approach to major health problems than MLD.

Naturopathic care and MLD are natural allies since the only focus of this method is to encourage normal tissue drainage, so meeting a primary objective – enhancing function without burdening the system with additional adaptive demands.

Further reading

1. Foldi M, Strossenreuther R 2003 Foundations of manual lymph drainage, 3rd edn. Mosby, St Louis
2. Chikly B 1997 Lymph drainage therapy study guide level II. Chickly and UI Publishing, Palm Beach Gardens, Florida
3. Wittlinger H, Wittlinger G 1982 Textbook of Dr Vodder's manual lymph drainage, vol 1: basic course, 3rd edn. Karl F Haug, Heidelberg

Massage

Indications/description

Based on the huge range of conditions that have been shown to benefit from therapeutic massage (see below under heading 'Validation of efficacy') it might be judged that the 'indication' for massage is that the individual is unwell (or wishes to remain well). There are few modalities that are more naturopathic, since in its most generic form massage is non-invasive, almost totally safe, and virtually without contraindications (see below). However, when massage incorporates techniques based on soft tissue manipulation, or when it becomes 'deeper' and has specific goals (deactivation of trigger points, reduction of fibrosis, etc.), universal suitability is reduced and cautions are required – for example, where serious pathology (cancer, arthritis), active inflammation and/or vulnerability (osteoporosis for example) are current.

Methodology

Massage application involves touching the body to manipulate the soft tissue, influence body fluid movement and stimulate neuroendocrine responses. How the physical contact is applied is considered to incorporate the *qualities of touch*.

The discussion earlier in the chapter regarding 'load' features should be recalled when considering the effects of the application of massage.

The mode of application (e.g. gliding/effleurage, kneading/petrissage, compression) provides the most efficient means of applying variations of load. Each method can be modified, depending on the desired outcome, by adjusting depth of pressure, drag (amount of tensile force applied), direction, speed, rhythm, frequency and duration.

The constituent elements that make up massage strokes include the following:

- *Petrissage* involves wringing and stretching movements, across the fiber direction of muscles.
- *Kneading* where the hands shape themselves to the contours of the area being treated. The tissues between the hands are lifted and pressed downwards and together.
- *Inhibition* involves application of pressure directly to the belly or origins or insertions of contracted muscles or to local soft tissue dysfunction for a variable amount of time or in a 'make-and-break' (pressure applied and then released) manner to reduce hypertonic contraction or for reflexive effects.
- *Effleurage* is a relaxing technique that is used, as appropriate, to initiate or terminate other manipulative methods. Pressure is usually even throughout the strokes, which are applied with the whole hand in contact.
- *Vibration and friction* contacts are used near origins and insertions and near bony attachments for relaxing effects on the muscle as a whole and to reach layers deep to the superficial tissues. It is performed by small circular or vibratory movements, with the tips of fingers or thumb. The heel of the hand may also be used.
- *Roulomont* involves skin lifting and rolling, which, as with most massage methods, can be used diagnostically as well as therapeutically.
- *Transverse or cross-fiber friction* is performed along or across the belly of muscles using the heel of the hand, thumb or fingers applied slowly and rhythmically or vigorously, depending upon the objectives.
- *Tapotement* involves percussive tapping, clapping, drumming and vibrating activities, involving fingertips or the ulnar borders of the hands.

Safety

There are few, if any, safety issues if cautions listed below are observed.

Validation of efficacy = 5 (see Table 7.2)

Following courses of massage:

- aggressive youngsters were less aggressive (Diego et al 2002)
- agitated physical behavior in Alzheimer patients was reduced (but not verbal aggression) (Rowe & Alfred 1999)
- peptic ulcer symptoms improved (Aksenova et al 1999, Bei 1993)
- symptoms of anxiety were significantly reduced (Shulman & Jones 1996)
- pain reduction and improved functionality were evident in patients with rheumatoid arthritis (Field & Hernandez-Reif 1997)
- there was significantly enhanced forced expiratory flow in asthmatics (Field et al 1997a)
- stereotypical behavior was reduced in autistics, and there was more socializing and fewer sleep problems (Escalona et al 2001)
- breast cancer patients demonstrated reduced anxiety, reduced depression, increased urinary dopamine, serotonin values, increased natural killer cell numbers and lymphocytes (Hernandez-Reif et al 2004)
- bulimia patients reported immediate reductions in anxiety and depression (Field et al 1998)
- there was a reduction of arm pain and discomfort following lymph node dissection in patients with breast cancer (Forchuk & Baruth 2004)
- massage treatment of trigger points reduced blood pressure significantly (systolic and diastolic) and decreased heart rate, as well as resulting in improvement in emotional state and muscle tension (Delaney et al 2002)
- chronic fatigue syndrome patients reported reduced depression and somatic symptoms, as well as improved sleep (Field et al 1997b)
- people with constipation had more normal bowel function and reduced incidence of soiling (Bishop et al 2003)
- compliance with insulin and food regulation improved and glucose levels decreased from 159 mg/dL to within normal range in diabetics over a 30-day period (Field et al 1997c)
- there was immediate decreased anxiety and depressed mood, long-term increased sleep hours and decreased sleep movements in fibromyalgia patients; substance P levels dropped as did pain ratings (Field et al 2002)
- HIV patients had enhanced immune system cytotoxic capacity (Ironson et al 1996)
- diastolic pressure reduced significantly in hypertensives (Hernandez-Reif et al 2000)
- mood improved as did white blood cell and neutrophil counts in leukemic patients (Field et al 2001)

- numerous studies as well as systematic review show benefit greater than acupuncture and self-care in cases of low back pain (Ernst 1999)
- multiple sclerosis patients demonstrated reduced anxiety and depression, improved self-esteem and social functioning (Hernandez-Reif et al 1998)
- numerous studies show enhanced tolerance to pain, raised pain threshold and improved function in a variety of settings, including chronic and postoperative pain (Walach et al 2003)
- Parkinson's disease patients showed improved daily living activities, less disturbed sleep (Hernandez-Reif et al 2002).

Alternatives

It may be hypothesized that forms of hydrotherapy (neutral bath, constitutional hydrotherapy for example) and various relaxation approaches (autogenic training for example) might produce similar benefits to that delivered by massage (Field et al 1996). As with studies showing benefits related to reflexology (Oleson & Flocco 1993) and aromatherapy (Cooke & Ernst 2000), it may also be hypothesized that much of the benefit deriving from massage relates to anti-arousal, anxiety-reducing influences that allow self-regulating processes to operate more efficiently. Although much of the benefit of massage may relate to its relaxation benefits, this is not entirely the case. In a Cochrane review published in *Spine* (Furlan et al 2002), massage was shown to be superior to sham therapy, more effective than exercise, corsets, relaxation and acupuncture, but not as effective as manipulation, in treatment of low back pain.

Physiological effects

The biochemical influences of massage include altered stress hormone (cortisol) production (Field 2000). Perhaps surprisingly, massage fails to increase blood flow through muscle unless it is exceptionally vigorous (Shoemaker et al 1997); however, drainage efficiency is improved when light techniques are employed (Ikimi et al 1996). Pain perception is reduced by massage, possibly due to gating of impulses (Clelland et al 1987).

Massage additionally mechanically modifies soft tissue status (stretching, mobilizing, etc.) depending on the variations in load application (sustained pressure, shearing load, etc.). The colloids in fasciae that surround, support and invest all soft tissues respond to appropriately applied pressure and vibration by changing state from a gel-type consistency to a solute, which increases internal hydration and assists in the removal of toxins from the tissue (Oschman 1997).

Psychological effects include reduced arousal, calmer mood and modified perception of anxiety (Rich 2002).

Neurological influences include a transient reduction in motor neuron excitability during and following massage (Goldberg 1992).

Massage also produces a decrease in the sensitivity of the gamma efferent control of the muscle spindles and thereby reduces any shortening tendency of the muscles (Puustjarvi 1990).

Cautions

- In areas that have been recently traumatized (2–3 weeks) and which are in the remodeling phase (including surgery).
- When a person is fatigued the duration and depth of the application should be reduced.
- If a patient has a fragile bone structure, the depth of pressure should be modified.
- When the patient is agitated the rhythm should be modified to create a calming effect.

The same cautions list applied to manual lymph drainage (Wittlinger & Wittlinger 1982) can be applied to use of massage:

- Acute infections and acute inflammation (generalized and local)
- Thrombosis
- Circulatory problems
- Cardiac conditions
- Hemorrhage
- Malignant cancers
- Thyroid problems
- Acute phlebitis
- Prominent varicosities.

Naturopathic perspectives

Because of its almost universal applicability, massage represents a modality that can be incorporated into naturopathic care of a wide range of conditions. It makes little demand on adaptive reserves – with evidence of value in treatment ranging from the distress of cocaine-addicted babies (Wheeden et al 1993) to advanced cancer patients (Ferrell-Torry & Glick 1993).

Further reading

1. Fritz S, Grosenbach J 1999 Mosby's basic science for soft tissue and movement therapies. Mosby, St Louis

2. Lowe W 2003 Orthopedic massage. Mosby, St Louis
3. Cassar M 2003 Handbook of clinical massage. Churchill Livingstone, Edinburgh
4. Chaitow L, Fritz S 2007 A massage therapist's guide to lower back and pelvic pain. Churchill Livingstone, Edinburgh
5. Chaitow L, Fritz S 2006 A massage therapist's guide to understanding, locating and treating myofascial trigger points. Churchill Livingstone, Edinburgh

Mobilization (also known as articulation)

See also discussion in Chapter 8 on combinations of mobilization methods deriving from early naturo-pathic or osteopathic settings.

Indications/description

Mobilization is indicated for treatment of restricted joints, including spinal (Maitland 2001), and/or where soft tissue (myofascial) changes are a factor in the restriction, or to enhance joint play and increased range when an intra-articular feature restricts free movement.

Mobilization offers a low velocity, high amplitude (LVHA) alternative to HVLA and/or can be used in conjunction with (preparatory to) thrust manipulation.

Carefully applied mobilization can be employed in relatively acute conditions (see also 'Mobilization with movement' discussion later in this chapter) as a combined means of assessment and treatment – for example, using Maitland's intervertebral physiologi-cal and accessory active and passive motion testing. Mobilization frequently involves rhythmically applied movement – see discussion of oscillation below.

Methodology

Manipulative techniques can be defined as techniques involving a high-velocity thrust, while mobilization techniques involve low-velocity techniques (Kent et al 2005).

- Manipulation (HVLA – see above) calls for a high velocity, low amplitude sudden movement, possibly performed through pain, usually associated with an audible sound (a cavitation 'pop').
- Mobilization on the other hand calls for low velocity, graded movement, gradually introduced, where there is ongoing palpatory feedback, with little or no pain, and no audible sound.

Patriquin & Jones (1997) describe the essence of mobilization/articulation. They suggest that both patient and practitioner should be positioned so that application of passive motion through the complete range of motion of the joint is possible:

Move the affected joint to the limit of all ranges of motion. As the restrictive barrier is reached, slowly and firmly continue to apply gentle force against it to the limit of tissue motion or the patient's tolerance of pain or fatigue. Then return the articulation slowly to the neutral portion of its motion. Repeat the process several times, each time regaining range and improved quality of motion. Cease repetition of motion when no further response is achieved.

Morris (2006a) notes variations on this theme: 'Joint mobilization is a safe, gentle and effective alternative to manipulation, although they can at times be effec-tive allies in reaching the goal of improved function.' He suggests that mobilization of a joint should involve three to four repetitions, each lasting approximately 30 seconds, with both the number of repetitions, and the duration of each mobilization, reduced if pain is a feature.

Joints are moved slowly and rhythmically through their current ranges of motion, using variable ampli-tudes of movement, usually commencing with small amplitudes and increasing – to end of range – as the slow stretching effects allow greater freedom. Involve-ment of patient participation may be usefully intro-duced in a number of ways:

- Patient introduces movement against isometric resistance from practitioner for 5–10 seconds – after which either patient or practitioner mobilizes joint
- Practitioner introduces movement against isometric resistance from patient for 5–10 seconds – after which either patient or practitioner mobilizes joint
- Mobilization is performed against slight patient resistance (isotonic), so producing various effects on soft tissues – toning some, stretching others. If performed slowly and deliberately, a generalized increase in ROM is likely along with improved balance of associated musculature.

These isometric and isotonic variations are examples of muscle energy technique – described more fully below.

Safety

Because of its slow, gradually introduced, well-controlled means of application, mobilization is extremely safe, allowing it to be used even in conditions where arthritic change has occurred.

Validation of efficacy = 5 (Delitto et al 1993, Jayson et al 1981) (see Table 7.2)

Systematic reviews have demonstrated benefit over no intervention, or sham intervention, for low back pain, but that mobilization is no more effective than other therapies (Assendelft et al 2003, Ferreira et al 2003).

A randomized controlled trial found that there was no difference in within-treatment-session change in pain and physical impairment, irrespective of whether the mobilization techniques used in treatment of non-specific low back pain patients was 'therapist selected' or 'randomly selected' (Chiradejnant et al 2003).

The Spencer shoulder treatment (Spencer 1976) is a traditional osteopathic articulation/mobilization procedure that has in recent years been modified by the addition (described below) of MET.

Clinical research has validated application of the Spencer sequence in a study involving elderly patients (Knebl 2002).

- Twenty-nine elderly patients with pre-existing shoulder problems were randomly assigned to a treatment (Spencer sequence osteopathic treatment) or a control group.
- The histories of those in the two groups were virtually identical: ±76% had a history of arthritis, 21% bursitis, 21% neurological disorders, 10% healed fractures.
- 63% had reduced shoulder ROM as their chief complaint, and 33% pain (4% had both reduced ROM and pain).
- Treatment of the control (placebo) group involved the patients being placed in the same seven positions (see descriptions and Fig. 7.9 below) as those receiving the active treatment; however, the one element that was not used in the control group was MET (described as the 'corrective force') as part of the protocol. Home exercises were also prescribed.
- Over the course of 14 weeks there were a total of eight 30-minute treatment sessions. Functional, pain and ROM assessments were conducted during alternate weeks, as well as 5 weeks after the end of treatment.
- Over the course of the study both groups demonstrated significantly increased ROM and a decrease in perceived pain. However, after treatment: 'Those subjects who had received osteopathic manipulative treatment [i.e. muscle energy-enhanced Spencer sequence] demonstrated continued improvement in ROM, while the ROM of the placebo group decreased.'

The researchers concluded: 'Clinicians may wish to consider OMT [i.e. muscle energy technique combined with Spencer sequence] as a modality for elderly patients with restricted ROM in the shoulder.'

See also Box 7.2 listing many conditions in which mobilization (and manipulation) has been shown to be helpful in enhancing self-regulation.

Alternatives

Mobilization and HVLA manipulation appear to be equally useful, in appropriately selected cases (see discussion earlier in this chapter regarding staging and classification), particularly in relation to the study by Flynn et al (2002).

Physiological effects

Apart from the purely mechanical effects of increased warmth and relaxation of joints during mobilization, the passive movements of joints encourage lymph and blood flow, involving both deep and superficial tissues (Giudice 1990, Le Vu et al 1997, Schmid-Schonbein 1990).

During the various stages of tissue repair following trauma or surgery an environment for repair can be enhanced by creation of low tensional forces while also encouraging circulation and drainage. Mobilization achieves these effects, as do oscillatory methods described later in this chapter, and rhythmically applied soft tissue methods that incorporate compression (Lederman 2005c).

Gating of pain impulses from muscles, tendons, joints and ligaments is influenced by joint articulation/mobilization/oscillation methods (Zusman 1988, Zusman et al 1989).

Earlier in this chapter there was discussion of research validating the use of mobilization and other manual methods in enhancing fluid movement, adaptation responses, respiratory and digestive function, etc., as outlined in Chapter 8.

Cautions

- Advanced bone disease
- Fracture
- Disc fragmentation
- Direct nerve root impingement that would contradict spinal manipulative therapy, evidence of cord or caudal compression by tumor, ankylosis or other space-occupying lesion

- Spinal canal stenosis
- Acute localized infection or inflammation
- Repetitive movements involving the upper cervical region in rotation and/or extension should be performed with caution

Naturopathic perspectives

Mobilization has clear advantages over HVLA manipulation in terms of safety, particularly in the cervical region. Since studies show no clear advantage for HVLA apart from saving treatment time, the choice of one or the other approach remains entirely a matter of preference. Keeping in mind the dictum to 'do no harm', this approach to enhancing joint function would appear to have advantages.

Further reading

1. Greenman P 1996 Principles of manual medicine, 2nd edn. Williams & Wilkins, Baltimore
2. Lewit K 1999 Manipulative therapy in rehabilitation of the locomotor system, 3rd edn. Butterworth-Heinemann, Oxford
3. Morris C (ed) 2006 Low back syndromes: integrated clinical management. McGraw-Hill, New York
4. Murphy D 2000 Conservative management of cervical spine syndromes. McGraw-Hill, New York
5. Ward R 1997 Foundations for osteopathic medicine. Williams & Wilkins, Baltimore

---

Box 7.6 Mobilization exercises

Exercise 1: Cervical mobilization/articulation

Mobilization of the cervicothoracic junction (indicated if there is reduced range of flexion, extension, side-flexion or rotation, at that level):

1. Patient is side-lying (if problem is unilateral, affected side should be up).
2. Practitioner stands in front and supports patient's head and neck with cephalad hand and forearm.
3. The patient's tableside hand/arm should be flexed at shoulder and elbow, while the other arm is in extension and adduction, resting on the lateral thoracic cage.
4. Practitioner's caudad hand engages and stabilizes the spinous process of T1.
5. If the restriction involves an inability of C7 on T1 to fully flex, side-bend and rotate, the hand supporting the head/neck flexes, side-flexes and rotates it so that the hand in contact with T1 becomes aware of forces building at that level as the barrier of free motion is reached (at C7 on T1).
6. When the barrier has been engaged this should be held for 3–5 seconds before a return to neutral.
7. The range of motion is repeated, and the barrier re-engaged rhythmically, with pauses at the barrier for 3–5 seconds, until no further gain in range is achieved.
8. Once the barrier has been engaged, isometric variations can be added by having the patient attempt to return to neutral, or to push through the barrier, against the practitioner's resistance for 5 seconds, using minimal effort, and with no pain being produced, after which a new barrier should be achieved.

Exercise 2: Shoulder mobilization/articulation (Spencer method)

A. Spencer treatment of shoulder extension restriction

1. The practitioner's cephalad hand cups the shoulder of the side-lying patient, firmly compressing the scapula and clavicle to the thorax, while the patient's flexed elbow is held in the practitioner's caudad hand, as the arm is taken into extension towards the optimal 90° of extension.
2. The first indication of resistance to movement should be sensed, indicating the beginning of the end of range of that movement.
3. At that 'first sign of resistance' barrier the patient is instructed to push the elbow towards the feet, or anteriorly, or to push further towards the direction of extension – utilizing no more than 20% of available strength, building up force slowly.
4. This effort is firmly resisted by the practitioner, and after 7–10 seconds the patient is instructed to slowly cease the effort.
5. After complete relaxation, and on an exhalation, the practitioner moves the shoulder further into extension, to the next restriction barrier, and the MET procedure is repeated, possibly using a different direction of effort.

Continued

Box 7.6 Mobilization exercises continued

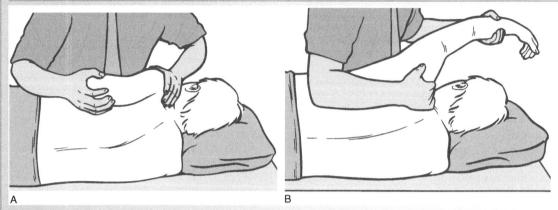

A   B

Figure 7.8 **A** Shoulder extension. Reproduced with permission from Chaitow (2006). **B** Shoulder flexion. Reproduced with permission from Chaitow (2006)

B. Spencer treatment of shoulder flexion restriction

1. The patient has the same starting position as in A, above.
2. The practitioner stands at chest level, half-facing cephalad. The practitioner's non-tableside hand grasps the patient's forearm while the tableside hand holds the clavicle and scapula firmly to the chest wall.
3. The practitioner slowly introduces shoulder flexion in the horizontal plane, as range of motion to 180° is assessed, by which time the elbow will be in extension.
4. At the position of very first indication of restriction in movement (palpated by the hand stabilizing the shoulder, and by the hand/arm moving the patient's arm toward the direction being assessed), the patient is instructed to pull the elbow towards the feet, or to direct it posteriorly, or to push further towards the direction of flexion – utilizing no more than 20% of available strength, building up force slowly.
5. This effort is firmly resisted by the practitioner, and after 7–10 seconds the patient is instructed to slowly cease the effort.
6. After complete relaxation, and on an exhalation, the practitioner moves the shoulder further into flexion, to the next restriction barrier, where the MET procedure is repeated.
7. A degree of active patient participation in the movement towards the new barrier may be helpful.

The Spencer sequence continues by sequentially introducing articulatory shoulder adduction and abduction, internal and external rotation, as well as circumduction movements (Chaitow 2006).

Exercise 3: Rib-raising mobilization

The example is given by Patriquin & Jones (1997) of an individual with viral pneumonia with a resistant chest wall in which all ribs are restricted in their range in both inhalation and exhalation. There is additionally paraspinal tenderness to even light pressure.

The articulation, or springing, method can be described as a low velocity, high amplitude (LVHA) approach in complete contrast to an HVLA thrust method.

1. The patient is bed-bound and is lying supine.
2. The practitioner stands at the head of the bed and reaches down under the patient's back, palms upwards so that the flexed fingertips can engage an upper pair of ribs (2nd ideally, or 3rd) as close to the angles on each side of the midline as possible.
3. A gentle cephalward pull is applied to help mobilize the costotransverse and costovertebral articulations, and to stretch both the intercostals and more superficial tissues.
4. The tension should be held for at least 10 seconds and then slowly released.
5. If the patient can cooperate, this process is enhanced by the patient inhaling as fully as possible, once the cephalad tension has been applied.
6. The same procedure is repeated on the same pair of ribs, until a sense is gained that no further freedom of movement can be achieved.

Box 7.6 Mobilization exercises continued

7. The next pair of ribs is then engaged and the process repeated.

8. Continue down as far as it is possible to achieve a degree of contact that allows the process to be carried out.

9. The practitioner then moves to the side of the bed at approximately hip level, facing the head of the table.

10. The non-tableside hand is placed under the patient, so that the slightly flexed fingertips can engage the superior surface of the 2nd rib, close to the angle of the ribs (one side treated at a time when the patient is supine).

11. A caudad drag should be introduced to move the rib inferiorly in relation to other thoracic structures,

with the effort being maintained for not less than 10 seconds in order to introduce a degree of intercostal stretch.

12. A slight degree of gentle 'springing' of the tissues against their barrier of resistance may also be usefully employed.

13. Once this appropriate degree of stretch has been achieved, and while this is still being maintained, the patient should be asked to inhale as deeply as possible.

14. The process should be repeated until a suitable degree of improved mobility/articulation has been achieved, at which time the next rib should receive the same treatment.

15. The other side is then addressed in the same way.

Muscle energy techniques (MET)/ proprioceptive neuromuscular facilitation (PNF) and variations

Note: MET and PNF are different in origin; however, over time, similarities have been emphasized and differences minimized, to the extent that in this text they are being considered as interchangeable terms.

As Fryer (2006) explains: 'Much of the research relevant to MET comes from the study of related techniques, such as Proprioceptive Neuromuscular Facilitation (PNF) stretching.' (See also discussion of stretching in Chapter 9).

Indications/description

- Mobilization of joints
- Preparation for the stretching/lengthening of shortened muscles, or for reducing tone in hypertonic muscles
- Introduction of controlled microtrauma in cases of fibrosis
- Toning inhibited/weakened muscles
- As part of an integrated sequence for deactivating myofascial trigger points (INIT – see below)
- Rehabilitation of motor control (using pulsed MET – see below)

Methodology

Muscle energy techniques are soft tissue manipulative methods in which the patient, on request, actively uses the muscles from a controlled position, in a specific direction, with mild effort, against a precise counterforce (Mitchell et al 1979).

The counterforce can:

- match the patient's effort (isometric contraction), subsequently resulting in a reduced sensitivity to stretching of the muscle (or its antagonist) (Magnusson S et al 1996)
- fail to match patient effort (concentric isotonic contraction). This produces an automatic toning of the contracting muscle, together with a simultaneous (very slight) inhibition of its antagonist(s), as well as a reduction in sensitivity to subsequent stretching (Lederman 2005c)
- overcome patient effort (eccentric isotonic contraction). If performed rapidly this creates controlled microtrauma of the contracting muscle (breaking minute adhesions, fibrosis – known as an isolytic contraction), whereas if performed slowly this produces a toning of the contracting muscle and a simultaneous (slight) inhibition of its antagonist(s), followed by a reduction in sensitivity to stretching (Liebenson 2006).

Depending upon the relative acuteness of the situation, the isometric or isotonic contractions commence from, or short of, a previously ascertained barrier of resistance. Barrier identification is an essential skill required if MET is to be used efficiently, calling for sound palpation expertise (see Chapter 6).

The most common forms of isometric stretching referred to in the literature are contract-relax (CR), where the muscle being stretched is contracted and then relaxed, agonist contract-relax (ACR), where contraction of the agonist (rather than the muscle being stretched) actively moves the joint into increased ROM, and contract-relax agonist-contract (CRAC), a combination of these two methods.

These techniques are commonly referred to as PNF stretching, but the similarity to MET methods for stretching muscles is obvious.

Researchers have used slightly different MET protocols (varying the force and duration of contraction and stretching, and number of repetitions, use of agonist contraction) and different methods of measuring hamstring length (active knee extension, passive knee extension, measurement of passive torque) to assess the effect of techniques on immediate changes to hamstring length.

Researchers have reported immediate hamstring length and ROM increases from 3° (Ballantyne et al 2003) to 33° (Magnusson S et al 1996) following MET or similar methods.

Numerous studies (Ferber et al 2002a) have demonstrated both short- and long-term increases in ROM using MET/PNF style protocols. The benefits do not seem to be age dependent. For example, Klein et al (2002) examined the effect of a 10-week flexibility program (including warm-ups, CR and cool-down exercises, twice a week) on various muscles in 11 assisted-living older adults (73–94 years). The researchers found that the subjects gained significant improvements in ankle flexion and shoulder flexion ROM, in isometric strength, and in balance and mobility for sit-to-stand.

The mechanisms involved in the benefits such as increased ROM offered by MET/PNF remain controversial.

For many years two primary concepts have been used to explain the increased ROM and improved ability to stretch, following use of MET-type isometric contractions:

- post isometric relaxation (PIR; Greenman 1996, Lewit & Simons 1984) producing neurological reflex muscle relaxation, and
- reciprocal inhibition (RI) produced by contraction of a muscle antagonist (Kuchera & Kuchera 1992).

Both of these have now been shown to offer only minimal contributions to MET benefits (Lewit & Simons 1984).

An additional explanation relates to changes in viscoelastic properties of tissues following isometric contractions. This concept has also been demonstrated to offer at best minimal contributions to increased ROM.

Researchers who have investigated the effect of passive stretching on hamstring extensibility using torque-controlled passive knee extension have found little evidence of any lasting change to tissue property (Magnusson M et al 1996).

The current explanation, which has as yet not clarified the neurological mechanisms involved, is expressed simply as 'an increased tolerance to stretch' following isometric contractions.

Stated simply, this explanation notes that it is possible to apply greater torque (force) following an isometric contraction, with reduced sensitivity/increased tolerance.

If, for example, an isometric contraction is introduced into shortened hamstring muscles, held at the end of range (i.e. at the level of pain tolerance), it will only be able to move to a new barrier (i.e. be lengthened/stretched following the contraction) if greater force is used, force that previous to the contraction would not have been tolerated (Magnusson S et al 1996).

A MET variation is the use of rapidly pulsing isometric contractions (Ruddy's method – a.k.a. pulsed muscle energy technique – described later in this chapter) (Ruddy 1962).

Safety

As with all modalities, inappropriate use, or employment of excessive force, is likely to result in negative outcomes and side-effects. Common errors made by the practitioner and/or the patient are listed below.

Patient errors during MET (Greenman 1996) (commonly based on inadequate instruction from the practitioner!)

- Contraction is too strong (remedy: give specific guidelines, e.g. 'use only 20% of strength', or whatever is more appropriate).
- Contraction is in the wrong direction (remedy: give simple but accurate instructions).
- Contraction is not sustained for long enough (remedy: instruct the patient/model to hold the contraction until told to ease off, and give an idea ahead of time as to how long this will be).
- The individual does not relax completely after the contraction (remedy: have them release and relax and then inhale and exhale once or twice, with the suggestion 'now relax completely').
- Starting and/or finishing the contraction too hastily (remedy: there should be a slow build-

up of force and a slow letting go; this is easily achieved if a rehearsal is carried out first to educate the patient into the methodology).

Practitioner errors in application of MET

- Inaccurate control of position of joint or muscle in relation to the resistance barrier (remedy: have a clear image of what is required and apply it).
- Inadequate counterforce to the contraction (remedy: meet and match the force in an isometric contraction; allow movement in an isotonic concentric contraction; overcome the contraction in an isolytic maneuver or slow eccentric isotonic contraction).
- Counterforce is applied in an inappropriate direction (remedy: ensure precise direction needed for best results).
- Moving to a new position too hastily after the contraction (there is usually at least 10 seconds of refractory muscle tone release during which time a new position can easily be adopted – haste is unnecessary and may be counterproductive; Moore & Kukulka 1991).
- Inadequate patient instruction is given (remedy: get the instructions right so that the patient can cooperate).
- Whenever force is applied by the patient in a particular direction, and when it is time to release that effort, the instruction must be to do so gradually. Any rapid effort may be self-defeating.
- The coinciding of the forces at the outset (patient and practitioner), as well as at release, is important. The practitioner must be careful to use enough, but not too much, effort, and to ease off at the same time as the patient.
- The practitioner fails to maintain the stretch position for a period of time that allows soft tissues to begin to lengthen (ideally 30 seconds, but certainly not just a few seconds) (Schmitt et al 1999).

Validation of efficacy = 4 (see Table 7.2)

Investigation of the effects of MET on spinal ROM (Lenehan et al 2003, Schenk et al 1994, 1997) and on clinical outcomes in symptomatic individuals shows noteworthy benefit. It is worth noting that MET is not commonly employed as a stand-alone technique (for instance, in the treatment of low back pain), but is frequently administered in combination with other manual approaches. In one clinical pilot study, MET – used as the sole intervention – was found to be significantly effective in treatment of acute low back pain (Wilson et al 2003).

As mentioned above, the distinction between PNF and MET is now largely historical, and PNF validation is well established (Carter et al 2000, Etnyre & Abraham 1986, Ferber et al 2002b, Godges et al 2003).

Alternatives

Stretching associated with prior, or simultaneous, use of isometric and/or isotonic contractions appears to offer major benefits when compared with passive or active stretching methods that do not employ these (Ballantyne et al 2003, Taylor et al 1997).

If mobilization is the objective, manipulation and mobilization methods (see above) are clearly alternatives. If lengthening shortened soft tissues is the objective, myofascial release and other stretching methods offer alternatives.

Physiological effects

MET and PNF stretching methods have been clearly shown to bring about greater improvements in joint ROM and muscle extensibility than passive, static stretching, both in the short and long term (Magnusson S et al 1996).

Cautions

- Acute arthritis and other inflammatory conditions (contraindicated during acute stages)
- Aneurysm
- Bone fractures or acute soft tissue injuries: wait for full healing (6–12 weeks)
- Hemophilia
- Hodgkin's disease
- Leukemia
- Malignancy with metastasis (or TB) involving bone
- Osteoporosis
- Pain production during procedure
- Patients on cortisone (wait 2–3 months)
- Patients with high fever
- Phlebitis
- Recent scar tissue
- Syphilitic articular or peri-articular lesions
- Uncontrolled diabetic neuropathy

- McArdle's syndrome (a rare glycogen storage disease characterized by exercise intolerance, myalgia and stiffness)

If pathology is suspected, MET should not be used until an accurate diagnosis has been established. Pathology (osteoporosis, arthritis, etc.) does not rule out its use; however, dosage of application needs to be modified accordingly (amount of force used, number of repetitions, stretching introduced or not, etc.).

DiGiovanna (1991) states that side-effects are minimal with MET:

MET is quite safe. Occasionally some muscle stiffness and soreness after treatment. If the area being treated is not localised well or if too much contractive force is used pain may be increased. Sometimes the patient is in too much pain to contract a muscle or may be unable to cooperate with instructions or positioning. In such instances MET may be difficult to apply.

Side-effects will be nil or limited if MET is used in ways that:

- stay within the very simple guideline which states categorically 'cause no pain when using MET'
- stick to light (20% of strength) contractions
- do not stretch over-enthusiastically, but only take muscles a short way past the restriction barrier when stretching
- have the patient assist in this stretch.

Naturopathic perspectives

MET can be used in acute and chronic modes – with or without stretching – to help mobilization of joints, to prepare joints for subsequent manipulation (HVLA), to encourage reduced tone where appropriate, or in its rhythmic pulsing (see below) or isotonic concentric modes, to assist in facilitating rehabilitation of injured or dysfunctional tissues. It therefore fits well with naturopathic care since it is capable of being used to remove obstacles to optimal adaptation, as well as encouraging enhanced functionality and self-regulating processes.

Variation: **Pulsed MET** (Ruddy's rapid resistive duction method)

Ruddy (1962) developed a method of rapid pulsating contractions against resistance which he termed 'rapid rhythmic resistive duction'. For obvious reasons the shorthand term 'pulsed muscle energy technique' is now applied to Ruddy's method (Chaitow 2001).

Its simplest use involves the dysfunctional tissue or joint being held at its restriction barrier, at which time the patient (or the practitioner if the patient cannot adequately cooperate with the instructions) introduces a series of rapid (two per second) tiny efforts. These miniature contractions toward the barrier are ideally practitioner resisted. The barest initiation of effort is called for with (to use Ruddy's term) 'no wobble and no bounce'.

The application of this 'conditioning' approach involves contractions which are 'short, rapid and rhythmic, gradually increasing the amplitude and degree of resistance, thus conditioning the proprioceptive system by rapid movements' (Ruddy 1962).

Ruddy suggests the effects are likely to include improved oxygenation, venous and lymphatic circulation through the area being treated. Furthermore, he believed that the method influences both static and kinetic posture because of the effects on proprioceptive and interoceptive afferent pathways, so helping to maintain 'dynamic equilibrium' which involves 'a balance in chemical, physical, thermal, electrical and tissue fluid homeostasis'.

Effects include:

- proprioceptive re-education
- strengthening facilitation of the weak antagonists
- reciprocal inhibition of tense agonists
- enhanced local circulation and drainage
- re-education of movement patterns on a reflex, subcortical basis.

Further reading

1. Chaitow L 2006 Muscle energy techniques, 3rd edn. Churchill Livingstone, Edinburgh
2. Greenman PE 1996 Principles of manual medicine, 2nd edn. Williams & Wilkins, Baltimore
3. DiGiovanna E, Schiowitz S (eds) 1991 An osteopathic approach to diagnosis and treatment. Lippincott, Philadelphia
4. Lewit K 1999 Manipulative therapy in rehabilitation of the locomotor system, 3rd edn. Butterworth-Heinemann, Oxford
5. Mitchell F Jr, Moran P, Pruzzo N 1979 An evaluation of osteopathic muscle energy procedures. Pruzzo, Valley Park, Missouri

Box 7.7 Muscle energy technique exercises

Exercise 1: MET treatment of a joint

When treating restricted joints using MET no stretching should be introduced following isometric contractions. The restriction barrier should be engaged and, following a 5- to 7-second isometric contraction involving no more than 20% of available strength, an attempt should be made to passively move to a new barrier, without force or stretching.

Unlike the period required to hold soft tissues at stretch (see next exercise), in order to achieve increased extensibility, no such feature is part of the protocol for treating joints.

Once a new barrier is reached, having taken out available slack without force after the isometric contraction, a subsequent contraction is called for and the process is repeated.

A variety of directions of resisted effort may prove useful (or, put differently, a range of different muscles should be contracted isometrically) when attempting to achieve release and mobilization of a restricted joint, including those where there is no specific muscular control over the joint, such as the sacroiliac, sternoclavicular and acromioclavicular joints.

Patient-directed isometric efforts towards the restriction barrier, as well as away from it, and using a combination of forces, often of a 'spiral' nature, may be experimented with if a joint does not release using the most obvious directions of contraction.

Additionally, Ruddy's pulsed MET approaches (described later in this chapter) are useful when attempting to release blocked joints.

Exercise 2: MET for shortness of lower hamstrings

To test the lower hamstrings for shortness the tested leg of the supine patient is taken into full hip flexion, helped by the patient holding the upper thigh with both hands (Fig. 7.9).

The knee is then straightened until resistance is felt, or bind is noted by palpation of the lower hamstrings.

If the knee cannot straighten with the hip flexed to 90°, this indicates shortness in the lower hamstring fibers, and the patient will report a degree of pull behind the knee and lower thigh.

MET treatment of this is carried out in the test position.

- The treated leg should be flexed at both the hip and knee, and then straightened by the practitioner until the restriction barrier is identified (one hand should palpate the tissues behind the knee for sensations of 'bind' as the knee is straightened).
- Depending upon whether it is an acute or a chronic problem, the isometric contraction against resistance

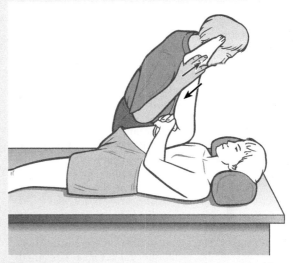

Figure 7.9 Assessment and treatment position for lower hamstring fibers. Reproduced with permission from Chaitow (2006)

is introduced at this 'bind' barrier (if acute) or a little short of it (if chronic). *Note:* These refinements as to position in relation to the barrier are not universally agreed and are based on the teaching of Janda (1978).

- The instruction might be something such as 'try to gently bend your knee, against my resistance, starting slowly and using only a quarter of your strength'.
- It is particularly important with the hamstrings to take care regarding cramp, and so it is suggested that no more than 20% of patients' effort should ever be used during isometric contractions in this region.
- Following the 7–10 seconds of contraction followed by complete relaxation, the leg should, on an exhalation, be straightened at the knee towards its new barrier (in acute problems) and through that barrier introducing a degree of stretch (if chronic), ideally with the patient's assistance.
- This slight stretch should be held for 30 seconds.
- Repeat the process until no further gain is possible (usually one or two repetitions achieve the maximum degree of lengthening available at any one session).
- Antagonist muscles can also be used isometrically by having the patient try to extend the knee during the contraction, rather than bending it, followed by the stretching procedure as described above.

Myofascial release methods (MFR)

Indications/description

A need to improve movement potential, and/or for the stretching/lengthening of shortened, contracted or fibrosed soft tissues, or for reducing tone in hypertonic muscles.

Fascia is a tough, fibroelastic, body-wide web of tissue that performs both structural and proprioceptive functions. Because of its contiguous nature, and its virtually universal presence in association with every muscle, vessel and organ, the potential influences of fascia are profound if shortening, adhesions, scarring or distortion occurs as a result of either slow adaptation (microtrauma) or trauma.

John Barnes (1996) writes: *'Studies suggest that fascia, an embryological tissue, reorganizes along the lines of tension imposed on the body, adding support to misalignment and contracting to protect tissues from further trauma.'* Having evaluated where a restriction area exists, MFR technique calls for a sustained pressure (gentle usually) which engages the elastic component of the elasticocollagenous complex, stretching this until it ceases releasing (this can take some minutes). Sustained or repetitive applications of load (pressure) are required when treating fascia because of its collagenous structure. There is no effective way of lengthening ('releasing') fascia rapidly (Hammer 1999).

Methodology

Myofascial release is a hands-on soft tissue technique that facilitates a stretch into the restricted fascia. A sustained pressure is applied into the tissue barrier; after 90 to 120 seconds the tissue will undergo histological length changes allowing the first release to be felt. The therapist follows the release into a new tissue barrier and holds. After a few releases the tissues will become softer and more pliable. (Barnes 1997)

Mock (1997) describes a hierarchy of MFR stages or 'levels':

1. Level 1 involves treatment of tissues without introducing tension. The practitioner's contact (which could involve thumb, finger, knuckle or elbow) moves longitudinally along muscle fibers, distal to proximal, with the patient passive.
2. Level 2 is precisely the same as the previous description but, in this instance, the glide is applied to muscle which is in tension (at stretch).
3. Level 3 involves the introduction to the process of passively induced motion, as an area of restriction is compressed while the tissues being compressed are taken passively through their fullest possible range of motion.
4. Level 4 is the same as the previous description but the patient actively moves the tissues through the fullest possible range of motion, from shortest to longest, while the practitioner/therapist offers resistance.

For example, the practitioner might apply moderate digital pressure to the involved tissue in a direction proximal to distal while the patient actively moves the muscle through its range of motion in both eccentric and concentric contraction phases. This modification of basic MFR has been called active release technique (ART) (Leahy 1999).

It can be seen from the descriptions offered that there are different models of myofascial release, some taking tissue to the elastic barrier and waiting for a release mechanism to operate and others in which active or passive force is applied to induce change.

Safety

The basic methodology of MFR requires that it should be applied slowly. Barriers of resistance are engaged and these are forced to retreat but by virtue of the steadily applied load. In this way the physiological responses of creep and hysteresis are produced, leading to lengthening. This is a non-violent, direct approach that has little potential for causing damage. When active or passive movements are combined with the basic methodology, caution is required, depending on the status of the patient and the tissues, to avoid excessive irritation. For example, enthesitis could occur if localized repetitive stretching combined with compression were applied close to an attachment (Simons et al 1999).

Validation of efficacy = 5 (see Table 7.2)

MFR is widely used and its value is referenced in numerous studies involving physical therapy, chiropractic and osteopathy (Hou et al 2002, Leahy & Mock 1992, Manheim & Lavett 1994, Roberts et al 2003, Souza 1994).

Alternatives

Since myofascial release is utilized to lengthen shortened soft tissues, all other methods that have this objective are alternatives, the most obvious being MET/PNF methods as described above. MFR does not incorporate isometric contractions into its methodology, although it is not difficult to conceive that such a tool could well be combined with MFR in order to reduce discomfort and encourage lengthening, so melding MET and MFR into a sequence.

Physiological effects

Shea (1993) explains:

The components of connective tissue (fascia) are long thin flexible filaments of collagen surrounded by ground substance. The ground substance is composed of 30–40% glycosaminoglycans (GAG) and 60–70% water. Together GAG and water form a gel . . . which functions as a lubricant as well as to maintain space (critical fiber distance) between collagen fibers. Any dehydration of the ground substance will decrease the free gliding of the collagen fibers. Applying pressure to any crystalline lattice increases its electrical potential, attracting water molecules, thus hydrating the area. This is the piezoelectric effect of manual connective tissue therapy.

By applying direct pressure (of the appropriate degree), at the correct angle (angle and force need to be suitable for the particular release required), a slow lengthening of restricted tissue occurs.

Slowly applied load causes the viscous medium to become more liquid ('sol') than would result from a rapidly applied pressure. As fascial tissues distort in response to pressure, the process is known by the shorthand term 'creep' (Twomey & Taylor 1982).

Hysteresis is the process of heat and energy exchange by the tissues as they deform (Dorland's Medical Dictionary 1985).

Fryer (2006) describes the effects as follows:

Connective tissues display mechanical properties relating to their fluid or gel components (viscous) and their elastic properties, called viscoelasticity. Connective tissue elongation is time and history dependent, and if a constant stretching force is loaded on a tissue, the tissue will respond with slow elongation or 'creep'. The tissue creep results in loss of energy (hysteresis), and repetition of loading before the tissue has recovered will result in greater deformation (Norkin & Levangie 1992). Additional loading may cause more permanent 'plastic' change, caused by micro tearing of collagen fibres (which would cause an immediate change in the stiffness of the tissue) and subsequent remodelling of fibres to a longer length (Lederman 1997c).

Cautions

- Acute arthritis and other inflammatory conditions (contraindicated during acute stages)
- Aneurysm
- Bone fractures or acute soft tissue injuries: wait for full healing (6–12 weeks)
- Hemophilia
- Hodgkin's disease
- Leukemia
- Malignancy with metastasis (or TB) involving bone
- Osteoporosis
- Pain production during procedure
- Patients on cortisone (wait 2–3 months)
- Patients with high fever
- Phlebitis
- Recent scar tissue
- Syphilitic articular or peri-articular lesions
- Uncontrolled diabetic neuropathy

Naturopathic perspectives

The same thoughts that apply to MET apply to MFR as a naturopathic modality. Used correctly, avoiding heavy stretching or the causation of pain, MFR is a useful, safe and efficient means of encouraging self-regulation by removing structural (and therefore functional) restrictions.

Further reading

1. Shea M 1993 Myofascial release – a manual for the spine and extremities. Shea Educational Group, Juno Beach, Florida
2. Lewit K 1999 Manipulative therapy in rehabilitation of the locomotor system, 3rd edn. Butterworth-Heinemann, Oxford

Mobilization with movement (MWM) – incorporating NAGs and SNAGs (natural apophyseal glides; sustained natural apophyseal glides)

Indications/description

Joint restrictions, or pain on movement involving a joint.

Because they involve simultaneous joint accessory mobilization with active movement, MWMs are used exclusively to treat movement-generated symptoms. They are not used where the patient complains of resting aches and pains, except perhaps where these are truly of minor significance to the patient, but are exacerbated by active movement. Significant resting symptoms are usually associated with a degree of underlying pathology far beyond that of relatively minor biomechanical abnormalities (Wilson 2007).

Methodology

A painless, gliding, translation pressure is applied by the practitioner, almost always at right angles to the plane of movement in which restriction is noted,

Box 7.8 Myofascial release exercises

Exercise 1: Longitudinal paraspinal myofascial release

- The practitioner stands to the side of the prone patient at chest level.
- The cephalad hand is placed on the paraspinal region on the contralateral side, fingers facing caudad.
- The caudad hand is placed, fingers facing cephalad, so that the heels of the hands (the arms will be crossed at this time) are a few centimeters apart, and on the same side of the torso.
- Light compression is applied into the tissues to remove the slack by separation of the hands, until each individually reaches the elastic barrier of the tissues being contacted.
- Pressure is not applied into the torso; instead, traction occurs on the superficial tissues, which lie between the two hands.
- These barriers are held for not less than 90 seconds, and commonly between 2 and 3 minutes, until a sense of separation of the tissues is noted.
- The tissues are followed to their new barriers, and the light, sustained separation force is maintained until a further release is noted.
- The superficial fascia will have been released and the status of associated myofascial tissues will have altered.

Exercise 2: Myofascial release of scar tissue contractures (Lewit & Olanska 2004) (repeated from Chapter 6)

- Palpate a scar, feeling the scar tissue itself and judge how the surrounding tissues – skin and deeper tissues – associate with it.
- Is there a sense of tethering, or does the scar 'float' in reasonably supple, elastic, local tissues?
- Can the scar be easily moved in all directions equally, or are there directions of movement for all, or part, of the scar that are limited, compared with others?
- If possible, palpate a recent and also a very old scar, and compare the characteristics.
- See if local tenderness or actual pain exists around the scar on pressure or distraction of attached soft tissues.
- Evaluate whether the skin elasticity alongside the scar varies.
- Can you release undue tension of the skin attaching to the scar by sustained painless stretching – holding it at its elastic barrier?
- This can be achieved in various ways – as in skin stretching, i.e. holding the skin at stretch for 15–90 seconds while stabilizing the scar with the other hand, or by means of pinching, compressing and/or rolling the scar tissue between the thumb and finger.

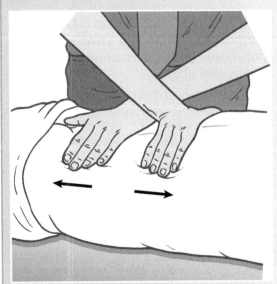

Figure 7.10 Cross-handed myofascial release. Reproduced with permission from Chaitow & Fritz (2006)

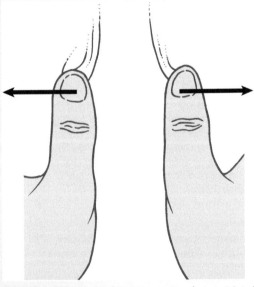

Figure 7.11 Holding skin (close to scar tissue) at stretch to begin process of trigger point deactivation. Reproduced with permission from Chaitow & Fritz (2006)

while the patient actively (or sometimes the practitioner passively) moves the joint in the direction of restriction, or the direction(s) that would produce painful symptoms.

Specific modifications are used for spinal mobilization (NAGs and SNAGs) in which a gliding of restricted facet (zygapophyseal) joints is introduced, as the patient performs previously restricted or painful movements (Mulligan 1992).

Most applications of SNAGs commence with the patient weight bearing, usually seated. SNAGs are movements that are *actively* performed by the patient, in the direction of restriction, while the practitioner *passively* holds an area in an anteriorly translated direction (in the cervical spine, it is the segment immediately cephalad to the restriction).

1. In the cervical spine the direction of translation is almost always directed along the plane of the facet articulation, i.e. toward the eyes.
2. In some instances, as well as actively moving the head and neck toward the direction of restriction while the practitioner maintains the translation, the patient may usefully apply 'overpressure' in which a hand is used to reinforce the movement toward the restriction barrier.
3. The patient is told that at no time should pain be experienced and that if it is, all active efforts should cease.
4. The reason for pain being experienced during use of MWM could be because:
   • light pressure along the plane of the facet joint may not have been correctly followed
   • the incorrect segment may have been selected for translation
   • the patient may be attempting movement toward the barrier with excessive force.
5. If a painless movement through a previously restricted barrier is achieved while the translation is held, the same procedure is performed several times more.
6. If correctly applied there should be an instant, and lasting, functional improvement.

Safety

In none of the MWM applications should any pain be experienced, although some residual stiffness/soreness is to be anticipated on the following day, as with most mobilization approaches.

Validation of efficacy = 5 (see Table 7.2)

Some examples of efficacy are summarized below.

• Konstantinou et al (2002) investigated the current use of MWMs for LBP management in the UK, involving 3295 practicing physiotherapists. Most respondents (51.4%) worked in a National Health Service setting. Over half used MWMs on at least a weekly basis, with 61.9% using MWMs primarily for mechanical LBP. Conclusion: MWM is widely and regularly used in the UK by physiotherapists in treatment of low back problems, in combination with other methods, with functional improvement and pain reduction as the main outcomes.
• Research by Paungmali et al (2004) has shown that Mulligan's MWM treatment technique for the elbow produces substantial *and immediate* pain relief in chronic lateral epicondylalgia (48% increase in pain-free grip strength).
• Collins et al (2004) investigated (double-blind randomized controlled trial) whether MWM improves talocrural dorsiflexion, a major impairment following ankle sprain, and relieves pain in subacute populations. Significant improvements in dorsiflexion occurred initially post-MWM ($F(2,26) = 7.82$, $p = 0.002$), but no significant changes in pressure or thermal pain threshold were observed, suggesting that MWM treatment for ankle dorsiflexion has a mechanical rather than hypoalgesic effect in subacute ankle sprains.
• Numerous research and case studies demonstrating efficacy using MWM are published annually in peer-reviewed journals worldwide (Abbott 2001, Hall et al 2000, Hearn & Rivett 2002, Horton 2002, Wilson 1994).

Alternatives

This mobilization approach has echoes of osteopathic positional release technique (PRT – see below) as well as McKenzie methodology (see discussion earlier in the chapter) and also of the blocking techniques used in sacro-occipital technique (SOT).

This is a particularly non-invasive mobilization approach that either works rapidly (usually instantly) or does not, in which case alternatives are available.

Physiological effects

The introduction of movement (joint play) that is outside of voluntary control appears to allow a retracking to occur, restoring normal function (Kaltenborn 1985).

Mulligan (2003) contends that many symptoms (pain, stiffness, weakness) result from joints with subtly malaligned biomechanics, and that these symptoms can be eliminated in many cases by equally subtle repositioning techniques, i.e. they assist in the restoration of biomechanical normality. The key word here is 'assist' – 'force' has no place in Mulligan's vocabulary.

That a normal joint will follow a normal 'track' or 'path' through any particular normal movement is axiomatic (Kapanji 1987). This articular track – incorporating spin, slide, glide, rotation, etc. – is a genetic inheritance and is dependent upon the shape of joint surfaces and articular cartilage, and upon the orientation and attachments of capsule, ligaments, muscles and tendons. To facilitate controlled, free movement while minimizing compressive forces is the overall aim of such a design. Any anomalies in the recruitment or coordination of the sequential elements of the movement pattern will be signaled to the central nervous system (CNS), which may well seek to inhibit that inappropriate movement by pain, stiffness or weakness. Thus the therapist is guided as to what is normal movement by its symptom-free status.

Cautions

- Fractured or dislocated joints
- Acute inflammatory conditions associated with joints
- Pain on use of MWM procedures

Naturopathic perspectives

As with many other procedures discussed in this chapter, MWM is seen to be essentially naturopathic inasmuch as its focus is restoration of normal function via use of minimally invasive procedures.

Further reading

1. Kaltenborn F 1985 Mobilization of the extremity joints. Olaf Norlis Bokhandel, Oslo
2. Mulligan B 1992 Manual therapy: NAGs, SNAGs, MWMs, etc., 2nd edn. Plane View Services, Wellington, New Zealand
3. Mulligan B 2003 Manual therapy: NAGs, SNAGs, MWMs, etc., 5th edn. Plane View Services, Wellington, New Zealand

Neural mobilization of adverse mechanical or neural tension

Indications/description

Maitland (1986), as well as Butler & Gifford (Butler 1991a, Butler & Gifford 1989), have described mechanical restrictions that impinge on neural structures in the vertebral canals and elsewhere as *the mechanical interface* (MI) – the tissues surrounding neural structures.

Among the negative influences on nerves are: 'deformations such as compression, stretching, angulation and torsion' in their passage over highly mobile joints, through bony canals, intervertebral foramina, fascial layers and tonically contracted muscles (e.g. posterior rami of spinal nerves and spinal extensor muscles) (Korr 1981).

Stewart (2000) notes that neural damage can result from all or any of the following: laceration, crush, stretch, rupture, compression and angulation, and that nerves can also be affected negatively by ischemia, hemorrhage, tumors, infection, autoimmune conditions, vasculitis, irradiation and marked temperature change such as intense cold.

Chemical or inflammatory causes of neural tension also occur, resulting in 'interneural fibrosis', leading to reduced elasticity and increased 'tension' that may be revealed during tension testing.

Any structural changes or pathology in the MI can produce abnormalities in, or interference with, free nerve movement within its mechanical interface, resulting in tension on neural structures leading to unpredictable effects.

Common examples of MI pathology are nerve impingement by disc protrusion or osteophyte contact, and carpal tunnel constriction.

Any symptoms resulting from mechanical impingement on neural structures will be more readily provoked in tests that involve movement, rather than passive tension.

When pain is produced by one or another element of a test that puts a nerve under tension it indicates that there exists abnormal mechanical tension (AMT) somewhere in the nervous system, *and not that this is necessarily at the site of reported pain*.

1. A positive tension test (see examples in Chapter 6, Exercises 6.27 and 6.28) is one in which the patient's symptoms are reproduced by the test procedure – for example, during straight leg raising (SLR).
2. Where these symptoms can be altered by 'sensitizing maneuvers' this adds weight to, and confirms, the initial diagnosis of AMT. For example, during the upper limb tension test (ULTT – see Chapter 6), when cervical movement is added as a sensitizing assessment, cervical lateral flexion away from the tested side causes increased arm symptoms in 93% of people, and cervical lateral flexion towards the tested side increases symptoms in 70% of cases.
3. Precise symptom reproduction may not be possible, but the test is still possibly relevant if other abnormal symptoms (pain, weakness, paresthesia, etc.) are produced during the test

and its accompanying sensitizing procedures. Comparison with the test findings on an opposite limb, for example, may indicate an abnormality worth exploring.

4. Altered range of movement during a test is another indicator of abnormality, whether this is noted during the initial test position or during sensitizing additions.

5. To achieve neural mobilization, oscillating, to-and-fro movements are used to increase and reduce tensions, so releasing neural tissues from restricting mechanical interference.

Testing for, and treating, abnormal mechanical tensions in neural structures offers an alternative method for dealing with some forms of pain and dysfunction, since such adverse mechanical tension is often a major cause of musculoskeletal dysfunction (carpal tunnel syndrome is a good example) (Butler & Moseley 2000).

Morris (2006b) notes: 'Restricted neural mobility can occur anywhere along the neuraxis, nervous tissue and supporting structures housed within the axial skeleton, and also continuing into the periphery.'

Maitland et al (2001) suggest that we consider this form of assessment and treatment as involving 'mobilization' of the neural structures, rather than stretching them, and that these methods be reserved for conditions that fail to respond adequately to normal mobilization of soft and osseous structures (muscles, joints).

Methodology

Two examples of testing for AMT (along with explanations) are described in Chapter 6 – see Exercises 6.27 (straight leg raising test) and 6.28 (upper limb tension test).

Additional AMT tests include:

- the slump test – suggested for use in all spinal disorders, most lower limb disorders and some upper limb disorders (especially those which seem to involve the nervous system) (Fig. 7.12)
- passive neck flexion (PNF) test (see Box 7.9) – for all spinal disorders, headache, arm and leg pain
- prone (or side-lying) knee bend (PKB) – for hip, thigh, lumbar and knee symptoms.

Neural tension tests selectively tension, compress and attempt to glide tissue along a selected nerve tract, from the central neural axis out to the distal end of the extremity. By adding and subtracting various differentiating movements it may be possible to infer the relationship that part of the nervous system has with its interfacing structures.

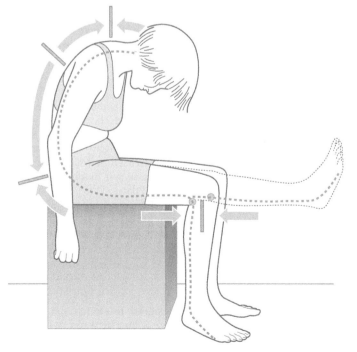

Figure 7.12 The slump test position stretches the entire neural network from pons to feet. Note the direction of stretch of the dura mater and nerve roots. As the leg straightens, the movement of the tibial nerve in relation to the tibia and femur is indicated by arrows. No neural movement occurs behind the knee or at levels C6, T6 or L4 (these are the tension points). Reproduced with permission from Chaitow (2003)

Questions that are being asked of the patient (or indeed, the tissues) when slack is being taken out during the process of placing neural structures, and their mechanical interfaces, under tension include:

1. *What do you feel?*
2. *Where do you feel it?*
3. *How long does the sensation last after the tension is released?*
4. *Are these symptoms that you recognize as being part of your problem?*

There are two broad classes of symptom produced by AMT:

1. When connective tissue elements, either external or internal to the nerve, are responsible for symptoms, these may produce local/general ache, and/or sensations of pressure and pulling.
2. When neural tissues are affected, sensations such as tingling, numbness and sometimes motor and/or autonomic effects may be reported.

Morris (2006b) explains variations possible when introducing the straight leg raising procedure:

*With regard to low back syndromes, the most important mobilization techniques involve variations of the supine SLR manoeuvre. Flexing, internally rotating, and/or adducting the hip, extending the knee, dorsiflexing and/or inverting the foot/ankle all cause a caudalward, or inferior, translation of the neuraxis and peripheral nerves. Superiorly, cervical extension reduces the length of the neural canal, allowing for greater neuraxial glide when combined with this SLR manoeuvre. Combinations of these manoeuvres therefore effectively increase the neural mobilization inferiorly, while the sequence in which joints are moved **isolates** the regional neural tensioning. Therefore, an SLR with internal hip rotation and hip adduction moves the neuraxis inferiorly, with increased isolation of tension at the exiting lumbar nerve roots and hip region. If the knee is then flexed this reduces nerve root and hip region tension, while ankle dorsiflexion and internal rotation will increase neural tension to the lower leg, allowing the clinician to isolate various target branches, as desired.*

If a superior neuraxial glide is desired combinations such as plantar flexion, reduced SLR and introduction of cervical flexion will accomplish this. Once the target neural tissues have been isolated and tensioned a repetitive, oscillating sequence of caudalward or cephalward movements creates the desired neural mobilization.

The therapeutic aspect of this approach requires that once mechanical interference has been established, the physiological barriers should be carefully engaged for a few seconds at a time. If no irritability is noted these engagements of barriers are repeated. The objective is to gradually increase free movement of neural structures within their mechanical interfaces, without creating additional irritation.

In order to create a more responsive environment for neural mobilization, muscles through which affected nerves are passing can be treated using MFR, MET, massage, etc., and associated joints mobilized.

Safety

Neural structures are vulnerable to irritation and damage requiring that these procedures are performed slowly, cautiously and responsively to reported symptoms.

If appropriate care is taken, the risk of causing neural irritation is small.

Validation of efficacy = 5 (see Table 7.2)

Butler & Gifford (1989) report on research indicating that 70% of 115 patients with either carpal tunnel syndrome or lesions of the ulnar nerve at the elbow showed clear electrophysiological and clinical evidence of neural lesions in the neck. This is, they maintain, because of a 'double crush' phenomenon, in which a primary and often long-standing disorder, perhaps in the spine, results in secondary or 'remote' dysfunction at the periphery.

This is probably a function of the nerve's physiology being altered as well as its biomechanics (Upton & McComas 1973).

Alternatives

There are no obvious alternatives that can be seen to specifically replace these methods; however, physical medicine approaches that help to restore normal function to joints and soft tissues might be expected to achieve some degree of increased neural mobility, as would well-designed exercise self-mobilization programs such as are found in Pilates, Thai yoga massage and yoga (as examples). Enhanced functionality that leads to reduced stress effects on somatic structures should also emerge from postural and breathing rehabilitation.

Physiological effects (Butler & Moseley 2000)

Neural stretching is designed to stretch and release adhesions within a nerve, either between fascicles or within a fascicle(s).

When a nerve is stretched, the wavy course of fascicles straightens. Connective tissue between and within the fascicles is tensioned and the axons themselves may be stretched. The mechanical forces exerted on the fascicles, and the increased pressure within the nerve, may alter conduction and gives rise to neurological symptoms. If the nerve is already compromised locally (and/or in other locations) it will respond in an irritable way to the manipulation. Therefore, before any stretch is performed as a treatment, the patient's level of sensitivity/irritability should be measured at an initial motion barrier to stretch for a few seconds.

Cautions (Butler 1991b)

- Recent onset of acute, or worsening of, neurological signs
- Cauda equina lesions
- Spinal cord injuries
- Disc pathology
- Any neural inflammatory condition
- Acute inflammatory infection
- Pain or other neural symptoms that persist after the first assessment of the effects of producing neural tension during tests
- Malignancy involving the nervous system
- Degenerative or progressive neural pathology (e.g. multiple sclerosis)

Naturopathic perspectives

In essence these approaches confront existing changes (fibrosis, scar tissue, etc.) that are unlikely to resolve in any other way. Therefore, if symptoms are the result, entirely or partially, of mechanical interference with neural structures, and if mobilization of these restrictions between the neural structure and its interface can be achieved by these methods, we have an example of the removal of an obstacle to self-regulation, and this is in line with naturopathic principles.

Further reading

1. Butler D 1991 Mobilisation of the nervous system. Churchill Livingstone, Edinburgh
2. Butler D 2000 The sensitive nervous system. Noigroup Publications, Adelaide

Neuromuscular techniques (NMT)

Indications/description

Neuromuscular technique, as the term is used in this text, refers to the manual application of specialized (usually) digital pressure and strokes, most commonly

---

Box 7.9 Exercise: Passive neck flexion (PNF) test (Butler 1991c)

This test allows movement of neuromeningeal tissues in relation to the spinal canal, which is its mechanical interface (MI).

In an industrial survey, 22% of patients with back and sciatic pain were shown to have a positive PNF test. This level rose to 35% of those referred for hospital attention (Troup 1981).

1. Patient lies supine, arms at the side and legs together.
2. The head and neck are supported as the head is lifted and the chin is taken toward the chest to its end of range.
3. In a normal neck the chin should approximate the sternum without force or symptoms.
4. If symptoms appear during this test, sensitizing movements or positions should be added to evaluate their effect on the symptoms (do the symptoms increase or decrease?).
5. Sensitizing elements might include (while the head is held in full neck flexion):
   - straight leg raising (one and then the other)
   - cervical side-flexion and/or rotation
   - knee flexion (prone knee bend) with patient in side-lying, neck fully flexed, or in full side-lying slump position.

Butler & Gifford (1989) report that if passive neck flexion reproduces back pain symptoms this implicates the nervous system (e.g. arachnoiditis or scarred dura) or a pathological feature involving structures through which the nerves pass, or to which they are attached.

---

applied by finger or thumb contact. These digital contacts can have either a diagnostic (assessment) or therapeutic objective and the degree of pressure employed varies considerably between these two modes of application.

Neuromuscular therapy in general, and neuromuscular technique in particular (both abbreviated as NMT), have among their key aims the removal of local and reflexogenic sources of pain and dysfunction. Modern pain research has demonstrated that a feature of the etiology of much chronic pain is the presence of areas of soft tissue dysfunction that promote pain and distress in distant structures (Lewit 1999, Melzack & Wall 1988, Mense et al 2000, Simons et al 1999). These are the loci known as myofascial trigger points.

Therapeutically, NMT aims to produce modifications in dysfunctional tissue, encouraging a restoration of functional normality, with a particular focus of deactivating focal points of reflexogenic activity, such as myofascial trigger points (Chaitow 2001, Chaitow & DeLany 2000).

An alternative focus of NMT application is toward normalizing imbalances in hypertonic and/or fibrotic tissues, either as an end in itself or as a precursor to joint mobilization or manipulation.

As discussed in Chapter 8, a general NMT assessment or treatment protocol exists in which a sequential assessment is made of all tissues, from the subocciput to the mid-thigh, in order to locate areas of dysfunction and, where appropriate, to treat these. This general NMT approach can be equated with other constitutional/whole-body approaches described in Chapter 8 (Chaitow 2001).

Neuromuscular therapy techniques emerged in both Europe and North America almost simultaneously over the last 50 years. The European version of NMT (where 'T' stands for technique, unlike the US version where it stands for therapy) was first developed by Stanley Lief ND DO DC and Boris Chaitow ND DC between the mid-1930s and early 1940. Trained in the USA in both chiropractic and naturopathy, these cousins developed integrated concepts partially based on the work of an Ayurvedic physician Varma (1937) as well as from physical culture approaches advocated by Macfadden (1916).

The use of NMT as a widely applicable sequential assessment and treatment tool was enhanced by the work of Raymond Nimmo DC (Nimmo 1957, Schneider et al 2001), whose work between the 1940s and 1980s overlapped and was influenced by the research into myofascial pain of Janet Travell MD and David Simons MD. Nimmo and his 'receptor-tonus' work seems to be a common link between European and American NMT.

European and American versions of NMT have subtle differences in their hands-on applications while retaining similar foundations in their theoretical platform. North American-style neuromuscular therapy uses a medium-paced thumb or finger glide to uncover contracted bands or muscular nodules, whereas European-style neuromuscular techniques use a slow-paced, thumb drag method of discovery (Youngs 1963). They also have slightly different emphasis on the method of application of ischemic compression in treating trigger points. Both versions emphasize a home care program and the patient's participation in the recovery process.

See Box 7.11, in which veteran naturopath/osteopath Brian Youngs offers recollections of the early use of NMT as part of a general naturopathic approach in the 1950s.

Methodology

Boris Chaitow ND DC (personal communication, 1983) has described the manual contact used in NMT:

To apply NMT successfully it is necessary to develop the art of palpation and sensitivity of fingers by constantly feeling the appropriate areas and assessing any abnormality in tissue structure for tensions, contractions, adhesions, spasms. It is important to acquire with practice an appreciation of the 'feel' of normal tissue so that one is better able to recognize abnormal tissue. Once some level of diagnostic sensitivity with fingers has been achieved, subsequent application of the technique will be much easier to develop. The whole secret is to be able to recognize the 'abnormalities' in the feel of tissue structures. Having become accustomed to understanding the texture and character of 'normal' tissue, the pressure applied by the thumb in general, especially in the spinal structures, should always be firm but never hurtful or bruising. To this end the pressure should be applied with a 'variable' pressure, i.e. with an appreciation of the texture and character of the tissue structures and according to the feel that sensitive fingers should have developed. The level of the pressure applied should not be consistent because the character and texture of tissue is always variable. The pressure should therefore be so applied that the thumb is moved along its path of direction in a way that corresponds to the feel of the tissues. This variable factor in finger pressure constitutes probably the most important quality a practitioner of NMT can learn, enabling him to maintain more effective control of pressure, develop a greater sense of diagnostic feel, and be far less likely to bruise the tissue.

Lief's basic spinal treatment followed a set pattern. The fact that the same order of tissue assessment is suggested at each session does not mean that the treatment is the same each time. The pattern suggests a framework and useful starting and ending points but the degree of therapeutic response offered to the various areas of dysfunction encountered varies, depending on individual features.

Safety

The same degree of safety applies to NMT as to massage. There have been no recorded cases of patient harm resulting from use of NMT therapeutically. The cautions and contraindications listed below should be followed.

Validation of efficacy = 3 (see Table 7.2)

There has been limited research into the use of NMT, although it forms an element of some clinical studies into treatment of myofascial and post-traumatic pain (commonly combined with MET and MFR methods), particularly in Europe (Fernández-de-las-Peñas et al 2005).

NMT in Europe has been in use since the mid-1930s and is taught at institutions such as the University of Westminster (as part of an undergraduate (BS) program on Therapeutic Bodywork), as well as at the British College of Osteopathic Medicine (BCOM) – formerly known as the British College of Naturopathy and Osteopathy, founded by the developer of European NMT, Stanley Lief ND DO DC in the 1930s.

In the age of 'evidence-based medicine' this length of time in use of NMT (or any other modality) is not in itself proof of usefulness or efficacy, since comprehensive research has not been conducted comparing NMT with other modalities, or evaluating clinical outcomes.

A number of small undergraduate studies have been undertaken as part of degree courses, and they offer a glimpse of what might be possible when more rigorous research is ever carried out. For example:

1. Patel (2002), as part of her undergraduate training at BCOM, compared the effects of neuromuscular technique and a muscle energy technique, on cervical range of motion. Forty asymptomatic female subjects aged between 20 and 25 years were randomly selected. The subjects were randomly placed into one of two possible groups.
   - Group 1 received neuromuscular technique on week one, followed by a 'rest' period on week two, followed by neuromuscular technique on week three.
   - Group 2 received muscle energy technique on week one, followed by a 'rest' period on week two, followed by neuromuscular technique on week three.
   - All treatments were a single application given to both scalene muscle groups (bilaterally) for 3 minutes.
   - Before and after treatment, measurements were taken of the cervical spine ranges of motion, with the cervical range of motion goniometer T-test analysis demonstrating that both neuromuscular technique and muscle energy technique significantly increased cervical range of motion in all planes of movement ($p < 0.05$).

   - MET was shown to be more effective in increasing range of motion than NMT.

2. Palmer (2002) noted that MET and NMT are used frequently in osteopathic practice to resolve muscle and joint dysfunction, but that there remains little scientific evidence to establish the efficiency of these techniques on muscle strength effect. She conducted a study to compare the effectiveness of MET and NMT on quadriceps muscle strength.
   - The study population comprised 30 (20 females and 10 males) asymptomatic subjects from the BCOM.
   - All subjects were free of injury and pathology to the knee, hip and lumbar spine.
   - The participants were randomly allocated to two groups of 15 subjects.
   - Group 1 was treated with MET while Group 2 was treated with NMT during the same week.
   - In the second week, Group 1 was treated with NMT while Group 2 was treated with MET.
   - Quadriceps strength of the dominant leg was determined, before and after the procedure, by means of a digital myograph (Myo-tech, model DM 2000).
   - T-test analysis of the results demonstrated that MET and NMT applied separately produced a statistically significant change on muscle strength ($p < 0.05$).

3. Tomlinson (2002) undertook a study to investigate whether or not two separate techniques (NMT and MET) used in clinical treatment at BCOM are effective in increasing ankle function in restricted dorsiflexion patients. The study included 21 subjects (12 females and 9 males) who were treated on three separate visits over 5 weeks.
   - After ascertaining the degree of ankle restriction in dorsiflexion, measuring passive ankle dorsiflexion range of motion using a universal goniometer, this feature was measured again both before and after treatment to the affected ankle.
   - The unaffected ankle was used as a control.
   - MET and NMT were applied to the plantar flexors, at two separate treatments, on two separate occasions, with a week of no treatment dividing the two.

- The final treatment included both techniques.
- T-test analysis demonstrated a significant increase in passive ankle dorsiflexion range of motion ($p < 0.05$) for both MET and NMT used alone, as well as for NMT and MET combined.
- There was no significant difference between the effectiveness of the two techniques used alone.
- One-way ANOVA analysis demonstrated a significant increase in passive ankle dorsiflexion range of motion ($p < 0.05$) using NMT and MET in combination compared to MET used in isolation.
- It was concluded that MET and NMT are effective methods for increasing passive ankle dorsiflexion range of motion when applied to the triceps surae muscle group, and that when both modalities are used together a greater ankle joint flexibility in dorsiflexion is attainable.

4. Rice (2002) investigated the effect of NMT to the diaphragm on cervical range of motion. In this study 24 students at the BCOM were selected, 13 females and 11 males.

- A within-subject or repeated measures design was used where each subject was exposed first to the control procedure and then received the intervention.
- Cervical range of motion was measured.
- Statistical analysis showed an increased range of motion following the application of NMT to the diaphragm ($p = 0.05$).
- There was no statistically significant difference in response to treatment between the male and female population ($p = 0.06$).
- There was no correlation between response to treatment and age of subjects ($p = 0.12$).
- This study provides quantitative evidence that NMT to the diaphragm can increase cervical range of motion, highlighting the importance of treating all factors involved in maintaining cervical spine dysfunction, both local and distant.

While the sort of evidence summarized above shows that NMT 'works', it says little about people with problems (apart from those with limited range ankle dorsiflexion described in study 3). In studies 1 and 2 the focus was to compare NMT and MET effectiveness in increasing range of motion in people who had no symptoms, whereas in study 4 an interesting remote effect was noted when NMT was applied to the diaphragm.

Until more rigorous research evaluates NMT in the real world of pain and dysfunction, we are left with its long history, many anecdotal case histories – and encouraging undergraduate studies such as these.

Alternatives

A variety of soft tissue manipulation modalities overlap, or are actually incorporated into neuromuscular therapy (the American version of NMT) which includes in its methodology all modalities and techniques that have the potential to beneficially induce change in the neuromuscular components of the body, such as massage, MFR, MET, PRT, etc.

European NMT has no obvious alternatives apart from the huge selection of individual manual palpation and treatment methods used in physical therapy and massage.

Physiological effects

Possibly the most distinctive element of NMT is its use of focused applied compression. In this it has similarities with what Simons terms 'trigger point release', and which used to be termed ischemic compression in osteopathic medicine.

The range of physiological effects resulting from sustained or intermittent compression (as used in neuromuscular therapy) includes:

- ischemia, which is reversed when pressure is released (Simons et al 1999)
- 'neurological inhibition', which results from sustained efferent barrage (Dowling 2000)
- a degree of mechanical stretching, which occurs when 'creep' of connective tissue commences (Cantu & Grodin 1992)
- piezoelectric effects, which modify the 'gel' state of tissues to a more solute ('sol') state (as in myofascial release, see above) (Barnes 1997)
- rapid mechanoreceptor impulses, which interfere with slower pain messages (gate theory) (Melzack & Wall 1994)
- pain-relieving endorphin, enkephalin and endocannabinoid release (Baldry 1993, Kiser et al 1983, McPartland et al 2005)
- Spontaneous release of taut bands associated with trigger points (Simons et al 1999)
- Traditional Chinese Medicine, which suggests modification of energy flow through tissues following pressure application (Zhao-Pu 1991)
- circulatory – blood and lymph – enhancement (fluid movement) (Lederman 1997a, Tamir et al 1999).

Cautions

- Deeply applied compression is contraindicated in tissues that have been recently traumatized or that are inflamed
- Acute arthritis and other inflammatory conditions (contraindicated during acute stages)
- Aneurysm
- Bone fractures or acute soft tissue injuries: wait for full healing (6–12 weeks)
- Hemophilia
- Hodgkin's disease
- Leukemia
- Malignancy with metastasis (or TB) involving bone
- Osteoporosis
- Pain production during procedure
- Patients on cortisone (wait 2–3 months)
- Patients with high fever
- Phlebitis
- Recent scar tissue
- Syphilitic articular or peri-articular lesions
- Uncontrolled diabetic neuropathy

Naturopathic perspectives

As explained above, NMT is the only soft tissue modality that is known to have evolved in a naturopathic setting in Europe. Designed initially as an assessment tool, its ability to revert to a therapeutic mode during assessment, particularly in relation to localized dysfunction, has made it, for many practitioners, a modality of choice in dealing with myofascial pain problems. An additional role is seen to relate to use of NMT prior to joint manipulation, preparing the tissues for this procedure. In its earlier incarnation, as part of Ayurvedic massage methodology (Varma 1937), NMT was used to 'normalize energy [prana] channels'.

Further reading

1. Chaitow L 2001 Modern neuromuscular techniques. Churchill Livingstone, Edinburgh
2. Chaitow L, Delany J 2008 Clinical applications of neuromuscular techniques, vol 1. Churchill Livingstone, Edinburgh

Nasal specific (craniofacial) technique

Indications/description

Chronic sinusitis and sinus headache, chronic head and/or facial pain, sleep apnea, allergic rhinitis relief, tinnitus.

Box 7.10 NMT exercise

See Figures 6.2, 6.3, 6.4 and 6.5A,B in Chapter 6.

- Begin to practice NMT by concentrating on your body position.
- Ensure that the treatment surface is of a height that will allow you to stand without hunching or stretching unduly. This should allow a straight arm position (when the thumb contact is being used), as well as the ability to transfer weight in order to increase pressure without arm muscle strength being used.
- After applying a light lubricant, position yourself and place your treating hand as shown in Figure 6.2 with your fingers acting as a fulcrum, thumb (medial tip) feeling through the tissues, slowly and with variable pressure.
- Practice this, in no particular sequence of strokes, until the mechanics of the body-arm-hand-thumb positions are comfortable and require no thought.
- Pay attention to varying the pressure, to meeting and matching tissues and to using bodyweight transferred through a straight arm to increase penetration when needed.
- Also practice the use of the finger stroke, especially on curved areas, by drawing the slightly hooked and supported (by one of its neighboring digits) finger toward yourself in a slow, deliberate, searching manner (see Fig. 6.3).
- Now apply these searching (and/or treating) strokes in a sequence such as that illustrated in Figure 6.5A,B. This uncomplicated series of strokes allows access to the soft tissues at the base and side of the cervical spine. Note that the direction of strokes need not follow arrow directions. The objective is to obtain information without causing discomfort to the patient and without stressing your palpating hands.

NMT in its treatment mode involves greater pressure in order to modify dysfunctional tissues but in these sequences you are designed for information gathering, not treating. In time, with practice, treatment and assessment meld seamlessly together, with one feeding the other.

Evaluate the ease of information gathering possible once you have mastered the concept of meeting, and not overriding, tissue tension with the palpating finger or thumb.

Methodology

A single case study (Folweiler & Lynch 1995) described treatment of chronic sinusitis and sinus headaches with spinal manipulation, massage and a technique called 'bilateral nasal specific' (BNS). The BNS procedure involves inflating small balloons (finger-cots

Box 7.11 Lief's neuromuscular technique: a recollection

Brian K. Youngs BSc(Lond) ND DO

Editor's note: Brian Youngs was (and remains in his ninth decade) a leading naturopathic/osteopathic practitioner in the UK. He was a colleague of both Stanley and Peter Lief (son of NMT's developer) and was for many years, from the 1950s, a leading tutor at the British College of Naturopathy and Osteopathy – now the British College of Osteopathic Medicine, founded by Lief. This short recollection of NMT, as it was practiced in its early years, is in response to a request by the editor.

This soft tissue technique, perhaps inappropriately named as neuromuscular technique (NMT), consisted of fairly heavily pressured movements, applied with the balls of the thumbs, and sometimes fingertips, over various soft tissue sites, followed by general (non-specific) manipulative procedures to the neck, thoracic spine and lumbar/pelvic areas. The soft tissue sites were mainly muscular attachments, viz. occipital insertions, spinal and pelvic origins and insertions. Where the belly of a muscle was treated, movements would be mainly transverse to the fibers.

Applied pressure was deeper than with regular massage, and although the treatment could be uncomfortable, it was common for patients to report that it was 'a hurt that's nice'! The manipulative procedures usually comprised a non-specific cervical rotation maneuver (supine); a thoracic extension procedure (seated with the practitioner standing behind), as well as bilateral lumbar rotation manipulations, to mobilize pelvic and spinal joints non-specifically. Anecdotal responses from patients, following a typical 15- to 20-minute NMT session, were usually that they 'felt looser' which, with repeated applications over time, was frequently maintained.

Specific structural problems would receive local attention, involving as part of the process the same NMT soft tissue procedures described above.

Usually accompanying this physical approach would be recommendations for dietary changes, exercise, breathing re-education, relaxation and short fasting episodes, as appropriate to the individual's needs. In this way long-term benefit, deriving from the physical procedures, would be supported and modified by responses resulting from the accompanying nutritional and lifestyle changes. This approach represented a package of non-specific interventions, designed to impact on total health – a veritable personalized holistic recipe!

The physiological effects of the NMT procedures were, in many ways, akin to those resulting from exercise, setting in train improved physiological function. There was an increase of general mobility; head on neck, on shoulders; increased flexion/extension of spinal movements; increased lung capacity – all of which would continue to improve if accompanying exercise advice was adhered to.

It was considered that resulting enhanced circulatory efficiency would not only benefit the cardiovascular system, but could also improve metabolic function via optimized hepatic circulation, especially if the liver region received NMT attention over its overlying protective rib cage. Here again the physical treatment would be enhanced by naturopathic dietary and other advice.

But what were the physiological changes at the tissue or cellular level?

Suggestions made then were purely speculative, based on the knowledge available in that era (1930s to 1950s) but included interpretations that subsequent research has largely validated – for example:

- Increased physical movement and muscular comfort might be associated with fluctuations in collagen deposition and removal, caused by fibroclastic/fibroblastic activity, responding to increased/decreased oxygen tension locally (Langevin et al 2005).

- Selye's general adaptation syndrome had just been promulgated and it was suggested that NMT treatment might act as a stressor, activating a hypothalamic/pituitary/adrenal response, leading to an immune response with corticoid hormones gathering at the site of 'injury', followed by appropriate tissue 'improvement'. See Chapter 2 for details of Selye's work, and the influence this has had on naturopathic thinking (Dhabhar & Viswanathan 2005, Selye 1971).

- Also in evidence in the thinking at that time was the concept of viscerosomatic reflexes, as well as somaticovisceral reflexes. Both these infer a neural reflex interaction between somatic structures and visceral components, operating out of the same spinal segmental level. Thus, for example, digestive problems could be helped by treating those spinal (osseous and soft tissue) areas that shared the same neural origin, i.e. both somatic and autonomic (Beal 1985).*

So, Lief's neuromuscular technique made its contribution – general and simplistic in its practice – as part of a wider naturopathic concept of health enhancement. It had, and has, its devotees on both sides of the treatment divide, practitioner and patient. It had its very considerable successes; its failures, in my experience, were few.

---

*See Box 2.2 in Chapter 2 on the topic of segmental facilitation, where the validity of these concepts is discussed (Kelso 1971, Korr 1976a). See also the discussion in Chapter 10 of the biology of physical (manual) medicine, where the evidence is explored more fully, with specific examples that validate the views of the early developers of NMT (Dhabhar & Viswanathan 2005, Khalsa et al 2006)

Box 7.12 Integrated neuromuscular inhibition technique (INIT) applied to trigger point deactivation

INIT involves using a combination of ischemic compression (NMT), positional release methods (PRT) and muscle energy technique (MET) in a logical sequence designed to produce trigger point deactivation.

It employs a position of ease as part of a sequence which commences with the location of a tender/trigger point, followed by application of ischemic compression (optional – avoided if pain is too intense or the patient too sensitive), followed by the introduction of positional release. After an appropriate length of time, during which the tissues are held in 'ease', the patient is guided to introduce an isometric contraction into the tissues housing the trigger point, after which these tissues are stretched locally. A whole muscle stretch is then introduced following an isometric contraction.

A subsequent facilitating sequence can then be taught, involving rhythmic contractions of the antagonist to the muscle housing the trigger point, resulting in an inhibitory effect on excessive tone in the affected muscle(s). This sequence is described below in detail.

INIT method

In an attempt to develop a treatment protocol for the deactivation of myofascial trigger points, a sequence has been developed (Chaitow 1994).

1. A trigger point is identified by palpation methods (see Chapter 6).
2. Ischemic compression is applied in either a sustained or intermittent manner (see NMT notes above).
3. When referred or local pain begins to diminish, the tissues housing the trigger point are taken to a position of ease and held for approximately 20–30 seconds to allow neurological resetting, reduction in nociceptor activity and enhanced local circulatory interchange (see PRT notes below).
4. An isometric contraction focuses into the musculature around the trigger point followed by the tissues being stretched both locally and (where possible) in a way that involves the whole muscle (see MET notes above).
5. The patient assists in the stretching movements (whenever possible) by activating the antagonists and facilitating the stretch.

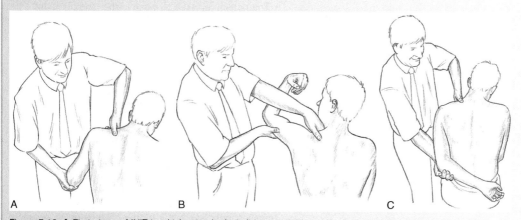

A   B   C

Figure 7.13 **A** First stage of INIT in which a tender/pain/trigger point in supraspinatus is located and ischemically compressed, either intermittently or persistently. **B** The pain is removed from the tender/pain/trigger point by finding a position of ease which is held for several seconds, following which an isometric contraction is achieved involving the tissues that house the tender/pain/trigger point. **C** Following this, the muscle housing the point of local soft tissue dysfunction is stretched. The whole muscle is then isometrically contracted and stretched. This completes the INIT sequence. Reproduced with permission from Chaitow & Fritz (2006)

attached to the bulb of a sphygmomanometer) within the nasal passages, creating a change of pressure and, theoretically, a realignment of nasal bones. Initial treatment of a 41-year-old woman with manipulation and massage for approximately 1 year had resulted in only temporary, mild relief. Her headaches resolved immediately following each treatment that included BNS, followed by increased amounts of postnasal dis-

charge and an improved sense of smell. At the end of two additional months of care, her headaches were reduced significantly in intensity and frequency.

Safety

The attachment of the finger-cot (mini-balloon) to the sphygmomanometer bulb has to be secure and inca-

Box 7.13 Spray and stretch techniques for trigger point deactivation

Chilling and stretching a muscle housing a trigger point rapidly assists in deactivation of the abnormal neurological behavior of the site. Both Travell and Mennel have described these effects in detail (Mennel 1975, Simons, Travell & Simons 1999). Simons et al (1999) have discouraged the use of vapocoolants because of environmental considerations relating to ozone depletion (newer versions are said to be 'ozone friendly'), and have instead urged the use of stroking with ice in a similar manner to the spray stream. The objective is to chill the surface tissues while the underlying muscle housing the trigger is simultaneously stretched.

- A container of vapocoolant spray with a calibrated nozzle which delivers a moderately fine jet stream, or a source of ice, is needed.
- The jet stream should have sufficient force to carry in the air for at least 3 feet. A mist-like spray is less desirable.
- Ice can consist of a cylinder of ice formed by freezing water in a paper cup and then peeling this off the ice. A wooden handle will have been frozen into the ice to allow for its ease of application, as it is rolled from the trigger towards the referred area in a series of sweeps.
- Whichever method is chosen, the patient should be comfortably supported to promote muscular relaxation.
- If a spray is used, the container is held about 2 feet away, in such a manner that the jet stream meets the body surface at an acute angle or at a tangent, not perpendicularly. This lessens the shock of the impact.
- For the same reason, the stream is sometimes started in air or on the practitioner's hand and is gradually brought into contact with the skin overlying the trigger point.
- The stream/ice massage/ice is applied in one direction, not back and forth. Each sweep is started at the trigger point and is moved slowly and evenly outward over the reference zone.
- It is advantageous to spray or ice-chill both trigger and reference areas, because secondary trigger points are likely to have developed within reference zones when pain is very strong. (The direction of movement is also in line with the muscle fibers towards their insertion.)

- The optimum speed of movement of the sweep/roll over the skin seems to be about 4 inches (10 cm) per second.
- Each sweep is started slightly proximal to the trigger point and is moved slowly and evenly through the reference zone to cover it and extend slightly beyond it.
- These sweeps are repeated in a rhythm of a few seconds on and a few seconds off, until all the skin over the trigger and reference areas has been covered once or twice.
- If aching or 'cold pain' develops, or if the application of the spray/ice/canister sets off a reference of pain, the interval between applications is lengthened. Care is taken not to frost or blanch the skin.
- During the application of cold or directly after it, the taut fibers should be stretched passively.
- The fibers should not be stretched in advance of the cold.
- Steady, gentle stretching is usually essential if a satisfactory result is to be achieved.
- As relaxation of the muscle occurs, continued stretch should be maintained for 20–30 seconds, and active motion is tested after each series of cold applications.
- The patient is asked to move in the directions that were restricted before spraying, or that were painful to activate.
- An attempt should be made to restore the full range of motion, but always within the limits of pain, as sudden overstretching can increase existing muscle spasm.
- The treatment is continued in this manner until the trigger points (often several are present, or a 'nest' of them) and their respective pain reference zones have been treated.

The entire procedure may occupy 15–20 minutes and should not be rushed. The importance of re-establishing normal motion in conjunction with the use of the chilling is well founded. It may be that the brief interruption of pain impulses is insufficient and that input of normal impulses must also occur for the obliteration of trigger points to be successfully achieved. Simple exercises that utilize the principle of passive or active stretch should be outlined to the patient, to be carried out several times daily, after the application of gentle heat (hot packs, etc.) at home. Usual precautions should be mentioned, such as avoiding the use of heat if symptoms worsen or if there is evidence of inflammation.

pable of spontaneous release, otherwise the inflated cot could conceivably be released, under great pressure, and become lodged in the sinuses or, more alarmingly, in the throat.

Validation of efficacy = 3 (see Table 7.2)

There is strong support for its use by those involved in regular clinical usage; however, there are only anecdotal accounts and a few single case studies to support application of this technique (Myers 2001).

Alternatives

Manual cranial and facial manipulation (Chaitow 2005, Von Piekartz & Bryden 2001).

Physiological effects

One explanation for the benefits noted may be the enhanced elimination of mucus from the nasal passages as a result of force from the inflated finger-cot, thus reducing pressure and pain and allowing increased sinus and nasal drainage.

Cautions

Patients need to be thoroughly evaluated before the treatment is undertaken, and forewarned that the process is uncomfortable, and that discomfort is probable afterwards.

According to Folweiler & Lynch (1995), it is common for the patient to hear 'cracking' or 'popping' sounds within the skull during application of the technique. Tenderness following treatment, along the median palatine suture and other facial sutures, is common, persisting for several days. Short-term epistaxis may occur.

Naturopathic perspectives

Doug Lewis ND (personal communication, 2001) has likened the effect of the inflating finger-cot to a high velocity thrust manipulation. If that modality is accepted as being a reasonable use of force to achieve a particular physiological benefit, then nasal specific technique might be regarded in the same light. It is certainly probable – for example, if relief is obtainable from chronic sinus problems via nasal specific use – that this same result might be obtainable over time with gentler drainage methods, along with the standard nutritional, hydrotherapeutic and botanical strategies that are likely to be employed in naturopathic care of patients with such problems.

Occupational and ergonomic therapies

Indications/description

In 1700 Ramazzini (1633–1714) wrote the first important book on occupational diseases and industrial hygiene *De Morbis Artificum Diatriba* (Diseases of Workers). In discussing the etiology, treatment and prevention of many diseases, Ramazzini often goes back to Hippocrates, Celsus and Galen, and, after summarizing their observations, relates his own experience.

When you come to a patient's house, you should ask him what sort of pains he has, what caused them, how many days he has been ill, whether the bowels are working and what sort of food he eats. So says Hippocrates in his work Affections. I may venture to add one more question: what occupation does he follow?

He even had a word for those using word processors:

The maladies that affect the clerks arise from three causes: first, constant sitting; secondly, incessant movement of the hand and always in the same direction; and thirdly, the strain on the mind . . . The incessant driving of the pen over paper causes intense fatigue of the hand and the whole arm because of the continuous . . . strain on the muscles and tendons.

More recently Wilson (2002, p. xi) observes:

Clinical Ergonomics is the art of managing the demands of the environment to enable people to comfortably meet these demands, and to enhance their capacity to meet the challenges of their environments, including the prevention, treatment and rehabilitation of musculoskeletal disorders.

In essence, the model of care offered in occupational and ergonomic therapeutics is in precise alignment with naturopathic thinking. It can also be shown to not deviate from the model described by Selye, since its objectives, as outlined by naturopath/osteopath Andrew Wilson, are to:

- reduce pain and dysfunction
- identify barriers to recovery (ergonomic, psychosocial and personal)
- assess people's ability to function in their environment
- improve people's ability to meet the demands of their environment
- reduce the demands of the environment to suit the individual and the population at risk
- minimize the risk of developing symptoms.

There is no attempt under this heading to provide the range of information covered in other modality topics, as the range of methods, techniques, systems and modalities employed in assessment and treatment within occupational and ergonomic therapy are as wide as the range of human activities.

Refer to Chapter 9 for a greater understanding of prevention and rehabilitation issues.

Further reading

1. Wilson A 2002 Effective management of musculoskeletal injury: a clinical ergonomics approach to prevention, treatment and rehabilitation. Churchill Livingstone, Edinburgh
2. Pope M, Andersson G 1991 Occupational low back pain. Mosby-Yearbook, St Louis

Oscillatory/vibrational rhythmic methods

Indications/description

Soft tissue and joint restrictions appear amenable to beneficial change in response to rhythmic oscillatory motion (Ramsey 1997), especially if this is persistent. A number of variations exist, variously dubbed 'harmonic techniquet' (Lederman 2000), Trager work (Blackburn 2004, Trager 1987) and facilitated oscillatory release (Comeaux 2002a).

Methodology

Morris (2006b) has noted three models of oscillatory methodology.

1. Proactive oscillatory methods are where the patient performs the movements while the practitioner/therapist offers resistance – either partially (isotonic) or totally (isometric). Variables include the arc of motion, as well as the speed, ranging from several oscillations per second to one oscillation every 3–4 seconds.
2. Reactive oscillatory methods involve the practitioner/therapist performing the movement, with the patient offering resistance. Very clear instructions need to be offered to the patient to ensure that the degree of force and the rhythm are what is called for.
3. Passive oscillatory methods involve the practitioner/therapist creating all the movements with the patient totally passive. The amplitude and rate of movements are therefore entirely under the control of the practitioner. It is this format that is described in the examples offered below.

Blackburn (2004) has described a Trager-style approach:

Movement is one of the key signatures of the Trager® *Approach. The client experiences rhythmical rocking motions much of the time during the tablework.*

Putting the client's body in motion has many advantages. Trager hypothesized that, when muscles that normally produce a movement are receiving movement, something unusual is happening in the neural feedback to the brain. The signals to the brain would be primarily receptive and would not include the usual impulses of muscle engagement and proprioception for that particular movement (Juhan 1989). The passivity of the body can allow the client to feel movements that would normally be blocked by muscle tension. In this way new movement possibilities may be instilled. There are also occasions when the client's body is still ... while being compressed, stretched or just supported. This stillness also includes intervals when the practitioner removes his/her hands and pauses. These pauses in movement and hand contact allow the client to assimilate the new movement possibilities.

Validation of efficacy = 4 (see Table 7.2)

Lederman & Brown (1996) and others (Takai et al 1991) have described the neurophysiology of harmonic technique, while clinicians such as Duval et al (2002) have described measurable changes with the Trager technique on muscle rigidity (e.g. in relation to the level of evoked stretch responses in patients with Parkinson's disease and rigidity). This and the widespread use of such methods for the best part of a century with no reported negative effects should provide adequate validation for the continued use of such methods, until further research offers definitive evidence.

Alternatives

Within this group of methods there are active and passive, as well as imposed and 'tuned into' models of oscillation/vibration, providing a range of alternatives to an approach that is itself an alternative to other mobilizing techniques.

Physiological effects

Comeaux (2004) has described the possible effects of facilitated oscillatory release (FOR) methods as follows:

A functionally appropriate rhythmic force may milk edema fluid from the area, may directly stretch tissue, may gently rearrange joint surfaces, or more to the point may induce, through entrainment, a functionally appropriate level of oscillatory neural coordination. In an articular or myofascial context, it may be an occasion to add energy to the system lost through trauma to reverse the deformation of fibrin through hysteresis.

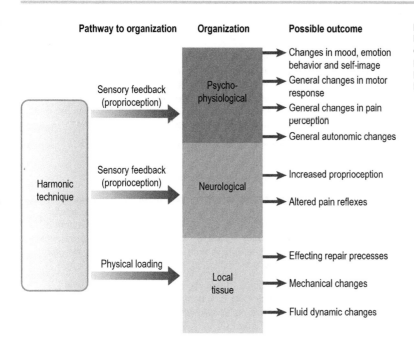

Figure 7.14 The physiological model of harmonic technique: the three organizational levels affected, possible pathways to these organizations and potential outcome. Reproduced with permission from Lederman (2000)

Lederman (2000) suggests that harmonic methods influence local tissue organization following trauma (influencing mechanical in addition to fluid dynamic properties), as well as neurological (providing proprioceptive stimulation in addition to gating of pain) and psychophysiological organization (reducing motor tone, inducing relaxation and enhancing integration).

Cautions

None noted apart from caution regarding rate and amplitude of rhythmic movements imposed on tissues under repair.

Naturopathic perspectives

There is something inherently naturopathic about bodily rhythms being employed to gently coax enhanced circulatory and drainage efficiency as well as neurological coordination and integration in distressed tissues.

Further reading

1. Lederman E 2000 Harmonic technique. Churchill Livingstone, Edinburgh
2. Comeaux Z 2002 Robert Fulford and the philosopher physician. Eastland Press, Seattle
3. Juhan D 1989 An introduction to Trager psychophysical integration and mentastics

movement education. Trager Institute, Mill Valley, California

Pilates methods

There is additional information in Chapter 9.

Pilates is an exercise system developed originally in the first half of the 20th century by Joseph H. Pilates (Anderson & Spector 2000). Pilates-based exercises can be performed on the floor, termed 'mat work', or on equipment, termed 'apparatus work'. A key piece of apparatus is the Reformer which comprises a single bed frame equipped with a sliding carriage that uses springs to regulate tension and resistance. Cables, bars, straps and pulleys are features of a variety of Pilates-based exercises, performed in multiple positions. Strength, endurance and flexibility of the major postural muscles involved in trunk (core) stability, particularly the abdominal group, receive focused attention (Mullhearn & George 1999). The 'core' is described as 'a box with the abdominals in the front, paraspinals and gluteals in the back, the diaphragm as the roof, and the pelvic floor and hip girdle musculature as the bottom' (Akuthota & Nadler 2004). In addition, Pilates-based exercise claims to improve both dynamic and static postural balance, even in the elderly (Hall et al 1999, Hutchinson et al 1998, Segal et al 2004).

Pilates has also been described as a mind–body fitness program (Pilates 1934, 1945). Validation of the

Box 7.14 Trager exercise (Blackburn 2004)

The Trager® practitioner at the table is . . . supporting body parts in various positional combinations of extension, flexion, rotation, torque, compression, and distraction. The movements happen within the safe confines of conditioned reflexes, creating a playful sense of letting go and trust in the client. The sensitivity of the practitioner determines the drop-catch response, fine-tuning it to the client's reflexive response – like tossing and catching the baby.

The rhythmical movement in Trager® creates a lulling relaxation, like floating on the sea, or swaying in a hammock. The practitioner can vary different parameters: frequency, amplitude, direction, hand contact, pattern, pause, position, stretch, or compression, while initiating movement from his/her feet, as the hands catch, nudge and anchor the motion. Like a ballroom dancer, the practitioner can take advantage of gravity, momentum, tensegrity, and tonus, while feeling for signs of impedance and flow. The client may also feel various types of resistances in his/her own body of which he/she was previously unaware.

The practitioner's intention to produce releases determines the ways in which the movements are produced. When resistance is felt, even a slight

reflexive arc that might precede muscle action, the practitioner can adjust the movement so that it falls within the range of least resistance. As the session proceeds the practitioner adjusts the parameters of movement in response to changes in resistance, relaxation and mobilization.

Exercise: Facilitated oscillatory release
(Comeaux 2004)

Comeaux (2004) suggests:

The stretch, cyclic afferent input, and articulatory movements associated with natural gait is a useful way of mobilizing restricted segments of the central axis. The Facilitated Oscillatory Release approach to the spine and sacrum attempts to replicate the gait cycle.

- *Beginning with the patient in a prone position, oscillation is initiated by gentle continuous rocking of the pelvis alternately from side to side using one hand.*
- *The heel of the other hand, reaching across the spine is placed over a transverse process of the vertebra.*
- *This hand is then set into motion rhythmically 180 degrees out of phase with the motion of the pelvis, creating torsion of the torso.*
- *In other words, as the hand on the pelvis moves away from the practitioner, the hand adjacent to the spine moves toward; at the end of that excursion, the directions are reversed in each hand.*
- *The uppermost hand adjacent to the spine will now be given a second role, of simultaneously assessing the quality of response to the motion.*
- *One can then move the sensing upper hand up and down the spine to localize this response at specific spinal segments.*
- *With practice one develops a sense of a normal rhythmic compliance.*
- *Comparison to segments above and below can isolate segments that are less than optimally compliant.*
- *Clinical correlation will help decide the involvement of such a segment with symptoms.*
- *This protocol involves passive motion testing and primarily the rotational phase, but assesses much more.*

If dysfunction is assessed in this manner, optimal resonance and freedom of motion can be facilitated by one of three strategies of application of rhythmic force:

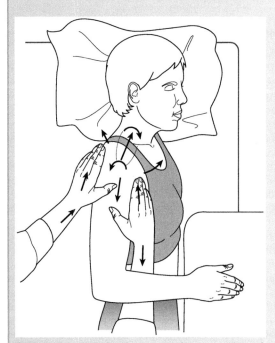

Figure 7.15 Holding shoulder: arrows indicate possibilities of movement and direction. Reproduced with permission from Blackburn J. *Journal of Bodywork and Movement Therapies* 2004;8(3):178–188

Box 7.14 Trager exercise continued

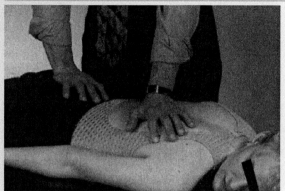

Figure 7.16 Application of facilitated oscillatory release to spine and pelvis. Reproduced with permission from Comeaux Z. *Journal of Bodywork and Movement Therapies* 2004;9(2):88–98

1. One strategy is to induce a stretch or articulation mobilization with a rapid exaggeration of the rotation of the segment in phase with the anticipated oscillation. This would represent a situation of constructive interference with the induced standing wave of force applied to the tissues.
2. A second more forceful strategy is to add the exaggerated rotation out of phase with the developed rhythm. This applies a destructive interference pattern to the established wave in the tissue by introducing more energy.
3. A third intervention strategy is to gently persist with the established wave pattern to soften tissue

by inducing any resistance in the tissue to accept the energy of the new wave pattern, allowing this rhythmic afferent input to entrain a more homeostatic endogenous rhythm of the neurons responsible for coordinating postural tone. In this application the intent would be to induce a relaxation pattern of baseline neuromuscular coordination and to entrain a more harmonic pattern.

Comeaux (2004) makes clear:

If a practitioner is applying these strategies to the spine, it is wise to begin with the patient in as gravity neutral a posture as possible, with access to the spine. The prone position is recommended. In this manner, a pattern of passive activity and afferent stimulation is reproduced that is equivalent to that during active walking, with its alternating pelvic rotation and counter torsion through the trunk. As the strategies are assimilated, it is possible to transfer most of these strategies to the seated position . . . Treatment in the lateral recumbent position is also possible.

In the prone position the thoracic and lumbar spine are treated by rotating the pelvis to develop a standing wave, and adding counter torsion of the trunk, with localization as is necessary. To diagnose in the pelvis and more particularly the sacrum, a reciprocal role of the two hands is used by rotating the trunk to generate momentum, and letting the sacral hand 'listen' to the quality and quantity of resonant tissue compliance, and to then making corrective suggestion.

---

efficacy of use of Pilates exists in a number of studies (Lange et al 2000, Segal et al 2004, Stanko 2002).

Further reading

1. Robinson L, Thomson G 1997 Body control: using techniques developed by Joseph H. Pilates. BainBridge Books, Philadelphia
2. Pilates J 1934 Your health. Presentation Dynamics, Incline Village, NV
3. Pilates J 1945 Return to life through contrology. Presentation Dynamics, Incline Village, NV

Positional release techniques (PRT)

Indications/description

Positional release techniques belong mainly to that class of modalities that *invite* change, rather than

forcing change, when treating dysfunctional tissues. By their nature they are indirect, i.e. the process almost always involves a disengagement from restriction barriers, rather than any direct attempt to engage and overcome such restrictions, as would be the case in HVLA, myofascial release or stretch methodology (Deig 2001).

As such, PRT methods are best suited to acute and subacute settings, although they are considered a useful aid in chronic conditions.

Simplistically, PRT methods attempt to create positions of 'ease' or 'comfort' for shortened and distressed tissues, commonly by taking already shortened (spasm, contracture, fibrosis, etc.) tissues into a supported degree of greater shortness, in the belief that a beneficial change will result, by means of mechanisms discussed in the 'Physiological effects' section below (D'Ambrogio & Roth 1997).

Methodology

There are two main PRT methods, with a number of variations, which have emerged out of osteopathic methodology.

1. Strain/counterstrain (SCS) utilizes a painful area in dysfunctional tissues (a 'tender point') as a monitor to guide the practitioner as tissues are positioned and fine tuned until the initial tenderness reduces from a pain score of 10 to 3 or less. The tissues are then held in this position for variable periods (90 seconds is a common recommendation) before being gently released to their resting state (Chaitow 2003, Jones 1981).

2. Functional technique uses palpation of distressed tissues or joints to position them into 'ease', without using pain sensitivity as a guide (as in 1 above). Functional approaches therefore rely on a skilled palpation sense (Johnstone 1997, Schiowitz 1990).

3. A variety of 'facilitating' methods are used to encourage functional and pain-reducing changes, including gentle compression, distraction or respiratory strategies (Goodheart 1984).

4. Physical therapy has evolved methods such as 'mobilization with movement' and 'unloading' taping that incorporate aspects of PRT. McKenzie exercise methods incorporate concepts of movement towards 'ease' that are also close to PRT concepts (Horton 2002, Long et al 2004, Morrissey 2002, Mulligan 1985).

5. In chiropractic, aspects of the use of sacro-occipital technique's 'blocking' methods incorporate placing tissues into an exaggeration of existing distortion (i.e. making whatever is short, shorter) and are also in line with PRT methodology (Blum et al 2003).

6. In craniosacral techniques much of the treatment involves indirect pressure, taking distortions into a 'crowded' state, so allowing change to take place spontaneously (Sergueef et al 2002).

Upledger & Vredevoogd (1983) give a practical explanation of indirect methods of treatment, especially as related to cranial therapy. The idea of moving a restricted area in the direction of ease is, they say, 'a sort of "unlatching" principle. Often in order to open a latch we must first exaggerate its closure'.

In normal tissues there exists in the mid-range of motion an area of 'ease' or balance, where the tissues are at their least tense. When there is a restriction in the normal range of motion of an area, whether of osseous or soft tissue origin, the now limited range will almost always still have a place, a moment, a point, which is neutral, of maximum comfort or ease, usually lying somewhere between the new restriction barrier in one direction and the physiological barrier in the other. Finding this balance point – also known as 'dynamic neutral' – is a key element in PRT.

Staying in this 'ease' state for an appropriate length of time (see below) offers restrictions a chance to 'unlatch', release, normalize.

In this way it can be seen that the positioning element of the process is the preparation for the treatment to commence, and that the 'treatment' itself is self-generated by the tissues (nervous system, circulatory system, etc.) in response to this careful positioning.

Safety

The nature of indirect approaches is essentially safe, since barriers are avoided and tissues are held in comfort.

Validation of efficacy = 5 (see Table 7.2)

Numerous studies demonstrate that these methods are safe as well as being effective (Cislo et al 1991, Ramirez 1989, Wong et al 2004a,b).

Hospital studies involving treatment of recently surgically traumatized tissue validate the essential safety of positional release methods (Dickey 1989).

Alternatives

Within the framework of positional release there are numerous alternatives, and the overall approach of indirect methodology offers an alternative to direct methods of treatment.

Physiological effects

Proprioception

Walther (1988) summarizes a 'strain' situation as follows:

When proprioceptors send conflicting information there may be simultaneous contraction of the antagonists . . . without antagonist muscle inhibition, joint and other strain results [and in this manner] a reflex pattern develops which causes muscle or other tissue to maintain this continuing strain. It [strain dysfunction] often relates to the inappropriate signalling from muscle proprioceptors that have been strained from rapid change that does not allow proper adaptation.

We can recognize such a pattern in an acute setting in torticollis, as well as in acute lumbago. It is also recognizable as a feature of many types of chronic somatic dysfunction in which joints remain restricted due to muscular imbalances of this type, occurring as part of an adaptive process.

This is a time of intense neurological and proprioceptive 'confusion', and is the moment of 'strain'. SCS appears to offer a means of quieting the neurological confusion and the excessive, or unbalanced, tone.

D'Ambrogio & Roth (1997) state that:

Positional release therapy (PRT) appears to have a damping influence on the general level of excitability within the facilitated segment. Weiselfish (1993) has found that this characteristic of PRT is unique in its effectiveness, and has utilized this feature to successfully treat severe neurologic patients, even though the source of the primary dysfunction arose from the supraspinal level.

Nociception

Bailey & Dick (1992) suggest that strain dysfunction is far more complex than the simple proprioceptive example:

Probably few dysfunctional states result from a purely proprioceptive or nociceptive response. Additional factors such as autonomic responses, other reflexive activities, joint receptor responses [biochemical features] or emotional states must also be accounted for. Nociceptive responses would occur (which are more powerful than proprioceptive influences) and these multisegmental reflexes would produce a flexor withdrawal, dramatically increasing tone in the flexor group.

Korr's (1976b) explanation for the physiological normalization of tissues brought about through positional release is that:

The shortened spindle nevertheless continues to fire, despite the slackening of the main muscle, and the CNS is gradually able to turn down the gamma discharge and, in turn, enables the muscles to return to 'easy neutral', at its resting length. In effect, the physician has led the patient through a repetition of the dysfunctioning process with, however, two essential differences. First it is done in slow motion, with gentle muscular forces, and second there have been no surprises for the CNS; the spindle has continued to report throughout.

Other hypotheses

Jacobson et al (1989) have suggested a circulatory hypothesis for the benefits of PRT. Another hypothe-

sis relates to the presumed effects of slackening fascial tissues during positional release.

D'Ambrogio & Roth (1997) summarize what may happen to the fascia, during PRT, as follows:

By reducing the tension on the myofascial system, the fascial components of dysfunction may be engaged. The reduction in tension on the collagenous cross-linkages appears to induce a disengagement of the electrochemical bonds and a conversion back [from the gel-like] to the sol [solate] state.

Whether proprioceptive, nociceptive, neurological, circulatory or fascial factors are involved in positional release effects remains a matter for further research.

Cautions

Used appropriately there appear to be no contraindications to use of positional release methods of treatment.

Naturopathic perspectives

In the realm of bodywork few if any methods would seem to be closer to basic naturopathic concepts than positional release methodology.

At its most basic, these are methods that allow self-regulation to operate by placing tissues in their most relaxed (ease) state. To this degree PRT may be seen to have philosophical and practical similarities to deep relaxation, therapeutic fasting, neutral (body temperature) bathing, and various psychotherapeutic approaches such as emotional experiencing and somatosensory psychotherapy.

In all these there is a 'detachment from barriers', provision of a 'safe place' ('position of ease'), a virtual 'granting of permission' or offering of an opportunity for self-regulation to operate.

Further reading

1. D'Ambrogio K, Roth G 1997 Positional release therapy. Mosby, St Louis
2. Chaitow L 2007 Positional release techniques, 3rd edn. Churchill Livingstone, Edinburgh
3. Doig D 2001 Positional release techniques. Butterworth-Heinemann, Boston
4. Johnston W, Friedman H, Eland D 2005 Functional methods. American Academy of Osteopathy, Indianapolis, Indiana
5. Jones L 1995 Strain–counterstrain. Jones, Boise, Idaho

Box 7.15 Exercise: Positional release skin on fascia

1. Locate an area of skin somewhere between your elbow and wrist, on the flexor surface. Place two or three finger pads onto the skin and slide it superiorly and then inferiorly on the underlying fascia.
2. To which direction does the skin slide more easily?
3. Slide the skin in that direction and, holding it there, test the preference of the skin to slide medially and laterally.
4. Which of these is the 'easier' direction?
5. Slide the tissue toward this second position of ease.
6. Now introduce a slight clockwise and anticlockwise twist to these tissues which are already being held ('stacked') in two directions of ease.
7. Which way does the skin feel most comfortable as it rotates?
8. Take it in that direction, so that you are now holding the skin in three positions of ease. Hold this final stacked position of ease for not less than 20 seconds.
9. Release the skin and retest; it should now display a far more symmetrical preference in all the directions that were previously restricted or 'tight'.
10. You have demonstrated that moving tissues away from their barriers or resistance, into ease, can achieve a release.
11. This is an example of a positional release technique (Chaitow 2007).

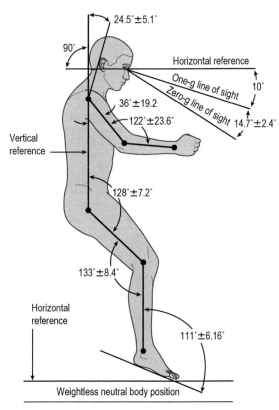

Figure 7.17 The position of the body in zero gravity, sometimes called astronauts' position or neutral body posture. Reproduced with permission from Cranz G. *Journal of Bodywork and Movement Therapies* 2000;4(3):155–165. Redrawn from NASA (National Aeronautics and Space Administration, USA)

Postural re-education (e.g. Alexander technique)

This topic is discussed in greater depth in Chapter 9.

Chapter 9 focuses on rehabilitation and has details of postural re-education methods, such as Alexander technique (Alexander 1996). Alexander technique encourages better (more efficient) use of the body, closely related to the approaches adopted in ergonomics (see earlier in this chapter). The process adopted by Alexander teachers (they do not regard themselves as therapists) is an educational one, a process during which old dysfunction-inducing habits are 'unlearned', being replaced over time by new, more efficient and balanced ones.

The concepts and methods used by such teachers are solidly based on well-researched anatomic and physiological principles. For example, Cranz (2000) has noted:

Standing tires the legs, and sitting tires the back, but halfway between sitting and standing is perching. This halfway posture is what Alexander (1984) called the 'position of mechanical advantage', and what marshal [sic] arts students recognize as the 'horse'. Figure 7.17 shows an astronaut in outer space in zero gravity; note the open angle (128° ± 7.2°) between trunk and thigh. The advantage of this posture is that it distributes the work of sitting upright evenly throughout the whole torso. Note also that perching on a high (27 inch) stool creates a similar leg–spine relationship. The Norwegian Balans chair, known variously as the posture, kneeling or computer chair, uses the same principle.'

Further reading

1. Alexander FM 1996 (originally 1910) In: Fisher JMO (ed) Man's supreme inheritance. Mouritz, London

Prolotherapy

Hal Brown ND DC RAc

The term prolotherapy refers to the proliferation that results when ligaments and tendons are injected at their attachment sites, resulting in the regrowth of those tissues. Dr Earl Gedney, an osteopath from Philadelphia, was the first to use an injection to strengthen sacroiliac ligaments. Dr George Hackett, a surgeon, active in the late 1950s, correlated pain patterns from strained ligaments with instability. He treated thousands of patients with ligament strengthening injections which he named prolotherapy (Patterson 2004a).

There is historical evidence that a version of this technique was first used by Hippocrates on soldiers with dislocated, torn shoulder joints. He would stick a heated poker into the joint, to encourage normal healing (Adams 1946). Of course, we don't use hot pokers today, but the principle is similar: get the body to innately repair itself.

Indications/description

The primary indication for the use of prolotherapy is lax or overstretched ligaments that are creating instability in the joints by not performing their primary structural task of holding the joints with firm integrity. Ligaments are rich in pain-sensitive fibers and excessive stress on these tissues can create local and/or referred pain (Hackett et al 2002a, Magnuson 1941, Meisenbach 1911, Mengert 1943).

A simple diagnostic indicator for a *ligamentous* pain pattern would be to consider whether the pain is worse when standing still or sitting in one place for any length of time. Once the patient gets up and moves around, there is relief. The same patient may also describe pain upon waking in the morning that is relieved once they begin to move. When the patient is at rest, the muscles relax and the ligaments support the structure; when the patient moves the muscles begin to hold the joints and there is relief. If the ligaments are lax, then there is more strain upon them and

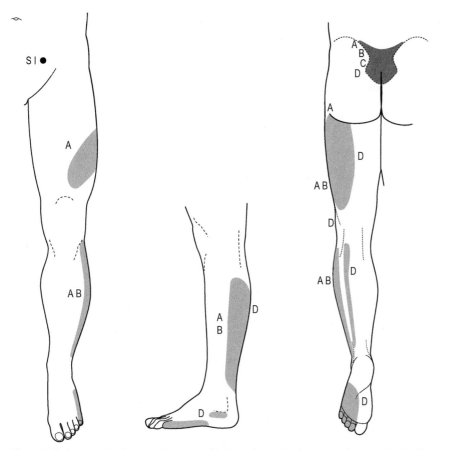

Figure 7.18 An example of pain patterns caused by injured sacroiliac ligaments discovered by Dr Hackett (Hackett et al 2002b). Reprinted by permission of Beulah Land Press

they are susceptible to producing pain. During physical examination, pain elicited by passive stretching of ligaments or firm pressure on ligament sites may also be indications for prolotherapy (Hackett et al 2002c).

Prolotherapy is also indicated for sprained or torn *tendons*. When *tendon attachments* onto bone (enthesis) are injured, the corresponding muscle groups react with hypertonicity and may develop *trigger points*. These muscles are commonly treated for spasm and tightness with trigger point therapies, stretching, massage or other methods. If the causative factor is the enthesopathy, then the focus of therapy on muscle may provide only temporary or partial relief. Often after prolotherapy injections, the trigger points will eventually disappear once the injured tendon attachment has remodeled. Frequently patients who are tight or stiff can gain a significant improvement in range of motion immediately after a treatment once the damaged tendon has been anesthetized and the hypertonic response reduced. Excessive tenderness at the tendon attachment site is an indicator that the causative factor may be in the tendon, rather than in the muscle, and would be an indication for prolotherapy (Hackett et al 2002d).

Prolotherapy can be useful for most *muscle and joint pain* problems. It can be used on any joint, tendon or ligament in the body except where contraindicated, and be useful with chronic and acute pain as well as arthritides, disc degeneration and herniation, dislocations, whiplash, tendonosis and many other conditions.

Methodology

Once the injured tendons or ligaments have been identified, they are usually treated by injection of a 12.5% dextrose solution diluted with 1% procaine (Hooper & Ding 2004, Reeves & Hassanein 2003, Topol et al 2005). Some practitioners use stronger solutions that include sodium morrhuate (Hackett et al 2002e) or PG2 (Hackett et al 2002f). The technique is dependent upon a good knowledge of anatomy including surface anatomy. The tissue to be injected is first palpated and the skin is marked with a sterile marking pen. The area is then sterilized. The needle is injected until the tip is felt to touch bone. The patient may often describe pain and/or a description of the referral pattern for that ligament or tendon. The solution is only injected while the needle is in contact with bone.

Injections may also be given intra-articularly in order to suffuse the entire joint and affect the capsular ligaments from inside the joint (Hackett et al 2002g).

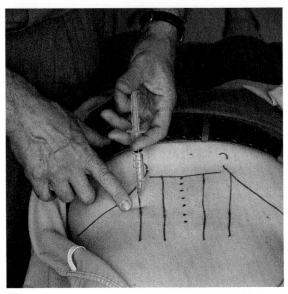

Figure 7.19 Markings for the lumbar spine and injection of the transverse process portion of the iliolumbar ligament

Safety

In studies, prolotherapy has not caused any serious injury. There is usually discomfort after each injection that lasts for a few minutes to several days, but this discomfort is seldom severe (Klein et al 1993). Research articles on prolotherapy do not report any problems related to safety.

Prolotherapy is safe in the hands of properly trained physicians. It is recommended that anyone wishing to learn this technique obtain training from institutions that are able to provide cadavers for training purposes. To avoid making mistakes it is prudent that the practitioner be trained by skilled experts who can provide hands-on guidance in the anatomy laboratory as well as appropriate instruction in the classroom.

There are risks, the most significant being nerve damage from an injection placed too close to a nerve (Schnirring 2000).

The risks associated with improper technique may include:

- injury to nerves or blood vessels
- piercing the dural membrane and producing a spinal headache
- injection into the spinal cord leading to permanent paralysis or death
- injection in the thoracic spine or on the ribs resulting in pneumothorax
- poor protocol resulting in injection into nerves
- the risk of infection if sterile procedures are not observed (Patterson 2004b).

Validation of efficacy = 5 (see Table 7.2)

Animal studies

- Prolotherapy has been performed on animal ligaments and tendons. Harvested tissue was compared to the non-treated side and it was found that the ligaments and tendons had increased bulk, width, tissue strength, and tissue to bone strength (Liu et al 1983, Maynard et al 1985).

- A study done at the University of Wisconsin (Jensen 2004) created a stretch injury in rabbit knees. The ligament injury was treated with prolotherapy at 14 days and at 21 days. At 28 days the animal was sacrificed. Results demonstrated that the mechanical properties of the ligaments were of greater strengthening, stiffening, enlargement and decrease of laxity. The effect was larger if the animal received two injections instead of one.

Human studies

- A study at the University of Kansas (Reeves & Hassanein 2003) concluded: 'Dextrose injection prolotherapy at 2- to 3-month intervals resulted in elimination of laxity by machine measure in 10/16 knees in the study population, with statistically significant laxity improvement by 6 injections, sustainable through 3 years with periodic injection.'

- Studies demonstrate statistically significant results in knees and finger joints (Reeves & Hassanein 2000a, 2003).

- Two low back studies revealed an impressive 60% sustained reduction in pain and disability after 12-month follow-up (Klein et al 1993, Ongley et al 1987).

- Topol et al's 2005 study in the *Archives of Physical Medicine & Rehabilitation* stated that dextrose prolotherapy showed marked efficacy for chronic groin pain in this group of elite rugby and soccer athletes.

- A study on fibromyalgia and prolotherapy demonstrated that the improvements in pain levels and functional ability after injection are supportive of tendon and ligaments being a major source of symptomatology in fibromyalgia (Reeves 1993).

- A retrospective case series on patients with chronic spinal pain showed that 91% of patients reported reduction in level of pain, 84.8% of patients reported improvement in activities of daily living, and 84.3% reported an improvement in ability to work. Conclusion: 'Dextrose prolotherapy appears to be a safe and effective method for treating chronic spinal pain' (Hooper & Ding 2004).

- A study in *Pain Physician* used intradiscal electrothermal treatment (IDET) in a control group, with the prolotherapy group demonstrating superior outcomes (Derby et al 2004).

- A study in the *Clinical Journal of Sports Medicine* concluded: 'Positive results compared with controls have been reported in nonrandomized and randomized controlled trials' (Rabago et al 2005).

- A study in *Pain Physician* concluded: 'This single blinded, randomized and cross-over study of prolotherapy was described as being a "minimally invasive" therapy with success rates of 80%' (Wilkinson 2005).

Alternatives

Dry needle tissue irritation may be an effective alternative for stimulation of inflammation and new growth. The acupuncture technique of 'bone-pecking' or 'osteopuncture' involves needle irritation at bony attachments of tendons and ligaments (Helms 1985, Lowenkopf 1976, Mann 1971).

There are many strategies available to achieve joint stability. The use of taping, tensor bandages or devices and splints to stabilize weakened ligaments may be helpful in reducing symptoms (Gatterman 1990b, Perrin 2005). Exercise for joints or core strengthening for the spine are effective in reducing pain and are useful in rehabilitation and maintenance (Rydeard et al 2006). There are forms of electrotherapy (Harvard Medical School 2006) and friction massage (Cyriax & Coldham 1984) that strengthen ligaments. Lee (2001), in conjunction with Vleeming, has developed the 'integrated model of joint function', a method which attempts to strengthen lax sacroiliac joints with specific muscle training. Surgery has been a standard medical practice and, more recently, growth factors and cell and gene therapies (Woo et al 2000) have been shown to be effective.

Physiological effects

The wound healing cascade is a process that begins with inflammation and proceeds to the proliferative and remodeling phases (Diegelmann & Evans 2004, Guyton & Hall 1997). Many injuries and degenerative processes do not fully heal on their own because of the inhibition of the initial inflammation phase by the common use of NSAIDs (Almekinders 1993, Elder et al 2001, Stanley & Weaver 1998). The prolotherapy

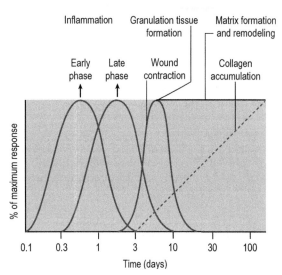

Inflammation　　Granulation tissue　　Matrix formation
　　　　　　　　　formation　　　　　and remodeling

Early　　Late　　Wound　　　　Collagen
phase　　phase　contraction　　accumulation

Figure 7.20 Schematic representation of the wound healing cascade. After Hackett et al (2002h)

injection is utilized to stimulate the spilling of inflammatory eicosanoids and other substances. This initiates a 3- to 5-day inflammatory cascade, followed by 2–4 weeks of fibroblast activity (Cockbill 2002, Reeves & Hassanein 2000b). This long understood principle of localized inflammation and tissue repair is the basis of how injuries self-repair. Prolotherapy, by irritating the injured site, initiates the natural inflammatory cascade that allows the body to bring fibroblasts and other cellular elements to the area which literally rebuild and grow newer and stronger ligaments and tendons through the natural proliferative and remodeling phases (Liu et al 1983, Reeves & Hassanein 2000a,b).

Cautions

- Diffuse myofascial pain – prolotherapy is indicated for localized pain
- If the problem is not a ligament or tendon
- Patient is taking coumadin, warfarin or blood thinners within 5 days
- Patient is taking anti-inflammatory medications or steroids
- Allergy to procaine
- Cancer patients
- Areas that are 'forbidden' by protocol such as the suboccipital region
- Areas that have been repaired by screws, plates or other hardware
- Needle phobic or high anxiety patient

Box 7.16 Exercise: Prolotherapy

It is not recommended that anyone attempt to perform prolotherapy injections without the proper training and licensure. To get a sense of the ligament diagnosis, find a patient with an unresolved sacroiliac pain. Motion palpation may reveal that one side is more mobile than the other. Consider that the problem may not be the restricted joint but perhaps a hypermobility in the other joint caused by ligament laxity. See if the symptom picture matches the indications outlined earlier in this section.

- A simple orthopedic test would be to fully flex the hip of the supine patient while placing a hand under the SI joint.
- Place pressure onto the knee so that you can feel the force into the passive hand under the patient.
- While in this position, internally rotate the femur while applying pressure towards the SI joint.
- If the patient describes pain with either of these tests, then turn the patient over and palpate the SI ligaments with firm pressure.
- If these ligament points are significantly tender, then consider this patient to be a candidate for prolotherapy (Ravin et al 2005).

Hypothesis

Form and force closure tests are also useful in identifying instability as described in Chapter 6. In the Vleeming/Lee model the force closure problem is addressed by increasing articular compression through the strengthening of specific muscle groups (Lee 1997). The one leg standing test and the active straight leg raise (ASLR) test that are utilized may also be good indicators of ligament laxity and could be integrated into a prolotherapy diagnostic process. Theoretically it would appear to be optimal to integrate both models, i.e. to stabilize joints through the ligament reconstruction of prolotherapy and the muscle tensegrity balancing of the integrated model of joint function. These tests might also assist in prioritizing treatment strategies.

- Not contraindicated in pregnancy or diabetes (Patterson 2004b)

Naturopathic perspectives

It has been shown that prolotherapy injections were more effective when combined with co-interventions concurrently (Yelland et al 2004). The integration with naturopathic methods may enhance the effectiveness of prolotherapy as a stand-alone therapy. By combining prolotherapy with manipulation, other manual therapies and exercise the patient should receive a more comprehensive treatment approach. The nutritional, lifestyle, biochemical and energetic aspects of the naturopathic practice will ensure that all perspectives of joint and tissue healing are addressed.

[Manual] pump techniques: lymphatics, liver or spleen (Arbuckle 1977)

Indications/description

Indications for the use of lymphatic pump techniques include all conditions that involve congestion, lymphatic stasis and infection (apart from those listed under 'Cautions').

Wallace et al (1997a) report:

Lymphatic pump techniques are designed to augment the pressure gradients that develop between the thoracic and abdominal regions during normal respirations.

Wallace et al also list the benefits of enhanced lymphatic movement – encouraged by the various 'pump' techniques described in this section – including:

- increased resorption of fluids
- increased circulation and respiration
- decreased proteins in the interstitium
- facilitation from a more beneficial pH balance.

Caution: It is important to make sure that the patient has no food, chewing gum or loose dentures in the mouth when these procedures are being applied.

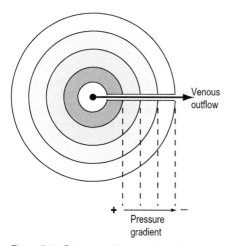

Figure 7.21 During muscle contraction, there is a pressure gradient with central high pressure (dark shading) to peripheral low pressure (light shading). Venous flow is down the pressure gradient. Reproduced with permission from Lederman (2005d)

Methodology

Lymphatic pump method description (Sleszynski & Kelso 1993)

- The patient lies supine, knees and hips flexed.
- The practitioner is at the head of the table with hands spread across the patient's chest, below the clavicles, with thumbs resting next to each other on the sternum, fingers spread laterally. The arms should be more or less straight for ease of transmission of force from the shoulder to the hands.
- Pressure is introduced by the practitioner, in a downwards and caudad direction, which is just sufficient to overcome resistance, by means of a repetitive, minimal, flexion and extension of the elbows.
- The patient continues to breathe normally and does not resist the repetitive pressure applied by the practitioner, which should be between a rate of 100 and 120 per minute.
- The patient breathes through the mouth, and the pumping action takes over the respiratory function.
- This should continue for at least 3 minutes, and for up to 5 minutes.
- In babies, the method can be used with one hand over the sternum, the other under the spine, with the baby cradled or seated on the practitioner's lap. The effect of this is to improve lymphatic drainage dramatically.
- This method is useful in all cases of edema and infection. It also has a beneficial effect on immune function (Hoag 1969).

Note: This is one example only; there are many other methods for enhancing lymphatic drainage, including direct 'pumping' of the lower thorax, exaggerated repetitive dorsiflexion during deep breathing by the patient, etc. Deep diaphragmatic breathing itself enhances lymphatic flow.

Safety

If normal precautions are observed there seem to be no contraindications to use of lymphatic pump methods.

Validation of efficacy = 5 (see Table 7.2)

The use of these methods in numerous studies (mainly osteopathic), as outlined in Chapter 8, puts their clinical usefulness at a high level.

Alternatives

Manual lymphatic drainage, regular exercise, enhanced respiratory function, avoidance of sedentary habits.

Physiological effects

See notes earlier in this chapter on fluid movement and also notes on this topic included in the description of manual lymphatic drainage (MLD) techniques and mobilization effects on physiology (Foldi & Strossenreuther 2003, Lederman 1997a).

Cautions

- Malignant or other serious diseases of the lungs, liver, spleen or associated organs
- Recent abdominal or thoracic surgery
- Hepatitis
- Infectious mononucleosis
- Osteoporosis
- Fracture, dislocation or other painful dysfunction involving the joints of the thoracic cage or spine
- Avoid thoracic pump techniques where the patient has a reduced cough reflex

Naturopathic perspective

As with MLD, pump techniques are very much in harmony with the naturopathic principle of promoting function in acute and chronic disorders.

Further reading

1. Ward R (ed) 1997 Foundations for osteopathic medicine. Williams & Wilkins, Baltimore
2. Lederman E 2005 Science and practice of manual therapy, 2nd edn. Churchill Livingstone, Edinburgh, p 87–224

Rehabilitation methods

The topic of rehabilitation is discussed in greater depth in Chapter 9.

Evidence-informed protocols exist for rehabilitation of specific forms of dysfunction. In this section two common dysfunctional conditions are briefly outlined:

- low back rehabilitation
- breathing pattern disorder rehabilitation.

Rehabilitation implies returning the individual toward a state of normality which has been lost through trauma or ill-health. Issues of patient compli-ance and home care are key features in recovery and these have been discussed elsewhere in this text (see Chapters 8 and 9).

Low back rehabilitation

Norris (1999) advises the following guidelines for re-establishing back stability, using stabilization exercises for the different triage groups that may be involved in back pain/dysfunction:

- *Simple backache*: Begin stability exercises (see below) and continue until fully functional
- *Nerve root compression*: Begin exercise as pain allows but refer to specialist if there has been no improvement within 4 weeks
- *Serious pathology*: Use back stabilization exercises only after surgical or medical intervention.

Among the many interlocking rehabilitation features involved in any particular case are the following (most have been described earlier in this chapter):

- Normalization of soft tissue dysfunction, including abnormal tension and fibrosis. Treatment methods might include massage, NMT, MET, MFR, PRT and/or articulation/ mobilization and/or other stretching procedures, including yoga.
- Deactivation of myofascial trigger points, possibly involving massage, NMT, MET, MFR, PRT, spray and stretch and/or articulation/ mobilization. Appropriately trained and licensed practitioners might also use injection or acupuncture in order to deactivate trigger points.
- Strengthening weakened structures, involving exercise and rehabilitation methods, such as Pilates.
- Proprioceptive re-education utilizing physical therapy methods (e.g. wobble board) and spinal stabilization exercises, as well as methods such as those devised by Trager (1987), Feldenkrais (1972), Pilates (Knaster 1996), Hanna (1988) and others.
- Postural and breathing re-education (see below) using physical therapy approaches as well as Alexander, yoga, tai chi and other similar systems (Mehling et al 2005).
- Ergonomic, nutritional and stress management strategies, as appropriate.
- Psychotherapy, counseling or pain management techniques such as cognitive behavior therapy.

Box 7.17 Pump technique exercises

Exercise 1: Piriformis muscle pump method

Janda (1996) points to the vast amount of pelvic organ dysfunction to which piriformis can contribute due to its relationship with circulation to the area. Richard (1978) notes that a working muscle will mobilize up to 10 times the quantity of blood mobilized by a resting muscle. He points out the link between pelvic circulation and lumbar, ischiatic and gluteal arteries and the blood vessels of the internal iliac artery that can all be influenced by using repetitive pumping of the pelvic muscles (including piriformis).

- Patient is supine, knee flexed to 90°.
- Practitioner stands with a hand on the lateral aspect of the ankle, resisting the patient's effort to externally rotate the hip using minimal but sustained effort for 7–10 seconds.

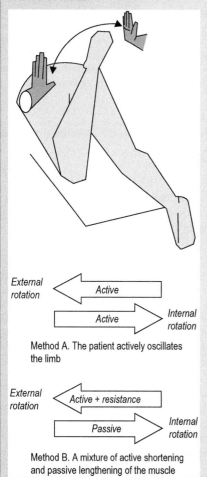

Method A. The patient actively oscillates the limb

Method B. A mixture of active shortening and passive lengthening of the muscle

Figure 7.22 Examples of different active muscle pump techniques. Reproduced with permission from Lederman (2005d)

- On relaxing this effort the practitioner takes the hip into internal rotation to its easy end of range.
- The patient performs the resisted contraction towards external rotation again, and the same process of relaxation and movement to internal rotation is performed.
- This process continues for 10–15 repetitions, or until the patient reports early signs of fatigue.
- No pain should be noted at any stage.

Lederman (2005a) observes:

A few cycles of muscle contraction against resistance can be used to initiate vascular changes (hyperemia) which will transiently 'open up' the blood flow in the muscle. Passive technique immediately follows, taking advantage of the hyperemia and the increase in flow.

Exercise 2: Pedal pump technique
(Wallace et al 1997b)

- Patient is supine.
- Practitioner stands at the foot of the bed and grasps both feet.
- Dorsiflexion or hyperdorsiflexion is introduced in a manner that initiates a degree of force and a wave-like motion in a cephalad direction.
- This is naturally followed by a caudad rebound (at which time the dorsiflexion is released).
- As the rebound wave reaches the feet, hyperdorsiflexion is again introduced, creating an oscillatory pump effect (see notes on oscillation and harmonic treatment earlier in this chapter).
- By observing the umbilicus the progression of the wave can most easily be noted.
- Once the oscillating rhythm has been established it is useful to introduce hyperplantarflexion as the wave is returning towards the feet. This adds a degree of fascial stretch of the anterior body surface.
- This repetitive process continues for several minutes to encourage lymphatic flow throughout the body.

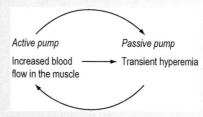

Figure 7.23 Alternate use of active and passive muscle pump techniques can be a potent stimulus to blood flow. Reproduced with permission from Lederman (2005d)

- Occupational therapy (see earlier in this chapter) which specializes in activating healthy coping mechanisms, determining functional capacity, increasing activity that will produce greater concordance than rote exercise and developing adaptive strategies to return the individual to a greater level of self-reliance and quality of life (Lewthwaite 1990).
- Appropriate exercise strategies to overcome deconditioning (Liebenson 1996b).
- A team approach to rehabilitation is called for where referral and cooperation allow the best outcome to be achieved.

Breathing rehabilitation

See Chapters 2, 4, 6, 9 and 10 for notes on additional aspects of breathing dysfunction.

There is good evidence that breathing rehabilitation is a useful method for achieving reduced anxiety/panic levels, and for improving postural control and a host of somatic complaints (Castro et al 2000, Mogyoros et al 1997).

Management of retraining includes assessment and treatment involving detailed explanations of breathing pattern disorders and building an individual integrated recovery program commonly based on:

- breathing retraining methods
- tension release through talk and relaxation
- stress perception and management
- enjoyable graduated exercise prescriptions
- rest/sleep guidance.

As many new patients present in a state of hyperarousal, the initial assessment and treatment programs require an emphasis on desensitizing through breathing retraining and relaxation.

Breathing rehabilitation has been shown to be most effective when it combines re-education, active (breathing) exercise protocols, and appropriate physical therapy aimed at mobilizing and normalizing somatic structures, particularly involving the thoracic cage (Aust & Fischer 1997, Han et al 1996, Lum 1984).

Further reading

1. Liebenson C (ed) 2006 Rehabilitation of the spine, 2nd edn. Lippincott Williams & Wilkins, Philadelphia
2. Chaitow L, Bradley D, Gilbert C 2002 Multidisciplinary approaches to breathing pattern disorders. Churchill Livingstone, Edinburgh

Shiatsu, acupressure, etc.

Indications/description

Shiatsu derives from an ancient form of Traditional Chinese Medicine that combines massage and acupressure.

Methodology

Shiatsu application includes point and meridian stimulation as well as use of a variety of manipulative techniques aimed at addressing structural features. The methodology includes stretching and rotation of body parts and tissues, possibly involving use of the practitioner's thumbs, hands, elbows and knees on the patient's body. Abdominal palpation is seen as an important aspect of diagnosis, with abdominal massage as required. Shiatsu is based on finding and treating areas of heightened neurological activity or apparent hypertonicity of the muscles (Beal 2000).

Conceptually, it is thought that imbalances, depletion or blockage of energy (chi) results in symptoms that are treated by application of firm, but not necessarily painful, pressure to key points and areas, in an attempt to restore balance (Mackay & Long 2003).

Safety

There is no evidence of risk in the literature from the use of shiatsu.

Validation of efficacy = 5 (see Table 7.2)

Numerous studies have demonstrated efficacy of shiatsu in treatment of musculoskeletal and other problems (Brady et al 2001, Galantino et al 2003).

Alternatives

The overlap between the methods of shiatsu and NMT which uses local ischemic compression is obvious. This should not be surprising since Lief's NMT was an evolution from Ayurvedic massage that incorporated a concept of 'energy (prana) blockages' being reduced by means of localized pressure techniques (Varma 1937).

Physiological effects

Whether or not 'energy' impedance exists in reality, as hypothesized by TCM and Ayurvedic medicine, is open to debate. What is known is that application of ischemic compression (also known as inhibitory pressure in osteopathic medicine) has a number of predictable physiological effects. As noted in Box 7.1, when compression is used locally to soft tissues, on release a rapid inflow of oxygenated blood to the tissues occurs (Simons et al 1999). The physiological changes that occur may also involve reduction of ischemia, as well as release of local endorphins, and possibly enkephalins (Baldry 1993, Kiser et al 1983). Mechanoreceptor stimulation affecting pain transmission also occurs (Melzack & Wall 1994). A combination of circulatory, endocrine and neurological changes therefore follow in response to applications of focused compressive loading of tissues.

Cautions

- Deeply applied compression is contraindicated in tissues that have been recently traumatized or that are inflamed
- Acute arthritis and other inflammatory conditions (contraindicated during acute stages)
- Aneurysm
- Bone fractures or acute soft tissue injuries: wait for full healing (6–12 weeks)
- Hemophilia
- Hodgkin's disease
- Leukemia
- Malignancy with metastasis (or TB) involving bone
- Osteoporosis
- Pain production during procedure
- Patients on cortisone (wait 2–3 months)
- Patients with high fever
- Phlebitis
- Recent scar tissue
- Syphilitic articular or peri-articular lesions
- Uncontrolled diabetic neuropathy

Naturopathic perspectives

Shiatsu has a methodology that encourages self-regulation, with explanations for its effects that can satisfy both the Western scientific mind and Oriental concepts.

Further reading

1. Zhao-Pu W 1991 Acupressure therapy. Churchill Livingstone, Melbourne
2. Jarney C, Tindall J 1991 Acupressure for common ailments. Gaia Books, London
3. Namikoshi T 1972 Shiatsu – Japanese finger-pressure therapy. Japan Publications, San Francisco

Somatic psychotherapy (a.k.a. body-centered psychotherapy, e.g. Hakomi)

Lisa Maeckel MA CHT

Somatic psychotherapies are based on the belief that the mind and body continuously inform one another, and they are primarily interested in this mind–body interface. The field of somatic psychology incorporates several basic concepts (Caldwell 1997):

1. Human beings are complex systems.
2. Any experience impacts the system at all levels: physical, emotional, cognitive and spiritual.
3. Pathology experienced at one level of the system is also experienced at the other levels.
4. The body is viewed as the blueprint for all experience.
5. Treatment consists of working experientially with the body in the present moment.

One form of somatic psychotherapy is the Hakomi Method of Experiential Psychotherapy. The Hakomi method was developed by Ron Kurtz and a team of therapists and educators in the late 1970s.

Influenced by Eastern philosophies, Kurtz believed Western psychological therapies to be violent and worked to create a method that facilitates change without force. The method has its roots in Buddhist and Taoist thought as well as general systems theory and body-centered therapies, including gestalt, psychomotor, Feldenkrais, focusing, Ericksonian hypnosis, neurolinguistic programming, bioenergetics and Reichian theory (Kurtz 1990).

Hakomi is a Hopi word that means 'Who are you?' and 'How do you stand in relation to these many realms?' Because human beings are continuously organizing their experiences into meaning, which ultimately shapes core beliefs and informs the way they view and navigate the world, Hakomi practitioners are interested in how people stand in relation to their many realms of experience. The Hakomi method focuses on the study of present experience in order to discover the psychological organization at work and answer the questions of who you are, how you came to be who you are, and how you can change.

Like other somatic therapies, the Hakomi method is both body-centered and experiential. Hakomi views the body as a doorway through which one can discover organizing material, which is typically hidden from awareness. It is in working with bodily experiences such as sensations, emotions, tensions and movements that the unconscious material is revealed. The Hakomi therapist looks for somatic indicators of unconscious material, not believed to be accessible through the intellect, then works in an experimental fashion with these indicators to access information regarding missing developmental experience and core wounding. Working with and through felt experience in the present moment, the method then seeks to provide the missing experience and heal the core material (Maurer-Groeli 1996).

At the core of the Hakomi method can be found the guiding principles of mindfulness, non-violence, mind–body holism, organicity and unity. Mindfulness – a relaxed and alert, self-observing state of consciousness – is employed by the therapist and the client in order to study present experience as it unfolds in the therapeutic session. Mindfulness allows the client to stay with experience as it deepens into core organizing material and ultimately bring this material into consciousness.

The principle of non-violence promotes working cooperatively with the system that is being studied. Force is never used in the Hakomi method. Working in alignment with this principle, the Hakomi therapist views the client's resistance as important and works to support it, rather than break through it or overcome it. Not only are defenses valued as an important protective function, they are viewed as a significant and valuable source of information about how the client has organized around core wounding.

The principle of mind–body holism recognizes that the mind and body are not separate; they continually interact and influence each other, and they jointly manifest whatever is experienced by the system. Evidence of core beliefs (how one views oneself and the world) exists both in the mind and the body; these beliefs not only determine thinking and behavior patterns, they also influence body structure and physiology. In Hakomi, the therapist and client are continually working the mind–body interface.

The principle of organicity refers to the fundamental wholeness, inherent wisdom and integrity of a system that is capable of self-regulating and self-correcting. This principle assumes that the client's process will unfold precisely according to the needs of the system, and the therapist's role is to facilitate and support that process. Rather than acting as healer, the therapist acts as a midwife to the client's self-discovery and innate capacity to heal.

The unity principle affirms that human beings are whole, composed of parts that serve the whole, all of which are interdependent on the other for health. Health of the human system depends upon the health of the communication between the parts of that system. The unity principle also recognizes the interdependence of human beings and, as such, assumes mutuality in the therapeutic relationship. The Hakomi practitioner works to dissolve the perceived barrier between self and other, and to promote an environment of loving presence in which healing can happen.

Further reading

1. Caldwell C 1997 Getting in touch: the guide to new body-centered therapies. Quest Books, Wheaton, Illinois
2. Kurtz R 1990 Body-centered psychotherapy: the Hakomi method. LifeRhythm, Mendocino, California
3. Levine P, Frederick A 1997 Waking the tiger: healing trauma: the innate capacity to transform overwhelming experiences. North Atlantic Books, Berkeley, California

Spondylotherapy (percussion techniques)

Indications/description

Percussion methods have obvious diagnostic/assessment value, where they can help to provide information in regard, for example, to localization of diseased lung tissue, such as pleural effusion = stony dull; atelectasis or consolidation = dull; pneumothorax = hyper-resonant; collapsed lung = dull, etc. (Pryor & Prasad 2002).

Percussion methods have also been used in naturopathic, osteopathic and chiropractic settings for well over a century, and in Traditional Chinese Medicine (TCM) for many centuries. One objective of Western percussion, particularly when applied spinally (spondylotherapy), is to stimulate visceral organs via the spinal pathways, or to influence the nervous system locally or more generally.

Cordingly (1924), in his text *Principles and Practice of Naturopathy*, states: 'Spondylotherapy is a method of eliciting reflexes at spinal nerve centers for the relief of morbid conditions in the body.' He also notes that, in addition to digital percussion, 'a mallet or plexo, and an applicator or pleximeter may be used'.

In addition, experts in the field of myofascial trigger points, Travell & Simons (1992a), suggest that these can be treated effectively using a series of percussive strokes (described below).

Over the past century in the USA, a number of mechanical methods of percussion have evolved, as have effective manual systems (Abrams 1922, Comeaux 2002b).

Methodology

To treat a trigger point using percussion:

1. The muscle is lengthened to the point of onset of passive resistance.

2. The clinician uses a hard rubber mallet, or reflex hammer, to hit the trigger point at exactly the same place, approximately 10 times.
3. This should be done at a slow rate of no more than one impact per second, but ensuring at least one impact every 5 seconds; slower rates are likely to be more effective than rapid ones.

Travell & Simons (1992a) suggest that this enhances, or substitutes for, intermittent cold with stretch ('spray and stretch') methods (discussed elsewhere in this chapter).

The trigger points in muscles that they list as benefiting most from percussion techniques include quadratus lumborum (Travell & Simons 1992b), brachioradialis, long finger extensors and peroneus longus and brevis.

Caution: It is specifically suggested that anterior and posterior compartment leg muscle *should not* be treated by percussion, owing to the risk of compartment syndrome, should bleeding occur in the muscle.

Western percussion

There a variety of opinions as to the ideal means of application of percussion to spinal tissues (spondylotherapy).

In Johnson's (1939) description, the middle finger is placed on the appropriate spinous process(es) while the other hand concusses the finger with a series of rapidly rebounding blows. This approach is known as spondylotherapy. One or two percussive repetitions are applied per second. Spondylotherapy percussion is usually applied to a series of three or four (or more) adjacent vertebrae.

An example of this is the treatment, as above, of the 5th thoracic spinous process, proceeding downwards to the 9th, in the case of liver dysfunction. Treatment would be applied only if the area is painful to palpating pressure. Similarly, concussion over the 10th, 11th and 12th thoracic spinous processes would be anticipated to stimulate kidney function.

In order to stimulate the organ or tissues using the spinal reflexes, percussion involves only a short amount of time: 15- to 30-second applications repeated three or four times, over approximately 4–5 minutes. A mild 'flare up' of symptoms and increased sensitivity in the area treated would normally indicate that the desired degree of stimulation had been achieved.

In order to inhibit function, or to produce dilation of local blood vessels, Johnson (1939) suggests that percussive repetitions be repeated for prolonged periods in order to fatigue the reflex.

A sound knowledge of spinal mechanics and neurological connections is a prerequisite to spondylotherapy usage.

Janse et al (1947) provide a variation on this approach, as follows:

For the purpose of stimulation the blows should be rapid and interrupted, e.g. percussion 10–15 strokes followed by an interval of rest for 1/4 of a minute – which is followed by 10–15 strokes again, and so on – the entire operation lasting 3 to 10 minutes.

On the other hand: 'Persistent rapid percussion will produce inhibition.'

As to location of application, this team of authors – who comprised two chiropractors and an osteopath (Wells) – note that percussion is most effective when applied 'to the area marking the junction of the transverse processes and the body of the vertebrae'.

TCM percussion

In recent years TCM methods involving percussion have added to our knowledge of the potential of these methods (Zhao-Pu 1991). It is worth noting that TCM percussion methods are based on the same theories as acupressure/acupuncture, and use the same points and meridians.

In TCM, percussion techniques involve one of three variations:

1. one-finger percussion, using the middle finger braced by the thumb and index finger
2. three-finger percussion, using the thumb, index and middle fingers
3. five-finger percussion, using the thumb and all fingers (Fig. 7.25).

The degree of force applied during percussion is also of three types:

1. light, which involves a movement of the hand from the wrist joint
2. medium, which involves a movement from the elbow joint with wrist fairly rigid
3. strong, which involves a movement of the upper arm, from the shoulder, with a rigid wrist.

Treatment may be offered daily, on alternate days or once every 3 days, and a course might involve 20 sessions. Patients often receive three courses or more. Professor Wang Zhao-Pu (whose work using this approach was based on his extensive experience as an orthopedic surgeon) describes remarkable clinical results involving patients with paralysis and cerebral birth injuries.

He states:

Box 7.18 Effects of Western percussion at various spinal levels

The influences of the various spinal levels are suggested (Schafer 1987) to be as follows:

- C3 – influences phrenic nerves influencing the diaphragm
- C4, 5 – stimulates reflex contraction of the lungs, therefore possibly helpful in those forms of asthma where dyspnea occurs during exhalation
- C6, 7 – has an influence on peripheral vasoconstriction and cardiomotor activity, therefore potentially useful in cases of hypotension
- T1, 2, 3 – stimulation dilates the lungs (inspiratory dyspnea); inhibits cardiac action; initiates gastric dilation reflex (therefore potentially useful in some forms of asthma, tachycardia and gastric hypermotility)
- T4 – initiates aortic and cardiac dilation; appears to ease viscerospasm
- T5 – pyloric and duodenal dilation (when right side stimulated)
- T6 – initiates gall bladder contraction (when right side stimulated)
- T7 – initiates slight visceromotor renal dilation, and stimulates hepatic function
- T8, 9 – gall duct dilation
- T10, 11 – initiates slight visceromotor renal contraction; enhances pancreatic secretion; relaxes intestines and colon; stimulates adrenals; when left side only stimulated, initiates splenic contraction
- T12 – initiates prostate contraction; tones bladder sphincter
- L1, 2, 3 – initiates uterine body, round ligament and bladder contraction; pelvic vasoconstriction; vesicular sphincter relaxation
- L4, 5 – initiates sigmoidal and rectal contraction; increases tone of lower bowel.

Parasympathetic tone can be encouraged by stimulation (moderate percussion/spondylotherapy) applied to C7 spinous process (Johnson 1977).

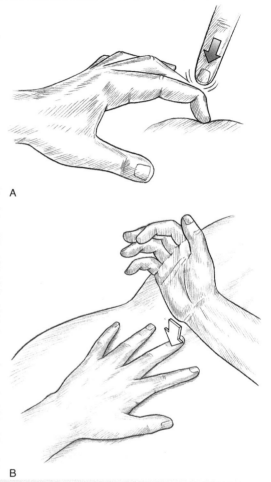

A

B

Figure 7.24 A Distal phalanx position held as vertical to the palpated surface as possible, described by Abrams, for percussion ('othopercussion') assessment. Reproduced with permission from Chaitow (2003). **B** Percussion technique (spondylotherapy) for reflexive effects or treatment of trigger points (slow percussion). Reproduced with permission from Chaitow (2001)

Research was carried out on the cerebral haemodynamics of patients with cerebral birth injury before and after acupressure (percussion as well as compression techniques) therapy. Scanning techniques were used in monitoring the short half-life radioactive materials through the cerebral circulation; in almost one-third of the patients the regional cerebral blood flow was increased after therapy ranging from 28 to 60 sessions. (Zhao-Pu 1991)

This approach is, therefore, not one that produces instant results, but that influences and gradually harnesses the potential for recovery and improvement that is latent in the tissues of the patient.

For more information on oriental bodywork approaches, a complete manual of Chinese therapeutic massage (with many aspects that echo NMT methodology), edited by Sun Chengnan (1990), is highly recommended.

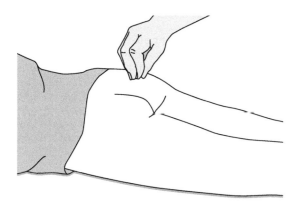

Figure 7.25 Five-finger percussion uses thumb and all fingers. Reproduced with permission from Chaitow (2001)

Safety

There seem no obvious risks from these methods, if cautions (below) are observed.

Validation of efficacy = 4 (see Table 7.2)

Based on anecdotal reporting (see citations in TCM percussion discussion above) and clinical experience.

Alternatives

Manual spondylotherapy complements NMT methodology (see above) by virtue of its reflex influences and its ease of application.

Physiological effects

In TCM, as well as hypothesized energy transmission, percussion is thought to 'stimulate circulation of blood . . . and improving conductivity of nerves' (Zhao-Pu 1991).

The mechanical stimulation of neural structures is a feature of many manual methods.

Schafer (1987) points out that 'neuroinhibition' is initiated by sustained pressure. He gives the example of a muscle spasm that can be released by placing the muscle in a position of functional rest followed by application of sustained pressure.

On the other hand, neurostimulation is most easily achieved by deep and rapid short-duration percussion at a rate of approximately 2 per second – interspersed with brief rest periods as suggested by Janse et al (above). If such percussion is prolonged, an inhibitory effect is likely.

Cautions

- Acute disease
- Severe heart disease
- Tuberculosis
- Malignant tumors
- Hemorrhagic disease
- Skin disease in area to be treated
- Poor constitutional states such as malnutrition or asthenia

Naturopathic perspectives

The use of percussion to stimulate or decrease visceral activity as part of a therapeutic intervention, where such outcomes seem to offer benefit to self-regulation, fits with naturopathic principles.

Thiele massage (for pelvic floor dysfunction)

Indications/description

High-tone pelvic floor dysfunction (PFD) that results in a variety of dysfunctional conditions including interstitial cystitis, stress incontinence, pelvic pain, dyspareunia, etc., has been treated using intra-anal or intravaginal massage of key muscles since the 1930s when Thiele described a successful manual approach to what he termed 'coccygodynia'.

High-tone PFD refers to the clinical condition of hypertonic, spastic pelvic floor musculature commonly associated with pelvic floor discomfort and the potential for resultant impairment of pelvic floor function. This was reported in 1937 by Thiele, in conditions in which coccygeal pain was accompanied by the presence of levator ani and coccygeus muscle spasm.

Methodology

There are a variety of protocols currently involving variations of Thiele massage. One typical protocol (Oyama et al 2004) is summarized as follows:

The technique consisted of massage from origin to insertion along the direction of the muscle fibers with an amount of pressure tolerable to the subject. The motion was performed 10 to 15 times during each session to each of the following muscles in order: coccygeus, iliococcygeus, pubococcygeus, and obturator internus. At the practitioner's discretion, 10 to 15 seconds of ischemic compression was applied to trigger points. A typical treatment lasted fewer than 5 minutes. Each massage was scheduled at least 2 days apart to allow for any inflammation or discomfort from the previous session to subside. Patients received two massages per week for a period of 5 weeks.

The researchers in this study noted that:

The technique is easy to learn and carries minimal risk. Nurses, or even the patient's partner, can learn and apply the technique, making this therapy accessible to patients unable to see a physical therapist.

Weiss (2001) used a slightly different approach in treating similar problems, in which patients received pelvic floor muscle compression, stretching, and right angle 'strumming', with the simultaneous use of external muscle stretching or heat application to facilitate greater muscle relaxation. This was followed by transvaginal or transrectal posterior traction with an isometric contraction of the pubovaginalis to help relax and elongate the muscle.

French osteopathic research (Riot et al 2005) has shown the value of Thiele massage in treating irritable bowel syndrome (IBS) problems in which there was a combination of massage of the coccygeus muscle, together with physical treatment of frequently associated pelvic joint disorders. The researchers noted that levator ani syndrome (LVAS) symptoms may be cured or alleviated with just one to two sessions of Thiele massage in 72% of the cases at 12 months, and since most of the IBS symptoms were relieved by such treatment, it is logical to suspect a mutual etiology, and to screen for LVAS in all IBS patients.

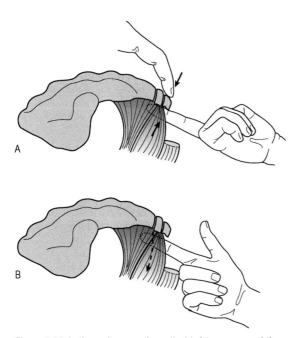

Figure 7.26 In these diagrams the patient is lying prone and the practitioner's finger is inserted into the rectum. The sacrum is on the left and the coccyx is on the right. A coccyx with two segments is shown here but coccyges can be in one, two, three or four segments. **A** Assessment of pelvic muscle tone. **B** Thiele massage in the direction of the fibers. Redrawn from Maigne & Chatellier (2001)

Safety

There are clear issues relating to the potential for inappropriate entry to anal and vaginal orifices, making it essential for informed consent, and the presence of a chaperon when these methods are used. Licensing and scope of practice issues are also of paramount importance. The treatment itself, if protocols are followed, is relatively painless, commonly successful in mitigating distressing symptoms, and carries little or no risk.

Validation of efficacy = 5 (see Table 7.2)

There are numerous validating examples of the safe and effective use of Thiele massage in treatment of coccydynia, interstitial cystitis (Holzberg et al 2001), pelvic pain, stress incontinence, high-tone pelvic floor problems, etc., and even chronic prostatitis (Anderson et al 2005). These conditions have been noted by some researchers to be frequently associated with sacroiliac dysfunction (Lukban et al 2001).

Alternatives

Cognitive behavioral therapy, used as part of manual therapy, is advocated by some researchers (McCracken & Turk 2002):

Our premise is that, in addition to releasing painful myofascial TrPs, the patient must supply the central nervous system with new information or awareness to progressively quiet the pelvic floor.

Surgery and a variety of electrical approaches (Caraballoa et al 2001) are used in treating such conditions.

Regrettably, since most such problems appear to involve excessive tone of the pelvic floor muscles, many such patients are referred for Kegel-type toning exercise, with predictably negative results.

A question also needs to be asked regarding inappropriate use of core-stability (Pilates) type exercises for such patients, who above all need to reduce tone rather than increase it.

Physiological effects

Removal of sensitized, local, pain-generating areas (trigger points) and normalization of high-tone muscles appears to allow normal function to be restored in many patients with apparently intractable pelvic problems.

Cautions

* Active inflammatory conditions or actual pathology involving the tissues of the region.

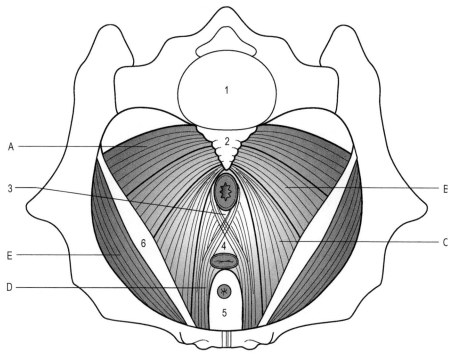

Figure 7.27 Schematic drawing of a cranial view of the pelvic floor. Muscles: A, coccygeus; B, iliococcygeus; C, pubococcygeus; D, puborectalis; E, obturatorius internus. Structures: 1, sacrum; 2, coccyx; 3, anus; 4, vagina; 5, urethra; 6. tendinous arch of the levator ani muscle. Redrawn from Pool-Goudzwaard et al (2004)

- Clearly since this approach is aimed at reducing tone it will be of little value in conditions associated with low-tone pelvic floor musculature – where toning exercises are more appropriate.

Visceral manipulation

Indications/description

Indirect approaches
Researchers such as the French osteopaths Barral & Mercier (1988) and the British osteopath Caroline Stone (1999) have documented the existence – in health – of symmetry in inherent axes of rotation (mobility and motility) in the motions of organs. With disease, these motions are claimed to be at variance with one another.

Influences on visceral motion include body movement, diaphragmatic activity, cardiac pulsations and peristaltic activity. Additionally, there exists an inherent organ motility, possibly relating to embryological development phases.

As an example, Barral & Mercier describe how, during the development of the fetus, the stomach rotates to the right in the transverse plane and clockwise in the frontal plane. The transverse rotation therefore orients the anterior lesser curve of the stomach to the right and the greater posterior curvature to the left. The pylorus is therefore rotated superiorly and the cardia inferiorly. These researchers suggest that these directions 'remain inscribed in the visceral tissues' with motion occurring around an axis, a point of balance, as it moves further into the direction of embryological motion and then returns to neutral.

The motility cycle is divided by Barral & Mercier into two phases which are termed *inspir* and *expir*, that are unrelated to the breathing cycle.

Inspir describes the inherent motion and *expir* the return to neutral afterwards (7–8 cycles per minute). An example of this is that the liver's inherent *inspir* phase involves rotation posterosuperiorly (its mobility, as influenced by inhalation's diaphragmatic movement, is almost exactly opposite, anteroinferior).

In palpation, it is claimed that it is usually easier to feel the *expir* phase (although *inspir* is more 'active', as there is less resistance to it), being a return to neutral.

Just as joints have articulations, so do viscera. These are made of sliding surfaces (meninges in the CNS, pleura in the lungs, peritoneum in the abdominal cavity and pericardium in the heart) as well as a system of attachments (including ligaments, intercavity pressure, various folds of peritoneal structures forming containment and supportive elements). Unlike most joints, few muscular forces directly move organs.

Stone has described the movement of organs:

Visceral biomechanics relate to the movements that the organs make against each other, and against the walls of the body cavities that contain them. The viscera 'articulate' by utilizing sliding surfaces formed by the peritoneal (and pleural or pericardial) membranes that surround the organs and line the body cavities. [Due to normal body movement including bending and locomotion, as well as body processes such as micturition] . . . as the body cavities distort and change their shape, so the individual organs must adapt to those changes, and they do so by slightly sliding over each other, given the constraints of their attachments and surrounds.

Direct approaches

Where adhesions have occurred, more direct, stretching methods have been employed, as discussed in Chapter 3 (Fielder & Pyott 1955). See also notes under subheading 'Validation of efficacy', below.

Naturopath and chiropractor Stanley Lief, developer of neuromuscular technique (see NMT description earlier in this chapter), utilized variations on the methods of 'bloodless surgery' described by Fielder & Pyott (1955).

Lief's cousin and collaborator, Boris Chaitow ND DC, described the value of this approach (personal communication, 1983) as follows:

It can be safely asserted that there is no one in middle age and older who has not, unfortunately, developed some of the tensions, contractions, adhesions, nerve and muscle spasms in various parts of the gastro-intestinal tract and abdominal cavity. All these would normally be outside the scope of the conventional manual therapist. But, with [this] technique, a practitioner can achieve almost dramatic benefits.

Lief devised a special technique for the abdomen known as 'bloodless surgery' – a method of breaking up deep-seated adhesions and contractions. This method also enables the practitioner to improve function and circulation related to female problems such as dysmenorrhoea, menorrhagia and amenorrhoea, fibroids.

Boris Chaitow described this method as follows:

*For the technique . . . palpate [the abdomen] with the tips of the fingers of the right hand, and having located the area of abnormal feel, place those four fingers as a group at the distal border of the lesioned area, and place the thumb of the left hand alongside the nails of the right fingers. Give a **sharp** flick with both hands simultaneously, the left hand thumb being twisted anticlockwise, and the fingers of the right hand clockwise (difficult if not impossible to describe on paper). This achieves an appreciable breaking-up, without trauma or hurt to the patient, of tensions, adhesions, congestions, etc., both on the wall of the abdomen and structures within the cavity. Obviously these flicks with the hands need to be repeated a number of times to feel a discernible difference in the lesioned tissue. Stanley Lief achieved dramatic changes in tissue structure and functional improvements in many types of abdominal stresses including digestive problems, gall bladder blockage, gall stones, constipation, spastic colon, colic, colitis, uterine fibroids, dysmenorrhoea, menorrhagia, small non-malignant abdominal tumours, postoperative adhesions, etc.*

(See Exercise 3 in Box 7.19, and Figure 7.32.)

Methodology

Indirect

The methodology of positional release is commonly utilized in visceral manipulation, i.e. the tissues are palpated and held towards their direction of greatest freedom of movement. See the exercises in Box 7.19, particularly Exercise 2, in which mesenteric restrictions are palpated and held in positions of 'ease' (preferred directions of movement).

Direct

Alternatively, more direct methods, involving stretching of perceived adhesions and restrictions, might be used (see under 'Validation of efficacy', below; Exercise 3 in Box 7.19; and Fig. 7.32).

Safety

The methods of indirect visceral manipulation are seldom invasive, replicating the methodology described in positional release, earlier in this chapter.

No pain should be noted during their application.

Direct approaches require caution and an accurate diagnosis, as fairly deep and invasive work is involved when attempting to alter adhesion status.

Validation of efficacy = 3 (see Table 7.2)

There is limited research validation, despite a wide range of clinical usage, particularly amongst osteopathic practitioners and those therapists using cranial ('craniosacral') manipulation.

In physical therapy (physiotherapy) settings more direct methods are employed. For example, Pierce & Webber (1996) report that:

Visceral manipulation is a treatment involving specific stretching techniques to the connective tissue around restricted organs. Using these techniques, a trained therapist is able to break down the adhesions formed between the connective tissue layers over individual organs. Studies have shown that adhesions are formed when the serous fluid between connective tissues thickens and becomes more viscous in nature during the inflammatory process. This phenomenon can occur after trauma such as motor vehicle accidents, direct blows to the rib cage, surgery, and some illnesses. In some fibromyalgia patients, visceral manipulation therapy may offer an important adjunctive therapy towards the restoration of efficient lateral-costal breathing. The data presented illustrates pre and post-treatment ETC.02 values (an increase from 30mmHg to 39mmHg) and a qualitative change in rib cage movement, after visceral manipulation therapy, in a 51 year old female patient with repetitive strain injury.

Alternatives

Mobilization methods (see earlier in this chapter as well as Chapter 8), massage and yoga asanas, as well as various osteopathic 'pump' techniques, should all be capable of non-specific visceral 'manipulation'; however, specific focused mobilization of organs that display restricted excursion in their normal movements would seem to be safely achieved by use of the visceral manipulation strategies outlined in this review.

Physiological effects

Enhanced mobility and motility would be anticipated to produce functional improvement, as well as enhanced circulation to, and drainage from, organs.

Cautions

- Malignant or other serious diseases of the lungs, liver, spleen or associated organs
- Recent abdominal or thoracic surgery
- Hepatitis
- Infectious mononucleosis
- Osteoporosis
- Fracture, dislocation or other painful dysfunction involving the joints of the thoracic cage or spine

Naturopathic perspectives

The methods employed in visceral manipulation fit well with naturopathic concepts of enhancing functionality without negative side-effects. As explained in Chapter 3, there is a long tradition of focused attention to the structures of the viscera. The less invasive evolutions of visceral manipulation, as well as the traditional direct methods – where necessary – should be part of the repertoire of NDs.

Further reading

1. Barral J-P, Mercier P 1988 Visceral manipulation. Eastland Press, Seattle
2. Stone C 1999 The science and art of osteopathy. Stanley Thornes, Cheltenham

---

Box 7.19 Visceral manipulation exercises

Exercise 1: Liver palpation

1. The person to be palpated should be supine.
2. You should be seated or standing on the right, facing the patient.
3. Place your right hand over the lower ribs, molding to their curve, covering the outer aspect of the liver. Your left hand should be laid over the right hand. Your mind should be stilled as you visualize the liver.
4. Ideally with eyes closed you are trying to assess the return to neutral (the expir phase of the motility cycle), which means that the direction of active motion would be the opposite to that palpated during this phase.
5. During the expir phase, three simultaneous motions may be noted:

- In the frontal plane, a counter-clockwise motion, from right to left, around the sagittal axis (of your hand and therefore the liver). This takes the palm of the hand towards the umbilicus (see Fig. 7.30).
- In the sagittal plane the superior part of the hand should rotate anteroinferiorly around a transverse axis through the middle of your hand.
- In the transverse plane, the hand rotates to the left around a vertical axis, bringing the palm off the body as the fingers seem to press more closely.

6. Each of these planes of movement can be assessed separately before they are assessed simultaneously, providing a clear picture of liver motility in the expir phase of the cycle (inspir is the exact opposite).
7. This palpation exercise should be performed with eyes closed.

Continued

Box 7.19 Visceral manipulation exercises continued

8. Periodically the patient should be asked to hold the breath for a 20-second period, to see whether this provides a less confused feeling of motion.

Exercise 2: Reducing visceral 'drag' and pelvic pain

Kuchera (1997) points to various ways in which pain and discomfort can arise in the pelvic and abdominal viscera, due to irritation or inflammation:

- A 'vague, gnawing, deep, poorly localized and mid-abdominal' pain may derive from irritation of contiguous peritoneal tissues and the abdominal wall.
- Or abdominopelvic pain may be due to reflex pain from different organs, or the spinal cord.
- Pain may also derive from a dragging force imposed on the mesentery (the double layer of peritoneal membrane that supports the small intestine) when organs and tissues have sagged (visceroptosis), irritating the peritoneal tissues (see Figs 7.30 and 7.31).

Kuchera suggests that tenderness and tension in the mesentery (see Fig. 7.30) can be palpated for tension, and treated as follows:

- Place the extended fingers flat over the lateral margin of the ascending or descending colon and, moving the viscera toward the midline of the body, monitor for changes in resistance to this movement.
- The mesentery of the sigmoid colon is moved toward the umbilicus (see Fig. 7.30A).
- Palpate the mesentery, along with the small intestines, by placing the extended fingers carefully into the lower left abdominal quadrant to make indirect contact with as much of the small intestines as possible.
- This is moved toward the upper right quadrant of the abdomen (see Fig. 7.30B).

To treat restrictions noted in such palpation:

- The patient lies supine, with knees flexed and feet flat on the table.

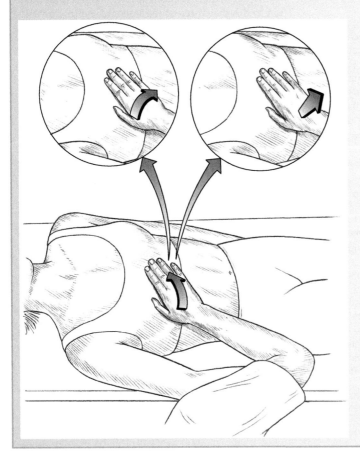

Figure 7.28 Palpation of the liver in which frontal, sagittal and transverse planes of motion are sequentially accessed. Reproduced with permission from Chaitow (2003)

Box 7.19 Visceral manipulation exercises continued

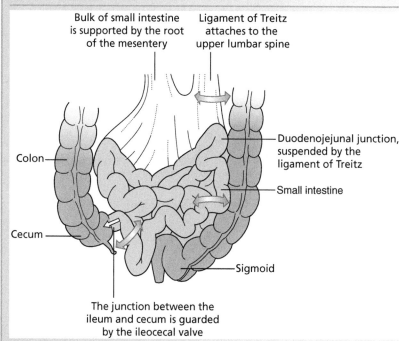

Bulk of small intestine is supported by the root of the mesentery

Ligament of Treitz attaches to the upper lumbar spine

Colon

Cecum

Duodenojejunal junction, suspended by the ligament of Treitz

Small intestine

Sigmoid

The junction between the ileum and cecum is guarded by the ileocecal valve

Figure 7.29 Suspensory mesenteric ligaments supporting the small intestine attach to the spine. Reproduced with permission from Chaitow (2003)

- The therapist's fingers are extended and placed flat over the lateral margin of the mesentery (to be treated) (see Fig. 7.31).
- Medial pressure is then applied to the 'restricted' section of bowel, at right angles to its posterior (mesenteric) abdominal wall attachment.
- The tension is held as the patient takes a half-breath and holds it.
- No pain should be produced by this.
- After release of the breath the tissues being held should be gently 'turned' clockwise and anticlockwise, to sense their position of greatest tissue freedom.
- The tissues are then held for not less than 90 seconds, or until a sense of relaxation is noted.
- When breathing resumes after this positional release approach, the tissues should be re-palpated.

Exercise 3: 'Breaking adhesions' (Chaitow 1980)
(modified from Lief's method as described earlier)

1. Having located an area of contracted (often sensitive) tissue, the middle finger locates the point of maximum resistance and the tissues are drawn towards the practitioner, to the limit of pain-free movement.
2. The middle finger (right hand) and its neighbors should be flexed, fairly rigid, and be imparting force

in two directions at this stage, i.e. downwards (towards the floor, into the tissues being treated) and towards the practitioner. (In 'bloodless surgery' techniques, the right hand is always 'on' the 'adhesion', and the other in contact with the organ to which the lesion is attached, as far as this is possible.)

3. With the fingers maintaining the above position, the thumb of the left hand is placed almost touching – no more than $1/4$ inch (6 mm) away – adjacent to the middle finger of the right hand, in such a way that a downward pressure (towards the floor) will provide a fulcrum point against which force can be applied via the right hand, in order to stretch or reduce the degree of contraction in the tissue (or indeed to break or 'peel' adhesions).
4. The thumb should also be flexed, and the contact can be via its tip or its lateral border, or a combination of both.
5. The idea of a fulcrum is important because the two points of contact are both on soft tissue structures, and the effect of the manipulation is achieved, not by pulling or twisting these apart, but by a combination of movements that impart torsional and shear forces in several directions at the same time.
6. This is accomplished by an *extremely rapid* clockwise movement of the right hand (middle finger

Continued

Box 7.19 Visceral manipulation exercises continued

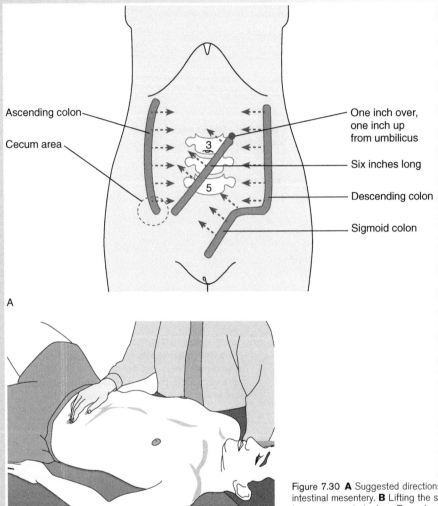

Ascending colon

Cecum area

One inch over,
one inch up
from umbilicus

Six inches long

Descending colon

Sigmoid colon

A

B

Figure 7.30 **A** Suggested directions of movement in treating intestinal mesentery. **B** Lifting the small intestine/sigmoid colon to ease mesenteric drag. Reproduced with permission from Chaitow (2001)

contact) against the stabilizing anchorage of the left thumb (see Fig. 7.32).

7. Synchronous movement of the thumb, during this release, is not essential or necessary. However, a degree of additional torsional force can be achieved by *rapidly* releasing the thumb contact in an anticlockwise direction at the moment of manipulation.

8. With both hands in contact, as described, and the contact digits flexed and rigid, the practitioner should be so positioned as to lean over the affected area, knees lightly flexed, with the legs separated for stability, and elbows flexed and separated to a point of 180° separation. The force

that will be present at the point of contact is a downward one, to which is added a slight separation of the hands, which increases the tension on the affected tissues. The manipulative force is imparted by a rapid (high velocity) flicking of the right thumb contact in a clockwise direction, whilst maintaining the left thumb contact (or taking it equally rapidly in an anticlockwise direction).

9. The effect of the right hand movement would be to snap the right elbow towards the practitioner's side. If a double release is performed, then both elbows will come rapidly to the sides.

10. The amount of force imparted should be controlled so that no pain is felt by the patient.

Box 7.19 Visceral manipulation exercises continued

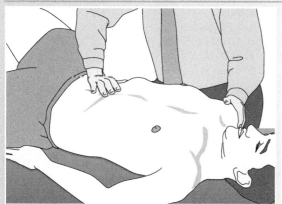

Figure 7.31 Lifting the cecum to ease mesenteric drag. Reproduced with permission from Chaitow (2001)

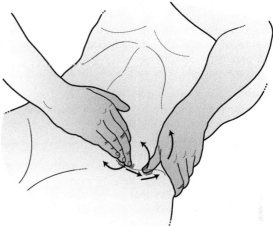

Figure 7.32 Specific release technique for adhesions

The essence of this technique is the speed with which it is applied. This very high velocity release involves tissues that have been 'wound up' by being taken in at least three directions of distraction – compression, separation and a degree of torsion – and its success depends upon this as much as the correct positioning of the hands and the exact location of the area of tissue dysfunction.

The same procedure can be repeated several times on the same area, and the release of a number of such areas of contracted or indurated tissue at any one treatment is usual. The same thumb contact is often maintained whilst variations in the direction of tissue

tension are dealt with by slightly altering the angle of the right hand contact and manipulative effort.

If, after manipulation, no objective improvement is noted on palpation, the angle of the contacts should be varied. Nothing will be gained, however, by attempting to use excessive force in order to achieve results. As the degree of soft tissue trauma to the patient is minimal, the after-effects should not include bruising or much discomfort. Any such after-effect would indicate undue pressure or force.

Other areas: Precisely the same technique can be usefully applied to the tensor fascia lata to reduce extreme contraction and induration.

Yoga

This topic is discussed in greater depth in Chapter 9.

Yogic therapies are based on self-regulation. The practice and study of yoga are claimed to help bring about a natural balance of body and mind in which optimal health can more readily manifest (Galantino et al 2000, Raub 2002).

Yoga aims to help to keep the spine flexible, muscles strong and bones dense (Birkel 1998). Research studies have shown that through the practice of yoga it is possible to learn to beneficially influence blood pressure, heart rate, respiratory function, metabolic rate, skin resistance, brain waves, body temperature and other bodily functions (DiCarlo et al 1995, Tran et al 2001). In treatment of orthopedic problems Garfinkel et al (1998) have demonstrated the usefulness of yoga in treating carpal tunnel syndrome.

The energy centers of the human body are referred to in yoga as 'chakras' ('wheel'). These are conceived as vortices of subtle energy operating through the autonomic nervous system (Gerber 1988, Hunt 1978).

Yogic approaches emphasize somatopsychic functioning in the present and not with past psychological history, differentiating yoga from most current psychotherapeutic techniques (Garde 1972).

Historical and theoretical perspective (Singh 2006)

The yoga system traditionally belongs to the Six system or 'shad-darsanas' of classical Hindu philosophy. The Sanskrit term yoga means 'the union of the individual self with transcendental self'. Compiled comprehensively by Patanjali, the system of yoga forms a bridge between the philosophy of ancient India and the fully developed Buddhism in the transcendental dimension of spiritual consciousness. Yogic approaches involve self-evolution and are claimed to act as a vehicle for successfully controlling pathological expression of biological psychic and social parameters of illness.

There are multiple yoga variations, including:

1. Kriya yoga: a preparatory yoga
2. Karma yoga: a means to attain enlightenment through everyday social activities
3. Hatha yoga: one of the most popular approaches where attainment of higher self is achieved by physical, physiological and psychological training, often involving complicated postures that are practiced for therapeutic purposes
4. Bhakti yoga: involves veneration of personified 'deities'
5. Jnana yoga: philosophical contemplation
6. Mantra yoga: special words are chanted
7. Raja yoga: emphasizes attaining mental development, mental self-control
8. Tantric yoga: utilizes the mystic but physiological notions of increasing the psychic power based on power called kundalini.

The path of yoga involves eight factors:

1. Yama – abstentions, or extinction of bad habits
2. Niyama – virtue or moral purification; gradual construction of positive behaviors
3. Asana – meditation postures or dynamic position of the human body statically maintained for a certain length of time.
4. Pranayama – control of vital breath
5. Pratyahara – channeling of mental activities
6. Dharana – concentration of the mind – focusing on ever fewer objects until aware of only one
7. Dhyana – concentrated meditation
8. Samadhi – transcendental super-consciousness.

Yoga is a vast topic and there is no attempt at a comprehensive summary of its methods and concepts in this text.

The value of the application of yogic practice is clearly demonstrated in Chapter 10, where its benefit has been shown in treatment of patients with numerous conditions and pathologies.

A summary of conditions in which yoga has been shown to have value in research studies (see Box 10.6, Chapter 10) includes the following:

- Anxiety (Selvamurthy 1994)
- Bronchial asthma (Faling 1986, Manocha et al 2002)
- Cardiovascular disease (Harinath et al 2004) related to diabetes (Malhotra et al 2002, Singh et al 2004)
- Chronic sinusitis (Telles et al 1994)
- Depression (Khumar et al 1993, Pilkington et al 2005)
- Epilepsy (Ramaratnam & Sridharan 2000)
- Headache (Latha & Kaliappan 1992)
- Hypertension (Patel & North 1975)
- Insomnia in cancer patients (Cohen et al 2004) and the elderly (Manjunath & Telles 2005)
- Irritable bowel syndrome and gastritis (Taneja et al 2004)
- Low back pain (Galantino et al 2004)
- Menstrual disorders (Chen 2005, Sridevi & Krishna-Rao 1996)
- Multiple sclerosis (Oken et al 2004)
- Peptic ulcer (Bhole 1983)
- Psychosomatic conditions (Goyeche & Ikemi 1977, Singh 2006)
- Stress-related symptoms in epilepsy (Panjwani et al 1995).

Zero balancing

Roger Newman Turner ND DO BAc

Indications/description

The creator of zero balancing (ZB), Dr Fritz Frederick Smith, prefers not to describe it as a technique so much as an approach to harmonizing of energy and structure in the body (Zero Balancing Health Association). Zero balancing – the name derives from the description of one of Smith's patients of a session she had just received – consists of a series of held stretches and manual fulcra applied at articulations and bony landmarks. It focuses on groups of joints in the body that are involved in the smooth transmission of the forces through the weight-bearing skeleton. The holding of a fixed point allows what is said to be an energetic change to take place and encourages natural realignment (Zero Balancing Association UK).

The very gentle manual procedures of ZB work in conformity with the naturopathic principle of facilitating self-regulation and it is particularly suited to elderly or hyper-reactive patients and those in acute pain for whom more vigorous physical therapy is too uncomfortable.

Methodology

After initial assessment of coordination and range of movement while walking and sitting, treatment is usually applied with the patient supine and, since tactile sensation is not critical to assessment, the patient may remain clothed. The intention is to engage with the energy of the patient by a series of contacts known as fulcra. Smith (1994) describes this as:

> . . . putting a pressure in the body which needs to be greater than the pressure holding the tissue in its current form. We lift the body, for example by placing our hands under a person's back when they are lying down, and we hold the body in a state of balance.

Lauterstein (1994) describes the process as follows:

> The ZB fulcrum is built by the therapist in such a manner that his or her energy and structure is brought into contact with, 'interfaces', with the energy and structure of a client. In addition to this structural/energetic interface at least two other dimensions are added to the fulcrum. This will result in a complicated geometric form through which to affect the client. The therapist may, for instance, take up the slack then traction and rotate at a joint. Or one may cradle the head and neck, then lift up in a graceful arc. Or, making contact with the ribs, gently press into them summarizing two or more vectors of force. Once this complex touch is achieved, it is held. Noting that 'a person cannot not react', Dr. Smith observed that a fulcrum, when sustained, will often stimulate a deep reaction within the being. Holding this space open is akin to quiet forms of meditation.

Once slack is taken up, energy is engaged by moving the joint into a second or third plane where it is held for a few seconds until signs of energy change are noted in the patient by the therapist. These usually take the form of a sigh, rapid eye movement or audible borborygmus. Fulcra are applied in specific sequence to key points and areas of energetic significance, especially the foundation joints. While the best results may be achieved by applying the full sequence as taught by instructors of ZB, it is possible to apply the approach to specific areas of restriction, such as the cervical spine or sacroiliac region. To be able to apply ZB effectively, however, it is essential to undergo training to a certification level because of the important experiential nature of the procedures.

Safety

Because the contact of ZB works only to the natural point of resistance of the patient's tissues, the risk of adverse events is minimal. Having been developed a little over 30 years ago, very little published material has found its way to the peer-reviewed literature and no adverse events have been reported.

Validation of efficacy = 2 (see Table 7.2)

Most accounts of ZB focus on its general application rather than specific conditions and any published reports are anecdotal.

Lauterstein (1994) gives a good account of the scope of its application:

> Because the proper function of the skeletal system is one of the theoretical bases for ZB and the literal basis underlying the muscles and fascia of the body, soft-tissue pain and dysfunction are often relieved through ZB. Headaches, neck and shoulder pain, low back dysfunction and many other physical symptoms may be dramatically affected by the application of the various fulcrums. Similarly, alignment will be improved through the attention paid to the foundation joints. Clients report the experience of a new uprightness and enhanced relationship of their body to gravity. Feelings of being taller and lighter with a greater fluidity to each of one's everyday movements are commonly reported. Although more difficult to prove, it is certainly hoped that ZB, as it brings the deepest structures and energetic domains of the body into graceful balance, has an ameliorative impact on disease and degenerative processes in the body.

The author can corroborate much of this from clinical experience using ZB as an adjunct to osteopathic manipulation and naturopathic soft-tissue procedures.

Alternatives

ZB bears certain similarities to positional release technique, strain/counterstrain and myofascial release, and these would be suitable (although sometimes more challenging) alternatives in cases of hypersensitivity.

Physiological effects

According to Smith's premise, ZB works through the body structure to harmonize function (Smith 1986). He describes the structural body as the bones, muscles and organs whilst the energy body is expressed through the movement of muscles, fluids, and cellular and molecular vibrations. The densest energy is conveyed through the skeletal system and it is through the bony articulations that the ZB fulcra are believed to exert their greatest effect.

The joints of the body are categorized according to their range of movement and motor control:

- *Foundation joints* – have no voluntary control and a small range of movement, e.g. cranial bones, symphysis pubis, carpals, tarsals
- *Semi-foundation joints* – have limited voluntary movement and this is collective rather than individual, e.g. intervertebral articulations and costovertebral and sternocostal joints
- *Freely moveable joints* – these may be moved voluntarily to varying degrees.

ZB fulcra are held to the endpoints of motion of the freely moveable joints but also applied to foundation and semi-foundation joints where appropriate.

Patterns of restriction may become established by postural stress or trauma that can be disruptive without obvious signs of physical injury. This may call for the application of a stronger force field to overcome the tension pattern. Smith describes a case in which a patient had been involved in a road traffic accident 13 months prior to treatment. Under medical care he was found to have no significant bodily injuries other than bruising.

When I examined the background energy field, however, I found a strong twisting current extending from the right side of his chest to the left side of his abdomen. This flow through the trunk represented the imprinting from the twisting force to which the body was subjected as the car rolled down the embankment.

Once I felt the torquing energy currents, I remained in touch with that field and exerted a slightly stronger force field through his body by increasing my traction on his legs. Holding this stronger field, I had the sensation of a rebounding effect along the energy imprint itself. By anchoring the new field, I let the rebounding subside. When it was complete, I gradually released my hold in the energy body, then the physical body, and then rested his legs on the table. Immediately after this Zero Balancing, the man felt a great sense of grounding and quietness. When I examined him again two days later, he reported he had been free of pain since the treatment and felt internal calm and well being. Checking the energy field, I found that the twisting currents were gone. I know from experience that stronger patterns are imprinted

---

Box 7.20 Exercise: Zero balancing (see Fig. 7.33)

The following exercise in assessment of bone, described by Dr F.F. Smith in his book *Inner Bridges*, is a useful way of developing the sense of energy in structure.

Assessment of the bone

Reading energy currents and flows within the bone itself can most easily be demonstrated by evaluating the long bones of the body. There is a general axiom that no one is symmetrical. No two forearms will energetically feel the same. This can easily be demonstrated: Take hold of a person's forearm above the wrist and below the elbow, and gently put a bending or 'bow' movement into the arm.

After taking up the slack of the physical body and soft tissues, the resistance of the bone itself will be encountered. Make a bowing motion in one direction and then gently release this tension; then make a bowing motion in the opposite direction. Try this several times, once with the eyes open, and once with the eyes closed. Repeat the exercise on the person's other forearm and compare the findings.

In a 'normal' uninjured extremity, the arm may bow more easily in one direction than the other; one bow may feel obstructed; or the bow may have the suggestion of a twisting motion. Similarly, one forearm may feel like a steel bar while the other may feel like rubber.

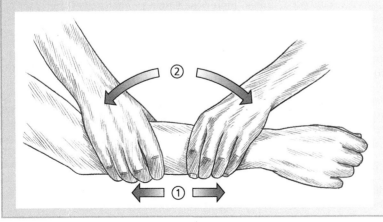

Figure 7.33 Smith's palpation exercise to assess the interface between the physical and the 'energetic' structures of the arm. Reproduced with permission from Chaitow (2003)

in different degrees of indelibility, and that a number of balancing sessions are often required for their improvement.

Cautions

- Acute arthritis and other inflammatory conditions
- Bone fractures or acute soft tissue injuries
- Recent prosthetic surgery, i.e. hips, knees
- Hemophilia
- Hodgkinson's disease
- Malignancy with metastasis (or TB) involving bone
- Pain production during procedure
- Phlebitis

Naturopathic perspectives

In common with other minimally intrusive techniques, ZB conforms very well with naturopathic objectives of restoring homeostasis. Although principally achieving this 'transformation through stillness' (Smith 1994) at a structural level, ZB can help to bring the body into balance on many levels.

Further reading

1. Smith FF 1986 Inner bridges: a guide to energy movement and body structure. Humanics New Age, Atlanta, Georgia
2. Smith FF 2005 The alchemy of touch: moving towards mastery through the lens of zero balancing. Complementary Medicine Press, Taos, New Mexico
3. Hamwee J 1999 Zero balancing – touching the energy of bone. Francis Lincoln, London

Conclusion

The summaries of modalities outlined in this chapter are far from comprehensive. They do, however, provide a background to many of the methods used in NPM, and offer an outline of what is possible in terms of health provision via manual individual methodologies. In the next chapter constitutional models of manual medicine are explored.

References

Abbate G 2004 Chiropractic neck manipulation linked to woman's death. Globe and Mail, Toronto, Ontario, January 17. Online. Available: www.globeandmail.com/servlet/story/RTGAM.20040117.wchiro0117/BNStory/Front/

Abbott JH 2001 Mobilization with movement applied to the elbow affects shoulder range of movement in subjects with lateral epicondylalgia. Manual Therapy 6(3):170–177

Abrams A 1922 New concepts in diagnosis and treatment. Physioclinical Co., San Francisco

Adams F 1946 (translator) The genuine works of Hippocrates. Williams & Wilkins, Baltimore, p 212–214

Aina A, May S, Clare H 2004 The centralization phenomenon of spinal symptoms – a systematic review. Manual Therapy 9(3):134–143

Aksenova AM, Teslenko OI, Boganskaia OA 1999 [Changes in the immune status of peptic ulcer patients after combined treatment including deep massage] [article in Russian]. Voprosy Kurortologii, Fizioterapii, Lechebnoi Fizicheskoi Kultury 2:19–20

Akuthota V, Nadler S 2004 Core strengthening. Archives of Physical Medicine and Rehabilitation 85(3 Suppl 1):S86–92

Alexander FM 1984 (originally 1932) The use of the self. Centerline Press, Downey, CA

Alexander FM 1996 (originally 1910) In: Fisher JMO (ed) Man's supreme inheritance. Mouritz, London

Almekinders L 1993 Anti-inflammatory treatment of muscular injuries in sports. Sports Medicine 15:139–145

American Stroke Association 2007 Stroke risk factors. Online. Available: www.strokeassociation.org/presenter.jhtml?identifier=4716

Anderson BD, Spector A 2000 Introduction to Pilates-based rehabilitation. Orthopaedic Physical Therapy Clinics of North America 9:395–410

Anderson R, Wise D, Sawyer T et al 2005 Integration of myofascial trigger point release and paradoxical relaxation training treatment of chronic pelvic pain in men. Journal of Urology 174(1):155–160

Andersson G, Lucente T, Davis A et al 1999 A comparison of osteopathic spinal manipulation with standard care for patients with low back pain. New England Journal of Medicine 341(19):1426–1431

Arbuckle B 1977 Selected writings of Beryl Arbuckle. National Osteopathic Institute and Cerebral Palsy Foundation

Assendelft W, Morton S, Yu E et al 2003 Spinal manipulative therapy for low back pain. A meta-analysis of effectiveness relative to other therapies. Annals of Internal Medicine 138:871–881

Aust G, Fischer K 1997 Changes in body equilibrium response caused by breathing. A posturographic study with visual feedback. Laryngorhinootologie 76(10):577–582

Bachman T, Lantz C 1991 Management of pediatric asthma and enuresis. In: Proceedings of National Conference on Chiropractic Pediatrics. International Chiropractic Association, Arlington, VA, p 14

Bailey M, Dick L 1992 Nociceptive considerations in treating with counterstrain. Journal of the American Osteopathic Association 92(3):334, 337–341

Baldry P 1993 Acupuncture, trigger points and musculoskeletal pain. Churchill Livingstone, Edinburgh, p 91–103

Ballantyne F, Fryer G, McLaughlin P 2003 The effect of muscle energy technique on hamstring extensibility: the mechanism of altered flexibility. Journal of Osteopathic Medicine 6(2):59–63

Barnes J 1996 Myofascial release in treatment of thoracic outlet syndrome. Journal of Bodywork and Movement Therapies 1(1):53–57

Barnes M 1997 The basic science of myofascial release. Journal of Bodywork and Movement Therapies 1(4):231–238

Barral J-P, Mercier P 1988 Visceral manipulation. Eastland Press, Seattle

Beal M 1985 Viscerosomatic reflexes review. Journal of the American Osteopathic Association 85:786–800

Beal M 2000 Acupuncture and oriental bodywork. Traditional and biomedical concepts in holistic care: history and basic concepts. Holistic Nursing Practice 14:69–78

Bei Y 1993 Clinical observations on the treatment of 98 cases of peptic ulcer by massage. Journal of Traditional Chinese Medicine 13(1):50–51

Bergman T 1993 Various forms of chiropractic technique. Chiropractic Techniques 5(2):53–55

Bhole M 1983 Gastric tone as influenced by mental states and meditation. Yoga Mimansa 22(1–2):54–58

Birkel DAG 1998 Activities for the older adult: integration of the body and the mind. Journal of Physical Education 69:23–28

Bishop E, McKinnon E, Weir E et al 2003 Reflexology in management of encopresis and chronic constipation. Paediatric Nursing 15:20–21

Blackburn J 2004 Trager® at the table – part 3. Journal of Bodywork and Movement Therapies 8(3):178–188

Blum CS, Esposito V, Esposito C 2003 Orthopedic block placement and its effect on the lumbosacral spine and discs. Three case studies with pre- and post-MRIs. Journal of Chiropractic Education 17:48–49

Bockenhauer S, Julliard K, Sing K et al 2002 Quantifiable effects of osteopathic manipulative techniques on patients with chronic asthma. Journal of the American Osteopathic Association 102(7):371–375

Boesler D, Warner M, Alpers A et al 1993 Efficacy of high velocity, low amplitude manipulative technique in subjects with low back pain during menstrual cramping. Journal of the American Osteopathic Association 93:203–214

Bogduk N, Twomey L 1991 Clinical anatomy of the lumbar spine, 2nd edn. Churchill Livingstone, Edinburgh

Bolton P, Stick P, Lord R 1989 Failure of clinical tests to predict cerebral ischemia before neck manipulation. Journal of Manipulative and Physiological Therapeutics 12(4):304–307

Borkan JM, Koes B, Reis S et al 1998 A report from the second international forum for primary care research on low back pain: reexamining priorities. Spine 23:1992–1996

Brady L, Henry K, Luth J et al 2001 The effects of Shiatsu on lower back pain. Journal of Holistic Nursing 19(1):57–70

Braem T 1994 The organs of the human anatomy – the lymphatic system. Bryan Edwards, Anaheim

Brennan G, Fritz J, Hunter S et al 2006 Identifying subgroups of patients with acute/subacute 'nonspecific' low back pain: results of a randomized clinical trial. Spine 31(6):623–631

Bronfort G, Assendelft W, Evans R et al 2001 Efficacy of spinal manipulation for chronic headache: a systematic review. Journal of Manipulative and Physiological Therapeutics 27(7):457–466

Brown B, Tissington-Tatlow W 1963 Radiographic studies of the vertebral arteries in cadavers. Radiology 81:80–88

Buratovich N, Cronin M, Perry A et al 2006 AANP Position Paper on Naturopathic Manipulative Therapy. American Association of Naturopathic Physicians, Washington, DC

Butler D 1991a Mobilisation of the nervous system. Churchill Livingstone, Edinburgh

Butler D 1991b Mobilisation of the nervous system. Churchill Livingstone, Edinburgh, p 104–105

Butler D 1991c Mobilisation of the nervous system. Churchill Livingstone, Edinburgh, p 137

Butler D, Gifford L 1989 Adverse mechanical tensions in the nervous system. Physiotherapy 75:622–629

Butler D, Moseley L 2000 The sensitive nervous system. Noigroup Publications, Adelaide

Caldwell C 1997 Getting in touch: the guide to new body-centered therapies. Quest Books, Wheaton, IL

Cantieri MS 1997 In-patient osteopathic manipulative treatment; impact on length of stay. American Academy of Osteopathy Journal 7(4):25–29

Cantu R, Grodin A 1992 Myofascial manipulation. Aspen Publications, Gaithersburg, MD

Caraballoa R, Bologna R, Whitmore K 2001 Sacral nerve stimulation as a treatment for urge incontinence and associated pelvic floor disorders at a pelvic floor center: a follow-up study. Urology 57(6 Suppl 1):121

Carey PF 1993 A report on the occurrence of cerebral vascular accidents in chiropractic practice. Journal of the Canadian Chiropractic Association 57(2):104–106

Carter AM, Kinzey SJ, Chitwood LF 2000 Proprioceptive neuromuscular facilitation decreases muscle activity during the stretch reflex in selected posterior thigh muscles. Journal of Sport Rehabilitation 9:269–278

Castro P, Larrain G, Pérez O 2000 Chronic hyperventilation syndrome associated with syncope and coronary vasospasm. American Journal of Medicine 109(1):78–80

Chaitow L 1980 Neuromuscular technique. Thorsons, Wellingborough, p 72–73

Chaitow L 1994 Integrated neuromuscular inhibition technique. British Journal of Osteopathy 13:17–20

Chaitow L 2001 Modern neuromuscular techniques, 2nd edn. Churchill Livingstone, Edinburgh

Chaitow L 2007 Positional release techniques, 3rd edn. Churchill Livingstone, Edinburgh

Chaitow L 2003 Palpation and assessment skills, 2nd edn. Churchill Livingstone, Edinburgh

Chaitow L 2005 Cranial manipulation: theory and practice, 2nd edn. Churchill Livingstone, Edinburgh

Chaitow L 2006 Muscle energy techniques, 3rd edn. Churchill Livingstone, Edinburgh

Chaitow L, DeLany J 2000 Clinical applications of neuromuscular techniques, vol 1: the upper body. Churchill Livingstone, Edinburgh

Chaitow L, Fritz S 2006 A massage therapist's guide to understanding, locating and treating myofascial trigger points. Churchill Livingstone, Edinburgh

Chen L-X 2005 Curative effect of yoga exercise prescription in treating menstrual disorders. Chinese Journal of Clinical Rehabilitation 9(4):164–165

Chengnan S (ed) 1990 Chinese bodywork. Pacific View Press, Berkeley, CA

Chikly B 1997 Lymph drainage therapy study guide level II. Chickly and UI Publishing, Palm Beach Gardens, FL

Chikly B 1999 Clinical perspectives: breast cancer reconstructive rehabilitation. Journal of Bodywork and Movement Therapies 3(1):11–16

Chiradejnant A, Maher C, Latimer J et al 2003 Efficacy of 'therapist-selected' versus 'randomly selected' mobilisation techniques for the treatment of low back pain: a randomised controlled trial. Australian Journal of Physiotherapy 49:223–241

Cinzia S, Rastenyte D, Cepaitis Z et al 2000 International trends in mortality from stroke, 1968 to 1994. Stroke 31:1588–1601

Cislo S, Ramirez M, Schwartz H 1991 Low back pain: treatment of forward and backward sacral torsion using counterstrain technique. Journal of the American Osteopathic Association 91(3):255–259

Clelland J, Savinar E, Shepard K 1987 Role of physical therapist in chronic pain management. In: Burrows G, Elton D, Stanley GV (eds) Handbook of chronic pain management. Elsevier, London, p 243–258

Cockbill S 2002 Wounds: the healing process. Hospital Pharmacist 9:255–260

Cohen L, Warneke C, Fouladi R et al 2004 Psychological adjustment and sleep quality in a randomized trial of the effects of a Tibetan yoga intervention in patients with lymphoma. Cancer 100:2253–2260

Collins N, Teys P, Vicenzino B 2004 The initial effects of a Mulligan's mobilization with movement technique on dorsiflexion and pain in subacute ankle sprains. Manual Therapy 9(2):77–82

Comeaux Z 2002a Facilitated oscillatory release. American Academy of Osteopathy Journal 12(2):24–35

Comeaux Z 2002b Robert Fulford and the philosopher physician. Eastland Press, Seattle

Comeaux Z 2004 Facilitated oscillatory release – a dynamic method of neuromuscular and ligamentous/articular assessment and treatment. Journal of Bodywork and Movement Therapies 9(2):88–98

Cooke B, Ernst E 2000 Aromatherapy for anxiety: a systematic review. British Journal of General Practice 50:493–496

Cordingley EW 1924 Principles and practice of naturopathy. Health Research, Mokelumne Hill, CA. Reprint 1971

Cordingley EW 1925 Principles and practice of naturopathy: a compendium of natural healing. O'Fallon, Bazan, CA

Cote P, Kreitz B, Cassidy JD, Thiel H 1996 The validity of the extension-rotation test as a clinical screening procedure before neck manipulation; a secondary analysis. Journal of Manipulative and Physiological Therapeutics 19:159–164

Coulter I, Hurwitz E, Adams A et al 1996 The appropriateness of manipulation and mobilization of the cervical spine. Rand, Santa Monica, CA

Cranz G 2000 The Alexander technique in the world of design: posture and the common chair. Part II: Body-conscious design for chairs, interiors and beyond. Journal of Bodywork and Movement Therapies 4(3):155–165

Cyriax J, Coldham M 1984 Textbook of orthopaedic medicine, vol E: treatment by manipulation, massage and injection, 11th edn. Baillière Tindall, London

D'Ambrogio K, Roth G 1997 Positional release therapy. Mosby, St Louis

Deig D 2001 Positional release technique. Butterworth-Heinemann, Boston

Delaney J, Leong K, Watkins A et al 2002 Short-term effects of myofascial trigger point massage therapy on cardiac autonomic tone in healthy subjects. Journal of Advanced Nursing 37:364–371

Delitto A, Cibulka M, Erhard R et al 1993 Evidence for use of an extension-mobilization category in acute low back syndrome: a prescriptive validation pilot study. Physical Therapy 73:216–222

Delitto A, Erhard RE, Bowling RW 1995 A treatment-based classification approach to low back syndrome: identifying and staging patients for conservative management. Physical Therapy 75:470–479

Derby R, Eek B, Lee S-H et al 2004 Comparison of intradiscal restorative injections and intradiscal electrothermal treatment (IDET) in the treatment of low back pain. Pain Physician 7(1):63–66

Dhabhar F, Viswanathan K 2005 Stress-induced enhancement of leukocyte trafficking to sites of surgery or immune activation. Brain, Behavior and Immunity 19(4 Suppl 1):e15

DiCarlo L, Sparling P, Hinson B et al 1995 Cardiovascular, metabolic, and perceptual responses to hatha yoga standing poses. Medicine, Exercise, Nutrition and Health 4:107–112

Dickey J 1989 Postoperative osteopathic manipulative management of median sternotomy patients. Journal of the American Osteopathic Association 89(10):1309–1322

Diegelmann R, Evans M 2004 Wound healing: an overview of acute, fibrotic and delayed healing. Frontiers in Bioscience 9:283–289

Diego M, Field T, Hernandez-Reif M 2002 Aggressive adolescents benefit from massage therapy. Adolescence 37:597–607

DiGiovanna E 1991 Treatment of the spine. In: DiGiovanna E, Schiowitz S (eds) An osteopathic approach to diagnosis and treatment. Lippincott, Philadelphia

DiGiovanna E, Schiowitz S 1991 An osteopathic approach to diagnosis and treatment. Lippincott, Philadelphia

Dishman J, Ball K, Burke J 2002 Central motor excitability changes after spinal manipulation: a transcranial magnetic stimulation study. Journal of Manipulative and Physiological Therapeutics 25(1):1–9

Dorland's Medical Dictionary 1985 26th edn. WB Saunders, Philadelphia

Dowling DJ 2000 Progressive inhibition of neuromuscular structures (PINS) technique. Journal of the American Osteopathic Association 100(5): 285–297

Duval C, LaFontaine D, Herbert J et al 2002 The effect of Trager therapy on the level of evoked stretch responses in patients with Parkinson's disease and rigidity. Journal of Manipulative and Physiological Therapeutics 25(7):455–464

Dynamic Chiropractic 2002 Coroner's Inquest in Canada. Dynamic Chiropractic August 16, 200, Vol 20, Issue 17. Online. Available: www.chiroweb.com/archives/20/17/05.html

Elder C, Dahners L, Weinhold P 2001 A cyclooxygenase-2 inhibitor impairs ligament healing in the rat. American Journal of Sports Medicine 29(6):801–805

Eliska O, Eliskova M 1995 Are peripheral lymphatics damaged by high pressure manual massage? Lymphology 28(1):21–30

Ernst E 1999 Massage therapy for low back pain. A systematic review. Journal of Pain and Symptom Management 17:65–69

Ernst E 2001 Prospective investigations into the safety of spinal manipulation. Journal of Pain and Symptom Management 21(3):238–242

Ernst E 2004 Musculoskeletal conditions and complementary/alternative medicine. Best Practice and Research Clinical Rheumatology 18(4):539–556

Ernst E, Canter P 2006 A systematic review of systematic reviews of spinal manipulation. Journal of the Royal Society of Medicine 99:189–193

Escalona A, Field T, Singer-Strunk R et al 2001 Improvement in behavior of children with autism. Journal of Autism and Developmental Disorders 31:513–516

Etnyre BR, Abraham LD 1986 H-reflex changes during static stretching and two variations of proprioceptive neuromuscular facilitation techniques. Electroencephalography and Clinical Neurophysiology 63(2):174–179

Evans D 2002 Mechanisms and effects of spinal high-velocity low-amplitude thrust manipulation. Journal of Manipulative and Physiological Therapeutics 25(4):251–262

Faling L 1986 Pulmonary rehabilitation physical modalities. Clinical Chest Medicine 7:599–618

Fallon J 1997 The role of chiropractic adjustment in the care and treatment of 332 children with otitis media. Journal of Clinical Chiropractic Pediatrics 2:167

Fallon J, Lok B 1994 Assessing efficacy of chiropractic care in pediatric cases of pyloric stenosis. In: Proceedings of National Conference on Chiropractic Pediatrics. International Chiropractic Association, Arlington, VA, p 72

Feldenkrais M 1972 Awareness through movement. Harper & Row, New York

Ferber R, Gravelle D, Osternig L 2002a Effect of proprioceptive neuromuscular facilitation stretch techniques on trained and untrained older adults. Journal of Aging and Physical Activity 10:132–142

Ferber R, Osternig LR, Gravelle DC 2002b Effect of PNF stretch techniques on knee flexor muscle EMG activity in older adults. Journal of Electromyography and Kinesiology 12:391–397

Ferezy J 1988 Neural ischemia and cervical manipulation: an acceptable risk. ACA Journal of Chiropractic 22:61–63

Fernández-de-las-Peñas C, del Cerrob L-P, Carneroa J 2005 Manual treatment of post-whiplash injury. Journal of Bodywork and Movement Therapies 9:109–119

Fernández-de-las-Peñas C, Alonso-Blanco C, Fernández-Carnero J, Miangolarra-Page J 2006 The immediate effect of ischemic compression technique and transverse friction massage on tenderness of active and latent myofascial trigger points: a pilot study. Journal of Bodywork and Movement Therapies 10:3–9

Ferrandez J, Laroche J, Serin D 1996 Lymphoscintigraphic aspects of the effects of MLD. Journal des Maladies Vasculaires 5:283–289

Ferreira M, Ferreira P, Latimer J et al 2003 Efficacy of spinal manipulative therapy for low back pain of less than three months' duration. Journal of Manipulative and Physiological Therapeutics 26:593–601

Ferrell-Torry AT, Glick OJ 1993 The use of therapeutic massage as a nursing intervention to modify anxiety and the perception of cancer pain. Cancer Nursing 16:93–101

Fiaschi E, Francesconi G, Fiumicelli S et al 1998 MLD for chronic post-mastectomy lymphoedema treatment. Panminerva Medica 40(1):48–50

Field T 2000 Touch therapy. Churchill Livingstone, Edinburgh

Field T, Hernandez-Reif M 1997 Juvenile rheumatoid arthritis benefits from massage therapy. Journal of Pediatric Psychology 22:607–617

Field T, Grizzle N, Scafidi F et al 1996 Massage and relaxation therapies' effects on depressed adolescent mothers. Adolescence 31:903–911

Field T, Henteleff T, Hernandez-Reif M 1997a Children with asthma have improved pulmonary functions after massage therapy. Journal of Pediatrics 132:854–858

Field T, Sunshine W, Hernandez-Reif M 1997b CFS: massage therapy effects depression and somatic symptoms. Journal of Chronic Fatigue Syndrome 3:43–51

Field T, Hernandez-Reif M, LaGreca A et al 1997c Massage therapy lowers blood glucose levels in children with diabetes mellitus. Diabetes Spectrum 10:237–239

Field T, Schanberg S, Kuhn C et al 1998 Bulimic adolescents benefit from massage therapy. Adolescence 33:555–563

Field T, Cullen C, Diego M et al 2001 Leukemia immune changes following massage therapy. Journal of Bodywork and Movement Therapies 5:271–274

Field T, Diego M, Cullen C et al 2002 Fibromyalgia pain and substance P decreases and sleep improves following massage therapy. Journal of Clinical Rheumatology 8:72–76

Fielder S, Pyott W 1955 The science and art of manipulative surgery. American Institute of Manipulative Surgery Inc. Carr Printing, Bountiful, UT

Flynn T, Fritz J, Whitman J et al 2002 A clinical prediction rule for classifying patients with low back pain who demonstrate short-term improvement with spinal manipulation. Spine 27:2835–2843

Foldi M, Strossenreuther R 2003 Foundations of manual lymph drainage, 3rd edn. Mosby, St Louis

Folweiler D, Lynch O 1995 Nasal specific technique as part of a chiropractic approach to chronic sinusitis and sinus headaches. Journal of Manipulative and Physiological Therapeutics 18(1):38–41

Forchuk C, Baruth P 2004 Postoperative arm massage. Cancer Nursing 27:25–33

Fritz JM, Delitto A, Erhard RE 2003 Comparison of classification-based physical therapy with therapy based on clinical practice guidelines for patients with acute low back pain: a randomized clinical trial. Spine 28:1363–1372

Fritz J, Whitman J, Flynn T et al 2004 Factors related to the inability of individuals with low back pain to improve with a spinal manipulation. Physical Therapy 84:173–190

Fryer G 2006 Muscle energy technique: efficacy and research. In: Chaitow L (ed) Muscle energy techniques, 3rd edn. Churchill Livingstone, Edinburgh

Furlan A, Brosseau L, Imamura M et al 2002 Massage for low-back pain – a systematic review within the framework of the Cochrane Collaboration back review group. Spine 27:1896–1910

Galantino ML, Iglarsh AZ, Richardson JK 2000 Orthopaedic physical therapy clinics of North America. Complementary Medicine 9(3):351

Galantino M, Boothroyd C, Lucci C 2003 Complementary and alternative medicine interventions for the orthopedic patient: a review of the literature. Seminars in Integrative Medicine 1(2):65–79

Galantino M, Bzdewka T, Eissler-Russo J et al 2004 The impact of modified hatha yoga on chronic low back pain: a pilot study. Alternative Therapies in Health and Medicine 10(2):56–59

Gallai V, Caso V, Paciaroni M et al 2001 Mild hyperhomocysteinemia: a possible risk factor for cervical artery dissection. Stroke 32:714–718

Gamber R, Shores J, Russo D et al 2002 Osteopathic manipulative treatment in conjunction with medication relieves pain associated with fibromyalgia syndrome. Results of a randomized clinical pilot study. Journal of the American Osteopathic Association 102(6):321–326

Ganong WF 1981 Dynamics of blood and lymph flow. In: Ganong WF (ed) Review of medical physiology. Lange Medical Publications, Los Altos, CA, p 470–484

Garde K 1972 Principles and practice of yoga therapy. DB Taraporevala, Bombay

Garfinkel MS, Singhal A, Katz WA et al 1998 Yoga-based intervention for carpal tunnel syndrome. Journal of the American Medical Association 280:1601–1603

Gatterman M 1990a Chiropractic management of spine related disorders: complications and contraindications to spinal manipulative therapy. Lippincott Williams & Wilkins, Baltimore, p 55–57

Gatterman M 1990b Chiropractic management of spine related disorders: disorders of the pelvic ring. Lippincott Williams & Wilkins, Baltimore, p 115

Gemmell H, Jacobson B 1989 Chiropractic management of enuresis: a time-series descriptive design. Journal of Manipulative and Physiological Therapeutics 12:386

Gerber R 1988 Vibrational medicine. Bear, Santa Fe, New Mexico, p 128, 130, 131

Gibbons P, Tehan P 1998 Muscle energy concepts and coupled motion of the spine. Manual Therapy 3(2):95–101

Gibbons P, Tehan P 2000a Manipulation of the spine, thorax and pelvis: an osteopathic perspective. Churchill Livingstone, Edinburgh

Gibbons P, Tehan P 2000b Manipulation of the spine, thorax and pelvis: an osteopathic perspective. Churchill Livingstone, Edinburgh, p 17–22

Giesen J, Center DB, Leach RA 1989 An evaluation of chiropractic manipulation as a treatment of hyperactivity in children. Journal of Manipulative and Physiological Therapeutics 12(5): 353–63

Giroud M, Fayolle H, Andre N et al 1994 Incidence of internal carotid artery dissection in the community of Dijon [letter]. Journal of Neurology, Neurosurgery and Psychiatry 57(11):1443

Giudice M 1990 Effects of continuous passive motion on the oedematous hands of two persons with flaccid hemiplegia. American Journal of Occupational Therapy 48(5):914–921

Glossary Review Committee 2005 Sponsored by Educational Council on Osteopathic Principles of the Association of Colleges of Osteopathic Medicine, Chevy Chase, MD

Godges JJ, Mattson-Bell M, Thorpe D et al 2003 The immediate effects of soft tissue mobilisation with proprioceptive neuromuscular facilitation on glenohumeral external rotation and overhead reach. Journal of Orthopaedic and Sports Physical Therapy 33:713–718

Goldberg J 1992 Effect of two intensities of massage on H-reflex amplitude. Physical Therapy 72(6)449–457

Goodheart G 1984 Applied kinesiology workshop procedure manual, 21st edn. Privately published. Detroit

Goyeche J, Ikemi Y 1977 Yoga as potential psychosomatic therapy. Asian Medical Journal 20(2):26–32

Graham IM, Daley LE, Refsum HM et al 1997 Plasma homocysteine as a risk factor for vascular disease: the European Concerted Action Project. Journal of the American Medical Association 1997; 277: 1775–1781

Greenman P 1989 Principles of manual medicine. Williams & Wilkins, Baltimore

Greenman P 1996 Principles of manual medicine, 2nd edn. Williams & Wilkins, Baltimore

Guiney P, Chou R, Vianna A et al 2005 Effects of osteopathic manipulative treatment on pediatric patients with asthma: a randomized controlled trial. Journal of the American Osteopathic Association 105(1):7–12

Guyton A, Hall J 1997 Inflammation and function of neutrophils and macrophages. In: Human physiology and mechanisms of disease, 6th edn. WB Saunders, Philadelphia, p 284–286

Hackett G, Hemwall G, Montgomery G 2002a Ligament and tendon relaxation treated by prolotherapy, 5th edn. Beulah Land Press, Oak Park IL, p 3–14

Hackett G, Hemwall G, Montgomery G 2002b Ligament and tendon relaxation treated by prolotherapy, 5th edn. Beulah Land Press, Oak Park IL, p 28

Hackett G, Hemwall G, Montgomery G 2002c Ligament and tendon relaxation treated by prolotherapy, 5th edn. Beulah Land Press, Oak Park, IL, p 14–18, 25

Hackett G, Hemwall G, Montgomery G 2002d Ligament and tendon relaxation treated by prolotherapy, 5th edn. Beulah Land Press, Oak Park IL, p 18–19

Hackett G, Hemwall G, Montgomery G 2002e Ligament and tendon relaxation treated by prolotherapy, 5th edn. Beulah Land Press, Oak Park IL, p 179, 259, 291, 292

Hackett G, Hemwall G, Montgomery G 2002f Ligament and tendon relaxation treated by prolotherapy, 5th edn. Beulah Land Press, Oak Park IL, p 180, 291

Hackett G, Hemwall G, Montgomery G 2002g Ligament and tendon relaxation treated by prolotherapy, 5th edn. Beulah Land Press, Oak Park IL, p 191–194, 197–201, 207, 213, 220, 226, 227, 234, 235, 238, 241, 249, 253, 269, 272, 319, 320

Hackett G, Hemwall G, Montgomery G 2002h Ligament and tendon relaxation treated by prolotherapy, 5th edn. Beulah Land Press, Oak Park IL, p 288

Haldeman S 1980 Modern developments in the principles and practice of chiropractic. Appleton-Century-Crofts, New York, p 377–378

Haldeman S, Chapman-Smith D, Peterson D (eds) 1993a Guidelines for chiropractic quality assurance and practice parameters. Aspen Publishers, Gaithersburg, MD, p 175

Haldeman S, Chapman-Smith D, Petersen D (eds) 1993b Guidelines for chiropractic quality assurance and practice parameters. Aspen Publishers, Gaithersburg, MD, p 170–172

Haldeman S, Carey P, Townsend M, Papadopoulos C 2001 Arterial dissections following cervical manipulation: the chiropractic experience. Canadian Medical Association Journal 165(7):905–906

Haldeman S, Kohlbeck F, McGregor M 2002a Unpredictability of cerebrovascular ischemia associated with cervical spine manipulation therapy: a review of sixty-four cases after cervical spine manipulation. Spine 27(1):49–55

Haldeman S, Kohlbeck FJ, McGregor M 2002b Stroke, cerebral artery dissection and cervical spine manipulative therapy. Journal of Neurology 249:1098–1104

Hall DW, Aguilar E, Larkam E 1999 Effects of Pilates-based training on static and dynamic balance in an elderly population. Medicine and Science in Sports and Exercise 31:S388

Hall T, Cacho T, McNee C, Riches J, Walsh J 2000 Efficacy of the Mulligan SLR technique. In: Singer KP (ed) Proceedings of the 7th Scientific Conference of the IFOMT in conjunction with the Biennial Conference of the MPAA. Perth, Australia, 9–10 November, p 185–109

Hammer W 1999 Functional soft tissue examination and treatment by manual methods. Aspen Publishing, Gaithersburg MD, p 535–540

Han J, Stegen K, De Valck C et al 1996 Influence of breathing therapy on complaints, anxiety and breathing pattern in patients with hyperventilation syndrome and anxiety disorders. Journal of Psychosomatic Research 41(5):481–493

Hanna T 1988 Somatics. Addison-Wesley, New York

Harinath K, Malhotra AS, Pal K et al 2004 Effects of Hatha yoga and Omkar meditation on cardiorespiratory performance, psychologic profile, and melatonin secretion. Journal of Alternative and Complementary Medicine 10(2):261–268

Harris R, Piller N 2004 Three case studies indicating effectiveness of MLD on patients with primary and secondary lymphedema. Journal of Bodywork and Movement Therapies 7(4):213–222

Harvard Medical School 2006 InteliHealth. Physical therapy: medications and other treatments. Online. Available: www.intelihealth.com/IH/ihtIH?d =dmtContent&c=339554&p=~br,S|~st,9339|~r,WSS|~b,*|#pt

Haynes M, Cala L, Melsom A et al 2002 Vertebral arteries and cervical rotation: modelling and magnetic resonance angiography studies. Journal of Manipulative and Physiological Therapeutics 25(6):370–383

Hearn A, Rivett DA 2002 Cervical SNAGs: a biomechanical analysis. Manual Therapy 7(2):71–79

Helms J 1985 Acupuncture energetics: a clinical approach for physicians. Eastwind Books, Berkeley, CA

Henderson D, Cassidy J 1988 Vertebral artery syndrome. In: Vernon H (ed) Upper cervical syndrome: chiropractic diagnosis and treatment. Williams & Wilkins, Baltimore, p 195–222

Hernandez-Reif M, Field T, Theakston H 1998 Multiple sclerosis patients benefit from massage therapy. Journal of Bodywork and Movement Therapies 2:168–174

Hernandez-Reif M, Field T, Krasnegor J et al 2000 High blood pressure and associated symptoms reduced by massage therapy. Journal of Bodywork and Movement Therapies 4:31–38

Hernandez-Reif M, Field T, Largie S et al 2002 Parkinson's disease symptoms reduced by massage therapy. Journal of Bodywork and Movement Therapies 6:177–182

Hernandez-Reif M, Ironson G, Field T et al 2004 Breast cancer patients have improved immune functions following massage therapy. Journal of Psychosomatic Research 57(1):45–52

Herzog S 2002 Internal forces sustained by the vertebral artery during spinal manipulative therapy. Journal of Manipulative and Physiological Therapeutics 8:504–510

Herzog W 2002 Testimony at Lewis Inquest, Coroner's Court, Toronto, November 26, 2002

Hill M 2003 Cervical artery dissection, imaging, trauma and causal inference. Canadian Journal of Neurological Sciences 30:302–303

Hoag J 1969 Osteopathic medicine. McGraw-Hill, New York

Holzberg A, Kellog-Spadt S, Lukban J et al 2001 Evaluation of transvaginal Theile massage as a therapeutic intervention for women with interstitial cystitis. Urology 57(6 Suppl 1):120

Hondras MA, Long CR, Brennan PC 1999 Spinal manipulative therapy versus a low force mimic maneuver for women with primary dysmenorrhea: a randomized, observer-blinded, clinical trial. Pain 81:105–114

Hooper R, Ding M 2004 Retrospective case series on patients with chronic spinal pain treated with dextrose prolotherapy. Journal of Alternative and Complementary Medicine 10(4):670–674

Horton SJ 2002 Acute locked thoracic spine: treatment with a modified SNAG. Manual Therapy 7(2):103–107

Hou C-R, Tsai L-C, Cheng K-F 2002 Immediate effects of various physical therapeutic modalities on cervical myofascial pain and trigger-point sensitivity. Archives of Physical and Medical Rehabilitation 83:1406–1414

Hovind H, Nielsen S 1974 Effect of massage on blood flow in skeletal muscle. Scandinavian Journal of Rehabilitation Medicine 6:74–77

Hoyland J, Freemont A, Jayson M 1989 Intervertebral foramen venous obstruction. Spine 14(6):558–568

Hunt A 1978 Electronic evidence of auras, chakras in UCLA study. Brain/Mind Bulletin 3:9

Hurwitz E, Haldeman S 2004 Manual therapy including manipulation for acute and chronic neck pain. In: Fischgrund J (ed) Neck pain. Monograph Series #27. American Academy of Orthopedic Surgeons, Rosemont, IL

Hurwitz E, Aker P, Adams A et al 1996 Manipulation and mobilization of the cervical spine: a systematic review of the literature. Spine 21(15):1746–1760

Hurwitz E, Morgenstern H, Vassilaki M, Chiang L 2005 Frequency and clinical predictors of adverse reactions to chiropractic care in the UCLA neck pain study. Spine 30:1477–1484

Hutchinson MR, Tremain L, Christiansen J et al 1998 Improving leaping ability in elite rhythmic gymnasts. Medicine and Science in Sports and Exercise 30(10):1543–1547

Ikimi F, Hunt J, Hanna G et al 1996 Interstitial fluid plasma protein, colloid, and leukocyte uptake into initial lymphatics. Journal of Applied Physiology 81(5):2060–2067

Ironson G, Field T, Scafidi F et al 1996 Massage therapy associated with enhancement of immune systems cytotoxic capacity. International Journal of Neuroscience 84:205–217

Jacobson EC, Lockwood MD, Hoefner VC et al 1989 Shoulder pain and repetition strain injury to the supraspinatus muscle: etiology and manipulative treatment. Journal of the American Osteopathic Association 89(8):1037–1045

Janda V 1978 Muscles, central nervous motor regulation, and back problems. In: Korr IM (ed) Neurobiologic mechanisms in manipulative therapy. Plenum, New York

Janda V 1996 Evaluation of muscular imbalance. In: Liebenson C (ed) Rehabilitation of the spine. Williams & Wilkins, Baltimore

Janse J, Houser R, Wells B 1947 Chiropractic principles and technic. National College of Chiropractic, Chicago, p 515–516

Jarmel ME, Zatkin JL, Charuvastra E et al 1995 Improvement of cardiac autonomic regulation following spinal manipulative therapy. In: Cleveland C, Haldeman S (eds) Conference Proceedings of Chiropractic Centennial Foundation, Davenport, Iowa, p 359

Jaskoviak P 1980 Complications arising from manipulation of the cervical spine. Journal of Manipulative and Physiological Therapeutics 3:213–219

Jayson M, Sim-Williams H, Young S et al 1981 Mobilization and manipulation for low-back pain. Spine 6:409–416

Jensen K 2004 University of Wisconsin, Department of Orthopedics & Department of Biomedical Engineering. Presented at the Hackett Hemwall Foundation Annual Prolotherapy Conference 2004. The University of Wisconsin Department of Family Medicine, Madison, WI

Johansseon K, Lie E, Ekdahl C et al 1998 Randomized study comparing MLD with sequential pneumatic compression for treatment of postoperative arm lymphoedema. Lymphology 31(2):56–64

Johnson A 1939 Principles and practice of drugless therapeutics. Straube, Los Angeles

Johnson A 1977 Chiropractic physiological therapeutics. Published by the author. Palm Springs CA, p 44–45

Johnstone W 1997 Functional technique. In: Ward R (ed) Foundations for osteopathic medicine. Williams & Wilkins, Baltimore

Johnston WL, Kelso AF 1995 Changes in presence of a segmental dysfunction pattern associated with hypertension: a long-term longitudinal study. Journal of the American Osteopathic Association 95:315–318

Jones L 1981 Strain and counterstrain. Academy of Applied Osteopathy, Colorado Springs, CO

Juhan D 1989 An introduction to Trager psychophysical integration and mentastics movement education. Trager Institute, Mill Valley, CA

Jull G, Janda V 1987 Muscles and motor control in low back pain. In: Twomey L, Taylor J (eds) Physical therapy for the low back. Clinics in physical therapy. Churchill Livingstone, New York

Kaltenborn F 1985 Mobilization of the extremity joints. Olaf Norlis Bokhandel, Oslo

Kapanji IA 1987 The physiology of the joints, vols 1, 2 and 3. Churchill Livingstone, Edinburgh

Keating J Jr 1992 Toward a philosophy of the science of chiropractic. Stockton Foundation for Chiropractic Research, Stockton, CA, p 189

Kelso A 1971 A double-blind clinical study of osteopathic findings in hospital patients. Journal of the American Osteopathic Association 70:570–592

Kenna C, Murtagh J 1989 Back pain and spinal manipulation, 2nd edn. Butterworth-Heinemann, Oxford

Kent P, Marks D, Pearson W et al 2005 Does clinician treatment choice improve the outcomes of manual therapy for nonspecific low back pain? A metaanalysis. Journal of Manipulative and Physiological Therapeutics 28(5):312–322

Kessinger R, Boneva D 1998 Changes in visual acuity in patients receiving upper cervical specific chiropractic care. Journal of Vertebral Subluxation Research 2(1):43–49

Khalsa P, Eberhart A, Cotler A et al 2006 The 2005 Conference on the Biology of Manual Therapies. Journal of Manipulative and Physiological Therapeutics 29(5):341–346

Khumar S, Kaur P, Kaur S 1993 Effectiveness of Shavasana on depression among university students. Indian Journal of Clinical Psychology 20(2):82–87

King H, Tettambel M, Lockwood M et al 2003 Osteopathic manipulative treatment in prenatal care. A retrospective case control design study. Journal of the American Osteopathic Association 103(12):577–582

Kiser RS, Khatami MJ, Gatchel RJ et al 1983 Acupuncture relief of chronic pain syndrome correlates with increased plasma met-enkephalin concentrations. Lancet 2:1394–1396

Klein D, Stone W, Phillips W et al 2002 PNF training and physical function in assisted-living older adults. Journal of Aging and Physical Activity 10:476–488

Klein RG, Eek BC, DeLong W et al 1993 A randomized double-blind trial of dextrose-glycerin-phenol injections for chronic low back pain. Journal of Spinal Disorders 6(1):23–33

Klougart N, Nilsson N 1989 Infantile colic treated by chiropractors: a prospective study of 316 cases. Journal of Manipulative and Physiological Therapeutics 12:281–291

Klougart N, Leboeuf-Yde C, Rasmussen L 1996 Safety in chiropractic practice. Part 1: The occurrence of cerebrovascular accidents after manipulation to the neck in Denmark from 1978–1988. Journal of Manipulative and Physiological Therapeutics 19:371–377

Knaster M 1996 Discovering the body's wisdom. Bantam, New York

Knebl J 2002 The Spencer sequence. Journal of the American Osteopathic Association 102(7):387–400

Ko D, Lerner R, Klose G et al 1998 Effective treatment of postoperative arm lymphedema. Lymphology 31(2):452–458

Konstantinou K, Foster N, Rushton A et al 2002 The use and reported effects of mobilization with movement techniques in low back pain management; a cross-sectional descriptive survey of physiotherapists in Britain. Manual Therapy 7(4):206–214

Korr IM 1976a Spinal cord as organizer of disease processes. Academy of Applied Osteopathy Yearbook, Newark, OH

Korr I 1976b Collected papers of I.M Korr. American Academy of Osteopathy, Newark, OH

Korr I 1981 Axonal transport and neurotrophic function in relation to somatic dysfunction. In: Korr I (ed) Spinal cord as organizer of disease processes, Part 4. Academy of Applied Osteopathy, Newark, OH, p 451–458

Kuchera W 1997 Lumbar and abdominal region. In: Ward R (ed) Foundations of osteopathic medicine. Williams & Wilkins, Baltimore, p 581–599

Kuchera WA, Kuchera ML 1992 Osteopathic principles in practice. Kirksville College of Osteopathic Medicine Press, Kirksville, MO

Kurz I 1986 Textbook of Dr Vodder's manual lymph drainage, vol 2: therapy, 2nd edn. Karl F Haug, Heidelberg

Kurz I 1987 Introduction to Dr Vodder's manual lymph drainage, vol 3: therapy II (treatment manual). Karl F Haug, Heidelberg

Kurtz R 1990 Body-centered psychotherapy: the Hakomi method. LifeRhythm, Mendocino, CA

Lange C, Unnithan V, Larkam E et al 2000 Maximizing the benefits of Pilates-inspired exercise for learning functional motor skills. Journal of Bodywork and Movement Therapies 4(2):99–108

Langevin H, Sherman K 2006 Pathophysiological model for chronic low back pain integrating connective tissue and nervous system mechanisms. Medical Hypotheses 68(1):74–80

Langevin H, Bouffard N, Badger G et al 2005 Dynamic fibroblast cytoskeletal response to subcutaneous tissue stretch ex vivo and in vivo. American Journal of Physiology, Cell Physiology 288:C747–756

Larsson S, Bodegard L, Henrikssn K et al 1990 Chronic trapezius myalgia: morphology and blood flow. Acta Orthopaedica Scandinavica 61(5):394–398

Laslett M, Oberg B, Aprill CN, McDonald B 2005 Centralization as a predictor of provocation discography results in chronic low back pain, and the influence of disability and distress on diagnostic power. Spine 5(4):370–380

Latha D, Kaliappan K 1992 Efficacy of yoga therapy in the management of headaches. Journal of Indian Psychology 10:41–47

Lauterstein D 1994 What is zero balancing? Massage Therapy Journal 33(1):28–35

Le Vu B, Dumortier A, Guillaume M et al 1997 Efficacy of massage and mobilization of the upper limb after surgical treatment of breast cancer. Bulletin of Cancer 84(10):957–961

Leahy M, Mock L 1992 Myofascial release technique and mechanical compromise of peripheral nerves of the upper extremity. Chiropractic Technology 6:139–150

Leahy P 1999 Active release techniques. In: Hammer W (ed) Functional soft tissue examination and treatment in manual methods, 2nd edn. Aspen, Gaithersburg, MD

Lederman E 1997a Fundamentals of manual therapy. Churchill Livingstone, Edinburgh, p 23–25

Lederman E 1997b Fundamentals of manual therapy. Churchill Livingstone, Edinburgh, p 3

Lederman E 1997c Fundamentals of manual therapy. Churchill Livingstone, Edinburgh

Lederman E 2000 Harmonic technique. Churchill Livingstone, Edinburgh

Lederman E 2005a Science and practice of manual therapy, 2nd edn. Churchill Livingstone, Edinburgh, p 87–224

Lederman E 2005b Science and practice of manual therapy, 2nd edn. Churchill Livingstone, Edinburgh, p 277–293

Lederman E 2005c Science and practice of manual therapy, 2nd edn. Churchill Livingstone, Edinburgh, p 71–72

Lederman E 2005d Science and practice of manual therapy, 2nd edn. Churchill Livingstone, Edinburgh, p 43, 44

Lederman E, Brown S 1996 Effects of active and passive oscillation technique of the knee joint on the stretch reflex. Unpublished study. British School of Osteopathy, London

Lee D 1997 Instability of the sacroiliac joint. In: Vleeming A, Mooney V, Dorman T, Snijders C, Stoeckart R (eds) Movement, stability and low back pain. Churchill Livingstone, Edinburgh, p 231–235

Lee D 2001 An integrated model of 'joint function and its clinical application'. Presented at the 4th Interdisciplinary World Congress on Low Back Pain and Pelvic Pain, Montreal, Quebec, November 8–10, 2001

Lee KP, Carlini WG, McCormick GF, Walters GW 1995 Neurologic complications following chiropractic manipulation: a survey of California neurologists. Neurology 45(6):1213–1215

Lenehan KL, Fryer G, McLaughlin P 2003 The effect of muscle energy technique on gross trunk range of motion. Journal of Osteopathic Medicine 6(1):13–18

Levine P, Frederick A 1997 Waking the tiger: healing trauma: the innate capacity to transform overwhelming experiences. North Atlantic Books, Berkeley, CA

Lewit K 1999 Manipulative therapy in rehabilitation of the locomotor system, 3rd edn. Butterworth-Heinemann, Oxford

Lewit K, Olanska S 2004 Clinical importance of active scars: abnormal scars as a cause of myofascial pain. Journal of Manipulative and Physiological Therapeutics 27(6):399–402

Lewit K, Simons D 1984 Myofascial pain: relief by post-isometric relaxation. Archives of Physical Medicine and Rehabilitation 65:452–456

Lewthwaite R 1990 Motivational considerations in physical therapy involvement. Physical Therapy 70(12):808–819

Liebenson C 1996a Rehabilitation of the spine. Williams & Wilkins, Baltimore

Liebenson C 1996b Active rehabilitation protocols. In: Liebenson C (ed) Rehabilitation of the spine. Williams & Wilkins, Baltimore

Liebenson C 2006 Rehabilitation of the spine, 2nd edn. Lippincott Williams & Wilkins, Philadelphia

Ligeros K 1937 How ancient healing governs modern therapeutics. GP Putnam, New York, p 402

Liu Y, Tipton C, Matthes R et al 1983 An in situ study of the influence of a sclerosing solution in rabbit medial collateral ligaments and its junction strength. Connective Tissue Research 11:95–102

Long A, Donelson R, Fung T 2004 Does it matter which exercise? A randomized controlled trial of exercise for low back pain. Spine 29:2593–2602

Lowenkopf A 1976 Osteopuncture. Medical Arts Press, Santa Barbara, CA

Lukban J, Whitmore K, Kellog-Spadt S et al 2001 The effect of manual physical therapy in patients diagnosed with interstitial cystitis, high-tone pelvic floor dysfunction, and sacroiliac dysfunction. Urology 57(suppl 6A):121–122

Lum L 1984 Hyperventilation and anxiety state [editorial]. Journal of the Royal Society of Medicine Jan:1–4

Macfadden B 1916 Macfadden's encyclopedia of physical culture, 5 vols. Physical Culture Publishing, New York

Mackay H, Long A 2003 The experience and effects of Shiatsu: findings from a two country exploratory study. University of Salford, Health Care Practice Research and Development Unit. Report Number 9. Online. Available: www.fhsc.salford.ac.uk/hcprdu

Magnuson P 1941 Differential diagnosis of causes of pain in the lower back accompanied by sciatic pain. Annals of Surgery 119:878–891

Magnusson M, Simonsen EB, Dyhre-Poulsen P et al 1996 Viscoelastic stress relaxation during static stretch in human skeletal muscle in the absence of EMG activity. Scandinavian Journal of Medicine and Science in Sport 6(6):323–328

Magnusson S, Simonsen E, Aagaard P et al 1996 Mechanical and physiological responses to stretching with and without pre-isometric contraction in human skeletal muscle Archives of Physical Medicine and Rehabilitation 77:373–377

Maigne J-Y, Chatellier G 2001 Comparison of three manual coccydynia treatments: a pilot study. Spine 26: E479–483; discussion E484

Maigne R 1972 Orthopaedic medicine: a new approach to vertebral manipulation. Thomas, Springfield, IL

Maitland G 1986 Vertebral manipulation, 5th edn. Butterworths, London

Maitland G 2001 Maitland's vertebral manipulation, 6th edn. Butterworth-Heinemann, Oxford

Maitland G, Hengeveld E, Banks K et al 2001 Maitland's vertebral manipulation, 6th edn. Butterworth-Heinemann, London

Malhotra V, Singh S, Singh KP et al 2002 Study of yoga asanas in assessment of pulmonary function in NIDDM patients. Indian Journal of Physiology and Pharmacology 46(3):313–320

Malone D, Baldwin N, Tomecek F et al 2002a Complications of spinal manipulation: a comprehensive review of the literature. Journal of Family Practice 42:475–480

Malone D, Baldwin N, Tomecek F et al 2002b Complications of cervical spine manipulation therapy: 5-year retrospective study in a single-group practice. Neurosurgical Focus 13(6):1–11

Manheim C, Lavett D 1994 The myofascial release manual. Slack, Thorofare, NJ

Manjunath N, Telles S 2005 Influence of Yoga and Ayurveda on self-rated sleep in a geriatric population. Indian Journal of Medical Research 121(5):683–690

Mann F 1971 Acupuncture: the ancient Chinese art of healing and how it works scientifically. Vintage Books, New York

Manocha R, Marks G, Kenchington P et al 2002 Sahaja yoga in the management of moderate to severe asthma: a randomised controlled trial. Thorax 57(2):110–115

Mathew J, Yates D 1988 Treatment of sciatica. Lancet 1:352

Maurer-Groeli Y 1996 [Body-centered psychotherapy] [article in German]. Therapeutische Umschau 53(3):217–224

Maynard J, Pedrini V, Pedrini-Mille A et al 1985 Morphological and biochemical effects of sodium morrhuate on tendons. Journal of Orthopedic Research 3:236–248

McCracken L, Turk D 2002 Behavioural and cognitive behavioral treatment for chronic pain: outcome, predictors of outcome, and treatment process. Spine 27:2564–2573

McGregor M, Haldeman S, Kohlbeck FJ 1995 Vertebrobasilar compromise associated with cervical manipulation. Topics in Clinical Chiropractic 2(3):63–73

McKenzie R 1981 The lumbar spine: mechanical diagnosis and therapy. Spinal Publications, Waikanae, NZ

McKenzie R, May S 2003 The lumbar spine: mechanical diagnosis and therapy. Spinal Publications, Waikanae, NZ, p 553–563

McPartland JM, Giuffrida A, King J et al. 2005 Cannabimimetic effects of osteopathic manipulative treatment. Journal of the American Osteopathic Association 105:283–291

Meade T, Dyer S, Browne W et al 1990 Low back pain of mechanical origin. Randomized comparison of chiropractic and hospital outpatient treatment. British Medical Journal 300:1431–1437

Mehling WE, Hamel KA, Acree M, Byl N, Hecht FM 2005 Randomized, controlled trial of breath therapy for patients with chronic low-back pain. Alternative Therapies in Health and Medicine 11(4):44–52

Meisenbach RO 1911 Sacro-iliac relaxation with analysis of eighty-four cases. Surgery, Gynecology and Obstetrics 12:411–434

Melzack R, Wall P 1988 The challenge of pain, 2nd edn. Penguin, Harmondsworth, Middlesex

Melzack R, Wall P (eds) 1994 Textbook of pain, 3rd edn. Churchill Livingstone, London, p 201–224

Mengert W 1943 Referred pelvic pain. Southern Medical Journal 36:256–263

Mennel J 1975 The therapeutic use of cold. Journal of the American Osteopathic Association 74(12):1146–1158

Mense S, Simons DG, Russell IJ 2000 Muscle pain: understanding its nature, diagnosis and treatment. Lippincott Williams & Wilkins, Philadelphia

Michaud T 2002 Uneventful upper cervical manipulation in the presence of a damaged vertebral artery. Journal of Manipulative and Physiological Therapeutics 25(7):472–483

Mitchell F Jr, Moran P, Pruzzo N 1979 An evaluation of osteopathic muscle energy procedures. Pruzzo, Valley Park, MO

Mock L 1997 Myofascial release treatment of specific muscles of the upper extremity (levels 3 and 4). Clinical Bulletin of Myofascial Therapy 2(1):5–23

Mogyoros I, Kiernan K, Burke D et al 1997 Excitability changes in human sensory and motor axons during hyperventilation and ischaemia. Brain 120(2):317–325

Moore M, Kukulka C 1991 Depression of Hoffman reflexes following voluntary contraction and implications for proprioceptive neuromuscular facilitation therapy. Physical Therapy 71(4):321–329

Mootz R, Dhami M, Hess J 1994 Chiropractic treatment of chronic episodic type headache in male subjects: a case series analysis. Journal of the Canadian Chiropractic Association 38(3):152–159

Morris C (ed) 2006a Low back syndromes: integrated clinical management. McGraw-Hill, New York, p 638–639

Morris C (ed) 2006b Low back syndromes: integrated clinical management. McGraw-Hill, New York, p 636–637

Morrissey D 2002 Unloading and proprioceptive taping. In: Chaitow L (ed) Positional release techniques, 2nd edn. Churchill Livingstone, Edinburgh

Mullhearn S, George K 1999 Abdominal muscle endurance and its association with posture and low back pain: an initial investigation in male and female elite gymnasts. Physiotherapy 85:210–216

Mulligan B 1985 Manual therapy: NAGs, SNAGs, MWMs, etc. Plane View Services, Wellington, NZ

Mulligan B 1992 Manual therapy: NAGs, SNAGs, MWMs, etc., 2nd edn. Plane View Services, Wellington, NZ

Mulligan B 2003 Manual therapy: NAGs, SNAGs, MWMs, etc., 5th edn. Plane View Services, Wellington, NZ

Murphy D 2000 Conservative management of cervical spine syndromes. McGraw-Hill, New York

Myers T 2001 Some thoughts on intra-nasal work. Journal of Bodywork and Movement Therapies 5(3):149–159

Nimmo R 1957 Receptors, effectors and tonus. Journal of the American Chiropractic Association 27(11):21

Noll D, Shores J, Gamber R et al 2000 Benefits of osteopathic manipulative treatment for hospitalized elderly patients with pneumonia. Journal of the American Osteopathic Association 100(12):776–782

Norkin C, Levangie P 1992 Joint structure and function: a comprehensive analysis, 2nd edn. FA Davis, Philadelphia

Norris CM 1999 Functional load abdominal training. Journal of Bodywork and Movement Therapies 3(3):150–158

Norris JW, Beletsky V, Nadareishvilli ZG 2000 Sudden neck movement and cervical artery dissection: Canadian Stroke Consortium. Canadian Medical Association Journal 163(1):38–40

Oken B, Kishiyama S, Zajdel D et al 2004 Randomized controlled trial of yoga and exercise in multiple sclerosis. Neurology 62:2058–2064

Oleson T, Flocco W 1993 Randomized controlled study of premenstrual symptoms treated with ear, hand, and foot reflexology. Obstetrics and Gynaecology 82:906–911

Ongley MJ, Klein RG, Dorman TA et al 1987 A new approach to the treatment of chronic low back pain. Lancet 2(8551):143–146

Oschman J 1997 What is healing energy? Pt 5: gravity, structure, and emotions. Journal of Bodywork and Movement Therapies 1(5):307–308

O'Sullivan P 2005 Diagnosis and classification of chronic low back pain disorders. Manual Therapy 10(4):242–255

Oyama I, Rejba A, Lukban A et al 2004 Modified Thiele massage as therapeutic intervention for female patients with interstitial cystitis and hightone pelvic floor dysfunction. Urology 64(5):862–865

Palmer BJ 1934 The subluxation specific – the adjustment specific. Palmer School of Chiropractic, Davenport, IA

Palmer D 2002 Comparison of a muscle energy technique and neuromuscular technique on quadriceps muscle strength. Online. Available: www.osteopathic-research.com/cgi-bin/or/Search1.pl?show_one=30704

Panjabi M, Yamomoto I, Oxland T et al 1989 How does posture affect coupling in the lumbar spine. Spine 14(9):1002–1011

Panjwani U, Gupta HL, Singh SH et al 1995 Effect of Sahaja yoga practice on stress management in patients of epilepsy. Indian Journal of Physiology and Pharmacology 39:111–116

Patel C, North W 1975 Randomised controlled trial of yoga and biofeedback in management of hypertension. Lancet 2:93–95

Patel P 2002 Comparison of neuromuscular technique and a muscle energy technique on cervical range of motion. Online. Available: www.osteopathic-research.com/cgi-bin/or/Search1.pl?show_one=30175

Patriquin D, Jones J 1997 Articulatory techniques. In: Ward R (ed) Foundations for osteopathic medicine. Williams & Wilkins, Baltimore, p 764–765

Patterson J 2004a History of prolotherapy. Presented at the Hackett Hemwall Foundation Annual Prolotherapy Conference 2004. University of Wisconsin Department of Family Medicine, Madison, WI

Patterson J 2004b Prolo pearls: safety, safety, safety. Presented at the Hackett Hemwall Foundation Annual Prolotherapy Conference 2004. University of Wisconsin Department of Family Medicine, Madison, WI

Paungmali A, O'Leary S, Souvlis T, Vicenzino B 2004 Naloxone fails to antagonize initial hypoalgesic effect of a manual therapy treatment for lateral epicondylalgia. Journal of Manipulative and Physiological Therapeutics 27(3):180–185

Penning L, Wilmink J 1987 Rotation of the cervical spine: a CT study in normal subjects. Spine 12(8):732–738

Perrin D 2005 Taping and bracing, 2nd edn. Human Kinetics, Champaign, IL

Peterson D, Bergmann T 2002 Chiropractic technique: principles and procedures, 2nd edn. Mosby, St Louis, p 107

Pezzini A, Del Zotto E, Archetti S et al 2002 Plasma homocysteine concentration, C677T MTHFR genotype, and 844-ins68bp genotype in young adults with spontaneous cervical artery dissection and atherothrombotic stroke. Stroke 33(3):664–669

Pierce L, Webber J 1996 Visceral manipulation therapy. Biological Psychology 43(3):267

Pikalov A, Kharin V 1994 Use of spinal manipulative therapy in treatment of duodenal ulcer. Journal of Manipulative and Physiological Therapeutics 17:310–313

Pilates J 1934 Your health. Presentation Dynamics, Incline Village, NV

Pilates J 1945 Return to life through contrology. Presentation Dynamics, Incline Village, NV

Pilkington K, Kirkwood G, Rampe H 2005 Yoga for depression: the research evidence. Journal of Affective Disorders 89(1–3):13–24

Plaugher G 1993a Textbook of clinical chiropractic. Williams & Wilkins, Baltimore

Plaugher G 1993b Upper cervical spine. In: Plaughter G (ed) Textbook of clinical chiropractic. Williams & Wilkins, Baltimore, p 308

Pool-Goudzwaard A, Hoek van Dijke G, van Gurp M et al 2004 Contribution of pelvic floor muscles to stiffness of the pelvic ring. Clinical Biomechanics 19(6):564–571

Poppen J 1945 The herniated intervertebral disc on analysis of 400 verified cases. New England Journal of Medicine 232:211–215

Protopapas M, Cymet T 2002 Joint cracking and popping: understanding noises that accompany articular release. Journal of the American Osteopathic Association 102(5):283–287

Pryor J, Prasad S 2002 Physiotherapy for respiratory and cardiac problems, 3rd edn. Churchill Livingstone, Edinburgh, p 353

Puustjarvi K 1990 Effects of massage in patients with chronic tension headaches. Acupuncture and Electrotherapeutics Research 15:159–162

Rabago D, Best T, Beamsley M, Patterson J 2005 A systematic review of prolotherapy for chronic musculoskeletal pain. Critical review. Clinical Journal of Sport Medicine 15(5):E376

Ramaratnam S, Sridharan R 2000 Yoga for epilepsy. Cochrane Database of Systematic Reviews (1):CD001524

Ramirez M 1989 Low back pain – diagnosis by six newly discovered sacral tender points and treatment with counterstrain technique. Journal of the American Osteopathic Association 89(7):905–913

Ramsey S 1997 Holistic manual therapy techniques. Primary Care 24(40):759–786

Raub J 2002 Psychophysiologic effects of hatha yoga on musculoskeletal and cardiopulmonary function: a literature review. Journal of Alternative and Complementary Medicine 8(6):797–812

Ravin T, Cantieri M, Pasquarello G 2005 Course notes: Prolotherapy below the waist. University of New England College of Osteopathic Medicine, Biddeford, Maine

Reeves K 1993 Treatment of consecutive severe fibromyalgia patients with prolotherapy. Journal of Orthopaedic Medicine 16:3

Reeves KD, Hassanein K 2000a Randomized, prospective, double-blind, placebo-controlled study of dextrose prolotherapy for osteoarthritic thumb and finger (DIP, PIP, and trapeziometacarpal) joints: evidence of clinical efficacy. Journal of Alternative and Complementary Medicine 6(4):311–320

Reeves K, Hassanein K 2000b Randomized, prospective, double-blind, placebo-controlled study of dextrose prolotherapy for knee osteoarthritis with or without ACL laxity. Alternative Therapies in Health and Medicine 6(2):68–80

Reeves KD, Hassanein K 2003 Long term effects of dextrose prolotherapy for anterior cruciate ligament laxity: a prospective and consecutive patient study. Alternative Therapies in Health and Medicine 9(3):58–62

Rice G 2002 The effect of a NMT to the diaphragm on cervical range of motion. Online. Available: www.osteopathic-research.com/cgi-bin/or/Search1.pl?show_one=30707

Rich GJ 2002 Massage therapy: the evidence for practice. Churchill Livingstone, Edinburgh

Richard R 1978 Lésions ostéopathiques du sacrum. Maloine, Paris

Riot F-M, Goudet P, Moreaux J-P 2005 Levator ani syndrome, functional intestinal disorders and articular abnormalities of the pelvis, the place of osteopathic treatment. Presse Medicale 33(13):852–857

Roberts E, Cremata E, Collins S 2003 Fibrosis release procedures, including manipulation under anesthesia: a handbook defining the mobilization, myofascial release, and spinal adjustive procedures for the primary and secondary doctor of chiropractic. Fremont Chiropractic Group, Fremont, CA

Rome P 1999 Perspectives: an overview of comparative considerations of cerebrovascular accidents. Chiropractic Journal of Australia 29(3):87–102

Rosner A 2003 Fables or foibles: inherent problems with RCTs. Journal of Manipulative and Physiological Therapeutics 26:460–467

Rothwell D, Bondy S, Williams I 2001 Chiropractic manipulation and stroke. Stroke 32:1054–1060

Rowane W, Rowane M 1999 An osteopathic approach to asthma. Journal of the American Osteopathic Association 99(5):259–264

Rowe M, Alfred D 1999 Effectiveness of slow-stroke massage in diffusing agitated behaviours in individuals with Alzheimer's disease. Journal of Gerontology and Nursing 25:22–34

Rozmaryn L, Dovelle S, Rothman E et al 1998 Nerve and tendon gliding exercises and the conservative management of carpal tunnel syndrome. Journal of Hand Therapy 11(3):171–179

Ruddy T 1962 Osteopathic rapid rhythmic resistive technic. Academy of Applied Osteopathy Yearbook, Carmel, CA, p 23–31

Rydeard R, Leger A, Smith D 2006 Pilates-based therapeutic exercise: effect on subjects with nonspecific chronic low back pain and functional disability: a randomized controlled trial. Journal of Orthopedics and Sports Physical Therapy 36(7):472–484

Sackett D 2002 Testimony at Lewis Inquest, Coroner's Court, Toronto, November 20, 2002

Sandoz R 1976 Some physical mechanisms and effects of spinal adjustments. Annals of the Swiss Chiropractic Association 6:91–141

Sarti C, Tuomilehto J, Sivenius J et al 1994 Declining trends in incidence, case-fatality and mortality of stroke in three geographic areas of Finland during 1983–1989. Results from the FINMONICA stroke register. Journal of Clinical Epidemiology 47:1259–1269

Schafer R 1987 Clinical biomechanics: musculoskeletal actions and reactions, 2nd edn. Williams & Wilkins, Baltimore, p 436–437

Schenk RJ, Adelman K, Rousselle J 1994 The effects of muscle energy technique on cervical range of motion. Journal of Manual and Manipulative Therapy 2(4):149–155

Schenk RJ, MacDiarmid A, Rousselle J 1997 The effects of muscle energy technique on lumbar range of motion. Journal of Manual and Manipulative Therapy 5(4):179–183

Schiowitz S 1990 Facilitated positional release. American Osteopathic Association 90(2):145–156

Schmid-Schonbein G 1990 Microlymphatics and lymph flow. Physiological Review 70(4):997–1028

Schmitt GD, Pelham TW, Holt LE 1999 From the field. A comparison of selected protocols during proprioceptive neuromuscular facilitation stretching. Clinical Kinesiology 53(1):16–21

Schneider M, Cohen J, Laws S 2001 The collected writings of Nimmo and Vannerson, pioneers of chiropractic trigger point therapy. Self-published, Pittsburgh

Schnirring L 2000 Are your patients asking about prolotherapy? Physician and Sportsmedicine 28(8):15–17

Segal NA, Hein J, Basford J 2004 The effects of Pilates training on flexibility and body composition: an observational study. Archives of Physical Medicine and Rehabilitation 85:1977–1981

Sejersted O, Hargens A, Kardel K et al 1984 Intramuscular fluid pressure during isometric contraction of human skeletal muscle. Journal of Applied Physiology 56:287–295

Selvamurthy W 1994 Yoga and stress management: physiological perspective. Indian Journal of Physiology and Pharmacology 38:46–47

Selye H 1971 Hormones and resistance. Journal of Pharmaceutical Sciences 60:1

Selye H 1978 The stress of life, revised edn. McGraw-Hill, New York

Senstad O, Leboeuf-Yde C, Borchgrevink C 1996 Predictors of side-effects to spinal manipulative therapy. Journal of Manipulative and Physiological Therapeutics 19:441–445

Senstad O, Leboeuf-Yde, C, Borchgrevink C 1997 Frequency and characteristics of side effects of spinal manipulative therapy. Spine 22(4):435–440

Sergueef N, Nelson K, Glonek T 2002 The effect of cranial manipulation on the Traube–Hering–Mayer oscillation as measured by laser-Doppler flowmetry. Alternative Therapies in Health and Medicine 8(6):74–76

Shea M 1993 Myofascial release – a manual for the spine and extremities. Shea Educational Group, Juno Beach, FL

Shekelle PG, Adams AH, Chassin MR et al 1992 Spinal manipulation for low back pain. Annals of Internal Medicine 117(7):590–598

Shievink WT, Mokri B, Whisnant JP 1993 Internal carotid artery dissection in a community: Rochester, Minnesota, 1987–1992. Stroke 24(11):1678–1680

Shievink WT, Mokri B, O'Falion WM 1994 Recurrent spontaneous cervical-artery dissection. New England Journal of Medicine 330(6):393–397

Shoemaker J, Tiidus P, Mader R 1997 Failure of manual massage to alter limb blood flow: measures by Doppler ultrasound. Medicine and Science in Sports and Exercise 29(5):610–614

Shulman K, Jones G 1996 Effectiveness of massage therapy intervention on reducing anxiety in the workplace. Journal of Applied Behavioral Science 32:160–173

Shustova N, Maltsev NA, Levkovitch Y et al 1985 Hyperemia in capillaries of gastrocnemius muscle following stretching. Fiziologicheskii Zhurnal SSSR 71(5):599–608

Simons D, Travell J, Simons L 1999 Myofascial pain and dysfunction: the trigger point manual, vol. 1: upper half of body, 2nd edn. Williams & Wilkins, Baltimore

Singh AN 2006 Role of yoga therapies in psychosomatic disorders. Proceedings of the 18th World Congress on Psychosomatic Medicine, Kobe, Japan, 21–26 August 2005. International Congress Series 1287, p 91–96

Singh S, Malhotra V, Singh K et al 2004 Role of yoga in modifying certain cardiovascular functions in type 2 diabetic patients. Journal of the Association of Physicians of India 52:203–206

Sleszynski S, Kelso A 1993 Comparison of thoracic manipulation with incentive spirometry in preventing postoperative atelectasis. Journal of the American Osteopathic Association 93(8):834–838

Smith FF 1986 Inner bridges: a guide to energy movement and body structure. Humanics New Age, Atlanta

Smith FF 1994 Interviewed by Brown S, Summer 1994. Caduceus Magazine, p 22–24

Souza T 1994 General approach to musculoskeletal complaints. In: Souza TA (ed) Differential diagnosis and management for the chiropractor, 2nd edn. Aspen, Gaithersburg, MD

Spencer H 1976 Shoulder technique. Journal of the American Osteopathic Association 15:2118–2220

Sridevi K, Krishna-Rao P 1996 Yoga practice and menstrual distress. Journal of the Indian Academy of Applied Psychology 22:47–54

Stanko E 2002 The role of modified Pilates in women's health physiotherapy. Journal of the Association of Chartered Physiotherapists in Women's Health 90:21–32

Stanley K, Weaver J 1998 Pharmacologic management of pain and inflammation in athletes. Clinical Sports Medicine 17(2):375–392

Stevinson C, Ernst E 2002 Risks associated with spinal manipulation. American Journal of Medicine 112(7):566–571

Stewart J 2000 Focal peripheral neuropathies, 3rd edn. Lippincott Williams & Wilkins, Philadelphia

Stone C 1999 The science and art of osteopathy. Stanley Thornes, Cheltenham

Strong J, Unruh A, Wright A, Baxter G 2002 Pain: a textbook for therapists. Churchill Livingstone, Edinburgh

Sung P, Kang Y, Pickar J 2005 Effect of spinal manipulation duration on low threshold mechanoreceptors in lumbar paraspinal muscles. Spine 25(1):115–122

Szuba A, Achalu R 2002 Decongestive lymphatic therapy for patients with breast carcinoma-associated lymphedema. Cancer 95(11):2260–2267

Takai S, Woo SL, Horibe S et al 1991 Effect of frequency and duration of controlled passive mobilization on tendon healing. Journal of Orthopaedic Research 9(5):705–713

Tamir L, Hendel D, Neyman C et al 1999 Sequential foot compression reduces lower limb swelling and pain after total knee arthroplasty. Journal of Arthroplasty 14(3):333–338

Tanaka S, Martin C, Thibodeau P 1998 Clinical neurology. In: Anrig C (ed) Pediatric chiropractic. Williams & Wilkins, Baltimore, p 608

Taneja I, Deepak K, Poojary G et al 2004 Yogic versus conventional treatment in diarrhea-predominant irritable bowel syndrome: a randomized control study. Applied Psychophysiology Biofeedback 29(1):19–33

Taylor D, Dalton J, Seaber A et al 1990 Viscoelastic properties of muscle-tendon units – the biomechanical effects of stretching. American Journal of Sports Medicine 18(3):300–309

Taylor D, Brooks D, Ryan J 1997 Visco-elastic characteristics of muscle: passive stretching versus muscular contractions. Medicine and Science in Sports and Exercise 29(12):1619–1624

Telles S, Nagarathna R, Nagendra H 1994 Breathing through a particular nostril can alter metabolism and autonomic activities. Indian Journal of Physiology and Pharmacology 38(2):133–137

Terrett A 1996a Vertebrobasilar stroke following manipulation. National Chiropractic Mutual Insurance Company, Des Moines, IA, p 8

Terrett A 1996b Vertebrobasilar stroke following manipulation. National Chiropractic Mutual Insurance Company, Des Moines, IA, p 13–16

Terrett A 1996c Vertebrobasilar stroke following manipulation. National Chiropractic Mutual Insurance Company, Des Moines, IA, p 15

Terrett A 1996d Vertebrobasilar stroke following manipulation. National Chiropractic Mutual Insurance Company, Des Moines, IA, p 32

Terrett A 1996e Vertebrobasilar stroke following manipulation. National Chiropractic Mutual Insurance Company, Des Moines, IA, p 34

Thiel H, Wallace K, Donat J, Yong-Hing K 1994 Effect of various head and neck positions on vertebral artery blood flow. Clinical Biomechanics 9:105–110

Thiele G 1937 Coccygodynia and pain in the superior gluteal region. Journal of the American Medical Association 109:1271–1275

Tissington-Tatlow W, Bammer H 1957 Syndrome of vertebral artery compression. Neurology 7:331–340

Tomlinson K 2002 Comparison of neuromuscular technique and muscle energy technique on dorsiflexion range of motion. Online. Available: www.osteopathic-research.com/cgi-bin/or/Search1.pl?show_one=30795

Toole J, Tucker S 1960 Influence of head position upon cerebral circulation: studies on blood flow in cadavers. Archives of Neurology 2:616–623

Topol GA, Reeves KD, Hassanein K 2005 Efficacy of dextrose prolotherapy in elite male kicking-sport athletes with chronic groin pain. Archives of Physical Medicine and Rehabilitation 86:697–702

Trager M 1987 Mentastics: movement as a way to agelessness. Station Hill Press, Barrytown, New York

Tran M, Holly R, Lashbrook J 2001 Effects of hatha yoga practice on the health-related aspects of physical fitness. Preventive Cardiology 4(4):165–170

Travell J, Simons L 1992a Myofascial pain and dysfunction: the trigger point manual, vol. 2: the lower extremities. Williams & Wilkins, Baltimore, p 10

Travell J, Simons L 1992b Myofascial pain and dysfunction: the trigger point manual, vol. 2: the lower extremities. Williams & Wilkins, Baltimore, p 73

Troup J 1981 Straight-leg raising and the qualifying tests for increased root tension. Spine 6:526–527

Twomey L, Taylor J 1982 Flexion, creep, dysfunction and hysteresis in the lumbar vertebral column. Spine 7(2):116–122

UK BEAM Trial Team 2004 UK back pain exercise and manipulation randomized trial. British Medical Journal 329(7479):1381–1385

Upledger J 1978 The relationship of craniosacral examination findings in grade school children with developmental problems. Journal of the American Osteopathic Association 77(10):760–776

Upledger J, Vredevoogd J 1983 Craniosacral therapy. Eastland Press, Seattle

Upton A, McComas A 1973 The double crush in nerve entrapment syndromes. Lancet 2:359–362.

Vallone S, Fallon J 1997 Treatment protocols for the chiropractic care of common pediatric conditions: otitis media and asthma. Journal of Clinical Chiropractic Pediatrics 2:113–115

van Wingerden JP, Vleeming A, Kleinrensink GJ, Stoeckart R 1997 The role of the hamstrings in pelvic and spinal function. In: Vleeming A, Mooney V, Dorman T, Snijders CJ, Stoeckart R (eds) Movement, stability and low back pain – the essential role of the pelvis. Churchill Livingstone, Edinburgh, p 207–210

Varma D 1937 The human machine and its forces: pranotherapy. Health for All Publishers, London

Vernon H, Dharmi I, Howley T et al 1986 Spinal manipulation and beta-endorphin. Journal of Manipulative and Physiological Therapeutics 9:115–123

Vleeming A, Mooney V, Snjiders C, Stoekart R (eds) 1977 Movement, stability and low back pain. Churchill Livingstone, New York

Von Piekartz H, Bryden L (eds) 2001 Craniofacial dysfunction and pain. Butterworth-Heinemann, Oxford

Walach H, Guthlin C, Konig M 2003 Efficacy of massage therapy in chronic pain – a pragmatic randomized trial. Journal of Alternative and Complementary Medicine 9:837–846

Wallace E, McPartland J, Jones J et al 1997a Lymphatic manipulative techniques. In: Ward R (ed) Foundations for osteopathic medicine. Williams & Wilkins, Baltimore

Wallace E, McPartland J, Jones J et al 1997b Lymphatic manipulative techniques. In: Ward R (ed) Foundations for osteopathic medicine. Williams & Wilkins, Baltimore, p 956–957

Walsh M, Polus B 1998 A randomized placebo controlled clinical trial on the efficacy of chiropractic therapy on premenstrual syndrome. In: Proceedings of International Conference on Spinal Manipulation, Vancouver, BC, July 16–19 1998

Walther D 1988 Applied kinesiology. SDC Systems, Pueblo, CO

Ward R 1997 Foundations for osteopathic medicine. Williams & Wilkins, Baltimore

Weiselfish S 1993 Manual therapy for the orthopedic and neurologic patient. Regional Physical Therapy, Hertford, CT

Weiss J 2001 Pelvic floor myofascial trigger points manual therapy for interstitial cystitis and the urgency–frequency syndrome. Journal of Urology 166:2226–2231

Wells M, Giantonoto S, D'Agate D et al 1999 Standard osteopathic manipulative treatment acutely improves gait performance in patients with Parkinson's disease. Journal of the American Osteopathic Association 99(2):92–98

Wheeden A, Scafidi A, Field T et al 1993 Massage effects on cocaine-exposed preterm neonates. Developmental and Behavioral Reviews 21:1–10

Wilkinson H 2005 Injection therapy for enthesopathies causing axial spine pain and 'the failed back syndrome': a single blinded, randomized and cross-over study. Pain Physician 8:167–176

Williams P 1988 Effect of intermittent stretch on immobilised muscle. Annals of Rheumatic Disease 47:1014–1016

Williams P, Catanese T, Lucey E et al 1988 The importance of stretch and contractile activity in the prevention of accumulation in muscle. Journal of Anatomy 158:109–114

Wilson A 2002 Effective management of musculoskeletal injury: a clinical ergonomics approach to prevention, treatment and rehabilitation. Churchill Livingstone, Edinburgh

Wilson E 1994 Peripheral joint mobilisation with movement and its effects on adverse neural tension. Manipulative Physiotherapist 26(2):35–39

Wilson E 2007 The Mulligan concept: NAGs, SNAGs, MWMs. In: Chaitow L (ed) Positional release techniques, 3rd edn. Churchill Livingstone, Edinburgh

Wilson E, Payton O, Donegan-Shoaf L et al 2003 Muscle energy technique in patients with acute low back pain: a pilot clinical trial. Journal of Orthopaedic and Sports Physical Therapy 33:502–512

Wittlinger H, Wittlinger G 1982 Textbook of Dr Vodder's manual lymph drainage, vol 1: basic course, 3rd edn. Karl F Haug, Heidelberg

Wong C, Schauer-Alvarez C 2004a Effect of strain/counterstrain on pain and strength in hip musculature. Reliability, validity and effectiveness of strain/counterstrain techniques. Journal of Manual and Manipulative Therapy 12(2):107–112

Wong C, Schauer-Alvarez C 2004b Effect of strain/counterstrain on pain and strength in hip musculature. Journal of Manual and Manipulative Therapy 12(4):215–223

Woo SL, Vogrin TM, Abramowitch SD 2000 Healing and repair of ligament injuries in the knee. Journal of the American Academy of Orthopedic Surgeons 8(6):364–372

Yates H, Vardy T, Kuchera M et al 2002 Effects of osteopathic manipulative treatment and concentric and eccentric maximal effort exercise on women with MS. Journal of the American Osteopathic Association 102(5):267–275

Yates RG, Lamping DL, Abram NL, Wright C 1988 Effects of chiropractic treatment on blood pressure and anxiety. A randomized controlled trial. Journal of Manipulative and Physiological Therapeutics 11:484–488

Yelland MJ, Del Mar C, Pirozzo S et al 2004 Prolotherapy injections for chronic low-back pain. Cochrane Database of Systematic Reviews (2): CD004059

Youngs B 1963 The physiological background of neuromuscular technique. British Naturopathic Journal and Osteopathic Review 5:176–178

Zero Balancing Association UK information leaflet. Zero Balancing Association, London

Zero Balancing Health Association, Columbia, MD. Online. Available: www.zerobalancing.com

Zhao-Pu W 1991 Acupressure therapy. Churchill Livingstone, Melbourne

Zusman M 1988 Prolonged relief from articular soft tissue pain with passive joint movement. Journal of Manual Medicine 3:100–102

Zusman M, Edwards B, Donaghy A 1989 Investigation of proposed mechanism for relief of spinal pain with passive joint movement. Journal of Manual Medicine 4:58–61

8

Integrated Naturopathic (Manual) Physical Medicine Protocols

Leon Chaitow ND DO

With contributions from:
Eric Blake ND
Douglas C. Lewis ND

CHAPTER CONTENTS

As discussed in Chapters 3 and 7 there exist a number of general ('universal'), constitutional manual approaches to health care, several of which emerged from a background of naturopathic medicine in the first half of the 20th century. As explained in this chapter, other general approaches have been developed by the osteopathic profession, and the research validation of these offers a useful supporting element to those used in naturopathic settings.

The purely naturopathic protocols are:

1. Collins' universal naturopathic tonic technique (Cordingley 1925) – also known as general naturopathic tonic technique, abbreviated to UNTT and GNTT
2. Lief's (1963) neuromuscular technique, abbreviated to NMT (see Chapter 7 for description).

In addition, general (whole-body, wellness, constitutional) massage can also be shown to offer the potential to assist homeostatic functions, irrespective of the nature of the symptoms, and should therefore be incorporated into this discussion (Fritz et al 1999). In the section covering massage in Chapter 7, page 223 (under the subheading 'Validation of efficacy'), see the lengthy list of conditions in which precisely this form of 'general massage' (i.e. non-specific) has shown itself capable of offering significant benefit almost universally in dozens of named conditions (Field 2006).

As explained later in this chapter (as well as in Chapter 10), osteopathic medicine has also evolved a number of integrated therapeutic manual protocols – using combinations of modalities also commonly employed in naturopathic practice (Wernham 1996). These methods, which usually include gentle rhythmic movements of the spine and extremities (Lederman 1999), have been shown in both hospital and office settings to effectively enhance the individual's adaptive potential and self-regulating functions, as evidenced by a reduction in time required to remain in hospital before recovery from a variety of conditions, including pneumonia, pancreatitis and surgery of various types.

While there are some differences between these protocols and methods (see below), they contain a number of essential similarities, making it possible to suggest that almost all patients, whether hospitalized or seen in an office setting, can benefit from what may be termed general, non-specific, whole-body, often rhythmic/oscillatory mobilization, using simple, non-invasive, modalities and techniques (see previous chapter), in combination with each other, as outlined in this chapter.

Evidence and opinion

Lederman (2005a) has diligently compiled evidence explaining the effects of particular manual approaches, and some of this information is summarized in Chapter 7, in particular relating to fluid movement and adaptation. See also the evidence relating to manual treatment and enhanced homeostasis and adaptation potential, in Chapter 10.

Lederman points out that:

Techniques that stimulate fluid flow play an important therapeutic role in manual therapy. These techniques are largely aimed at assisting the repair process and homeostasis in different tissues.

From a naturopathic perspective there could be little that is more important than encouraging self-regulation.

UNTT and NMT

Universal (general) naturopathic tonic technique (UNTT or GNTT) is a constitutional, virtually generally applicable method, developed in the early part of the 20th century by Frederick Collins MD ND, and described by Cordingley in 1925.

UNTT offers naturopaths (and others) the opportunity to evaluate biomechanical changes, and to modulate these as appropriate, in the context of a general mobilizing treatment. According to Cordingley, the total time required to perform Collins' GNTT is 7–10 minutes.

UNTT can be used as a means of offering a non-specific, general, 'loosening'/mobilizing process, during which areas of mild restriction may normalize, while offering an opportunity for the practitioner to evaluate levels of compensation, adaptation, restriction, dysfunction, discomfort and asymmetry. This leads to enhanced circulatory (blood and lymph), neurological and mobility functions,

benefiting the individual's adaptive potential. A description of a modified GNTT protocol is given later in this chapter while its historical context is described in Chapter 3.

Lief's NMT

In its general application, Lief's NMT offers a similar, non-specific, global, whole-body opportunity for the practitioner to simultaneously evaluate, assess and (if appropriate) treat dysfunctional biomechanical (possibly viscerosomatic in origin) patterns that represent evidence of failed or failing adaptation, or of actual pathology (Chaitow 2002).

Peter Lief ND DC, son of the primary developer of NMT Stanley Lief ND DC, noted: 'NMT is a type of specific soft tissue treatment which is followed [or accompanied] by a general mobilising articular manipulation' (Lief 1963).

Boris Chaitow ND DC, cousin of Stanley Lief and co-developer of NMT, has observed (Chaitow B 1980):

The body's integrity and its functional efficiency depends not only on its chemistry, influenced by the food and drink we ingest, but also on effective nerve and blood circulation, free of mechanical and functional obstructions. To this purpose there is no formula devised by the osteopathic or chiropractic professions that will more effectively achieve the optimum result than . . . the technique [NMT] devised by Stanley Lief.

Clinically, an average NMT treatment involving general mobilization of the spine, pelvis and extremities takes approximately 15 minutes.

(See fuller descriptions of Lief's NMT in Chapters 6 and 7, and also the notes in Chapter 7 by Brian Youngs ND DO, a veteran of the early years of NMT usage in the UK, who describes its application in the context of naturopathic care of patients.)

In terms of modifying structure to enhance function, these approaches can be seen to represent a means whereby adaptive changes can frequently be recognized (and potentially modified if appropriate) in the context of a non-specific therapeutic encounter (see Chapter 2 for an in-depth discussion of adaptation features).

Guidelines, not instructions

In essence, the constitutional approaches described comprise an integrated use of several of the individual modalities described in the previous chapter –

including neuromuscular techniques (NMT), massage and joint mobilization methods. The formulae/protocols outlined below are therefore suggested as being broad blueprints, guidelines, not necessarily to be followed blindly, or as firm instructions.

More realistically, what both Lief's NMT and Collins' GNTT/UNTT suggest is that naturopathic health care should offer *each and every patient* a degree of biomechanical release from held patterns of restriction, as part of the treatment process. This should be the case whatever the named condition may be, and whatever the age or state of health of the person, since all the constituent elements (modalities), including applied compression, stretching, mobilization, etc., can readily be modulated to being applied extremely gently, or more robustly, depending upon the vitality and needs of the individual.

Comparison with constitutional hydrotherapy

In this way it is easy to reflect that constitutional manual approaches such as NMT, GNTT and massage should, in all particulars, be considered in the same way as constitutional hydrotherapy (CH) (see Chapter 11).

In use of CH the standard towel application (potentially involving variations in the degree of contrast of temperatures and/or other variables including amount of water in applied towels, length of time in contact with the skin, etc.) provides the foundation of the treatment.

Along with the towel application, physical therapy electrical modalities can provide both a standard application and the potential for individualized treatment – for example, the location of the front electrode during abdominal electromuscular stimulation treatment (see Chapter 12) can be directed to the stomach, as in the standard approach, or over the umbilicus to treat the small intestine, etc. Additional phases of treatment, involving different physiotherapy modalities, can focus the treatment to individual needs even further.[1]

In bodywork the variables relate to the degree of stimulus offered. The notes on force loading, in

Chapter 7, describe the different forces that can be employed in physical medicine, and it is obvious that a few ounces/grams of digital pressure will have quite a different effect, and will engender quite a different response, as compared with pounds or kilos of pressure.

The notes that discuss manual methods of assisting adaptation, fluid flow and neurological influences in Chapter 7 offer further information as to the potential benefits of a general, constitutional, mobilization approach.

The degree of mechanical input, duration and speed, and the rhythm employed, will all modify what could superficially be seen to be a predetermined set of mechanical maneuvers, where every patient receives the same series of modalities and manipulations. Instead, what emerges is a veritable orchestration of the variables to meet the particular needs of the individual.

All symphonies are not the same, even though they involve (more or less) use of the same instruments, and no two NMT sessions, GNTT sessions or massage treatments are the same, despite more or less following the same sequence, and utilizing similar therapeutic instruments.

Osteopathic evidence

In considering what support exists for the use of an integrated formulation of non-specific modalities and manual methods, it is useful to reflect on the evidence that has emerged from various osteopathic clinicians and researchers.

In all the examples listed below the term 'OMT' is used to describe a range of approaches including muscle energy technique, myofascial release, positional release (strain/counterstrain), high velocity, low amplitude methods, as well as a number of specific methods that focus on lymphatic and respiratory function ('lymphatic pump').

All these methods are discussed or described in this chapter, in Chapter 7 or in Chapter 9.

For example, Clark & McCombs (2006) have described a selection of basic techniques designed to support respiration, circulation, ventilation and perfusion in hospitalized patients, in order to augment recovery following a surgery.

They note that there are numerous examples where osteopathic manipulative treatment (OMT) has been shown to have a positive impact on the length of hospital stay for patients with a variety of diagnoses.

They refer to studies by Stiles (1979), Radjieski et al (1998), Cantieri (1997), Noll et al (1999, 2000), Sleszynski & Kelso (1993) and others – all of which

---

[1]*Editorial note:* In earlier years this type of electrical stimulation was offered by sine-wave machines (see Chapter 12). However, as Doug Lewis ND points out, 'Nowadays, if one were to go looking for a sine-wave machine, most equipment suppliers will not know what is being asked for. Most newer devices do not actually produce a sine wave; rather they produce a square or rectangular wave that is modulated via a square, triangular ramp, or sometimes a sine wave.'

show that recovery time from various conditions and situations can be reduced, and length of stay in hospital minimized, when combinations of modalities, clustered under a general heading of osteopathic manipulative (or manual) treatment (or therapy), abbreviated as OMT, are used. It should be emphasized that although some of the OMT combinations, discussed in this chapter, may have emerged from osteopathic medicine, most of the modalities incorporated into these general integrated sequences are used universally by physical medicine practitioners of all schools.

Clark & McCombs note that:

- Radjieski et al's (1998) randomized controlled study demonstrated that in cases of pancreatitis, length of hospital stay was reduced by about one half when OMT involving 10–20 minutes daily of a standardized protocol (using myofascial release, soft tissue and strain/counterstrain techniques) was given, together with standard medical care. Patients who received OMT averaged significantly fewer days in the hospital before discharge (mean reduction, 3.5 days) than control subjects.
- Noll et al (1999, 2000) applied osteopathic manual methods to elderly hospitalized patients with pneumonia, and the result was that the length of stay in the hospital was reduced from a mean of 8.6 days without OMT, to 6.6 days with OMT. Additional benefits in this study, for those receiving OMT, included reduced length of use of intravenous antibiotics.
- Stiles (1979) demonstrated that patients' average length of hospital stay was reduced by roughly one day when appropriate general osteopathic methods (see Chapter 7) were used on bed-ridden patients with a variety of health problems ranging from congestive heart failure to obstetric and surgical conditions. Stiles (1977) observed: 'In many cases patients with chronic problems thought to be neurotic were relieved. In other cases surgical measures were avoided as a result of structural examination and manipulation.'
- Cantieri's (1997) study involving hospitalized patients with a variety of diagnoses, demonstrated that OMT, combined with normal medical care, reduced the length of hospital stay by an average of half a day, compared to normal medical care alone.
- A study by Sleszynski & Kelso (1993) compared thoracic pump technique (see Chapter 7) to incentive spirometry techniques in the prevention of postoperative atelectasis. Thoracic pump was used twice daily while spirometry was used three to four times a day. Both treatments were effective in reducing atelectasis from a 50% occurrence rate to a 5% occurrence rate; however, the manual methods achieved the result with half the number of treatments, and patients' recovery, as measured by pulmonary function tests, occurred more rapidly.
- Nicholas & Oleski (2002) utilized a four-step protocol composed of rib raising, treatment of the thoracic inlet, respiratory diaphragm and pelvic diaphragm in treatment of postoperative pain. They report that: 'Patients who receive morphine preoperatively and OMT postoperatively tend to have less postoperative pain and require less intravenously administered morphine. In addition, OMT and relief of pain lead to decreased postoperative morbidity and mortality and increased patient satisfaction. Also, soft tissue manipulative techniques and thoracic pump techniques help to promote early ambulation and body movement.' (See Chapter 7 for details of thoracic pump methods.)
- O-Yurvati et al (2005) documented the physiological effects of postoperative OMT following a coronary artery bypass graft (CABG) to determine the effects on cardiac hemodynamics. Ten subjects undergoing CABG surgery were recruited for postoperative OMT. The primary assessment compared pre-OMT versus post-OMT, measurements of thoracic impedance, mixed venous oxygen saturation and cardiac index. Immediately following CABG surgery OMT was provided to alleviate anatomic dysfunction of the rib cage caused by median sternotomy, and to improve respiratory function. This adjunctive treatment occurred while subjects were completely anesthetized. Results suggested improved peripheral circulation and increased mixed venous oxygen saturation after OMT. These increases were accompanied by an improvement in cardiac index ($p \leq 0.01$). The authors conclude that OMT has immediate, beneficial hemodynamic effects after CABG surgery when administered while the patient is sedated and pharmacologically paralyzed.
- In Chapter 10 evidence is offered of the value of a non-specific osteopathic and soft tissue

protocol, in treatment of chronic fatigue syndrome (Perrin et al 1998).

Clark & McCombs (2006), whose perspective derives from osteopathic medicine, observe that the natural sequelae of the cumulative insults to physiology that occur during surgery:

> . . . are seen daily in every hospital in America: atelectasis, ileus and venous stasis (edema, deep venous thrombosis, skin ulcerations). Allopathic medicine offers incentive spirometry, early ambulation, continuous passive motion equipment, anticoagulation drugs, and skilled nursing practices to counteract the effects described.

They suggest that early intervention with physical (osteopathic) medicine strategies may avert or reduce such adverse outcomes.

Their objectives in suggesting the physical medicine protocol summarized below are to:

1. restore the cranial rhythmic impulse to its full rate and excursion
2. restore ventilation to full capacity
3. maintain and/or restore peristalsis
4. restore the third space fluid (lymph) to the circulation.

They suggest that various techniques can be used to achieve each of these four goals, and that some of the techniques overlap, and meet multiple goals.

Clark & McCombs' osteopathic protocol

Observing that the results reported by Noll et al (2000) were achieved by using a similar protocol (see below), Clark & McCombs list a seven-step sequence based on osteopathic manipulative techniques, all of which are discussed in this chapter, in Chapter 7 or in Chapter 9.

The methods employed by Noll et al, where these are different from those selected by Clark & McCombs, are listed subsequent to this list:

1. Condylar decompression (using a lateral approach if the head of the bed is inaccessible). This technique was also utilized by Noll et al.
2. Sphenobasilar decompression (using a lateral approach if the head of the bed is inaccessible).
3. Correction of cervical spine dysfunctions utilizing soft tissue technique and, if appropriate, HVLA techniques. This approach was also utilized by Noll et al.
4. Bilateral rib-raising. This was also utilized by Noll et al.

5. Re-doming of the diaphragm. This was also utilized by Noll et al.
6. Lumbosacral decompression and balancing of the pelvic diaphragm, as indicated.
7. Lymphatic pump, such as the pedal pump (not suitable in cases of deep vein thrombosis, if there are central venous lines, the patient is intubated or if the leg is immobilized in a cast or other fixation device). Noll et al employed thoracic lymphatic pump methods (see Chapter 7).

The techniques employed by Noll et al (2000) in treating elderly, hospitalized patients with pneumonia, which differed from the Clark & McCombs' protocol, included use of:

1. bilateral spinal inhibition techniques
2. myofascial release of the anterior thoracic inlet
3. thoracic lymphatic pump methods (Kuchera & Kuchera 1990).

Within the framework of this protocol a great deal of flexibility was encouraged, directed by what was assessed in the individual patient. For example, Noll et al report that:

> The application of each technique was fitted to each individual's unique somatic dysfunction found on structural examination. For example [those] giving the standardized protocol were able to spend more time applying muscle inhibition, or rib raising, on those paraspinal segments with somatic dysfunction, and less on those relatively free of somatic dysfunction. Where appropriate, attempt was made to achieve local tissue texture changes, myofascial release, or segmental function, before going on to the next region or technique.

In addition to the standardized protocol, Noll et al note:

> To address somatic dysfunction not adequately treated by the standardized protocol, each patient was seen by an OMT specialist, who was allowed to use any technique he felt appropriate to address specific somatic dysfunction.

The variability demonstrated in this example, in which individual needs are recognized within a framework of a general approach, re-emphasizes the message mentioned earlier, that although the pattern remains the same, this is *not* a standardized, 'one size fits all' approach.

This focus on individuality was also the case in the 1920s, when naturopaths employed the UNTT approach (as described earlier). Cordingley (1925) proposed that the general UNTT should be given, followed by treatment of specific 'lesions', together with use of spondylotherapy (see Chapter 7) and dietetic counseling.

Rationale for selection of techniques used in the Clark & McCombs' protocol

Clark & McCombs report that the techniques listed were chosen because they are easily administered. Their objective was to suggest that even supervised students could administer these relatively simple methods, with very low risk to the patients, and a high probability of successful outcome.

They note that the Noll et al (2000) protocol was administered by second-year students who had received specific training in use of the protocol for treatment, designed to be administered to postoperative patients.

Clark & McCombs observe that:

- The condylar decompression technique was selected to offset the hyperextension necessitated by intubation, as well as possibly reducing compression and irritation of the vagus nerve pathway through the jugular foramen, so reducing the possibility of postoperative ileus.
- The sphenobasilar synchondrosis (SBS) decompression technique is also suggested to offer benefits in reducing the postoperative effects of anesthesia and intubation. Both condylar and SBS decompression can be applied from a lateral position if a hospital bed position precludes access from the head end.
- Treatment to the cervical spine is suggested to be beneficial since the phrenic nerve originates at C3, C4 and C5, providing as it does innervation to the diaphragm. Neck extension during intubation stresses this area. They note that, anecdotally, 'many patients with postoperative singulitis (intractable hiccup) have dysfunctions of C3, 4, or 5'. Manual treatment to this area may help normalize nerve supply to the diaphragm and eliminate the singulitis.
- Rib-raising techniques were included in the protocol because of their ease of application and their extremely lengthy use in osteopathy (since 1890). Rib raising improves inhalation function, and helps restore autonomic balance. In addition, it encourages lymphatic drainage through the thoracic duct, and can be beneficial in maintaining and restoring peristalsis.

- Re-doming of the diaphragm improves respiratory function, stimulates peristalsis and improves lymphatic flow.
- Willard (1998) has shown that the diaphragm has significant lymphatic collection structures on its inferior surface, so that the rise and fall of the diaphragm accelerates the collection of ascitic accumulations in the abdomen, returning them to lymphatic circulation.
- Lumbosacral decompression and balancing of the pelvic floor muscles may assist in the maintenance and restoration of peristalsis and urinary function.

Noll et al's (2000) technique selection

In a pilot study in 1999, Noll et al described the use of OMT in treating seriously ill, elderly, hospitalized patients with a combination of conventional (intravenous antibiotics) and manual methods.

The manual methods used were provided twice weekly as follows:

- Bilateral paraspinal inhibition
- Bilateral rib raising
- Diaphragmatic myofascial release
- Condylar decompression
- Cervical soft tissue technique
- Bilateral myofascial release of the anterior thoracic inlet
- Thoracic pump methods.

They noted:

All patients were treated while they lay supine in bed. The individuals giving the treatment would sit or stand on one side of the patient and administer paraspinal muscle inhibition and rib raising to the closest side. Then this individual would move to the opposite side of the patient and again administer paraspinal inhibition and rib raising. Next myofascial release would be given to the diaphragmatic area. Then the practitioner would move to the head of the bed and administer condylar decompression, cervical soft tissue technique, and bilateral myofascial release of the thoracic inlet and the thoracic lymphatic pump. Each standardized protocol treatment was administered for a duration of 10 to 15 minutes, twice daily on Monday through Friday, and once at each weekend. The protocol continued until one of the endpoints for the study were reached [normalization of fever, leukocytosis].

In this 1999 pilot study, Noll et al demonstrated reduced need for antibiotic use (oral and intravenous) and length of hospital stay when OMT was added to normal medical care.

At this point it is worth repeating (see Chapter 7) some of Lederman's (2005b) compilation of evidence for the usefulness of manual therapy in various settings:

- Enhancement of local circulation and drainage (Foldi & Strossenreuther 2003, Hovind & Nielsen 1974)
- Reduction of swelling and improved washout of inflammatory chemicals (Tamir et al 1999, Wittlinger & Wittlinger 1982)
- Assistance in normalization of trigger point myalgia (Larsson et al 1990)
- Modification of neural irritation caused by local edema (Hoyland et al 1989, Rozmaryn et al 1998)
- Assistance in postsurgical recovery (Cantieri 1997)
- Encouragement of optimal regeneration and repair, particularly during the remodeling phase of tissue recovery (Williams 1988, Williams et al 1988).

How do osteopathic protocols compare with those for GNTT and NMT?

As discussed above, the two most fully described, and studied, osteopathic protocols in recent years are those of Noll et al and Clark & McCombs.

It is possible to compare those approaches with very early general naturopathic (see later in this chapter) and osteopathic protocols – for example, the approach described by Barber in 1898 (see Box 8.1).

When asked whether delivery of a general osteopathic treatment to patients meant that they all received the same methodology, Mary LeClere DO observed (in 1922):

I have been asked to describe my typical general treatment. I might reply that there is no such thing as a typical general treatment. Each patient is a law unto himself, and the treatment must be adapted to his particular needs and characteristics.

The objectives of osteopathic integrated interventions – currently and for over 100 years – include enhanced respiratory, digestive, cardiovascular and circulatory (including lymphatic) functions – with a broad health enhancement outcome, as evidenced by a variety of studies demonstrating enhanced recovery from surgery and serious illness.

The description of Collins' general naturopathic tonic technique (GNTT) by Cordingly (1925) includes the following elements.

Box 8.1 General osteopathic treatment
(as described by Barber 1898)

1. Place the patient on the side; beginning at the upper cervicals, move the muscles upward and outward, gently but very deep, the entire length of the spinal column, being very particular in all regions which appear tender to the touch, have an abnormal temperature, or where the muscles seem to be in a knotty, cord-like or contracted condition. Treat the opposite side in a similar manner.

2. With the patient on the back, place the hand lightly over the following organs, vibrating each for 2 minutes, respectively: lungs, stomach, liver, pancreas and kidneys.

3. Flex the lower limbs, one at a time, against the abdomen, abducting the knee and abducting the foot strongly as the limb is extended with a light jerk.

4. Grasping the limb around the thigh with both hands, move the muscles very deeply from side to side the entire length of the limb. Treat the opposite limb in a similar manner.

5. Place one hand on the patient's shoulder, pressing the muscles down toward the point of the acromion process; with the disengaged hand grasp the patient's elbow, rotating the arm around the head.

6. Holding the arm firmly with one hand, with the other rotate the muscles very deeply, the entire length of the arm; also grasp the hand, placing the disengaged hand under the axilla, and give strong extension. Treat the opposite arm in a similar manner.

7. Place one hand under the chin, the other under the occiput, and introduce gentle but strong extension/traction.

8. Place one hand under the chin, drawing the head backward and to the side; with the disengaged hand manipulate the muscles [that are under tension]. Treat the opposite side in a similar manner. Also manipulate/mobilize, thoroughly and deeply, the muscles in front of the neck.

9. Place the patient on a stool; the operator places the thumbs on the angles of the 2nd ribs, an assistant raises the arms slowly but strongly above the head, as the patient inhales; press hard with the thumbs as the arms are lowered with a backward motion; the patient relaxes all the muscles and permits the elbows to bend; move the thumbs downward to the next lower ribs; raise the arms as before; and repeat, until the fifth pair of ribs have been treated in a similar manner.

GNTT (modified)

Note: Different descriptions of the GNTT list variations in the sequence of modality application, and of the areas involved. Clearly the objective was to cover the territory as efficiently and effectively as possible, utilizing soft tissue, mobilization and manipulation methods, as appropriate. The opportunities the use of these methods offered when used this way, to both evaluate and treat the patient, were very similar to those associated with Lief's neuromuscular technique, as described earlier.

1. With the patient lying prone, the articulations of the spine should be mobilized by beginning at the vertebra prominens (seventh cervical) and working downward. The articulations of the spine should also be mobilized ('opened'), beginning at the fifth lumbar and working upward. For example, L2 and 3 are 'opened' by placing the heel of the hand against the superior and inferior aspects of the spinous processes, respectively, and then delivering a light thrust, springing movement.

2. Standing at the left side of the patient, the right hand should be placed on the posterior crest of the right ilium, while the left hand cups the underside of the acromion process. The right hand pushes downwards at the same time that the left hand lifts in a cephalad direction, so opening the articulations of the intercostals on the left.

3. The right hand is then placed on the left posterior crest of the ilium, and the left hand cups the right acromion process, so that the procedure can be repeated, in order to open up the articulations of the intercostals on the right side.

4. Muscular contractions between the ribs are then released inferiorly, beginning at the 1st rib and working downward, by making contact with the heel of each hand on each side of the spine, contacting the superior surfaces of the ribs at their angles and springing these in an oblique direction, caudally and toward the floor.

5. The articulations of the ribs are then mobilized superiorly, beginning at the 10th pair of ribs, and working upward.

6. Still standing on the left side of the prone patient, the circulation of the trapezius, and other back muscles, should be enhanced by placing the right hand on the contralateral anterior crest of the ilium, with the left hand on the right scapula. Mobilization and stretching (or rhythmic rocking) can be achieved by holding the scapula towards the floor while lifting the pelvis. The opposite side is then treated by changing position to stand on the right.

7. The sternocleidomastoid muscle is stretched (along with the scalenes and upper trapezius) by having a heel of hand contact on the first three upper thoracic vertebrae while the head is rotated one way and then the other.

8. Apply 'the famous S-move' (rotating the first two fingers or thumbs deeply in the muscle mass) on the laminae of the thoracic and lumbar spines.

9. The patient lies supine with knees and hips flexed. The colon is then treated, beginning at the sigmoid flexure. Deep kneading of the colon is performed – up the left side of the abdomen, then across the transverse colon, and over the ascending colon on the right side.

10. The abdominal muscles are stretched from the hip to the shoulder on each side by lifting the pelvis while pushing down just beneath ribs, and vice versa.

11. Flex each knee and hip and rotate outward and inward.

12. Stretch the neck muscles and mobilize the cervical region.

Notes
- Item 1 would have similar effects to those noted in osteopathic paraspinal inhibition.
- Items 2, 3, 4 and 5 would achieve very much the same effect as that noted in osteopathic rib raising.
- Items 6 and 7 address soft tissue stiffness, and to some extent influence the thoracic inlet, as in the osteopathic protocol described earlier.
- Item 8 would have a similar effect to inhibitory pressure used in the OMT protocol, and would also have a general mobilizing influence.
- Item 12 replicates what is done in OMT.

Eric Blake ND has provided a commentary on the GNTT that elaborates on what is being achieved – or aimed for – during the various stages of the treatment protocol (Box 8.2).

GNTT and OMT compared

When GNTT is compared with OMT protocols as described earlier in this chapter, the following differences emerge:

Box 8.2 Anatomy of a tonic treatment

Eric Blake ND MSOM Dipl Ac

Note: Some of the methods and sequencing of this description differ from those outlined earlier in this chapter. As noted at the start of that previous description of GNTT, there was no absolute uniformity or pattern in use of this, apart from an attempt to efficiently, comprehensively and effectively mobilize tissues, while gathering information.

1. To begin, each of the thoracic and lumbar vertebrae is superiorly and inferiorly mobilized in a graded mobilization fashion. A light HVLA thrust may be introduced if appropriate to the patient's needs. Graded mobilization allows palpation of motion, and a stretch or thrust provides a treatment option. Often cavitation will occur as graded mobilization is gently introduced.

2. The second movement is a passive stretching/mobilization of the intercostal muscles, as a preparation for manipulation of the costovertebral joints.

3. The third movement involves mobilization of the costotransverse joints, and is similar mechanically to the first movement along the spine. Again there is a superior and inferior mobilization of the joint in a graded mobilization fashion, with the option of a grade 5, HVLA thrust.

4. The fourth movement is a passive stretching and rotational mobilization of the thorax, this time in a transverse plane in a direction opposite to the second movement. This also incorporates kneading of the trapezius and rhomboids along the scapular border on the relevant side.

5. The fifth movement is a passive stretching movement to the sternocleidomastoid. An optional thrust manipulation may be introduced. The object of the initial passive stretch is a traction of the cervical soft tissues, as well as a mobilization of the cervical vertebrae. The positioning of the final thrust is quite similar to the modern HVLA bedside technique, more accurately described as rotation gliding, patient prone, operator at side (Gibbons & Tehan 2000).

6. The sixth prone movement is of interest. It ultimately introduces a rotational movement of the entire thoracic column, as well as the first two lumbar segments. The movement employed is referred to as 'the famous S-move'.

Commentary to this stage of the GNTT

Chaitow has offered a description of the objectives of the 'S' technique:

This technique should be applied along the course of particularly tense and hard unyielding

tissues . . . The same procedure may be used, but with a flicking action . . . to complete the stroke, once effective tension has been created . . . This 'springing' has the effect of stimulating local circulation most effectively, and if the tissues are not too sensitive, may be effective in breaking down infiltrated or indurated tissues.

Elsewhere he gives credit to Lewit's (1999) application of similar approaches, and continues: 'This technique can be applied on inflexible tissues particularly spastic and hard' (Chaitow 2002).

The relevance of these modern observations of the possible effect of the technique is important, because the longitudinal spinal erector muscles of many patients are so frequently extremely tense.

An additional effect of the 'S' contact along the spine, aside from the soft tissue effects, appears to be the rotational mobilization of the spinal segments. Again a thrust is offered as an option. Thus the effect may involve soft tissue manipulation, passive stretch, and HVLA rotational mobilization of the thoracic and first two lumbar segments. While performing the 'S' technique, simultaneous diagnosis and treatment are performed, with time preferentially spent at diagnosed segments that are indurated, tense or hyperexcitable (Chaitow L 1980).

The 'S' move along the spine contains yet another layer of significance.

Inhibition

The movement can be classified according to the 'inhibitive' manipulation of Lindlahr's neurotherapy (Lindlahr 1981). The effect of inhibition along the spinal segments as they exit the foramina is to diminish or exhaust temporarily the hyperexcitable nervous and reflex activity. Inhibition is introduced by heavy steady pressure. For example, in the case of someone with gastritis, inhibition could be selectively applied to the segments innervating the stomach (T4, T5, T6). In cystitis this would include the sacral segments.

Wendel describes a similar approach to the spine in his naturopathic spinal manipulative technique, published in the early 1950s. Wendel, third president of the American Naturopathic Association, and Lust's handpicked successor if Collins declined the nomination, dedicated his booklet describing his technique to Dr Collins' memory. Wendel's approach similarly incorporated a general mode of mobilization, along with the specific joint manipulation.

Wendel's method incorporates a vibratory motion that Collins did not (see discussion of rhythmic oscillation methods earlier in this chapter).

Continued

Box 8.2 Anatomy of a tonic treatment continued

Item 6 above concludes the series of prone movements of the series.

At this point it may be well worth reviewing the cumulative scope of the movements thus far.

- It can be seen that all of the spinal segments have been in some way mobilized.
- The twisting motions of the passive stretches, along a transverse plane, in some way address the segments not thoroughly individually treated.
- The segments individually treated will have been mobilized in a superior, inferior and rotational fashion.
- These segments will also have been treated for relevant restrictions (somatic dysfunction, 'lesions', 'subluxations').
- The musculature of the posterior shoulder girdle and cervicothoracic region will have been stretched and kneaded.
- The costothoracic joints will have been mobilized as an aspect of the rotational passive stretching, as well as individually in an inferior-oblique and superior-oblique fashion.
- Finally, inhibitory neurotherapy will have been applied along almost the entire length of the spinal column.

Chiropractic influences

The tremendous role that the chiropractic profession affords spinal mobility should be reflected upon here, as by this stage (Item 6) the whole spine will have been assessed and to a certain extent treated, albeit non-specifically. Particular restrictions should have been identified, with the option for these to be treated more specifically at a later point in the treatment. More importantly, an experienced practitioner would have begun to evaluate a larger pattern of tissue dynamics, due to the important region that will have been surveyed. The relative importance of the individual somatic restrictions could then be evaluated, as part of a broader assessment. The amount of time required for an experienced practitioner to reach this point of the general treatment is claimed by Collins to be approximately 3–4 minutes.

7. The seventh movement of the series begins with the patient's dorsal portion of the GNTT. This movement involves a passive stretching of the cervical muscles and prepares the lymphatic cervical chain for drainage in the next (eighth) movement.
8. The eighth movement involves lymphatic drainage of the cervical chain.
9. The ninth movement is a general mobilization of the upper limbs.
10. The tenth movement incorporates a series of movements to manipulate the contents of the abdomen. The description of the movement includes a light manipulation of the spleen, liver, kidneys, and the cecum in particular. The practitioner is instructed to break up adhesions in each of the relevant areas. Finally, the kidneys are manipulated in a rotational fashion with varying pressure.

Comment on visceral approaches

The instruction to manipulate the internal organs illustrates the evolution of professional lexicon over the past 100 years. While manipulation is today commonly associated with the HVLA thrust, it is actually a more broadly encompassing term. Manipulation can have a variety of meanings and, in this case, manipulation is to be more clearly understood as comparable to the contemporary osteopathic organ (visceral) manipulation (Barral 1993). This technique is, in reality, a gentle massage of the organs. The breaking up of adhesions is another manipulative technique pioneered in the first half of the 20th century as 'bloodless surgery'.

Fielder & Pyott (1955) compiled a rigorous academic work in 1952, renaming the approach *manipulative surgery*. While manipulative surgery was a very extensive technique, GNTT is a more general one, scanning for particularly gross adhesions. The final rotational portion of the movement, over the kidneys, is said to affect all of the abdominal viscera. The movement certainly subjects a large area of the abdomen to a rotational traction and undulating pressure. The effect can be seen as a logical result of the pumping action induced by rotation and stretching of the vascular and lymphatic tissues, and the pressure applied to the organ parenchyma.

11. The eleventh movement involved a passive stretching of the abdomen that included kneading along the length of the sartorius.
12. The twelfth and final movement stretched and mobilized the lower limbs.

The total time for the GNTT, from beginning to end, takes approximately 6–8 minutes, during which time almost every portion of the body will have received attention.

- Unlike OMT usage, diaphragmatic release is not a part of the GNTT protocol; however, much of the thoracic mobilization and the direct abdominal work would have some influence on this structure.
- Thoracic inlet release is less specific in GNTT than OMT; however, a number of the movements are likely to assist in 'opening' this drainage channel.
- Specific lymphatic pump methods are not a part of GNTT, although the mobilizations described in its repertoire can undoubtedly assist in lymphatic movement.
- Specific paraspinal inhibitory pressure is not included in GNTT, although the 'S' bend method (Item 8 in the GNTT sequence) would to some extent mimic this.
- Condylar and/or sphenobasilar decompression are not included in GNTT.

Would GNTT achieve the objectives set out by Clark & McCombs to:

1. restore the cranial rhythmic impulse to its full rate and excursion
2. restore ventilation to full capacity
3. maintain and/or restore peristalsis
4. restore the third space fluid (lymph) to circulation?

The first objective is unlikely to be modified by GNTT; however, the other three would probably be beneficially influenced by this general mobilization approach.

A chiropractic perspective – and dysponesis

Unlike osteopathic approaches, chiropractic interventions tend to be more localized, albeit with an intent (and it is claimed an effect) that is far more widespread, as outlined below. In truth, much that is foundational in both osteopathy and chiropractic has a familiar ring to the ears of naturopaths.

A basic concept in chiropractic was, and for many still is, that of *innate intelligence*.

As Masarsky & Todres-Masarsky (2001a) observe:

*Assessment of autonomic tone was an integral part of chiropractic analysis from the earliest years of the profession . . . Disturbed tone was considered the most readily observable manifestation of **dis-ease**. [This] was understood as a failure of [the] organism to adapt optimally to internal and external stressors because of loss of contact with the inherent organizing principle,*
*or innate intelligence, found in every living organism . . . that originated from the ancient idea of **vis medicatrix naturae**, or the healing power of nature.*

See Chapter 2 for a deeper evaluation of failing adaptation that results in just such a sequence.

The term *dysponesis* is now used in chiropractic to describe reversible physiopathological states, consisting of unnoticed, misdirected neurophysiological reactions to various agents (environmental events, bodily sensations, emotions and thoughts), and the repercussions of these reactions throughout the organism.

These adaptive changes, which are capable of producing functional disorders, consist mainly of covert errors in action-potential output from the motor and premotor areas of the cortex, and the consequences of that output.

The concept of dysponesis was first described by Whatmore & Kohli (1968), who stated their belief that:

Most diseases consist of physiologic reactions that lead to organ dysfunction. These physiologic reactions constitute the response of the organism to some noxious agent, whether microbial, chemical, or mechanical.

This sounds remarkably like Selye's hypothesis of adaptation exhaustion, which fits well with naturopathic thinking, since it incorporates the concept of being reversible.

As Kent & Gentempo (1994) explain:

*Dysponesis relates to human health as a functional whole, rather than a sum of independent parts. It is philosophically and scientifically appropriate for a chiropractor to diagnose a patient with dysponesis, secondary to a **vertebral subluxation complex** (VSC).*

Masarsky & Todres-Masarsky (2001b) note that modern chiropractic envisages the subluxation as being a complex, sometimes termed the *vertebral subluxation complex* (VSC) in which resulting neural disturbance may lead to hypo-sympatheticotonia, including inappropriate vasodilation. Associated neurodystrophy involves disturbed axoplasmic flow and eventual immunosuppression (Cleveland 1997).

Normalization ('correction') of the 'subluxation', or the VSC, then becomes the chiropractic key to restoring homeostasis, via focused manipulative methods, usually HVLA, rather than the generalized protocols suggested by those employing OMT, where HVLA might or might not be employed, subsequent to (or instead of) general mobilization.

Examples abound in the chiropractic (and to an extent osteopathic) literature of key areas of dysfunction ('subluxations') being manipulated as a precursor to rapid self-regulating processes manifesting, as a variety of health problems – ranging from pediatric pyloric stenosis to nocturnal enuresis, hypertension, perimenopausal symptoms, headaches, premenstrual syndrome, and more – respond and improve.

In chiropractic thinking such responses represent examples of self-regulating ('vis' or 'innate') processes operating (Alcantara 2002, Biomerth 1994, Connelly & Rasmussen 1998, Fallon 1994, Fitz-Ritson 1990, Mootz & Dhami 1994, Walsh & Polus 1998, Weber & Masarsky 1996).

Additional changes associated with VSC might include facilitation (hypertonia) of visceral pain pathways, resulting in 'simulated visceral disease' (see Box 2.2 for a discussion on the concept of facilitation from an osteopathic perspective).

Masarsky & Todres-Masarsky conclude with these thoughts:

Two aspects of the neurological component of the VSC model . . . are critically important. One is the possible disturbance of the anterior, lateral, or posterior horn of the spinal cord [implying] disturbance of tone throughout the body. The other critical aspect is the concept of abnormal articular nociception and mechanoreception leading to hypertonic or hypotonic autonomic function . . . a possible source of systemic errors in energy expenditure (dysponesis).

Chiropractors do not – as a rule – offer a selection of general mobilization and soft tissue methods that equate with those described in OMT (above), or in earlier naturopathic protocols such as GNTT (although there are undoubtedly exceptions to this generalization).

Instead, much mainstream chiropractic usually operates on the assumption that spinal dysfunctions (vertebral subluxation complexes) have widespread influences on health, correctable by manipulation. Whether these ideas can be fully, or only partially, reconciled with naturopathic beliefs is an open question; however, in one essential they do totally agree, since all benefits are ascribed not to the manipulation, but to self-regulatory responses (innate) that follow from appropriate manipulation.

How would Lief's NMT methods compare with the OMT protocols?

Lief's NMT covers the territory from the cranial base to the mid-thigh, anteriorly and posteriorly, in its assessment mode, and incorporates methods such as muscle energy technique, myofascial release, positional release techniques, inhibitory pressure, rhythmical oscillatory motions and a number of the lymphatic pump techniques, as well as joint mobilization and, if necessary, HVLA manipulation, in order to balance and normalize any dysfunctional patterns uncovered during the assessment.

It therefore has the potential to offer – depending entirely on what dysfunctional patterns are elicited during assessment – all of the therapeutic inputs described in the OMT studies earlier in this chapter, and possibly a number not described. (See the protocol description of Lief's NMT in Chapter 7.)

And what about massage?

The list of conditions that have been shown to be helped by means of application of non-specific ('Swedish' or 'wellness') general massage (see Chapter 7) is so comprehensive that it is safe to say that this is a form of therapeutic input that should/could be offered to all patients, of whatever age or gender, or level of well-being or illness.

The very nature of massage ensures that, if applied with thought, compassion and appropriate intent, it can/must:

- improve circulation and drainage
- reduce levels of anxiety, so improving autonomic function
- encourage enhanced respiratory and digestive function
- in general ensure that self-regulatory activities operate more effectively.

The naturopathic context

In the context of a naturopathic therapeutic encounter, in which biomechanical, biochemical and psychosocial influences on health are being considered in relation to the patient's health concerns, a general, non-specific manual protocol may be seen to have a great deal to offer.

Irrespective of the foundational causes of the health problem, there is commonly going to be a requirement for enhancement of respiratory, digestive, circulatory, drainage and/or immune function.

The fact that evidence exists for such approaches being successfully and beneficially applied, and that there are studies validating integrated selections of modalities (as in the OMT studies listed earlier in the chapter), offers confidence for routine inclusion of such methods in naturopathic practice.

The basic naturopathic injunctions to work with nature, to encourage self-regulation, and to do no harm, are all met by the appropriate application of NMT, 'wellness' massage and/or GNTT – or one or other of the OMT protocols outlined above – all of which can be seen to be thoroughly naturopathic.

The next chapter takes these themes forward, as rehabilitation processes are evaluated in a naturopathic context.

References

Alcantara J 2002 Chiropractic care of a patient with temporomandibular disorder and atlas subluxation. Journal of Manipulative and Physiological Therapeutics 25(1):63–70

Barber E 1898 Osteopathy complete. Hudson-Kimberly Publishing, Kansas City, MO, p 306–307

Barral J-P 1993 Visceral manipulation. Eastland Press, Seattle

Biomerth P 1994 Functional nocturnal enuresis. Journal of Manipulative and Physiological Therapeutics 17:335–338

Cantieri MS 1997 In-patient osteopathic manipulative treatment; impact on length of stay. American Academy of Osteopathy Journal 7(4):25–29

Chaitow B 1980 Personal communication to the author. In: Chaitow L (1985) Neuromuscular technique. Thorsons, Wellingborough

Chaitow L 1980 Neuromuscular technique: a practitioner's guide to soft tissue manipulation. Thorsons, Wellingborough, p 90–179

Chaitow L 2002 Modern neuromuscular techniques. Churchill Livingstone, Edinburgh

Clark R, McCombs T 2006 Postoperative osteopathic manipulative protocol for delivery by students in an allopathic environment. American Academy of Osteopathy Journal 16(20):19–21

Cleveland C 1997 Neurobiological relations. In: Redwood D (ed) Contemporary chiropractic. Churchill Livingstone, New York, p 45

Connelly DM, Rasmussen SA 1998 The effect of cranial adjusting on hypertension: a case report. Chiropractic Technique 10(2):75–78

Cordingley A 1925 Principles and practice of naturopathy: a compendium of natural healing. O'Fallon, Bazan, CA

Fallon J 1994 Assessing the efficacy of chiropractic care in pediatric cases of pyloric stenosis. International Chiropractic Association: Proceedings of National Conference of Chiropractic and Pediatrics, Arlington VA, p 72

Field T 2006 Massage therapy research. Churchill Livingstone, Edinburgh

Fielder S, Pyott W 1955 The science and art of manipulative surgery. American Institute of Manipulative Surgery Inc. Carr Printing, Bountiful, UT

Fitz-Ritson D 1990 The chiropractic management and rehabilitation of cervical trauma. Journal of Manipulative and Physiological Therapeutics 13:17–25

Foldi M, Strossenreuther R 2003 Foundations of manual lymph drainage, 3rd edn. Mosby, St Louis

Fritz S, Paholsky K, Grosenbach MJ 1999 Mosby's basic science for soft tissue and movement therapies. Mosby, St Louis

Gibbons P, Tehan P 2000 Manipulation of the spine, thorax and pelvis: an osteopathic perspective. Churchill Livingstone, Edinburgh, p 131–141

Hovind H, Nielsen S 1974 Effect of massage on blood flow in skeletal muscle. Scandinavian Journal of Rehabilitation Medicine 6:74–77

Hoyland J, Freemont A, Jayson M 1989 Intervertebral foramen venous obstruction. Spine 14(6):558–568

Kent C, Gentempo P 1994 Dysponesis: chiropractic in a word. Chiropractic Journal. Online. Available: www.worldchiropracticalliance.org/tcj/1994/sep/sep1994d.htm

Kuchera M, Kuchera A 1990 Osteopathic considerations in systemic dysfunction. Kirksville College of Osteopathic Medicine Press, Kirksville, MO, p 33–52

Larsson S, Bodegard L, Henrikssn K et al 1990 Chronic trapezius myalgia. Morphology and blood flow. Acta Orthopaedica Scandinavica 61(5):394–398

LeClere ML 1922 Technic of a general treatment. Journal of Osteopathy. Online. Available: www.meridianinstitute.com/eamt/files/articles/artlecle.htm

Lederman E 1999 Harmonic technique. Churchill Livingstone, Edinburgh

Lederman E 2005a Science and practice of manual therapy, 2nd edn. Churchill Livingstone, Edinburgh, p 31–66

Lederman E 2005b Science and practice of manual therapy, 2nd edn. Churchill Livingstone, Edinburgh, p 277–293

Lewit K 1999 Manipulative therapy in rehabilitation of the locomotor system, 3rd edn. Butterworth-Heinemann, Oxford

Lief P 1963 Neuromuscular technique. British Naturopathic Journal and Osteopathic Review Autumn, p 304

Lindlahr H 1981 Natural therapeutics, vol 2: practice. Edited and revised by JCP Proby. CW Daniel, Saffron Walden, Essex

Masarsky C, Todres-Masarsky M 2001a Somaticovisceral considerations in the science of tone. In: Masarsky C, Todres-Masarsky M (eds) Somatovisceral aspects of chiropractic. Churchill Livingstone, New York, p 3

Masarsky C, Todres-Masarsky M 2001b Somaticovisceral considerations in the science of tone. In: Masarsky C, Todres-Masarsky M (eds) Somatovisceral aspects of chiropractic. Churchill Livingstone, New York, p 4

Mootz R, Dhami M 1994 Chiropractic treatment of chronic episodic tension type headaches. Journal of the Canadian Chiropractic Association 38(3):152–159

Nicholas A, Oleski S 2002 Osteopathic manipulative treatment for postoperative pain. Journal of the American Osteopathic Association 102(9 Suppl 3):S5–S8

Noll D, Shores J, Bryman P et al 1999 Adjunctive osteopathic manipulative treatment in the elderly hospitalized with pneumonia: a pilot study. Journal of the American Osteopathic Association 99(3):143–152

Noll D, Shores J, Gamber R et al 2000 Benefits of osteopathic manipulative treatments for hospitalized elderly patients with pneumonia. Journal of the American Osteopathic Association 100(12):776–782

O-Yurvati AH, Carnes MS, Clearfield MB et al 2005 Hemodynamic effects of osteopathic manipulative treatment immediately after coronary artery bypass graft surgery. Journal of the American Osteopathic Association 105(10):475–481

Perrin R, Edwards J, Hartley P 1998 Evaluation of the effectiveness of osteopathic treatment on symptoms associated with myalgic encephalomyelitis. A preliminary report. Journal of Medical Engineering and Technology 22(1):1–13

Radjieski J, Lumley M, Cantieri M 1998 Effect of osteopathic manipulative treatment on length of stay for pancreatitis: a randomized pilot study. Journal of the American Osteopathic Association 98:(5):264–272

Rozmaryn L, Dovelle S, Rothman E et al 1998 Nerve and tendon gliding exercises and the conservative management of carpal tunnel syndrome. Journal of Hand Therapy 11(3):171–179

Sleszynski S, Kelso A 1993 Comparison of thoracic manipulation with incentive spirometry in preventing postoperative atelectasis. Journal of the American Osteopathic Association 93(8):834–838

Stiles E 1977 Osteopathic manipulation in a hospital environment. Yearbook of the American Academy of Osteopathy, Colorado Springs, CO, p 17–32

Stiles E 1979 Somatic dysfunction in hospital practice. Osteopathic Annals 7(1):35–38

Tamir L, Hendel D, Neyman C et al 1999 Sequential foot compression reduces lower limb swelling and pain after total knee arthroplasty. Journal of Arthroplasty 14(3):333–338

Walsh M, Polus B 1998 A randomized placebo controlled clinical trial on the efficacy of chiropractic therapy on premenstrual syndrome. In: Proceedings of International Conference on Spinal Manipulation, Vancouver, BC, July 16–19 1998, p 92–95

Weber M, Masarsky CS 1996 Cervicothoracic subluxation and hot flashes in a perimenopausal subject – a time-series case report. Journal of Vertebral Subluxation Research 1(2):33–38

Wendel P c.1950 Naturopathic spinal manipulative technique. Wendel, Brooklyn, NY, p 1–15

Wernham J 1996 Applied osteopathic therapeutics. Institute of Classical Osteopathy, Maidstone, Kent

Whatmore G, Kohli D 1968 Dysponesis: a neurophysiologic factor in functional disorders. Behavioral Science 13:102–124

Willard F 1998 Anatomy of the lymphatics. American Academy of Osteopathy Convocation presentation

Williams P 1988 Effect of intermittent stretch on immobilised muscle. Annals of Rheumatic Disease 47:1014–1016

Williams P, Catanese T, Lucey E et al 1988 The importance of stretch and contractile activity in the prevention of accumulation in muscle. Journal of Anatomy 158:109–114

Wittlinger H, Wittlinger G 1982 Textbook of Dr Vodder's manual lymph drainage, vol 1: basic course, 3rd edn. Karl F Haug, Heidelberg

Rehabilitation and Re-education (Movement) Approaches

Matthew Wallden ND DO

Continued

Before starting to read this chapter, it should be recognized that the style is one of a story – a story of evolution and of how the human locomotor apparatus arrived at this point in history. This, it is proposed, allows for a better understanding of how human biomechanics are supposed to function based on the stresses to which they have been exposed and to which they have adapted in order to survive their environment. This approach also contextualizes the many different rehabilitation approaches available – each with its own merits and shortcomings.

Consequently, if you wish to use this chapter in more of a textbook, reference style, the contents list will help to guide you. However, if you wish to understand a bigger picture, and still want to use the chapter as a reference source, the mindmap (Fig. 9.2) will help you to find the relevant links to their topic(s) of interest.

In this chapter you will learn how consideration of naturopathic philosophy can be integrated into rehabilitation and re-education (movement) approaches to enhance the outcome.

Various models are presented – some established, some adapted and some new. In the production and presentation of new concepts, there is always potential for controversy. The logical progression of the discussion presented here is designed to allow you to feel at ease with these concepts, and to fit them into your current understanding of the functional human organism.

As stated above, the primary objective of this chapter is to provide a broader contextual framework within which you may fit current and future knowledge in the field of rehabilitation and movement re-education approaches. A secondary objective of this chapter is to provide useful applicable information to allow naturopaths and other health care providers to coach patients back to optimal function using foundational corrective exercise principles. This latter objective is as broad as the combined knowledge base and imaginations of all those involved in rehabilitation – and therefore is an ever-expanding task – impossible to fit into any textbook, let alone chapter.

In writing this chapter, it is fully recognized and should be emphasized that these are simply useful clinical models – and do not purport to be an ultimate truth. In this context then, it is hoped that you can develop your own truth, utilizing what fits with your own model and leaving what does not.

Most importantly, the naturopathic triad – which is the cornerstone of naturopathic medicine – is referred to and its links with movement approaches will be emphasized (see notes on psychosocial, biochemical and biomechanical influences on health in Chapter 1, as well as Figure 1.2).

Introduction

The importance of movement approaches to naturopathic patients

Movement approaches are a critical part of almost any rehabilitation program; they are not only a natural approach to re-instigate health into the tissues, but are also of great importance from a psychological and an efficacy perspective.

Much of manual therapy embodies the concept that a trained practitioner can detect what needs to be done to correct dysfunction in joints, muscles and other tissues of the body. This has a level of validity. However, the effects of passive manual interventions have a lower level of validity – particularly when

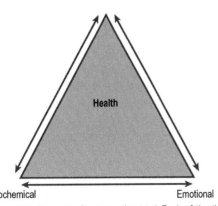

Biomechanical

Health

Biochemical   Emotional

Figure 9.1 Diagram of naturopathic triad. Each of the three components of the naturopathic triad must be in balance to achieve health. Adapted from Newman Turner (1990)

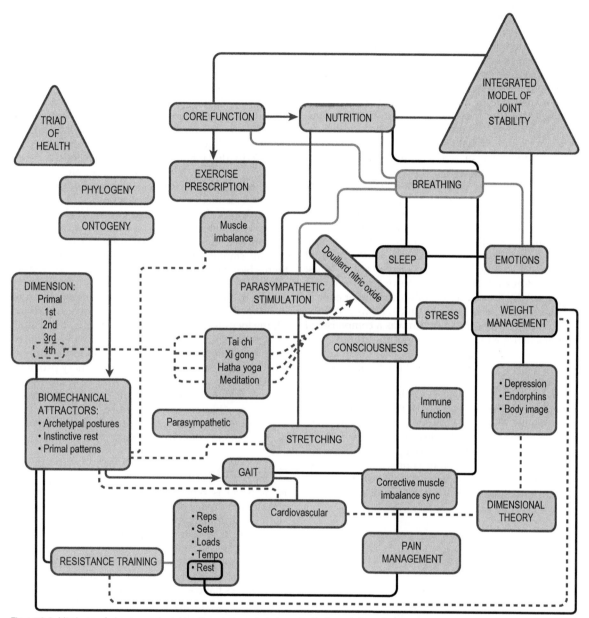

Figure 9.2 Mindmap of chapter content. Use the mindmap to help navigate through the information in this chapter and to see the integrated nature of the information presented

long-term effects are measured. As Lederman (1997) argues, this is because most manual interventions affect the patient at the peripheral reflexive level. At this level, little or no motor learning occurs, so the movement dysfunction which brought about the tissue stress and dysfunction in the first instance may not be addressed. Instead, traditional manual techniques have to rely on the hope of a homeostatic response which allows the patient to recognize that they are now in a better postural position or functional state. This is what is sometimes called 'the parking lot test' – does the patient's postural or functional correction last as far as the parking lot? If yes, then perhaps what we hoped would happen, has happened. Many times, unfortunately, this is not the case.

Lederman (1997) states that an active event (e.g. an exercise intervention) implicitly requires the patient to go through a cognitive phase of motor learning, which results in an associative phase (where the patient may associate a given movement pattern with a sport or activity) followed by the autonomous phase. At this point a new motor pattern is stored. However, a passive event (e.g. massage, mobilization or manipulation) works at an automatic peripheral reflexive level, and results in only a transient motor event.

Active movement or rehabilitation approaches, by their very nature, must affect the patient at the central level. The central nervous system has to be consciously engaged in order to achieve prescribed movement, in contradistinction to manual treatment, where tissues are, in the main, addressed passively by the clinician (Lederman 1997). In addition to such motor learning prerequisites, etiological features – which may fall outside of the immediate motor learning remit – must also be addressed. For example, through appropriate local rehabilitation, proprioception and motor control may be returned to a sprained ankle. However, if the original cause of the ankle sprain was a compensated Trendelenburg gait pattern, the motor learning at the ankle is of little significance, as it is likely to be sprained again until this dysfunctional gait pattern is addressed.

One of the key models to understand how pain patients come to be in pain is Panjabi's model of joint stability (Fig. 9.3). In order for any moving joint to have biomechanical stability, it must have a functional passive support system of ligaments, joint capsules, discs, fascia and other connective tissues. As Gracovetsky (2004) points out, a passive support system is useless without an active muscle subsystem controlled by a neural subsystem. Gracovetsky explains:

If you were to knock out the brain nullifying the neural subsystem, control of the active system is lost. How long thereafter will the person stay standing?

Of course there are far more subtle effects that a neural subsystem may have on the supporting muscles, some of which are discussed later in the chapter. Additionally, the active subsystem may be further divided into two systems, the deepest muscles typically having a stabilizer dominance and the more superficial muscles having a mobilizer dominance – again this is discussed further below.

In order to effectively diagnose and subsequently prescribe an effective corrective exercise program, the practitioner must first understand which components of joint stability are affected (usually all three) and then – based on the case history, the onset and nature of symptoms – reason which system is the primary symptom generator. From this point, a strategy can be developed to return the joint(s) to optimal function.

If the focus is purely – or even primarily – on manual treatment techniques, clinical practice will be limited (and proportionally clinical success) to those patients who have tissue restriction as their primary problem, thereby neglecting all of those who have instability or motor control deficits as their primary etiological factor. As this chapter progresses it will become apparent that the latter equates to a higher proportion of pain patients than the former.

Stress and strain

Hans Selye is reported to have said 'the complete absence of stress is death'. Within the natural homeostatic environment of the body we expect to have stresses to challenge the regulatory functions of the organism (see Chapter 2). From a movement and rehabilitation perspective, Liebenson (2002a) and Sahrmann (2002) explain that both too much and too little tissue stress have a detrimental effect on tissue integrity. Hence it is important to understand the relevant levels of therapeutic stress to which the client should be exposed, which includes training them to survive their environments, taking into account the cumulative effect of other stressors in their life, and how further stress in the form of exercise may affect overall function. If exposed to too little stress, the required beneficial adaptation is not attained. Too much stress and the tissue, the system or the organism becomes 'strained'. These considerations are explored throughout this chapter and have been discussed in earlier chapters, particularly Figures 2.2 and 2.3 in Chapter 2.

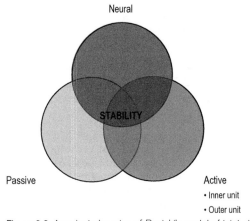

Figure 9.3 An adapted version of Panjabi's model of joint stability. Each of the three components of the joint control system must be functioning correctly for optimal joint stability and control

Table 9.1 Prescribing versus coaching

Giving a fish	Teaching how to fish
Manual treatment methods, 'this for that' nutritional remedies, pharmaceutical prescription	Corrective exercise, corrective stretching, biomechanical attractors, fundamental health principles, naturopathic 'dealing with causes'

Benefits of movement re-education

As Liebenson (1999) describes, the benefits of a rehabilitation/movement re-education approach are that, aside from working in a similar manner to manual treatment to decrease pain, it can also directly or indirectly enhance performance, can be used preventively, and most importantly is proactive and therefore empowering. Benefits of movement re-education include:

- decreased pain
- increased performance
- preventive
- proactive/empowering.

These benefits have very important ramifications for patients, and in particular for chronic pain patients, with the emphasis being placed on the patient to take responsibility for their own health, rather than looking for the magic bullet or the magic therapist who can 'magic them better'. This more common disarming approach is not only psychologically questionable but may be ineffective and, given our current level of knowledge, possibly even unethical. It is the difference between giving a fish, and teaching how to fish. It is also the difference between a naturopathic approach and an allopathic one (Table 9.1). Giving a hungry person a fish is an act of kindness and temporary empowerment – and may even save that person's life. Although it may be enough to set that person on the right track to 'finding more food', it will likely only provide a short-term remedy to their predicament as their behavior has not been modified – it has been sustained, perhaps even reinforced. Teaching someone to fish is an act of empowerment, and provides a life-long tool for survival within their environment.

The story of human movement

To provide a natural insight into rehabilitation and re-education movement approaches, it is important to first analyze how 'natural' movement emanated.

To gain a clear understanding of how and why specific exercise methodologies should be employed by the naturopath, it is the clinician's responsibility, using the best scientific evidence available, to provide an overall context to help cut through the dogma of fad-based exercise approaches, rife in today's therapeutic arena. This will take some significant introductory background but, as will become clear, it will reaffirm that what is being prescribed and why it is being prescribed is in optimal alignment with nature and therefore naturopathic philosophy.

As Astrand et al (2003) point out, close to 100% of our biological heritage was dominated by 'outside' activities. This should give some useful cues with regard to how the body evolved and why it evolved as it did. Understanding such evolution is beneficial to the naturopathic clinician in particular, as his or her role should be to optimize the homeostatic mechanisms of the patient. Since movement has formed a significant component of the evolutionary lifetime of all species, they have developed means, in their natural environment, to remain balanced and in homeostasis. It is the rapidly devolving environment in which humans find themselves that is of such detriment to physical health.

MERRING

Anyone who has studied biology to a basic level knows that the acronym 'MERRING' describes the key criteria comprising a living organism, namely:

- **M**ovement
- **E**xcretion
- **R**eproduction
- **R**espiration
- **I**rritability
- **N**utrition
- **G**rowth.

Movement (or the ability to move) is the first defining component of a living organism. Hence even the most primitive of organisms were able to move; they had some level of motility.

Dimensional mastery

'Phylontogenetic' dimensions

Phylogeny is the development of species in general, while ontogeny concerns the development of the individual. It is a commonly stated that, as a loose rule, ontogeny recapitulates (or recaptures/mimics) phylogeny (Heglund & Schepens 2003). This concept is illustrated in any comparative anatomy or developmental biology text: 'ontogeny recapitulates phylogeny'.

Phylontogenetic dimensions can be defined as: 'The emergent movement patterns of the individual, in which the pattern of evolving dimensional mastery of species is reflected.'

The detail of how such emergent movement patterns reflect the dimensional mastery demonstrated throughout the fossil record, from single-celled life to lower mammals, is described in the following section 'Phylogeny: dimensional mastery'.

Phylogeny: dimensional mastery

Primal dimension

Cellular life – radial/multiplanar/direction non-specific

The most primal phylontogenetic dimension is that of radial contraction – a contraction and expansion of the outer borders of the organism without any necessary respect for direction. This was first the domain of the single-celled organism.

Remnants of single-celled organisms can be traced back in nearly the oldest sediments on the planet to around 3.5 billion years ago (Erwin et al 1997). And for nigh-on the next 3 billion years single-celled organisms were the predominant life form (multicellular grade algae have been traced back to near 1 billion years). Hence, there was some significant time for trial and error and adaptation.

The structure of cell walls includes myofilaments (animal) and cytoskeleton (plant) that are able to contract and produce the first form of space manipulation – a radial contraction. When such contraction is released we have a radial relaxation or relative expansion.

A key thought to hold in mind as the story of movement progresses is that ontogeny (the development of the individual), as a general rule, 'recapitulates' or follows in the same tracks as phylogeny (the development of species). In this example, it is interesting that radial contraction – which was the primal form of space manipulation, and is seen as the primary form of locomotion in many of the most ancient species left on the planet (bacteria, comb jellies, jelly fish and sea anemones) – is ontogenetically the first form of movement in the human fetus. This kind of contractile mastery is essential in the most fundamental of survival mechanisms: swallowing and breathing. Right from as early as 5 months in utero, the human fetus swallows amniotic fluid and even suckles on its thumb – thereby engaging its radial contractile field. Of course, the first thing that the baby does when it's born is to take a huge breath (again, a radial field action), and then search for the nipple of its mother to suckle.

Additionally, it should come as no surprise that much of the manual therapy literature of the last decade has focused on the fact that the primitive deep muscles (such as the transversus abdominis) should contract in advance of the more recently evolved outer unit musculature (such as arm and leg musculature) (Richardson et al 1999).

At the cellular level, radial contraction is multiplanar and therefore direction non-specific. This might be termed as movement in the 'primal dimension' – the first space manipulation – literally manipulating the space which the organism occupies, most likely to create pressure differentials encouraging diffusion into, or out of, the cell: a kind of primitive ingestion/excretion system. In more complex organisms, radial contraction is organized about skeletal structures, fascial sleeves, non-compressible visceral compartments and around complex pressure mechanisms associated with air, fluids and diaphragms. In this group of more complex organisms, to which we belong, radial contraction is direction specific – usually occurring primarily in the transverse plane.

At this point it might be pertinent to ask: 'Why didn't cells simply get larger rather than join together to form multicellular organisms?' The answer can be both philosophical and physiological:

- *From a physiological point of view*: Cells are small. This smallness is practical. Their size allows them to effectively diffuse nutriment across their membrane walls to support their organelles and ongoing health. If we take the example of oxygen, a hypothetical cell of 10 mm diameter would require an increase of atmospheric oxygen pressure to 25 times its current level to ensure adequate oxygenation of the cell (Astrand et al 2003).

- *From a philosophical point of view*: It appears that biophysical properties dictate that there is a huge drive for atoms, molecules and organisms to 'belong'. This may be paralleled in the macroscopic world with the herding instinct, with what drives tribal/family associations (1st chakra principles) in Ayurveda, or the grounding or Earth element principles in traditional Chinese medical philosophy. In such systems, these are foundational principles of health – to belong. Even subatomic particles, it seems, have an extraordinary drive to assemble (Bryson 2003).

This view, which touches on matters of spirituality, may be viewed as naturopathic inasmuch as it implies that 'God' is in everyone and in everything – omniscient, omnipresent and omnipotent. *Note*: Not necessarily omnipotent in the 'all powerful' way that many classic scriptures might be interpreted, but in the way that every atom in existence has potential. In this line of thinking, which has scientific foundation in quantum physics (McTaggart 2003), we all can be viewed as 'God' at the subatomic level – with extraordinary potency, in the same way that we are all a part of Mother Nature, no greater or lesser than the next cluster of atoms alongside us – and with lots of potential! The naturopath's role is to allow the patient to realize that potential.

Interestingly, breath work is most commonly utilized in disciplines with a spiritual leaning, such as meditation, yoga, tai chi, Xi gong and, according to Hartley (1995), primal dimensional mastery (or 'the cellular respiration pattern') is linked in to the mindset of 'being'.

How this pertains to human development and movement rehabilitation

Breathing and digestion are inextricably interlinked. When breathing is calm and relaxed, the parasympathetic nervous system is stimulated, sending messages to the gut to digest. Diaphragmatic excursion – a product of relaxed breathing – massages the digestive organs, stimulating further peristalsis.

As a primal consideration in the ontogenetic development of humans, each person must reflect his or her phylogenetic development by first learning to maneuver within the limited space in the womb. This will initially involve swallowing – which is almost certainly related to the primitive method of ingestion know as phagocytosis. Swallowing appears to reflexively activate the transversus abdominis muscle (Wallden & Patel 2007).

Since respiration is arguably more critical for survival in the moment than swallowing (Chek 1994), one might be forgiven for thinking that swallowing coming ahead of breathing seems a little out of phase. However, breathing occurs after swallowing in the ontogenetic development of the human as the amniotic sac provides an aquatic environment for the developing baby. This ontogenetic sequence follows the phylogenetic pattern, the first form of respiration in species being photosynthesis in water, then later being associated with various gill apparatus in sealife, and it was only at the stage when the organism moved from the water (read: *amniotic fluid*) to dry land (read: *birth*) was breathing, as we know it, acquired.

It is well established in naturopathic medicine that both functional respiratory patterns (Bradley et al 2002, Caine 2004, Chaitow 2004, Gilbert 1998) and

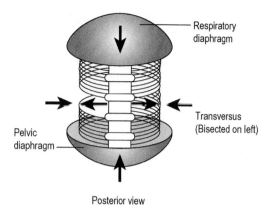

Figure 9.4 Diagram of lumbopelvic inner unit, including transversus abdominis, pelvic floor, respiratory diaphragm and lumbar multifidus. Reproduced with permission from Hodges (1999)

eating an appropriately proportioned, natural diet (Murray & Pizzorno 2000, Wolcott & Fahey 2000) are cornerstones of good health, and so these two factors are fittingly coupled with primal dimensional mastery. Movement in the primal dimension therefore is first about incorporation of nutriment from outside of the organism – truly a primary requirement for life.

From the early 1990s the manual therapy literature has thoroughly explored the concept of core stability, within which the transversus abdominis (TVA) has received particularly rigorous attention. Although still considered by some to be controversial (Siff 2003), the concept of core stability, motor control, and specifically the role of the transversus abdominis in maintaining optimal spinal function are now well established in the scientific literature. Implicated alongside the TVA in optimal motor control of the trunk are the respiratory and pelvic diaphragms (as well as the multifidus). Collectively, these active lumbopelvic support tissues are known as the inner unit (Lee 2004).

While the information available on this topic is vast and much beyond the scope of this chapter, it is nevertheless important to recognize the significance of having a functional inner unit (or local stability system). *Note*: The term *inner unit* can be applied to any joint complex – not just the spinal joints – as typically the deeper the muscle the higher the preponderance of slow twitch muscle fibers (Williams 1995) and the smaller the lever arm. Hence, deep inner unit muscles are more suited for postural use.

To have a functional inner unit means to have a co-contraction of the given muscle group in a feed-forward mechanism before engagement of the outer unit or global stability system musculature. This is achieved in part by the fact that low threshold motor neurons predominate in the nerve supply to these muscles (Kuno 1984). A low threshold to stimulus means only a small neural drive is required to activate the muscle, whereas high neural drive is required to activate higher threshold outer unit muscles.

To simplify things a little, the inner unit musculature – due to its approximation to the axis of rotation of joints (whether spinal or peripheral) – has very little potential for levering a joint but is more suited to compression (and therefore to provide stability) at the joint it spans. In contrast, outer unit muscles have a characteristic leverage that is better suited to mobilize the joint(s) over which they act – commonly using the deeper inner unit muscles in a way similar to sesamoid bones – to increase their mechanical advantage.

The relevance of this to the phylontogenetic discussion is that, just as our phylogenetic relations are reflected in the various layering and overlayering of the brain, so our biomechanical architecture reflects this process with deeper structures being of older phylogenetic origin – particularly at the spine (Kent & Carr 2001). This anatomic progression is similarly echoed physiologically in the motor control literature (Haynes 2003, Richardson et al 1999).

Multicellular life – radial/multiplanar/direction non-specific

Plant life

As described above, clustered cells, such as algae, emerged around 1 billion years ago, though they did not proliferate until around 565 million years ago, in what was known as the *Neoproterozoic*. Algae cells are one of the simplest cells in the plant kingdom and contain within their cell walls an architectural arrangement known as a cytoskeleton. The cytoskeleton is a set of small filaments that is found in the cytoplasm of eukaryotic cells (cells containing a nucleus). The purpose of the cytoskeleton is to maintain the cell's structural integrity. The cytoskeleton acts as both a skeleton and a muscle. There are three filaments that make up the cytoskeleton: actin filaments, microtubules and intermediate filaments. The cytoskeleton provides shape, support and movement. The sliding, assembly, and disassembly of actin and microtubules cause cell movement. The microtubules and the actin can move organelles about within a cell. The transportation method of endocytosis (drawing nutrition into the cell from the outside) requires the cytoskeleton. The cytoskeleton helps the cell acquire particles. For the process of phagocytosis, the cytoskeleton helps the cell move liquid into the cell (pinocytosis) and, in the process, the cytoskeleton helps the cell move large particles into the cell (Robinson 2006).

Hence we can see that nutrition and/or respiration was probably the primitive drive to develop the ability to move in the earliest plant species.

In animal cells, the cell wall contains myofilaments which are contractile – again allowing for phagocytosis and/or movement (space manipulation).

Animal life and body plans

To better understand how the organism functions it is important to first understand how it was built. The study of body plans or 'bauplans' allows us to see which body architectures were successful and therefore preserved through the evolutionary process. There are 37 known body plans shared across the entire animal kingdom. Of these 37, only four are prevalent (Erwin et al 1997). These four will be discussed below to demonstrate how natural selection may have prioritized certain features and have driven our biomechanical design. These basic animal body plans are half a billion years old. The commonality of anatomic features in these body plans cannot be ascribed to chance alone, and, moreover, those features are components of a deeply integrated shared pattern of development (Raff 1996).

Sponges are widely acknowledged, through morphological and molecular evidence, to be the most primitive of animal phyla and have been traced as far back as the Neoproterozoic (570 mya).

It was at this stage of evolution that multicelled organisms started to develop cells with specialized functions (Erwin et al 1997), rather than simply reproducing piece-meal. As cells began to differentiate, their roles became increasingly specialized. Three fundamental embryological categories exist, as outlined in Table 9.2 (Critchley 1990).

Sponges were the first animals to exhibit specialization of cells, though at this stage they were still only loosely differentiated. Although some authorities suggest that sponges do not have motility, they have high cellular motility (primal dimension movement) (Lorenz et al 1996), their larvae are motile and they commonly have flagella to draw in nutrients from the ocean (Oxford Park Academy 2006). Their ability to phagocytose foodstuffs (Leys & Eerkes-Medrano 2006), such as bacteria, demonstrates that radial contraction is still a key movement pattern in sponges.

As cellular differentiation became better defined, so the first of the major body plans arose, the diploblastic body plan (Fig. 9.5). The diploblastic body plan utilized radial contraction and consisted of a layer of ectoderm (nervous/sensory tissue) and a layer of endoderm (gut tissue) with a thin separating gelatinous layer of mesoglea. The diploblastic body plan is seen in primitive organisms such as comb jellies, sea

Table 9.2 Tissue specializations

Endoderm (inner)	Mesoderm (middle)	Ectoderm (outer)
Epithelial lining of respiratory system (bar the nose), almost entire alimentary system and glands supporting it, some ductless glands, prostate gland, urinary bladder and adjoining urethra	Muscle, bone, cartilages, fibrous connective tissues, gonads, the dermis, kidneys, upper genital and urinary ducts, spleen, adrenal cortex, and the connective tissue component of all organs and tissues, the whole cardiovascular and lymphatic systems	Skin (epidermis) and derivatives (including sweat glands, hair follicles, mammary glands), lining of mouth/nose, central and peripheral nervous systems, lens of the eye

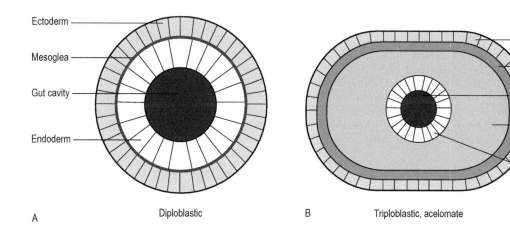

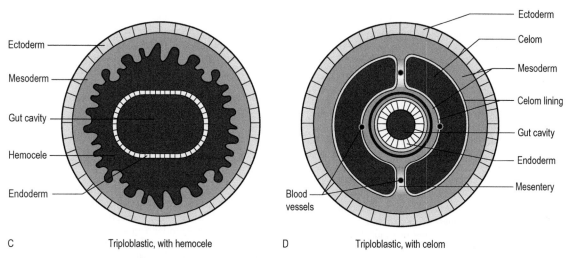

Figure 9.5 Diagram of the four major body plans. In modern times: **A** the diploblastic body plan is found in anemones and jellyfish; **B** the triploblastic acelomate body plan is found in flatworms; **C** the triploblastic, with hemocele plan is found in roundworms; and **D** the triploblastic with celom basic architecture is found in fish, amphibians, lizards and mammals all the way through to man

anemones and jelly fish – each of which exhibits this same radial contraction pattern as their primal dimensional mastery.

Such organisms often float on the currents and the direction of their efforts may be governed more significantly by outside influences than by their own conscious decision-making. Their movements may be seen as 'preconscious' or autonomic – reflecting their close association with respiration and digestion. This has relevance with regard to the ontogenetic development of movement. They are exposed to the natural rhythms and cycles of life and literally have to *go with the flow*.

How this pertains to human development and movement rehabilitation

Activation of the deep intrinsic muscles of the spine and the peripheral joints should be effortless and occur without the need for thought. It is for this reason that 'feeling' commands, instead of 'doing' commands (Lee 2003), should be utilized when retraining inner unit musculature (see below) and is also why repetition must be used so that the motor learning progresses from cognitive, to associative, to autonomous (see discussion under the subheading

'The importance of movement approaches to naturopathic patients' above).

The majority of body plans from the late Neoproterozoic are represented by the sponges or the comb jellies, jelly fish and sea anemones (Erwin et al 1997). Thirty-five million years later (around 530 mya), what is widely described as the 'Cambrian explosion', due to the proliferation of multicellular organisms, brought with it all of the basic architectures of animals. By the close of the Cambrian, some 490 mya, all body plans were established – and even migration from sea-based living to life on land brought with it only minor adaptations.

How this pertains to human development and movement rehabilitation

Our phylogenetically oldest muscles are ontogenetically the first we learn to use, both in utero and in the early months of postnatal life. This learning occurs early in life before volitional motor control and cause/effect learning have developed (see Table 9.3). This pattern is reflected in adult life by pre-contraction (or the feed-forward mechanism) of deep, intrinsic, inner unit musculature – providing stability before mobility.

Box 9.1 'Metamerism' or segmentation

Metamerism is the subdivision of the embryonic body into a series of segments. Such segmentation allows for sequential radial contraction and is the basis for the two largest animal groups on Earth, the vertebrates and the insects (Drews 1995).

Kent & Carr (2001) state that the immediately evident feature of axial muscles in fish and tetrapods is their metamerism. This primitive arrangement, in combination with a metameric vertebral column, allows fish and aquatic tetrapods to propel themselves forward by means of lateral undulation.

However, according to Kent & Carr (2001), this feature of metamerism became increasingly obscured as locomotion by lateral flexion was superseded by limbs. Disappearance of epaxial myosepta (literally meaning segmented back muscles) in amniotes gave rise to long, strap-like or pennate bundles disposed of dorsally to the transverse processes (erector spinae), leaving only a vestige of metamerism in the deepest bundles. Such bundles in modern-day humans would include the intertransversarii, the interspinales and the rotatores muscles; hence evolutionary progression is consistent, in part, with the concept of inner unit muscles and their pre-contraction.

Hypaxial myomeres (abdominal muscle segments) were gradually replaced by strata of broad muscular sheets. Intervertebrals are the deepest epaxial muscles and the only ones to retain their primitive metamerism. They extend between two successive transverse processes, neural spines, neural arches or zygapophyses. In humans, the only examples would be rectus capitis posterior minor, obliquus capitis superior, obliquus capitis inferior, interspinales, intertransversarii anteriores/posteriores/laterales/mediales, rotatores, and possibly levatores costarum. The deep, segmental fibers of the quadratus lumborum, being phylogenetically older than the abdominal sheet muscles (O'Reilly et al 1997), are also likely to be surviving remnants of primitive musculature involved in lateral flexion and frontal plane stability. *Note:* The intercostals would not be categorized – even though they are depicted as segmentally attached between ribs, which are a component of axial anatomy. This is because the intercostals, the scalenes and the entire abdominal wall are formed from one embryonic sheet and the ribs literally grow around from the spine and through this muscle sheet to artificially divide it. Functionally, of course, the intercostals respond in exactly the same way to loading as the abdominal obliques, assuming that the rib cage and costal cartilages maintain their flexibility.

Flatworms – radial/direction specific

The flatworm body plan (see Fig. 9.5B) would appear to be more advanced than the diploblastic plan of jelly fish and anemones, though more primitive than that of the roundworm (Erwin et al 1997). In the same way that cell size in Earth's environment is limited due to atmospheric oxygen pressure and the ability to oxygenate the cell (Astrand et al 2003), so flatworms needed to remain flat in order to diffuse oxygen across their gut walls to their inner tissue layer (Erwin et al 1997). This was mainly due to the fact that they lack the ability to 'carry' nutrients as they do not have a circulatory system (see Fig. 9.5).

Due to the soft bodies of flatworms there is, quite literally, no hard evidence for their evolution in the fossil record. However, molecular and morphological evidence indicates that flatworms formed in advance of roundworms (see below).

Flatworms exhibit a body plan similar to the diploblastic body plan of jelly fish inasmuch as they only have one orifice through which to engulf food and through which to excrete waste. Again, this wouldn't make for particularly efficient movement. For the flatworm to move forward through a sequential radial contraction – a peristaltic motion – would require, or at least imply, that it is concurrently digesting food in an inward direction. If the flatworm later wanted to excrete any waste products, it would have to go into a retroperistalsis (as humans experience during vomiting). This would imply a relatively inefficient movement mechanism – a kind of *one-step-forward, one-step-backward* motion, based on digestive and eliminative cycles.

Starfish are categorized as triploblastic acoelomates and, as such, can be viewed as further down the evolutionary road than jelly fish and anemones, and their behavior may be seen in human ontogenetic terms as the naval radiation pattern in the womb – where the central point of stability (or technically where the fetus is held in a 'closed chain' environment[1]) is via the umbilicus. At any point beyond 8 weeks in utero, the four limbs have formed and the head, forming the fifth point of the metaphorical star is proportionally far larger than it is in the adult. This results in formation of five approximately equal appendages radiating out from a central point of stability. This pattern is maintained throughout intrauterine development and into the outside world. The initial flailing of the arms and legs in the newborn infant is an example of the naval radiation pattern being used.

Flatworms were likely the first creatures to orchestrate sequential contraction and, as such, required greater computational power through an organized and complex nervous system. This nervous system would utilize as its mainframe a longitudinal cord of nervous tissue. This was the advent of the *chordates* (Raff 1996).

How this pertains to human development and movement rehabilitation

- *The appearance of chordates was the expression of the survival pressure for improved nervous system control of locomotor function.*

- *From an ontogenetic point of view, motor control in the infant is almost exclusively limited to primitive reflexive movements until about 1–2 months postnatally. It is only later (around 7 months postnatal) that more gross, volitional movements predominate (Goldfield 1995).*

- *In the same way that it cannot be assumed that an untrained person's muscles are as large as they would be if he or she had trained, it also cannot be assumed that an untrained person's nervous system has the best possible control of the muscles. Therefore, in the course of any rehabilitation or conditioning program, one might anticipate a training effect (adaptation) in both the muscles (increased size) and the nervous system (improved activation and coordination of muscles) (Sale 1988).*

- *Indeed, Bompa (1999) explains that neural adaptations to exercise are the primary reason for strength gains in the first 8 weeks of any new training program, and only after this period does hypertrophy predominate as the primary means of strength gain. This neuromuscular learning effect can be explained by the phenomenon of facilitation (see Box 9.2).*

Roundworms – radial/direction specific

The emergence of roundworms (see Fig. 9.5C). – still in the Neoproterozoic – brought with it changes in the digestive process. At this stage of development, roundworms now had a unidirectional gut tube, rather than the bidirectional gut tube of the diploblastic and acoelomate triploblastic body plans of earlier designs.

These were the first organisms capable of leaving traces of their existence through meandering trails, burrows and fecal pellets that could only have been left by creatures with a complete gut tube (Erwin et al 1997). Additionally, such movement patterns

---

[1]When the body is biomechanically in a closed chain it means that it cannot overcome the resistance against it. Therefore, in this example, the arms, legs and head are in an open chain environment as they can overcome resistance of the amniotic fluid, but the fixed point of the fetus – the point that cannot move – is its attachment to the uterine wall via the placenta and umbilical cord.

would require a 'soft skeleton' of fluid-filled spaces that could act using hydrostatic pressure between tissue layers. Many invertebrates use such hydrostatic systems to move, and many vertebrates use hydrostatic systems in localized body parts (O'Reilly et al 1997), such as the function of the human lumbopelvic inner unit (transversus, respiratory and pelvic diaphragms) or blood in the vertebrae contributing significantly to their compressive resistance (Bogduk 1997).

Now digestion and forward motion could be complementary – one facilitating the other. This would surely enhance efficiency. Active absorption of foodstuffs into a blood system (hemocele) meant that digestive efficacy was further enhanced and therefore metabolic efficiency optimized. This would allow for optimal delivery of nutriment to the working parts – whether this was the nervous system, the musculature or the digestive system itself. Such efficacy would allow the worm to evolve greater muscle mass as oxygen delivery to the tissues could now operate via the active vehicle of blood, rather than passive diffusion. In terms of competition, this would surely prove an advantage over the flatworm body plan (see Fig. 9.5).

Roundworms became the ultimate masters of the primal dimension – radial contraction. Longitudinally arranged musculature would also allow for some degree of flexion-extension (as seen in the caterpillar); however, without a bony spine the flexion-extension would be little more than a transient 'ripple' down the body segments.

How this pertains to human development and movement rehabilitation

In terms of motor control, this movement is exploiting transverse plane musculature in a more phasic way to provide a relatively inefficient means of mobilizing the organism. In humans, of course, the appendicular extensions (arms and legs) are also employed to facilitate movement. This may be seen as a caterpillar-like movement in babies when placed on their tummies in early infancy and is referred to by Hartley (1995) as the 'spinal push pattern'.

At this level of mastery, the ability to control radial contraction highlights the ability to decouple radial contraction with digestion and radial contraction with respiration. This has been demonstrated in work by Hodges et al (2001) in which they confirm Lewit's (1999) assertion that the diaphragm is a respiratory muscle with postural functions, while the transversus is a postural muscle with respiratory function. Research by Hodges and colleagues (2001) showed that human subjects, when under perturbation loads, would recruit both transversus and diaphragm to optimize

motor control at the spine at the expense of breathing. However, when the metabolic debt became too high – even under the same perturbation loading – the diaphragm would resume its respiratory function.

This research demonstrates that when a metabolic crisis is looming, higher functions such as breathing are prioritized over the health and stability of the lumbopelvic structures. However, until such time, lumbopelvic stability can be maintained through decoupling the respiratory role of the diaphragm (and transversus abdominis) from its natural rhythm.

Fish (1st dimensional mastery) – lateral flexion/direction specific

As the complexity of organisms increased, and the nervous control of this complexity became more fundamental to the organism's survival, bony encasement of the neural components became commonplace (Kardong 2002). The skull had already formed to protect the brain, but the longitudinal cord of nervous tissue had yet to develop a bony spinal encasement.

Whether this was the selective pressure that drove the development of a spine or whether it was for other reasons remains unclear; biomechanically, however, the effects of bony spinal development were that there was now a new movement option. Rather than sequential peristaltic contraction, there was now the option to contract the musculature down the entire length of the body on one side, then, using the stretch this induced in the spindle cells and the natural elasticity of the contralateral muscle mass, a reciprocal contraction could be executed. This would provide an efficient cyclical means of moving forward through water and made use of the viscoelastic properties of mesodermal (muscle) tissue.

How the development of a bony spine relates to this new ability to move through lateral flexion is that a bony strut would be required to prevent 'telescoping' of the body under the load of unilateral longitudinal contraction (Kardong 2002).

Naturally the spine would be segmented due to the developmental principle of metamerism (see above) – thereby allowing for segmental motion – which is, of course, how we clinically analyze spinal function today – 'the spinal motion segment'.

Now, with the inheritance of the hemocele from the roundworm bauplans, digestion became less dependent on movement and, in fact, with a decreased utilization of the peristaltic action of the body wall, would require a further functional separation of the digestive and movement systems. Therefore, any creature that has mastery of a movement pattern beyond a peristaltic forward creep, must have evolved a celomic cavity to allow gross movement without compromising digestive efficiency. Indeed this is what the fossil record and morphological studies suggest.

The earliest animals to truly master motion in the frontal plane (above and beyond the primal dimension) were fish. It is at this juncture in evolution (and in every vertebrate development after fish) that we find development of a celomic cavity.

In his paper on embryological development of the infra-umbilical abdominal wall, Glenister (1958) demonstrates that the celom, which goes on to become the muscular wall of the digestive system, forms from the same layer of embryological tissue (the lateral plate mesoderm) as the abdominal wall musculature (see Glenister 1958, p. 123, for illustration). The structure therefore is interrelated with the function. Good digestive function depends on good abdominal wall function and good abdominal wall function depends on good digestion (see 'Viscerosomatic reflexes' below).

How this pertains to human development and movement rehabilitation

- *In the infant human, and in many apes, lateral flexion is utilized as a primary trunk pattern in both gait and other gross movements – such as throwing in youngsters. One of the characteristics of early gait is a laterally directed arm swing (to compensate for frontal plane motion of the trunk), as opposed to the drive forward and backward in more accomplished sprinters (Haywood & Getchell 2005).*

- *Recognition of the laterality of the body – and therefore competent utilization of decussating muscle slings – does not reach a developing child's awareness until around the age of 4–5 years (Haywood & Getchell 2005).*

- *In adults, many exercises, and exercise equipment found in the gym environment, train the user primarily in the sagittal plane; hence frontal plane (and transverse plane) deconditioning is most commonly found on examination. (To identify frontal plane motor deficits, see the description of the stick test in Box 9.7.)*

Lizards (1st dimensional mastery) – lateral flexion/direction specific/ coupled rotation

From this point in the evolution of vertebrate design, we can turn to the work of Gracovetsky (1988) to provide a concise, insightful description of upcoming events.

Having mastered motion in the frontal plane in the water, the first amphibious pioneers brought this movement skill with them to swamps to clamber over debris in and out of the water (Ahlberg 2001). On land, however, this mastery brought with it some serious limitations.

Gracovetsky (1988) describes how any ground-lying objects, such as rocks, stones, fallen trees, would need to be circumnavigated by a creature whose spine had yet to develop flexion-extension in the sagittal plane. One solution to this would be to lift the limb high enough so that it was raised above and beyond the obstacle. This solution would result initially in axial rotation which, when coupled with lateral flexion, would culminate in motion in the sagittal plane. This sequence of events is corroborated by Kent & Carr (2001).

The mechanical properties of any rod (the spine included) are that, if laterally flexed and axially rotated, the rod has to move through the sagittal plane into flexion-extension. Gracovetsky (1988) believes that this provided a solution to both the ground-lying objects and the fact that, until this juncture, the mass of muscle responsible for moving the organism forward on land was intra-abdominal and therefore was competing for space with the vital viscera in the abdominal cavity. This seriously limited the potential for significant hypertrophy.

An alternative solution, Gracovetsky (1988) argues, was to develop effective flexion-extension of the trunk and limb which brought with it a number of benefits over lateral flexion:

- The creature could now progress by the length of its body plus the length of its limbs with each bound.
- The full capacity of the creature's bilateral muscle mass could now be utilized in one forward bound rather than alternating from left to right muscle mass. In a competitive and hostile environment, this would have been highly desirable.
- Simple lateral flexion does not allow the feet to pass over ground-level obstacles.

Gracovetsky (1988) suggests that it became inevitable that, at some point, sufficient strength would develop in the hip extensor mechanism that bipedalism could be achieved. Of course, the story is far more complex than this, but it does provide a general overview of our understanding of the evolution of vertebrate biomechanics – including our own – based on the fossil record. This then provides a greater insight to how human biomechanics have evolved and are designed to work. This understanding is fundamental to helping solve problems when the biomechanics break down.

Gracovetsky (1988) proposed progression based on mechanical principles and the fossil record:

Lateral flexion → Axial rotation → Flexion-extension

How this pertains to human development and movement rehabilitation

- *Lateral flexion and axial rotation (and the effective control of these motions) are the foundations upon which sagittal plane flexion-extension is built.*
- *Good motor control in these planes must be demonstrable before high speed, or heavily loaded tasks in the sagittal plane, are considered – for example, lifting tasks, sprinting, jumping or squatting with load.*
- *Since the spine is the mechanism from which movement emanates, optimal condition of the spine is key to optimal performance in the periphery. When compensation patterns are present, injury may occur either centrally at the spine or peripherally in a limb.*
- *Epicondylitis is a classic example of this, where – because the spine is deconditioned or muscles around the spine are compensating – correct force sequencing from the legs through the trunk and into the arms does not occur. The end result is an attempt to increase the power from the arm, increasing the tension locally through the arm and the grip required on the racket, club or other implement. Across a period of time, cumulative stress to the tendons of the extensor and/or flexor masses of the wrist will result in 'epicondylitis'.*

Mammals (2nd dimensional mastery) – flexion-extension/direction specific/coupled lateral flexion-axial rotation

What Gracovetsky (1988) only touches on within his evolutionary model is that motion in the transverse plane (axial rotation) can be viewed predominantly as an artifact of the mechanical motion coupling of the spine. True mastery of the transverse plane – or the 3rd dimension – requires significant nervous system development, which is why it has only really been mastered by the primates – although some cats and birds may also merit the award of transverse plane mastery. As has been pointed out (P Ahlberg, Professor of Evolutionary Organismal Biology, Uppsala University, Sweden, personal communication, 2000), rotation in the transverse plane does occur in certain lower vertebrates, including dinosaurs, lizards, snakes and birds. However, significant rotation would only appear to be limited to birds in the cervical portion and mammals, particularly cats, in the lumbar region. Primates have their greatest range of motion in the cervical spine – like the birds – although they have a significant degree of transverse plane rotation in the thoracic spine (reference range 30–50° in either direction). From this, Ahlberg (personal communication, 2000) agrees it can be inferred that, consistent with Gracovetsky's interpretation, axial rotation may be allowed (as a mechanical necessity) during evolution from lateral flexion to sagittal flexion-extension.

In contradistinction to – or perhaps just in greater detail than – Gracovetsky's description, Ahlberg (personal communication, 2000) suggests that true, finely-controlled, high-amplitude axial rotation is a specialization that has only evolved in animals that have already mastered sagittal flexion-extension.

Ahlberg's modification of Gracovetsky's interpretation of spinal evolution comprises:

Mastery (active) lateral flexion → (Coupled (passive) axial rotation) → Mastery (active) sagittal flexion extension → Mastery (active) axial rotation

Indeed, even in a human infant, it takes many years to gain a true mastery of the transverse plane, a reflection of the significant computational demands of decussating motor control and interlimb coupling in bipeds (see Schmidt & Wrisberg 2000 for more details and illustrations).

It is interesting to note that the only two true bipeds alive today are birds and humans, and that both of them have significant spinal rotation, and both are able to sing and generate rhythm. This is a factor that is believed to be intrinsic in the spinal cord circuitry of bipeds – to effectively generate rhythmic gait. A rhythmic pattern stored at the cord level is known as a central pattern generator (Allen 1990).

The astute observer may, at first, consider that a cat's reflexes, its ability to right itself, might be considered more advanced than human reflexes, and consequently may question the idea that human mastery of the transverse plane is greater than feline mastery. However, it only takes a few minutes watching the X-Games, the Olympics, or even a professional soccer match to recognize that no matter how much time was invested, a cat could simply not be taught to ride a bike, let alone jump a bike, somersault a bike, nor jump out of a helicopter with skateboard in hand to land in a 30-foot high half pipe performing all kinds of mind-bending tricks. Indeed, even picturing a leopard standing on its hind legs and flicking a football up with one paw and juggling it on the other paw is unthinkable – if amusing! The point is that, no matter how it is viewed, the human nervous system can be developed far above and beyond that of the average cat and it is this development, these kinds of abilities which the average person might consider 'extreme', that would have been part and parcel of survival pressures as recently as 20 000 years ago.

How this pertains to human development and movement rehabilitation

- *True mastery of the transverse plane requires significant computational demands, and this may be why learning difficulties (e.g. dyspraxia), intracranial bleeds or mild traumatic brain injury from head trauma or whiplash may result in decoupling of this transverse plane mastery.*

- *Exercises which use cross-patterning to stimulate both sides of the brain (such as those devised by the Brain Gym group – see below) can help to retrain integration of the two sides of the body and a return to efficient movement patterns.*

Primates (3rd dimensional mastery) – top-down voluntary axial rotation/direction specific

To brachiate is to move by using the arms to swing from branch to branch (Anderson 2000). To truly brachiate is a rare feature even within primates, though by and large all primates are able to rotate their upper (cranial) limbs through nearly 360° of motion – something felines and other mammals are unable to do. This, combined with the ability to grip, allows for a greater number of hunting and/or escape possibilities in an arboreal environment, than having claws and limited range of forelimb motion. For example, it allows for movement via vines and under branches, as well as on them.

Such quick-witted, highly coordinated, interlimb coupling, with trunk rotation in the transverse plane and the computational requirements to commandeer an arboreal environment, would require a significant and powerful processing system – the primate brain.

Nevertheless, predation from many of the big cats was presumably a problem for our ancestors – as it still is for our primate cousins today (Anderson 2000, Morgan 2001). As various commentators have suggested, the migration from the shrinking canopy to a more land-dwelling existence would have brought with it an increased risk of predation from our altogether larger, stronger and 'toothier' feline counterparts (Erwin et al 1997).

Did the aquatic environment of certain lakes and river systems – known to be prohibitive to most felines – provide a protective barrier for our ancestors from the cats that proved such a threat on the ground and in the trees?

As Morgan (2001) points out, although critics of the aquatic ape theory might suggest that the aquatic environment is altogether as dangerous as the savannah, many of the hominid fossils have been found around lakes whose crocodilian inhabitants – even to this day – are not man-eaters, since they have an abundance of other easier prey to satiate them. Attenborough (2002, 2003), De Waal & Lanting (1997) and Morris (1982) support the Homo aquaticus theory with observation of wading behavior in chimpanzees, while Holford (1997) suggests that life at the water's edge provides a cute explanation for how hominid brain development achieved such rapid growth through abundant nutritional availability of essential fatty acids in that environment.

Additionally, such an aquatic environment helps to explain a very fast shift from tetrapedalism to bipedalism and provides a mechanism by which the mastery of the transverse plane (3rd dimension) from the arms down was inverted to become mastery of the transverse plane from the feet up.

This provides a possible explanation for how Gracovetsky's (1988) model of gait – the spinal engine – could have developed, and the subsequent realization that movement emanates from the core (Cresswell et al 1992). Overcoming such aquatic resistance to forward propulsion of the lower limbs would necessitate development of spinal strength in the transverse plane during gait, which most primates lack. Instead, modern-day apes exhibit more lateral sway in the frontal plane. Indeed any actor trying to mimic an ape-like gait will always incorporate more of side-to-side gait sway, which is instantly recognizable as 'ape-like'. Experiments where chimpanzees have been trained to walk bipedally have sadly resulted in heart failure due to the massive demands on the chimpanzees' gluteus medius muscles (more akin to the gluteus maximus in man topographically and size-wise) and subsequent metabolic demands of the muscle (Vleeming 2003).

How this pertains to human development and movement rehabilitation

- *Efficient human bipedal gait requires strength in the upper limbs, the trunk and the legs. To help to retrain dysfunctional gait patterns, exercises which teach integration, while building strength in upper and lower limbs, may be useful (see 'Standing cable pull' below).*

- *In addition, pool-based aquatic rehabilitation may be useful both to help decompress and to provide transverse plane resistance for disc injured, lower limb injured, trunk injured and chronic pain patients.*

Humans (3rd dimensional mastery) – axial rotation/direction specific/bottom-up

Certainly, it would seem that controlled long-axis rotation of the spine from the finely controlled, high-amplitude axial rotation is a specialization that has only evolved in animals that have already mastered sagittal flexion-extension (P Ahlberg, personal communication, 2000).

This brought with it some significant advancements, including:

- increased efficiency in gait over long distances
- decreased surface area for the sun to strike, resulting in less energy wasted on thermoregulation
  - greater hunting opportunities (the big cats – as with all felines – are predominantly nocturnal hunters)
- the ability to carry things (weapons, water, prey)
- the ability to craft things (tools, weapons, shelter).

The rapid expansion of the human brain didn't begin until less than 2 million years ago – millions of years after Homo sapiens stood upright. Bipedalism therefore was the forerunner of neocortical development – rather than the result of it. Because human gait demands alternating contraction of the anterior oblique slings for forward propulsion (see sling systems below), across time this would have remolded the shape of the pelvic girdle to make it more of an oval shape rather than a narrow oblong.

In his classic paper on human gait, Lovejoy (1988) demonstrates how the pelvic anatomy has adapted over millions of years from our closest living relatives, the chimpanzees, through to 'Lucy' our first known bipedal ancestor, and on to modern-day human pelvic design (Fig. 9.6).

However, Lovejoy (2005, Lovejoy et al 2003) goes on to describe how it may not be correct to assume that evolutionary stressors remolded the musculoskeletal architecture. Lovejoy suggests that developmental biology may hold more accurate clues as to how our connective tissues have been determined principally, if not exclusively, by pattern formation during embryological development. In other words, the control of new anatomic designs may be purely down to genetically orchestrated biochemical events.

Form following function

To build on Lovejoy's commentary, the assertion that anatomic adaptation may be down to biochemical events at the genotypic and/or phenotypic level still does not explain what the stimulus was to drive these events – the implication, it seems, being that it is pure chance. This provides little useful information to the physician trying to understand how the human architecture arose and should optimally function.

Lovejoy et al (2003) go on to describe that within any given embryological field of development (limb, bone, muscle, tendon) each is controlled by a structured genetic subprogram. To bring about change in an adult structure – such as those we might anticipate if we could watch hominid evolution unfold – must therefore involve altering the positional information of the developmental field. Lovejoy et al (2003) suggest, then, that it is this 'field' – not the bone or the muscle – that is the selective force driving the adaptation. Expression, therefore, of new anatomies is not the result of the genes so much as the regulatory field. In other words, it's not the hardware (the structure), or the software (the genotype), but the software operator (the phenotypic expression) that results in adaptive progression of the locomotor apparatus. Activity within these fields determines not only which genes are expressed but also their timing and degree of expression (Lovejoy et al 2003). Such structural adaptations to use are discussed further in Chapter 2.

This is in line with Ingber's (1999) evidence that gene expression alters when structural features are modified as in the weightlessness affecting astronauts preventing normal metabolism in cells whose cytoskeleton tensegrity structures have warped in zero-gravity conditions.

Recent studies confirm that alterations in the cellular force balance can influence intracellular biochemistry within focal adhesion complexes that form at the site of integrin binding as well as gene expression in the nucleus. These results suggest that gravity sensation may not result from direct activation of any single gravioreceptor molecule. Instead, gravitational forces may be experienced by individual cells in the living organism as a result of stress-dependent changes in cell, tissue, or organ structure that, in turn, alter extracellular matrix mechanics, cell shape, cytoskeletal organization, or internal pre-stress in the cell-tissue matrix.

This seems to have implications for other forms of structural distortion via age, adaptation, etc., discussed in Chapter 2.

It is interesting then, to consider that, firstly, the period through which this process of field development occurs is the first 8 weeks of gestation. During this embryonic period, there is huge cellular differentiation and the developing embryo is relatively small and therefore freer to move within the womb (Bradley 2001). The implications of this are that:

1. under 'natural' conditions it is unlikely the mother would know she is pregnant at this early juncture

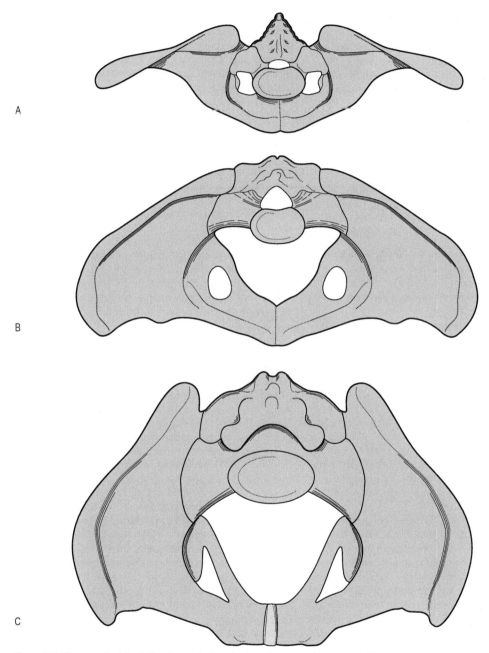

Figure 9.6 Diagram of pelvic girdles demonstrating structure–function relationship. **A** Chimpanzee pelvis, demonstrating mastery of the frontal and sagittal planes. **B** Australopithecine (AL-288-1) pelvis, demonstrating increasing mastery of transverse plane. **C** Human pelvis, demonstrating full mastery of transverse plane. Reproduced with permission from Lovejoy (1988)

2. the mother is, at this stage, not athletically compromised
3. mechanical stresses through connective tissues (growing or grown) create a piezoelectric charge, meaning embryonic development may be affected to some degree by the movements of the mother
4. embryonic tissues form around predetermined axes (Larsen 1988, O'Rahilly & Müller 2003), which will also be influenced by the mother's movement patterns
5. the course of neurological development – which is rapid prenatally (up to 4000 neurons proliferating per second; Haywood & Getchell 2005) – is very much affected by an interplay between both genetic and extrinsic factors.

The genes are more responsible for the hardware of the nervous system while extrinsic factors (such as the mother's movement patterns) contribute to the trillions of finer connections between nerve cells (Haywood & Getchell 2005).

In the first 8 weeks of intrauterine life (the embryonic period), over 90% of the full adult structure of the human being has developed (O'Rahilly & Müller 2003). This process includes, in its rudimentary state, the entire locomotor system. Hence, it is in this first 8 weeks of gestation that the pattern formation of the musculoskeletal system Lovejoy (2005, Lovejoy et al 2003) describes is at its most prolific and significant. It seems that as the cells of a body part – a limb, for example – begin to develop, each cell is able to recognize and respond to positional information within the limb which instructs it to proliferate, or to migrate, or to change shape, or to commit 'suicide' – cellular apoptosis (Lovejoy et al 2003).

This means that, even if a clump of cells is severed or removed from the developing limb, other cells in the locality are able to recognize the changes and fully restore the limb to its original, pre-specified dimensions (Lovejoy et al 2003). How the cells know their role is not yet fully understood, but is believed to be based on an informational map formed by deployment of chemical signals and cell-to-cell communication.

Interestingly, this assertion bears striking resemblance to observations made by physicists, such as Brennan (1988), who have used Kirlian photography to document the effects of severing or removing a portion of a leaf. The remaining portion of the leaf, and the area that the removed portion formerly occupied, remain intact on Kirlian photography, as if the energetic matrix holding the leaf together remains in place even when the physical leaf tissues have been removed or displaced. This has been termed the 'phantom leaf effect'. This etheric template may provide an explanation for how tissues in a severed embryo are able to regrow within a predetermined energetic lattice (Gerber 2000). Backster (2003) also describes similar processes involving identification of pulses in the unfertilized chicken egg – implicating an organizing energy field.

Research into the effects of movement on embryological development has been conducted in chicks (Bradley 2001). There are several similarities in behavior between the developing human and chick. For example, both initiate limb movements less than a quarter of the way through development – and, of course, this may reflect the fact that birds and humans are the only true bipeds in existence (Berrill 1954, Verma 1999). By halfway through the prenatal period, human fetuses can suck their thumbs and chicks chew their toes. Both begin to generate breathing movements in the final third-stage of prenatal development, and both as neonates can make alternating stepping movements, which correlates with these two species being the only two true bipeds.

The embryo is initially buoyant and its movements are relatively unconstrained; however, during the second half of development as body size increases, buoyancy diminishes, plus the rigid shell wall (similar, though not identical, to the muscular human uterine wall) increasingly constrains movement, eventually forcing the embryo into an extremely flexed posture. The human fetus experiences similar changes relative to its environment during development. Work by Bradley (2001) sought to determine whether these movement experiences play an instructive role as motor control is established.

Bradley's (2001) research has shown that parameters of embryonic movement are altered by environmental perturbations, such as a reduction in buoyancy and fixation of a single limb joint. Two lines of evidence were identified to suggest that alterations in motility patterns are attributable to more than transient mechanical phenomena: (1) mechanical constraint of leg motions significantly alters the patterns of wing movement, and (2) physical constraint can yield a net increase of activity.

Lovejoy and colleagues (2003) conclude their discussion by describing an important consequence of the genetic regulatory function in evolution – a phenomenon known as 'transcriptional heterochrony'. Raff (1996) concurs that the prevalent view is that heterochrony is the most common mechanism for evolutionary changes of animal form. In other words, small differences in timing and spatial expression patterns of developmental loci – as controlled by *cis*-regulatory architecture – can account for significant differences in the entire morphology of the organism.

Since it is the *cis*-regulatory elements (which are modular in construction) that have adaptive scope, while the genetic coding is relatively robust, it is most likely that an adaptation-inducing piezoelectric stressor from maternal movement patterns will affect the *cis*-regulatory elements. Simply put, it is the *cis*-regulatory elements that can influence phenotypic expression of the gene – and it is they that are most adaptable or 'plastic'.

When one considers that the entire organism is formed of interwoven chains of piezoelectric dipolar molecules – each capable of oscillation due to its spiral nature – it is of little surprise that alterations in the functional capacity of this three-dimensional, ubiquitous network may occur as a result of extrinsic forces (Barnes 1997). Indeed this is the premise for how manual techniques applied to adult tissues may facilitate change in the polarity potential of the tissue, producing a therapeutic effect (Oschman 2000, Schleip 2003a). It is therefore possible, if not likely, that these same piezoelectrically active molecules would respond to mechanical stressors, such as bipedal gait, based on the axes of motion about which bipedal gait were carried out.

Vital force and tissue organization

Discussing the properties of the living matrix of an organism – which would include the developing embryo – Oschman (2000) states that connective tissues form a mechanical continuum, extending through the animal body, even into the innermost parts of each cell. Each tension, each compression, each movement causes the crystalline lattice of the connective tissues to generate bioelectronic signals that are precisely characteristic of those tensions, compressions and movements.

Interestingly, a naturopathic slant on this discussion is that Claude Bernard, who famously stated that the terrain was more important than the seed, also had the foresight in 1839 to state: 'The genes create structures, but the genes do not control them; the vital force does not create structure, the vital force directs them' (Oschman 2000).

Ontogenic adaptive loads

In an ape, such as a chimp not proficient in bipedal gait, the side-to-side lurching would have a very different effect on the developing embryo than in a modern-day human, for example. The argument against looking at the bony or muscular arrangement of the human body to understand more about how Homo sapiens arrived at this juncture may be at least stalled, if not halted, by this way of viewing ontogenetic prenatal development.

Throughout this discussion, there is one other factor that remains unconsidered. If bipedalism brought with it some advantage – such as being able to intimidate potential predators, to hunt or gather more effectively, and to carry foods back to a home base (Lovejoy 1988) – then surely the first apes within a tribe (or troop) to hone this skill would be the most desirable for the opposite sex to befriend and to mate with. Since, in the world of sexual attraction it is known that like attracts like – an athletic male most commonly attracts an athletic female – in this way a simple precursor of bipedal gait may have driven mating selection and successful hunting, defending and reproduction.

In the same way it is said that 'to become an elite athlete requires that you pick your parents well', it is the expression (phenotype) of these genes that is dependent on what the individual is or isn't exposed to in their ontogenetic development. A child that doesn't crawl, is wheeled everywhere in a push-chair, is not fed an optimal diet, that is encouraged to stay in their room, play computer games and watch TV until late every night, is very unlikely to make the grade as a professional athlete, no matter how good the genes they inherited.

To summarize the above discussion, if a primitive hominid found itself able to stand upright and, with some practice, to walk, it doesn't mean that this skill is automatically encoded in that individual's genetic hardware. More likely, however, this skill may exert a mating preference (especially amongst those who desire or who have this skill) and may additionally result in phenotypic expression in progeny of females able to walk bipedally during pregnancy – similar to the wading chimps of the Congo delta (Attenborough 2002).

Benefits of bipedalism

Arguably, the most significant benefit of bipedal adaptation was the ability to be able to defend (and to hunt) from a distance. Tetrapods have to rely on teeth and claws – which are both somewhat found wanting in Homo sapiens. The ability to stand brought with it the ability to punch and with that, the ability to stab, and with that, the ability to throw. As Morris (1982) points out, that what started quite literally as an 'arms' race has simply grown metaphorically with slings, bows and arrows, guns and now long-range weaponry. Our arms have literally and metaphorically grown longer and/or bigger – putting a greater gap between us and our adversaries.

Table 9.3 Dimensional mastery, movement and consciousness level

Mastery of	Results in the ability to	Dominance	State of consciousness
Radial contraction (primal)	Manipulate body cavities: swallow, breathe, excrete, creep	Organismal stability	Preconscious
Lateral contraction (1st)	Swim, move with low efficiency on land	Organismal mobility	Periconscious*
Sagittal plane (2nd)	Moderate-high efficiency of gait on land	Organismal mobility	Conscious
Transverse plane (top-down) (3rd)	Brachiate	Organismal mobility	Conscious
Transverse plane (base-up) (3rd)	Walk efficiently bipedally, to throw, to carry, and to swim	Organismal mobility	Conscious

*See reflexlocomotion, under 'Instinctive sleep postures' below.

Inner unit function in pain conditions

Aside from the phylontogenetic relevance of the preconscious state, the significance to the clinician is that although research has shown that inner unit function is inhibited when a patient is in pain, there is little understanding of the mechanism for this. Aside from the physiological explanation regarding threshold to stimulus (see Table 9.3 above and 'Viscerosomatic reflexes' below), a further psychogenic explanation may be as follows: Pain induces a stress response. When the body is threatened, it has two options, to fight, or to flee. More figuratively, when challenged, the individual has two comparable options: to move forward into growth, or to retreat to safety (Morris 1985, Proctor 2003).

The former option – *move forward into growth* – may equate to the individual learning about his or her pain condition, what may have caused it and how to treat and prevent further episodes. The latter option – *retreat to safety* – is what most people under stress will opt for as an initial strategy, as reliable information may not be readily available – this normally takes the form of retreating into a surrender/fetal posture.[2] In such an instance, controlling the area in pain with the deep (phylogenetically old) intrinsic muscles is not an option since control of these muscles occurred developmentally (ontogenetically) in a preconscious state. In other words, learning to activate inner unit muscles occurs so early in infancy through various rolling and reflexlocomotion patterns (see below under 'Instinctive sleep postures') that it occurs prior to active *cause*

and *effect* cognition on the part of the infant. More gross motor movements based on intention, such as reaching for an object, or moving from position 'a' to position 'b' only become predominant after 7 months of postnatal life (Goldfield 1995).

Clinically, it is likely that, as a pain-avoidance strategy, the patient responds by retreating to 'what they know' and, in doing so, can only revert to muscle control that developed under conscious volitional conditions – the outer unit musculature.

This would explain why 'bracing' of the area occurs using the inefficient faster twitch, outer unit muscles and, subsequently, why it is these muscles that go on to develop trigger points (Lee 2003).

How this pertains to human development and movement rehabilitation

- *True mastery of the transverse plane has brought with it efficient gait, the ability to make tools, to hunt with more than what nature has provided, and to carry food, water and implements wherever we travel.*
- *Rearing up on our hind legs also makes us look larger to potential predators.*
- *Many of these factors that bipedalism has allowed are now acted out in the parks and playgrounds of the world and provide a steady stream of patients into the musculoskeletal rehabilitation centers of the world.*
- *Understanding a little more about the steps that species took to reach this point and the phases that the individuals seeking naturopathic health care took to reach this point, allows for a more complete understanding of why they're here, and how to return them, safely, to the environment of their lives.*

---

[2]Note also, the fetal posture is part of the flexor response to pain or threat. Since both the transversus abdominis and the multifidus exert an extensor moment on the lumbar spine, they may be shut down as part of the neural mechanisms involved in the flexor response.

Overriding extrinsic forces influencing evolutionary development

Compressive

The compressive effects of the water of the oceans would have been the first adaptive force imposed on the earliest single-celled living organisms – hence their ability to resist compression (i.e. viscous properties) and, based on the principle of specific adaptation to imposed demands (SAID), their ability to further manipulate their shape away from danger or toward nutriment meant that radial contraction would have been the most likely movement pattern to develop first.

Currents

Larger organisms that had a sense of desire to move against the lateral force of ocean currents (whether for food, to escape predators, to stay 'safe' within the pack, or to reach a spawning ground) adapted to the imposed demands of these extrinsic forces by developing musculature and sensory organs down the lateral aspects of the body. A dorsal fin developed – like the tail wing of an airplane – to minimize pitching and rolling of the body. Interestingly, their ability to breathe (gills) and their major sense organ – the lateral line, which in land dwellers is condensed into a lateralized sense organ 'the ear' (Radinski 1987) – are found on the lateral aspect of the body wall. This is a reflection of the extrinsic forces and adaptations to these forces developed by fish.

Gravitational

Moving onto land, lateral flexion was no longer the primary force acting on the body, as laterally there was only air, below was ground and above (colloquially, at least) was gravity. This meant that the next natural transition was mastery of the sagittal plane – or flexion-extension. The lateral line gradually lost its usefulness and became redesigned as an ear. The gills were converted into pharyngeal arches and the primary apparatus for breathing became the nose – a midline structure, inherently linked to flexion and extension of the organism (Radinski 1987). Indeed respiration itself became facilitated by, and coupled with, axial extension (inhalation) and axial flexion (exhalation).

Hence the primary adaptive strategy for resisting gravity was to literally meet it head-on through flexion and extension – as is seen in mammalia; however, there is only one species that effectively combats gravity in the transverse plane – and that is the species that has traveled the globe on foot and conquered virtually all terrains – Homo sapiens.

The efficiency of bipedalism, originally believed to be less efficient than tetrapedalism, is now broadly recognized as being the most efficient way to locomote on land (see 'Gait, Primal patterns' below). In many ways more efficient than the wheel, the unique arrangement of human biomechanics allows the body to move using elastic recoil (Gracovetsky 1997, 2001) as a series of wheel-like motions – yet without the constraints of having to remain on a fixed axis of rotation. A wheel, for example, would struggle to roll up a steep hillside laden with boulders and fallen trees, or to climb a tree or rock-face – yet these are not such significant barriers for a set of legs.

It is when the gravity-combating active subsystem (see Fig. 9.3) of the human organism becomes deficient or defective in some way that stress begins to be put on the joints and passive subsystem of the body. Most commonly, this takes the form of an upper or a lower crossed syndrome – see 'Muscle imbalance physiology' and 'Gravity patterns' below.

Spatial mastery and the 4th dimension

Having mastered the primal dimension of radial contraction, and the three spatial dimensions of the frontal, sagittal and transverse planes, the next dimension to consider, the 4th dimension, is *time*.

Of course, mastery of time is a concept familiar to the yogi and those experienced in meditation or shamanic journeying and so may very much have a place in this chapter. However, the proposed mechanisms for how one may truly master time are far too big and hypothetical a topic to broach in this chapter. For an accessible discussion of quantum aspects of the 4th dimension, see *The Field* by Lynne McTaggart (2003).

Nevertheless, for the scientist, the clinician, the pain patient and those rooted in concerns of the physical here and now, the 4th dimension of time still plays a critical role in our understanding of etiology, treatment strategy, exercise prescription and subsequent therapeutic success.

As Kapandji (2003) states, 'at every moment we are in a tri-dimensional cross-section of our being, in 4 dimensions'. Human mechanics are built with cells, a cellular system, whereas industrial mechanics are built with materials, a modular system. This is why in biological systems the whole is greater than the sum of the parts (Table 9.4).

Time and tissue damage etiology

Cumulative trauma/gravitational strain

What is commonly defined as the 4th dimension – time – is critical in our understanding of how joint restrictions, ligamentous contracture, myotonic

Table 9.4 Cartesian versus quantum systems

The whole is greater than the sum of the parts	The sum of the parts is equal to the whole
Living organism	Synthetic machine
Cellular	Modular
Holon (entire picture)	Pixel (part of whole)
Quantum	Newtonian/Cartesian

changes, fascial tensions and many other musculoskeletal aberrations may be brought about.

Posture

While it has been recognized for some time that posture and deportment are important in preventing injury, the actual process of injury has only recently been understood.

In very simplistic but practically useful terms, the recognition of the active process of specific adaptation to imposed demands (or the SAID principle) is key to understanding how biological tissues respond to the stresses of life. The entire musculoskeletal system is composed of various connective tissues, in varying proportions. Collagen is one such connective tissue that is the predominant tissue through the body's connective tissue matrix. Collagen is known to undergo the mechanical property called 'creep' when it is placed under load.

It is essential to understand that creep is both time dependent and load dependent. In other words, if a light load is applied many times to a given biological tissue, it can have the same effect as applying a heavier load just one or two times to that same tissue (McGill 2002).

It is easy to identify with the idea that a large or 'macro' impact to the body will create potential damage to the tissues of the body. Falling over onto the outstretched arm might be a good example – the scaphoid fracture being a relatively common outcome. Such an event is visible and easily discernible in its *cause and effect* nature.

However, it is a little more difficult to relate to the idea that someone typing at the computer for 20 years with wrists that are slightly too hyperextended may end up with a very debilitating condition – far worse prognostically than a scaphoid fracture. Yet no one observed what happened.

It is like the common scenario seen all too often in the clinical environment. The patient blames a lumbar disc herniation on bending over to tie a shoelace – as this is when he or she 'felt it go'. The fact that this individual has been sitting at a desk job for 25 years with poor ergonomics and poor posture is not considered as being causative, as the cumulative microtrauma to the annulus of the disc was relatively – if not completely – pain-free.

The concept of specific adaptation to imposed demands is essential in understanding how the human biomechanical design evolved, and what interventions the naturopathic practitioner can make to enhance biomechanics – whether through treatment, stretch programs or corrective or performance-based exercise.

Optimal instantaneous axis of rotation

When in optimal postural (biomechanical) alignment, the range of motion of the joints of the body remains optimal. When additional vectors of motion are added to the joint (whether they are primary, secondary or accessory motions), restriction of joint range of motion will occur. This fact means that suboptimal alignment both limits performance capabilities of the joint, as well as amplifying the risk of injury to structures of the passive stability subsystem of the joint (see Fig. 9.3 – Panjabi's model of joint stability).

In fact, it is this very principle that is employed by osteopaths, chiropractors, naturopaths and other joint manipulators to create a 'locking' of the joint, meaning that only a limited range of motion (low amplitude) need be thrust through to surpass the physiological barrier of joint range (Hartman 1997).

Therefore, if a joint has faulty posture, it has a limited range of motion through which it can move – which equates to earlier stress on the passive subsystem and decreased range through which power may be generated. Since power is calculated as acceleration multiplied by mass, and acceleration across distance results in speed, the outcome of joint restriction will be a decreased capacity to generate speed and power. In modern living this means that sporting competition may be hampered, though in bygone times such loss of power would have resulted in earlier demise due to predator–prey survival pressures.

Aside from sports and repetitive actions associated with activities of daily living, gravity – the single biggest, yet most underestimated physical stressor – is relentless (Kuchera 1997). Similar to buildings and bridges, the human architecture is stressed by any slight deviation from optimal posture and, in its natural or developmental environment, has a range of different postures – for example, archetypal rest postures (P Beach, Lecturer, British College of Naturopathy & Osteopathy, personal communication, 1994) and instinctive sleep postures (Tetley 2000, M Tetley,

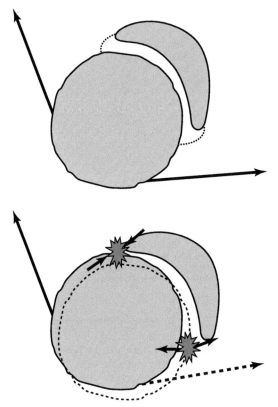

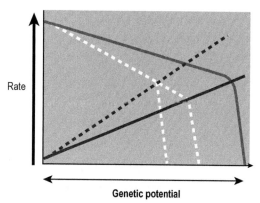

Figure 9.8 Cumulative microtrauma versus repair rate model. If rate of repair is good (gray line) throughout life, and the rate of cumulative microtrauma (black line) is kept mimimal through optimal mechanics, the rate of repair will exceed the rate of damage and the tissue, or organism, will fulfil its genetic potential. If the rate of repair is suboptimal (white dotted line) due to poor nutrition and lifestyle habits, and/or the rate of cumulative microtrauma is increased due to poor mechanics, the rate of damage will exceed the rate of repair earlier in life, and the tissue, or the organism, will fail before genetic potential is reached. If biomechanics are suboptimal, the rate of cumulative microtrauma will increase (black dotted line), surpassing the rate of healing at an earlier stage in life, and resulting in early tissue failure

Figure 9.7 Diagram of optimal instantaneous axis of rotation. Top, optimal pull from muscles in 'balance' with each other results in no disruption of the instantaneous axis of rotation and therefore no significant trauma to the joint. Bottom, a muscle imbalance where one muscle (solid arrow) is stronger than its antagonist (dotted arrow) results in compressive stress to one side of the joint, and distractive stress on the opposite side of the joint

personal communication, 2004; see below under 'Biomechanical attractors') – that it regularly adopts to avoid too much stress on any one specific structure.

Different from buildings and bridges, however, is the fact that a living organism has a cyclical (diurnal) hormonal rhythm. This rhythm means that during its waking hours the organism is predominantly in a breakdown, catabolic state, and when it sleeps it should be predominantly in a growth and repair, anabolic state (Chek 2003).

In a 'functional' environment, a motile living organism will always damage itself microscopically (and sometimes macroscopically) during its more active waking period(s), and will always repair itself during its resting period(s).

Problems only arise when the rate of damage begins to exceed the rate of repair. We can deduce that in clinical practice, cumulative microtrauma is the etiology of most pain conditions we see. Chek (2002) and Vleeming (2003) state that 85% of patients attending

for orthopedic consultation have an idiopathic onset to their pain condition. What this implies is that since most of these pain presentations were not brought on by a clear, traumatic event, it is likely they can be attributed to a cumulative microtrauma mechanism (Fig. 9.8), often a habitual and relatively innocuous pattern. For example:

- typing with poor (hyperextended) wrist posture
- sitting with a flexed lumbar spine 8 hours per day for 25 years
- femoral medial rotational instability on the weight-bearing phase of gait.

The implication for naturopaths, manual therapists and bodyworkers is that if 85% of patients presenting in orthopedic surgery clinics have cumulative microtrauma as part of the etiological matrix, then the percentage of conditions seen in naturopathic or manual therapy clinics that can be ascribed to cumulative trauma will be even higher.

Add to this the fact that cumulative microtrauma progressively undermines the tensile strength of the tissue (McGill 2002), and one arrives at the realization that even apparently 'macrotraumatic' events – such as a bad tackle in a football or rugby match which results in a rupture of a major ligament – may have been predisposed by previous microtrauma to the ruptured tissue (Fig. 9.9).

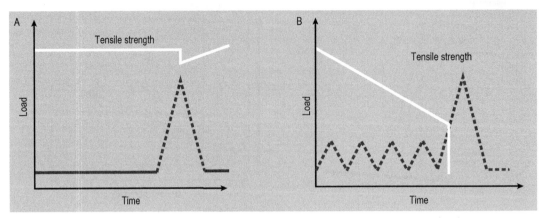

Figure 9.9 Cumulative microtrauma and tensile strength model: For example: Anterior cruciate ligament (ACL) from a healthy knee (**A**) versus ACL from a knee with pronation pattern (**B**); and respective loads they can bear before rupture. Whereas a knee that has good biomechanical function and relatively little load on the ACL (**A**, solid black line) and therefore good tensile strength (**A**, solid white line) may be able to tolerate a blow from a tackle or mistimed landing from a jump (**A**, dotted black line), an ACL that has undergone repetitive microtrauma (**B**, dotted black lines) from a pronation or gravity pattern will lose its tensile strength across time (**B**, solid white line) and therefore will not be able to resist this same load and rupture will occur. This principle applies to any tissue (e.g. Achilles tendon, patella tendon, disc, etc.). Adapted from McGill (2000)

Hence, we can confidently state that, in most cases, a dysfunction in the primal (radial – to include breathing and digestion), 1st (frontal), 2nd (sagittal) or 3rd (transverse) dimension, in the moment, is probably of little consequence, but when in the context of the 4th dimension (time) the impact may be profound.

This view is wholly naturopathic since it highlights both the need for minimization of biomechanical loading through avoidance of cumulative microtrauma, in concert with the need for maximization of tissue repair in the form of nutrition and lifestyle factors.

Clinical importance of the dimensional model

Current models of rehabilitation have correctly identified the deep intrinsic muscles of the spine and those muscles intrinsically involved in compartmental pressure regulation (radial field mastery) as those requiring first consideration in the rehabilitation setting. However, there are few suggestions in the literature explaining how nutrition and lifestyle factors may influence this mastery, nor how to progress these usually floor- or couch-based rehabilitation strategies into subsequent dimensional mastery (see 'Viscerosomatic reflexes' below).

Theories such as those propounded by Hodges (1999) literally take a one-dimensional approach – a necessary prerequisite in quantitative research settings. Hodges rationalized that the pre-contraction (or feed-forward mechanism) of the inner unit – described as a 'visceral cylinder' (see Fig. 9.4 above) – raises the intra-abdominal pressure, thereby creating a stiffen-

ing of the spine and therefore minimizing potential trauma to the tissues surrounding it.

However, there may be a fundamental flaw with this view – or at least the interpretation of it. Stiffness is defined as the change in tension per unit of change in length (Sahrmann 2002). The spine, when used to its maximum functional capability, is stretched throughout its full range of motion. Stiffness of the spine, therefore, may at first appear contradictory to full performance; however, the provision of stiffness by the inner unit will presumably be generated at the exact level required to maintain functional integrity of the passive subsystem, without compromising range of motion. An integral component of a muscle's capacity to generate stiffness is its number of sarcomeres in parallel (as opposed to in series). Since each myosin filament within the sarcomere has six titin proteins (titin being the primary intramuscular connective tissue), the more there are arranged in parallel, the more stiffness the muscle will have (Sahrmann 2002). Hunter (2005), who has studied hamstring strain in professional footballers, states that stiffness within the muscle seems to decrease with fatigue, and therefore cannot absorb as much energy, resulting in increased injury risk to the muscle. While metabolic fatigue is unlikely to occur in an inner unit muscle due to its preponderance of slow twitch fibers and its (typically) unisegmental action, the fatigue element to the series and parallel elastic components, resulting in creep, may ultimately create passive insufficiency in the muscle.

Hunter (2005) goes on to state that of eight players who had recurrent hamstring strain, six had had their hamstrings measured as the least 'stiff' in their club.

Table 9.5 Dimensional dysfunction and therapeutic intervention

Dimension	Example of intervention
Radial	Nutritional intervention Breath-based exercises Singing/voice work Prone transversus activation with biofeedback cuff 4-point transversus activation
Frontal (coronal)	Reptilian crawl Hanna 3-part side-flexion (Hanna 1988) Swiss ball side flexion Lateral lunge (skater's lunge) Standing single arm dumbbell work
Sagittal	McKenzie extension push-up Prone cobra (dorsal raise) Mammalian crawl Supine hip extension: • On ground • Feet on Swiss ball • Back on Swiss ball Squat Dead lift (bend pattern/stiff-legged)
Transverse	Rolling exercises (à la Feldenkrais) Single-leg lower abdominal exercises Lower Russian twist (feet on ball) Upper Russian twist (back on ball) Standing cable push Standing cable pull Woodchop Lunge Gait • Walk • Run • – Sprint

If the spinal range of motion is analyzed kinesiologically in any sport requiring power generation, not only does the spine typically go through its full rotation range of motion but also it usually ends up fully flexed. As Gracovetsky (1997) rhetorically enquires, why would nature select a spine that uses rotation and flexion – which maximally stress the annulus fibrosis – unless there was a selective advantage?

Clearly the evolutionary benefit of the combined spinal flexion-rotation is the fact that a relatively small creature (Homo sapiens) can recruit a greater numbers of muscle fibers via its muscular sling systems to execute movements that were intrinsically linked to survival. How far could a lion throw a javelin? Without brachiating shoulder joints and limited voluntary trunk rotation, the answer is clearly, 'not far' – despite its formidable power.

Although trunk flexion-rotation may thus be advantageous in a survival environment, it does not alter the fact that this motion is known to be most likely to damage the spinal discs, which similarly would be catastrophic for an early hominid.

Studying the applied anatomy of the abdominal wall and pelvis provides another suggestion. Firstly, the three layers of the abdominal wall – transversus abdominis, internal oblique and external oblique – are fashioned in such a way that they can slide over one another (Rizk 1980). Of course, the obliques, having the greatest lever arm of all trunk rotators and a higher ratio of fast twitch fibers, are prime movers in explosive rotation movements.

If there is a pre-contraction of the transversus abdominis, creating a visceral cylinder about which the obliques can pull, then:

- the power output will be significantly greater
- rotational control of the trunk will be dramatically enhanced (see below).

If the applied anatomy of the abdominal wall is scrutinized, then the internal oblique is observed to insert into the deep lamina of the posterior layer of the thoracolumbar fascia (see Vleeming et al 1997, p. 62, for illustration).

The biceps femoris also attaches into this same lamina. The relevance of this can be seen when considering sporting postures as metaphorical survival motor patterns.

The rate-limiting factor in movement

It is important to recognize that the brain will only accelerate a limb as fast as it can decelerate it; if this rule is broken, the passive subsystem is the first to become compromised (see Panjabi's model of joint stability, Fig. 9.3). Hence the rate-limiting factor is the functionality of the muscles responsible for deceleration and control.

In all of the instances given above, we have the sling from the biceps femoris of the dominant side, via the sacrotuberous and thoracolumbar fascia into the internal oblique of the contralateral side, via the abdominal aponeurosis into external oblique of the dominant side, and via the pectoralis major into the dominant arm, as the all-important deceleration sling.

This sling effectively controls the flexion-rotation motion of the trunk and therefore each factor along its path must function optimally for full performance and minimal risk of injury. Understanding this mechanism helps to illustrate how something as simple as shoulder pain, causing increased tone in the pectoral group, may ultimately result in hamstring strain, for example.

This description of the abdominal cylinder, essentially acting as a visceral fulcrum (visceral from 'viscous' meaning non-compressible), provides a

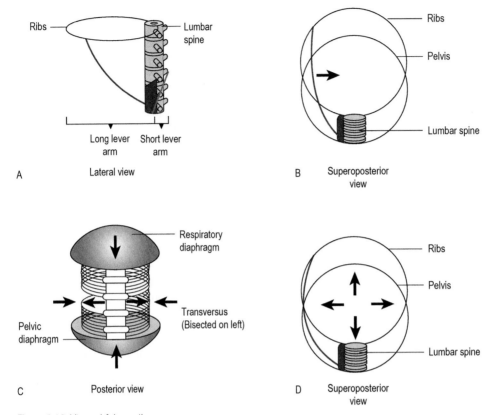

Ribs — Lumbar spine

Long lever arm   Short lever arm

A   Lateral view

Ribs

Pelvis

Lumbar spine

B   Superoposterior view

Respiratory diaphragm

Pelvic diaphragm

Transversus (Bisected on left)

C   Posterior view

Ribs

Pelvis

Lumbar spine

D   Superoposterior view

Figure 9.10 Visceral fulcrum theory

perhaps fuller, multidimensional explanation of why pre-contraction of the inner unit of the trunk is critical in stabilizing, controlling and protecting the low back.

Aside from the conventional view of the visceral cylinder, the deep intrinsic muscles of any body segment may, as a rule, be viewed as 'inner unit' and therefore more involved in proprioception and stabilization than in moving the joint. Examples include the gemelli, obturator internus and externus, quadratus femoris, gluteus minimus at the hip or vastus medialis, popliteus and biceps femoris' short head at the knee.

While such muscles have a stabilizer dominance and secondarily act as mobilizers, so the more superficial multijoint muscles typically serve a mobilizer dominance and act as secondary stabilizers.

Outer unit sling systems

Examples of key mobilizer systems (commonly termed 'sling systems'), which are also critical in providing (particularly dynamic) stability, include:

- posterior oblique sling
- anterior oblique sling

- deep longitudinal system
- lateral system
- deep diagonal sling
- posteroanterior power sling.

To lose sight of the inter-relationship between current research findings and the evolution of body plan design is to decontextualize the available knowledge base and disconnect the integration of systems of the organismal whole.[3]

The naturopath specializes in viewing the body, its systems and its overall health in an *integrated* manner; to look at it and treat it in any other way is to pursue *disintegration* of health. This is the polar opposite of naturopathic objectives.

Summary

In summary, as a basic model, the earliest movement patterns based on the known major body plans were

[3]To read further around the ontogenetic development mimics phylogenetic development, see *Wisdom of the Body Moving* by Linda Hartley (1995), *Amazing Babies* by Beverly Stokes (2002) and related texts.

that of radial contraction. Radial contraction is what we see in our most primitive reflexive functions: breathing and eating. Radial contraction is also known as a precursor to movement in the human organism, such as the transversus abdominis feed-forward mechanism (Richardson et al 1999). Singular radial contraction and expansion may initially have developed as a primitive means of phagocytosis. This may be termed the *primal dimension*, or the *first space manipulation*.

With multiple cells (or segments), one attached to the next, a sequenced radial contraction may result in a peristaltic wave that produces movement both within the body and movement of the body. This movement pattern eventually combined forward movement with digestion, where previously digestion was bidirectional and therefore would have compromised attempts at forward movement. Coordinated contraction clearly requires a nervous system to orchestrate it, leading to the advent of chordates.

The next stage of development appears to be a synchronous contraction of musculature down one side of the body of the organism to induce a lateral flexion – as found predominantly in fish and lizards. To prevent the body from telescoping in on itself, a rigid axel down the length of the organism was required. This brought about the dawn of vertebrates (Kardong 2002).

As stated above, having understood more about how body plans have evolved to adapt to extrinsic forces by mastering the three dimensions of space, it is important to consider what happens if any of these dimensions is not optimally controlled across the 4th dimension of time. If time is traversed with an imbalance or dysfunction in any of the three movement dimensions, or the primal contractile dimension, stability and movement control is jeopardized, usually resulting in cumulative trauma to the passive subsystem.

Muscle imbalance physiology

Muscle imbalance physiology was first described by the eminent muscle physiologist Vladimir Janda (1968, 1983). Muscle imbalance was mainly embraced by the physiotherapy community, though in recent years it has lost some of its popularity to the concept of core function and motor control. Nevertheless, this author considers identification and correction of muscle imbalance an invaluable clinical tool.

Perhaps one reason for the decline in interest in muscle imbalance is that, as with nearly all clinical entities, to find a 'textbook' case is less common than finding a partial case. This brings with it confusion.

Box 9.2 Central sensitization

Willard (1996a–c) explains that once a sensitization has occurred at a spinal segment, that facilitation can be maintained by just a very mild afferent input to the cord (and can perpetuate for several days after the initial stimulus has gone due to plastic changes within the nervous system).

So, for example, a person with a lateral epicondylitis will experience repetitive afferent drive from the extensor mass and periosteum of the lateral epicondyle which facilitates (or sensitizes) the C6 level of the spinal cord. Such sensitization will become more 'plastic' the longer the sensitization is maintained. After 2 or 3 months of pain (and cumulative afferent drive to the cord), that person may consult a therapist for treatment. At this point, even if the therapist were able to 'magic' the tissue trauma away, the patient would still feel pain at the site for a further few days. Equally, if that patient were to start to feel better and so use their wrist again in an unprotected way, only the mildest of microtrauma will evoke a significant pain response at the cord level, disproportionate to the level of tissue damage.

Hence, the focus should not be on the symptomology, but on a return to function. By optimizing the biomechanical function of the shoulder and the core (as well as taking some local protective measures, such as use of an epicondyle clasp), the patient can work to minimize stress through the soft tissues of the arm and, in the meantime, can embrace nutritional and lifestyle measures that optimize the healing rate of the tissues. This takes the focus away from the symptomology and concentrates it on the etiology and/or adaptive capacity. This is clearly in line with naturopathic principles as outlined in Chapter 1.

Commonly, the approach to diagnosing a muscle imbalance (for practical purposes) is based primarily on subjective assessment, such as observation of standing posture. While this approach may be time-effective and is not un-useful, it does mean that prescription of treatment – corrective stretching, corrective mobilization, corrective exercises and other nutrition and lifestyle advice – may be somewhat non-specific. Additionally, aside from subjective symptomology, progress is difficult to gauge with such subjective approaches.

As Liebenson (1999) states, to effectively manage pain patients, it is critical to provide a focus on returning function as opposed to getting rid of dysfunction. This means that a patient can make great strides towards a return of function, yet may still have a similar symptom profile. This phenomenon may be explained neurophysiologically through the process of central sensitization (see above). Hence, objectively

Table 9.6 Phasic versus tonic characteristics

Phasic	Tonic
Fast twitch preponderance	Slow twitch preponderance
Fatigue early	Fatigue late
High threshold to stimulus	Low threshold to stimulus
Mobilizer dominance	Stabilizer dominance
Superficial	Deep
Outer unit	Inner unit
Global stability	Local stability
Multi-articular	Mono-articular
Lengthen/weaken	Shorten/tighten

we may be able to see improvement – even though the patient may be able to feel little difference. Therefore, the means to assess joint position, joint range of motion and length–tension relationships objectively is critical, in order to manage patients effectively and provide ongoing motivation for a return toward function.

As reported in Chapter 5, an international panel of experts discussed the role of muscle imbalance and classification of muscle function in the *Journal of Bodywork and Movement Therapies* (Bullock-Saxton et al 2000). Interestingly, even among these experts, there was still some confusion regarding muscle classification. It may be that this confusion, which presumably would be greater in 'non-experts', could be part of the reason that muscle imbalance hasn't become a mainstay of clinical assessment for many manual therapists. Table 9.6 will hopefully provide some clarity. However, it is important to recognize that these are just useful clinical models, and like all models there are exceptions (particularly in the bottom two categories of the table).

Muscle imbalance in manual therapy may have lost some of its appeal, as to measure such length–tension relationships and joint ranges about both pelvic and pectoral girdles and to assess their impact on spinal mechanics through inclinometry takes longer than the average consultation usually allows. So, under traditional practice, we are only left with observationally assessing the condition then treating and making exercise recommendations to the client, which, in itself, has some serious shortcomings.

1. This approach depends on a very subjective assessment – which is wide open to bias.

2. Observation – or standing, seated or supine static examination – bears only limited relationship to the patient's active daily environment.

3. When under stress, the body will migrate to its position of greatest strength – which is why dynamically loading the patient can help to identify dysfunctional postural patterns.

4. This subjective assessment approach provides little incentive for the patient to perform prescribed corrective exercises – especially in the absence of pain.

In Chapter 4 there is some discussion of what constitutes 'dysfunction' of a somatic tissue and the point is made that pain does not have to present for a tissue to be dysfunctional. Hence, it is entirely possible that a patient may attend with a muscle imbalance (which represents a biomechanical dysfunction) yet have no pain. Nevertheless, any muscle imbalance disrupts the optimal axis of joint motion (a spatial or three-dimensional dysfunction) which will, over time, result in tissue damage (a 4th dimension dysfunction). The point at which the sufferer feels pain is the point at which the rate of damage exceeds the rate of repair (see Fig. 9.8).

Hence, it is strongly urged that to evaluate any muscle imbalance, clinical measurement tools, including, but not limited to, inclinometers, tape measures, 1st rib calipers, forward head calipers, plumb-line and digital camera and/or camcorder should be used (see Fig. 9.11). Additionally, to assess the body under load it is useful to have, at the very least, a Swiss ball, but ideally a cable column and a squat rack with barbell.

Further to the discussion of neurophysiology in Box 9.3, it is important to understand the clinical applications of the law of facilitation (Korr 1978), which states the following:

When an impulse has passed through one set of neurons to the exclusion of others, it will tend to take the same course on future occasions and each time it traverses this path the resistance will be smaller.

Janda classically used EMG to demonstrate that a facilitated lumbar erector would dysfunctionally fire when its antagonist – the rectus abdominis – was engaged in an abdominal curl (sit-up) (Chek 2001a, Cranz 2000, Janda 1978, Williams & Goldspink 1973, 1978). After stretching the facilitated lumbar erector (thereby inhibiting it), it would no longer fire with the rectus abdominis during the sit-up maneuver (Janda 1978). This is a classic example of facilitation and how it can create disrupted function at a range of joints (in this case joints of the lumbopelvic region).

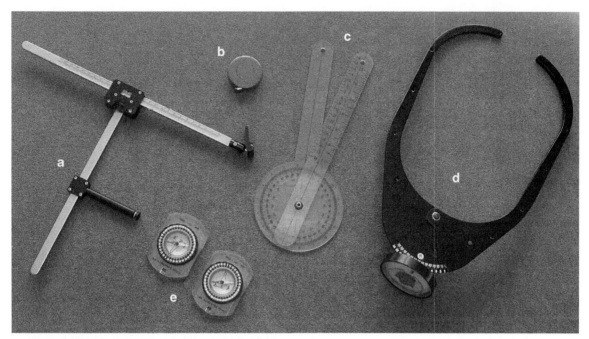

Figure 9.11 Clinical measurement tools: a, forward head caliper; b, tape measure; c, goniometer; d, first rib caliper; d, indinometers

---

Box 9.3 You are an athlete within your environment

An important concept to embrace is the idea that everyone is an athlete within their own environment. Hence the idea that someone is too old or too deconditioned to use any of these tools for assessment is, likely, unfounded. It is not uncommon to hear that a therapist works with a mainly elderly population, therefore a Swiss ball would be inappropriate.

In fact, the therapeutic truth is that, if a given individual is unable to sit on a Swiss ball (with three bases of support) then, theoretically, they should not be able to stand (two bases of support) and certainly should not be able to walk (one base of support for 80% of the gait cycle). To walk, therefore, is far more neurologically demanding than sitting on a Swiss ball.

Quite aside from the therapist's concerns, if a patient is unable to sit on a Swiss ball then is it more or less likely that they will fall on slippery ground? We know that 25% of elderly patients will die within 1 year of fracturing a hip (National Osteoporosis Foundation 2006) and that falling is the leading cause of death in those over 65 years of age (Chek 2004b); hence a naturopathic approach is surely to prevent such falls. Swiss ball training can condition the tilting reflex – something moving under the body. This is technically what happens when the interface between the ice and sole of the shoe meet – the water on the surface of the ice moves and the foot slips over it. Therefore, Swiss ball conditioning is ideal for training fall prevention in the elderly in a slippery (tilting) environment, whereas a discipline such as tai chi may be more beneficial in a non-slippery (righting) environment.

The importance of this phenomenon and the relevance of it to muscle imbalance is that if we have a group of muscles that are prone to overuse, tightening and shortening, they will be preferentially activated by the central nervous system via a facilitated pathway. Due to the plasticity of the nervous system, this makes correcting a muscle imbalance a potentially challenging task requiring a lot of repetitive contraction to facilitate new pathways to the inhibited antagonists.

Upper crossed syndrome (see Chapter 6, Fig. 6.33)

The upper crossed syndrome is an extremely common muscle imbalance. In fact, clinical experience suggests that it is extremely rare in the symptomatic population to find any patient that does not exhibit at least an aspect of the upper crossed syndrome.

Upper crossed syndrome, like lower crossed syndrome, is essentially a gravity pattern. It is what gravity would do to our skeletons if we had no musculature to hold them in place. This is also known as a pronation pattern. (See discussion of crossed syndrome patterns in Chapter 6.)

Muscles that are commonly considered to be short and tight (or stiff) in the upper crossed syndrome are as follows:

- Suboccipital group
- Sternocleidomastoid
- Upper fibers of trapezius
- Levator scapula
- Pectoralis minor
- Rectus abdominis (upper fibers).

Muscles that are commonly considered to be long and weak in the upper crossed syndrome are as follows:

- Deep cervical flexors
- Supra- and infrahyoid group
- Middle and lower fibers of trapezius
- Rhomboids
- Serratus anterior
- Thoracic erectors.

The classic osteokinematic coupling of an upper crossed syndrome is a forward head posture (ventral cranial glide), an increased 1st rib angle (dropped sternum), protracted shoulder girdle, flexed cervicothoracic junction and an increased thoracic kyphosis.

Arthrokinematically, this means that the cervical lordosis tends to flatten with a compensatory hyperextension in the upper cervical spine to maintain the eyes on the optic plane (horizon). The increased 1st rib angle creates a flexion stress onto the 1st thoracic vertebra rotating it forward into sagittal flexion – with the potential end result being a 'dowager's hump'. The dropped sternum means that the ribs are held in a flexed or 'exhalation' position. This may be problematic for those with athletic requirements or with breathing disorders. With the rib cage in exhalation, the thoracic spine moves into sagittal flexion and, across time, may develop an extension restriction due to contracture of the anterior longitudinal ligament, among other structures. The protraction of the shoulders, with or without thoracic extension restriction, disrupts the optimal instantaneous axis of rotation of the glenohumeral joint, and may result in impingement syndromes and/or capsular instabilities (see Fig. 9.12).

Lower crossed syndrome (see Chapter 6, Fig. 6.33)

Muscles that are commonly considered to be short and tight (or stiff) in the lower crossed syndrome are as follows:

- Lumbar erectors
- Iliopsoas
- Tensor fascia lata
- Rectus femoris
- Adductors (short – i.e. not spanning the knee).

Muscles that are commonly considered to be long and weak in the lower crossed syndrome are as follows:

- Rectus abdominis (lower)
- Gluteus maximus
- Hamstring group.

Osteokinematically, the pelvis is usually held in an anterior tilt in the lower crossed syndrome. At the lumbar spine, lordosis is enhanced, meaning that the low back is held in relative extension.

Arthrokinematically, the anteriorly tilted pelvis means that the hips are relatively in flexion and therefore in their loose-packed position (Lee 2004). Across time, this will lead to increased microtrauma, instability and pain in the hip joint, predisposing to degenerative change. Interestingly, lower crossed syndrome is more frequently observed in women – which may help explain the higher incidence of hip problems in elderly women (Baechle & Earle 2000). Since lordosis is increased in the lumbar spine, greater loading is placed through the facet joints (see discussion below under 'Neutral spine philosophy'), meaning that they are more prone to cumulative trauma and injury. Spinal pathologies, such as spondylolysis, spondylolisthesis, foraminal stenosis and spinal stenosis, are more common in the extended lumbar spine.

Layered syndrome

Muscles commonly considered short and tight in the layered syndrome are as follows:

- Hamstrings
- Gluteus maximus
- Thoracolumbar erectors
- Upper fibers of trapezius
- Suboccipitals.

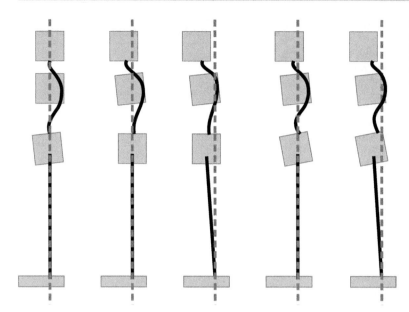

Figure 9.12 Silhouettes of the major muscle imbalances. From the left: optimal posture, layered syndrome, layered syndrome with a sway, lower-crossed and upper crossed syndromes, lower and upper crossed syndromes with a sway

Muscles commonly considered to be long and weak in the layered syndrome are as follows:

- Hip flexors (rectus femoris and iliopsoas)
- Lumbar erectors
- Thoracic erectors
- Lower/middle fibers of trapezius.

Osteokinematically, the pelvis is posteriorly tilted, and the lumbar spine is flat with extension at the thoracolumbar junction leading into a thoracic kyphosis and forward head posture. In layered syndrome, the posture of the upper quarter is very similar to – and, in some cases, indistinguishable from – an upper crossed syndrome (see Fig. 9.12 and Fig. 6.33 in Chapter 6).

Arthrokinematically, this means that the hip joints are held in relative extension (and therefore may feel and measure as being 'tight'), and the loading through the lumbar spine shifts more onto the discs and less through the facet joints. Consequently, this posture is commonly associated with lumbar disc injury clinically.

Western seated posture (WSP) and ergonomics (see also Alexander technique in Chapter 7, particularly Fig. 7.17)

The topic of rehabilitation and movement approaches couldn't be addressed without discussing the impact of the modern-day ergonomic environment on human biomechanics.

Since it is known that the body is reactive to its environment and will attempt to adapt to the demands placed upon it, it would seem logical that it should be adapting to the ergonomic environment of the modern workplace. This may hold very little truth, but also should be put into the context of evolution. Since chairs are known to have been used since 8000 BC (Cranz 2000) and it takes somewhere in the region of 100 000 years for the human genome to change by 0.01% (Chek 2001b), it is unlikely that adaptation to a life of sitting on chairs will be forthcoming for a minimum of 90 000 years yet!

How the body does adapt is by changing its length–tension relationships about the pelvis and trunk, the most common clinical adaptation being one towards a layered syndrome. As the rib cage approximates the pelvis, so the anterior oblique slings (of anterior internal oblique fibers through the linea alba to the contralateral external oblique) will be held in a shortened position. Reciprocally, the lumbar erector group will be held in a lengthened position.

From the work of Williams & Goldspink (1973, 1978) it is known that it takes around 1 week for there to be a laying down of sarcomeres in a muscle that is held in a lengthened position (Sahrmann 2002). Reciprocally, there is a taking up of sarcomeres in muscles that are consistently held in a shortened position.

A key concept to embrace here – as described above – is that each individual must train to survive his or her unique environments: 'we all are athletes within our own personal ecosystems'.

For example, the new mother who not only has to lift her baby and may spend long durations breast feeding and changing nappies (diapers) – all with a systemic overlay of relaxin compromising her passive control subsystem (see Panjabi's model of joint stability, Fig. 9.3) – simply must also have good motor control if she is to survive her environment pain-free and without compromising herself.

Another example is the office worker who likes to spend her weekends playing hockey. She must train her body to survive the relentless load of gravity on her back and neck during her seated work hours and still be well conditioned enough to not 'crash' her biomechanics when she suddenly takes on the highly competitive unpredictable environment of the hockey pitch at the weekend.

A further example would be the professional sportsman who, for his sport, has to constantly stay on his toes. In most ball sports this is an early skill to be taught as a prerequisite to moving the feet quickly in response to the opposition's play. Such a command, and habitual use of this stance, result in quadriceps dominance and a whole host of common sports injuries associated with such a posture – such as anterior cruciate ligament injury, meniscal tear, Achilles injury and plantar fasciitis (Wallden 2007). Hence, in conditioning to survive his sport, such a sportsman must use movement patterns and loading that help to redress the imbalance his sport creates. (Of course, the same premise holds true for sports that reinforce laterality patterns – such as racket and kicking sports, as well as track-based running.)

In summary, to think that anyone can get by in a conventional modern environment without training to survive it, is to dramatically increase risk of injury and to unquestionably doom that individual to suboptimal biomechanical function.

Note: This being said, many people 'get by' without optimal biomechanical function and remain asymptomatic; it just depends on the motivations and the objectives of each individual as well as their inherited and acquired characteristics, nutritional status, psychosocial factors and other factors – in other words, the context within which the naturopathic triad is embraced. If the objective of work in this field is to prevent injury and to realize potential as well as to treat injury, then what is stated above still holds true.

Structural length versus functional tone

One of the reasons that the popularity of evaluation of muscle imbalance may have dwindled in the manual therapy community – aside from the discussion above of objective measurement – is the fact that commonly clinical testing procedures may identify both the agonist *and* the antagonist as short or stiff.

The nomenclature for muscle imbalance has been discussed by Sahrmann (2002) and the use of the word 'tight' has been suggested to, perhaps rightly, be too nondescript and open to misinterpretation. The word 'stiff' denotes the mechanical property of the tissue (see Table 9.7), whereas something that is either short-

Table 9.7 Definitions of tissue properties

Term	Definition
Creep	The slow movement of a material that becomes viscous due to shear stresses
Stiffness	A material's resistance to deformation
Strain	The amount of deformation that occurs as a result of the applied force
Hysteresis	A measurement of permanent deformation of a viscoelastic material that does not retrace the force–length tension curve traced when the force was first applied. It is the energy lost from the tissue during this transaction
Elasticity	The property of a material to return to its original form or shape when a deforming force is removed
Viscosity	The measure of shear force that must be applied to a fluid to obtain a rate of deformation. It is time dependent. Viscous means non-compressible
Plasticity	The property of a material to permanently deform when it is loaded beyond its elastic range
Thixotropy	The property exhibited by materials such as muscle of becoming fluid when disturbed or shaken and of setting again when allowed to stand
Viscoelasticity	The property of being both viscous and elastic

After Lardner (2001).

ened or lengthened may, technically, be tight. In the past, this potential difficulty has be circumnavigated by describing 'short and tight' or 'long and taut' in the same phrase, but 'stiff' also implies that there is resistance to lengthening, something Sarhmann believes is a by-product of the series elastic components (such as titin) within the sarcomere. Hence the more sarcomeres in parallel, the more stiffness a tissue will have, whereas additional sarcomeres in series may result in little or no change to tissue stiffness.

The literature and clinical experience suggest that a further consideration to add to the picture should be *structural tension versus functional tone*.

Study of the microstructure of skeletal muscle tells us that the sarcolemma, t-tubule and sarcoplasmic reticulum provide a direct connection from the sarcomere to the endomysium, epimysium and perimysium (Williams 1995). In cases of traumatic scarring, or of long-term aberrant posture, tissues held in a shorted position will undergo contracture and a myofascial tension will prevent effective lengthening of that tissue. In such instances, contract–relax methodologies of muscle lengthening will be futile, since these techniques depend on changes in muscle tone as opposed to myofascial stretching. Instead, muscles that have been held in a shortened position across extended periods of time – also involving their associated fascial nets – will respond better to low load prolonged tensile forces, such as those deployed in myofascial release techniques (Schleip 2003a) and those associated with archetypal rest postures or instinctive sleep postures (see below).

So-called 'static stretching' (slow, prolonged holds) would seem to have an overall effect of relaxing the neuromyofascial system by stimulating the parasympathetic nervous system (Vaughn 2003). Since electron microscopy has demonstrated that fascia has smooth muscle cells embedded within it (Barnes 1997), we can see that, once again, the primitive vegetative nervous system intricately links the musculoskeletal system with digestive, respiratory and other primary functions in the body – which has important ramifications for the archetypal rest postures described below.

Thixotropic changes (where a tissue transforms from a more gel-like state to a more soluble state) have been shown to occur when connective tissues are held under long-term mechanical stress (Barnes 1997).

Muscle tone will be increased under any condition of aberrant loading or when under stress (Barlow 1959 and Selye 1976, cited in Chaitow 2001). Since being held in an inner range or an outer range creates adaptive stress on the musculoskeletal system, we can expect an increased tone. Indeed, commonly the patient perceives the greatest tone in the muscle being held in a lengthened position – in its outer range.

It is findings like those described in the clinical examples in Box 9.4 that may have confused many clinicians working on a short 20- or 30-minute model where they do not have time to assess all of the relevant findings and therefore conclude by rejecting the concept of muscle imbalance as being clinically unuseful. With a little closer attention, muscle imbalance physiology can be understood to have a profound influence on the human frame, its performance and its failure.

Static versus dynamic dysfunction

It is critical when assessing a patient to do so in a way that is representative of how that individual uses his

---

Box 9.4 Clinical examples

Example 1

A soccer player presented to our clinic complaining of hamstring tightness. Goniometric examination revealed both a short, tight hamstring group and a concomitant short tight iliopsoas and rectus femoris. On palpation, the hamstrings in particular felt very tight. A standing assessment revealed an anterior pelvic tilt of 11° (reference range 4–7° tilt for males) and an increased lumbar lordosis of 38° (reference range 30–35°). The player had experienced a number of hamstring strains in his career and recently an ankle inversion injury. He was constantly feeling the need to stretch his hamstrings. What was going on? How should we advise this client?

Without assessing pelvic tilt, or lumbar lordosis inclinometry, we would have no idea where to start advising the patient. He felt that his hamstrings were 'tight' and on palpation they felt tight; they also measured as being short or tight.

The clue that gave away the true etiology of the client's perceived hamstring tension was his lumbopelvic posture, which showed that he had a lower crossed syndrome. His quadriceps and iliopsoas were truly 'short', pulling his pelvis into anterior tilt and inducing a lumbar lordosis, while he perceived tension in his hamstrings because they were strung taut and therefore were exhibiting increased tone to try to hold the pelvis from going into further anterior tilt. Measuring his hamstrings goniometrically, they appeared 'short', but in

fact, the apparent shortness was purely due to parafunctional tone (see left-hand column of Fig. 9.13).

Ultimately, this patient's hamstring tension was alleviated by stretching the quadriceps, the iliopsoas and working the hamstrings in their inner range using functional exercise patterns.

Example 2

Perhaps the most classic example of altered tone being confused with altered length is the pain experienced by many seated workers in their rhomboid and middle trapezius region.

Many manual therapy students spend a great deal of time massaging each other's rhomboids, stretching the rhomboids and practicing other techniques on the rhomboids. Yet these muscles are commonly long and weak – and, far from requiring stretch-based work, they require corrective stretching to the antagonistic and shortened pectoralis minor, followed by corrective exercises to work the rhomboids and/or middle trapezius in its inner range.

It is a common perception that the rhomboids 'need' stretching as there is increased parafunctional tone in this group (and, as a result, more accumulation of metabolic waste). This is another example of the importance of assessing the patient rather than only listening to the patient's feelings as to his or her needs.

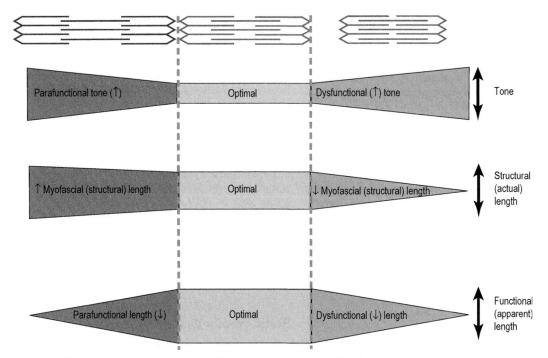

Figure 9.13 Functional tone versus structural length. Any deviation of structural length, whether long (left, dark gray column), or short (right, mid-gray column), results in increased tone. This may create an apparent or functional shortness in the muscle on length–tension assessment

or her body during activities of daily living (ADLs). This means assessment using functional movement patterns. Liebenson (2002a) states that exercises for conditioning and rehabilitation should closely resemble activities of daily living, and demands of employment or sports and recreational activities. Chek (2000a) describes functional exercise as encompassing all of the following characteristics:

1. Comparable reflex profile
2. Maintenance of center of gravity over base of support:
   - Dynamic
   - Static
3. Generalized motor program compatibility
4. Open/closed chain compatibility
5. Relevant biomotor abilities
6. Isolation to integration.

Some of these factors will be described below, but for further reading see Chek (2000a).

However, it is important not just to train in these movement patterns, but also to assess in these movement patterns. Most therapists will assess the client in standing, possibly in sitting and, thereafter, only in a recumbent position. However, consideration of motor

learning and performance highlights that such assessment strategies only provide a very limited view of the function of the human body.

Assessing a patient simply standing provides almost no insight into how that body will respond under load. Since it is load (either micro or macro) that is the primary cause of injury, it is imperative to observe how the body reacts under load – if we are both to treat and to prevent future injury in our clients. For example, many patients will present with a layered syndrome (lumbar flexion pattern) in their standing examination but when under load or when sprinting, they exceed their stabilization threshold and their spine switches into a lower crossed syndrome (lumbar extension pattern).

Neutral spine philosophy

The neutral spine philosophy is a concept that, essentially, is based on good motor learning physiology, the idea being to train the patient to maintain the spine in a neutral position during activities of daily living – such as bending, lifting, sitting, getting in and out of a chair or other familiar movement patterns.

This philosophy is based on the fact that the body will always move towards its position of strength

(Chek 2001b). It is not based on the idea that the spine should always remain in neutral, simply that in neutrality should be where the spine should be at its strongest.

This concept is supported by research from Richardson et al (1999) demonstrating that the transversus abdominis activates most effectively with the lumbopelvic region in 'neutral'.

What is a neutral spine?

According to Schaefer (1987), the optimal anteroposterior angulation of the spine should be in the region of 30–35°. Other researchers, such as Neumann (2002), suggest slight variations on these figures – but, in the main, these are due to methodological differences or to do with using an 'average' or 'normal' sample rather than an *optimal* sample. As an example, Boos et al (1995) carried out MRI scanning of a group of 46 symptomatic (low back pain) and 46 asymptomatic (age-, sex- and risk factor-matched) individuals. In those with low back pain, 96% were found to have concomitant structural disc defects on MRI. However, of the asymptomatic group, 76% of them had a posterior disc herniation. None of these individuals was in any pain or had any awareness of their dysfunction. In this circumstance, disc bulge could be said to be 'the norm', yet it is clearly not functional. Just because something is normal (forward head posture or upper crossed syndrome are also good examples) does not mean it is functional. We know, clinically, that posterior disc bulge is most commonly associated with a flattened lumbar lordosis (hypolordotic). Hence it is likely that approximately three-quarters of the group assessed by Boos et al (1995) had a flattened lumbar curve. This is not functional, but is the norm amongst sedentary populations. Liebenson (2002b) confirms epidemiological studies demonstrate that individuals with seated (Western seated posture) occupations have a heightened risk of disc herniation: *Just because something is 'normal' does not mean it is 'functional'.*

Kapandji (1974), Gracovetsky (1988, 1997, 2003) and McGill (2002) also discuss the concept of the neutral spine and all concur that a bias too much toward a kypholordotic or a flattened spine compromises function and therefore performance, and also predisposes to injury.

Though it is recognized that the spine is designed to move well outside of its range of neutral, as soon as the spine migrates to a position outside of neutral its risk of injury increases (see below). This is not to say that flexibility is a bad thing. The fact is that flexibility should be optimal in all ranges of motion, and should be properly controlled by the overlying muscular system.

The healthy spine has 6° of freedom (flexion-extension in three planes and translation in three planes). So, based on probability alone, your spine is unlikely to be neutral most of the time. Once again, the point of the matter is that if the spine is not able to maintain itself in an optimal alignment, its owner simply will not ever reach their full performance potential – and all the time they are trying to, they will be leaning ever-closer toward an upcoming episode of low back pain as adaptation-exhaustion approaches.

Kapandji (1974) described how the Delmas index calculates that if the spine has either too much or too little curve, this will disrupt the optimal transfer of load. Of course disruption in this way will result in increased injury risk and decreased performance. Kapandji (1974) also describes the tripod mechanism of the spine, showing how the compressive load of the head, arms and trunk is borne through the vertebral body (and discs) – the major anterior pillar, and through the facets (and facet compartments) – the minor posterior pillars.

Bogduk (1997) and Adams et al (2002) also describe weight-bearing through the spine and indicate that some early research suggested that the zygapophyseal (facet) joints carried approximately 20% of the load of the body and the disc 80%. More recent studies have suggested that the facet joints can bear up to 40% of the applied load, while other research has suggested that, in the lumbar spine at least, the facet surface orientation means that no weight can be borne through these structures (Bogduk 1997). However, the L4–5 and L5–S1 facets – the levels most commonly injured – are orientated in a position to weight-bear. Bogduk (1997) concludes that, for the facet joints to participate in weight-bearing, an aberration in their orientation must occur. A clinical example of just such an aberration may be the lower crossed syndrome.

One further consideration is that Bogduk's (1997) discussion is based on assessment of a static upright spine; however, as Gracovetsky shows, in simple everyday tasks such as walking, the spine naturally migrates between flexed and extended positions (see 'Gait' below).

The hypothetical ratios of weight-bearing at the lumbosacral facet joints correspond to the relative strength of the structures involved in the task. The disc, for example, is extremely strong and can withstand massive compressive stresses (more than the vertebrae themselves), while the size of the facets clearly indicates a significantly smaller role in weight-bearing of the head, arms and trunk – which equate to two-thirds of the body's total weight. This arrangement, therefore, is a good example of load-sharing between the disc and two facets so that there is not too much load on any given structure at any given time. Natural movements, such as the gait cycle, result in a switch of load from front to back and from left to right with every step taken – minimizing the effects of creep and optimizing fluid imbibition (see Gracovetsky 1988, 1997, 2001, 2003).

Evolutionary forces dictate how much strength a specific structure can withstand, and in this case, it is unlikely that the facets can withstand much more than would be expected in a neutral posture – and this is what is observed clinically. It is well documented that those patients with an increased lumbar or cervical lordosis (like Kapandji's dynamic spine) commonly suffer with inflammation, and later, degeneration, of the facet joints. Those whose occupations involve a lot of back or neck flexion or even just a 'flat spine' (like Kapandji's static spine) are candidates for disc injury.

Objections to the neutral spine philosophy

Objections to the neutral spine philosophy include the comment that we do not want to instigate a braced or mummified pain-avoidance behavior. This is true, and is exactly why full range stretches and/or non-axially loaded exercises should be introduced in the subacute phase of back pain rehabilitation. Nevertheless, we still require that the spine is at its strongest in its neutral position where it has the greatest range of movement options.

The neutral spine and martial arts

Most tai chi and Xi gong instructors suggest that failure to tuck the tail and flatten the lumbar spine will block chi flow and reduce strength. This line of enquiry is discussed in Box 9.5.

Box 9.5 The neutral spine and martial arts

In a recent forum Chek (2004a) suggests one should consider the following points regarding the neutral spine in martial arts:

1. The healthy, fully functional human spine has a 30–35° curve in the lumbar, thoracic and cervical spines, all in balance. Since this is the spinal alignment that affords optimal function, and therefore optimal expression of spirit (innate chi) through the body, it's debatable to say that reducing curves even further improves chi flow, particularly when most people will have to struggle by using the muscular system to flatten the curves beyond such a natural spine position if they are not quite supple to begin with. If one must make an exerted effort to reduce curves, then they are reducing blood flow through all the muscles they are exerting because they are now tasked posturally to hold the reduced spinal curves; thus, there will be a *reduction* in chi flow, since one of the primary forms of acquired chi comes through breath primarily and is delivered as paramagnetic energy (positive charge) via the heme of the red blood cells to the tissues of the body, which like water, is diamagnetic (negative charge). Therefore, anything that reduces blood flow reduces chi flow!

2. Chi is all intelligent life force. It knows what to do and where to go. Chi is consciously directed. The mere fact that one is focusing on chi brings it to any point of the awareness. You can easily tell where chi flow is being diminished because the quality of the tissues diminishes first, next they get a disease, and, finally, when you are out of chi, you are dead! Please consider that chi/prana/life-force may all be equated to aspects of the conscious mind, which gives its

commands to the subconscious mind; the subconscious then structures the chi forces in accordance with your commands . . . you are the God of your body and your life! Please read the law below, borrowed from *The Luck Factor* by Brian Tracy (1997), and simply replace the words 'subconscious mind' with 'Chi: the Law of (Chi) Subconscious Activity'.

Whatever thought or goal you hold in your conscious mind will be accepted by your subconscious mind as a command or as an instruction. Your subconscious, the seat of the Law of Attraction, will then go to work to bring into your life the goals you have set for yourself. Your subconscious mind will make all your words and actions (directed chi force!) fit a pattern consistent with your self-concept or your dominant thoughts and ideas about yourself.

3. Tai chi instructors know little at all about spinal mechanics; in fact, in one of the most respected books on the subject, *Warriors of Stillness* (Diepersloot 1997), they actually have the mechanics of breathing backward . . . just like the Pilates teachers often teach it! I have a responsibility to guide people in the public to a safe exposure to chi cultivation. When you consider Gracovetsky's research (2003, 2004) showing that some 76% of the general population has an undiagnosed disc bulge, I prefer the concept of minimizing stress on the spinal column while doing breathing squats because if a disc herniates and presses on a pain sensitive structure, there will be a large leak created in that persons chi bank account!'

Corrective exercise programming

There are many different ways to design an exercise program, some of which have greater efficacy than others per se, and others that fit into the patient's lifestyle better.

There is little doubt, for example, that an appropriately designed corrective stretching, mobilization and exercise program of a duration in the region of 40–50 minutes, completed three to four times a week, will bring about optimal adaptation in the average person. However, we rarely work with an 'average' person and, more importantly, it doesn't matter how good the exercise program is if the patient never does it.

Therefore, in advance of designing an exercise program for a patient, it is important to ascertain what they feel their major obstacles to success may be – time, money or energy. If it is the first or the last, the corrective exercise program must be adapted accordingly. If it is money, then you are literally looking to give the patient the 'biggest bang for their buck' (see 'big bang' exercises below).

The faulty healing model

For those patients who are unable to find time to do their corrective exercises, in reality it is not because they do not have the time, but because they do not prioritize their healing over other activities of daily living. They may fall under the classification of having a *faulty healing model* – reinforced by the tide of public perception regarding what medical care represents. Due to what is now known as the 'orthodox' pharmaceutical model (biomedicine) of health care, most patients seeking medical assistance believe that they are looking for someone (an expert) or something (usually a pill) to fix them. In other words, the onus for healing is placed on the practitioner and the patient abdicates responsibility for getting better. This notion has been cultivated through the common prescription of a pharmaceutical 'magic bullet' where a patient with a dysfunctional lifestyle which has resulted in, for example, a high cholesterol score, can carry on with the exact same lifestyle so long as they take a statin-based drug. Even if this is not the advice of the medical doctor, it is, by and large, the reality of the situation.

The magic bullet approach has its merits, such as the use of a pain killer to break a pain–spasm–pain cycle, or antibiotics for a burns victim, but it also has many flaws. It is, in general, a reactive approach to something which, in most cases, has taken a long time to arise. Similar to the cumulative microtrauma etiology of most musculoskeletal dysfunction described above, a comparable percentage of 'illness' as a whole will be due to cumulative microstresses on the systems of the body – the detoxifications system, the immune system, the cardiovascular system, the nervous system. The belief that a 'magic bullet' is going to fix, for example, the cumulative effects of dysbiosis across many years, which has culminated in constipation, is hardly a fair expectation to be placed on the medication (see discussions in Chapters 1 and 2 on this topic).

With corrective exercise and rehabilitation practices, a similar mechanism can come into play with the patient being quite willing to attend for assessment, diagnosis and exercise coaching, only then to go away and complain 3 or 4 weeks later when they don't feel any better. On being asked about the benefits of the exercise program, the patient may often honestly and somewhat bizarrely report back that they haven't yet started the program. Nevertheless, because money has been paid, an expectation exists that the symptoms should be improving. It is critical therefore to coach the patient regarding the importance of taking responsibility and confirm that this is the intention. Of course, this can be 're-framed' from the idea of taking responsibility – which sounds like a chore – to the fact that the corrective exercise program empowers the individual, so that he or she assumes a sense of being 'in control' of the symptoms and is not so dependent on the practitioner. Psychologically, this empowering approach is far superior and is a truism physically, mentally, emotionally and spiritually, and is inherently naturopathic.

Gravity patterns (see also discussion of gravity influences in Chapter 2)

Gravitational loading also brings with it patterns of biomechanical loading into the leg. Wallden (2008) identified that many hamstring strain injuries (the most common of sports injuries) are likely to be caused by a gravitational strain pattern. See also discussion of various stretching approaches in Chapter 7, and evidence of efficacy in Chapter 10.

In recognizing this mechanism of hamstring injury, Wallden (2008) also identified a number of other tissues that come under cumulative load when the body is stressed. He termed this the 'hamstring syndrome'. See Table 9.8 for further detail.

Corrective stretching (see also discussion of specific modalities in Chapter 7, particularly muscle energy, PNF and associated techniques)

To stretch or not to stretch?

Stretching remains one of the most controversial topics in manual therapy, sports care and sports performance. In almost all cases, stretching is viewed as

Table 9.8 Key injuries and mechanisms associated with 'the hamstring syndrome'

Injury	Mechanism
Lumbar facet impingement (and associated sequelae, e.g. spondylytic change/spondylolisthesis)	Gravity pattern → lumbar extension → impingement of facet joints under load
Lumbar disc injury	Lumbar extension/anterior pelvic tilt → SIJ instability and slackening of iliolumbar ligament → increased shear at LS junction → wear and tear (arthropathy, disc degeneration, spondylolysis/spondylolisthesis) compensatory upregulation of hamstring tone → short/stiff hamstrings (±posterior tilt of pelvis) → ↑ leverage/mobility at lumbar spine to compensate for ↓ hip flexion ROM
Lumbopelvic instability	As above, plus disc injury/degeneration → narrowing of disc space → compromise of local ligamentous support → loss of passive subsystem → dependent on active/neural subsystem → pain inhibits active/neural subsystem → further instability
Sacroiliac joint dysfunction	Gravity pattern → anterior pelvic tilt → relative counternutation of sacrum → loss of form closure while under load → dependence on active and neural subsystems If inner unit/local system shut down, outer unit global system will compensate → hamstring strain
Hip adduction/hypermobility syndrome	Anterior tilt at pelvis → relative flexion of hip → slackens hip ligaments cumulative stress to posterior hip joint capsule → loss of passive support system → dependent on deep/local active support system Pain switches off neural drive (neural system) to deep, local active support system → degenerative change in hip
Meniscal tear	Gravity pattern collapses leg into pronation (osteokinematically associated with anterior pelvic tilt) → medial rotational instability at the femur → rotary stress through menisci (lateral > medial)
Coronary ligament fibrosis	Meniscal rotation resisted by coronary ligaments binding menisci to tibial plateau
Medial collateral ligament strain/tear	Medial rotational instability (see above) results in an adduction moment at the knee every time weight is borne through the unstable leg → repetitive tensile stress to medial collateral
Anterior cruciate ligament (ACL) strain/tear	ACL resists medial rotation and anterior translation of tibia under femur Medial rotational instability places cumulative microtrauma on the ACL of the unstable leg, reducing tensile strength over time (see Fig. 9.9) Pronation pattern is associated with quadriceps dominance (over gluteal group) → ↑ stress to ACL and is associated with ↑ incidence of ACL tear (Elias et al 2003)
Patella tendinopathy	Pronation pattern/lower cross syndrome is associated with quadriceps dominance → ↑ quadriceps recruitment and ↑ load of patella tendon
Patella tracking problems	Medial rotation of the femur under the patella results in a relative lateral positioning of the patella and poor tracking through the femoral intercondylar notch
Osgood–Schlatter's disease	As above, plus ↑ loading of tendon → ↑ traction on developing tibial tuberosity
Chronic compartment syndrome	Pronation through limb → instability at ipsilateral SIJ → ↑ tone through deep longitudinal system (biceps femoris, tibialis anterior, peroneus longus) Pronation into the foot → collapse of medial longitudinal arch → attempt to correct by tibialis anterior → ↑ tonus and traction to/metabolic accumulation in lower leg compartments
Achilles tendinopathy	Pronation at the subtalar joint → traction to medial > lateral Achilles tendon → ↓ tensile strength in medial fibers over time
Inversion sprain	Pronation pattern through lower limb → compensated Trendelenburg → translation of body weight lateral to base of support during weight-bearing gait → ↑ risk of inversion sprain
Heel spur/traction apophysitis	Pronation through medial longitudinal arch of foot → cumulative tensile stress to plantar fascia → stress to their attachment on calcaneus → traction apophysitis
Plantar fasciitis	See above
Hallux valgus/bunion	Pronation → ↑ loading at toe-off through medial aspect of first digit → hallux valgus

a generalized treatment modality with little regard for specifics or individuality. Below is some discussion to help bring some clarity to this complex topic.

Stretching for the sake of stretching

There are certain general benefits to stretching, just as there are to strengthening. However, it should be recognized that most people migrate toward what they are good at, so the average yoga class is full of flexible (usually female) participants who don't really need to be there, while the gym is full of strong (usually male) athletic types, who would benefit more from going to yoga.

Benefits of stretching for stretching's sake

1. Endorphin release (Alter 2004, Elias et al 2003)
2. Increased body awareness (Alter 2004, Vaughn 2003)
3. Aids relaxation/parasympathetic stimulation (Vaughn 2003)
4. Allows 'self' time
5. Increased tissue tolerance to stretch (Alter 2004)
6. Greater range of motion in joints (Alter 2004):
   • May decrease injury risk
   • Should increase ability to generate power

Flaws of stretching for stretching's sake

1. Possible injury/microtrauma (Alter 2004, Lederman 1997, Schleip 2003a)
2. Increased risk of injury (decreased stiffness of active subsystem about joint)
3. Just end up 'looser' but with same muscle imbalance (Chek 2001b)
4. Increased stretch tolerance may leave little margin for error
5. Attracts those with good flexibility – migrate to what you're good at (Chek 2001b)
6. May make muscle less efficient (decreased/later elastic recoil) (Gleim & McHugh 1997, Herbert & Gabriel 2002)
7. Decreased stiffness results in early fatigue and increased injury rate (Hunter 2005)

The logic of stretching

Picture a primitive human – perhaps Australopithecus afarensis – who frequented the plains (and possibly the lakes) of Africa between 3.9 and 3 million years ago. He's out walking looking for berries or for a discarded kill of a big game animal – perhaps an antelope – killed by a big cat. Such scavenging was a common

means of gaining food for our early ill-equipped ancestors (Cordain 2002). However, unfortunately, A. afarensis reaches the kill at the same time as a new hungry big cat that had smelled a waft of the fresh kill on the wind and traced it to the discarded carcass. The clinical and perhaps cynical questions we need to ask are:

1. Does A. afarensis turn and run to the nearest tree and clamber high up in the branches where the big cat is unable to reach?, *or*
2. Does he stop and stretch his hamstrings, then his quadriceps and so on to make sure he doesn't pull a hamstring as he sprints off?

This should paint the picture of how ridiculous the concept of stretching before sports or combative situations really is – assuming a tuned or honed body pre-exists. The question for the naturopath and, moreover, the naturopath's patients, is how to tune the body's length–tension relationships (see 'Biomechanical attractors' below).

However, just because human ancestors wouldn't have stretched in the context described above doesn't mean that either we never stretched or stretching is not useful. It is unlikely, for example, that primitive men and women sat down on a chair-like structure at all, let alone for between 8 and 15 hours per day – like most of their modern-day counterparts do. In the same way that early Homo sapiens wouldn't have carried around a 2-liter bottle of mineral water with them – as we can survive on relatively little water – this does not necessarily 'prove' that to drink relatively little water (or to do no stretching) supports optimal health. We know it does not. (See 'Biomechanical attractors' below for further discussion.)

A meta-analysis of moderate quality stretching studies by Herbert & Gabriel (2002) concluded that neither pre-exercise nor post-exercise stretching provided protection from post-exercise soreness, while stretching before exercise does not provide any practically useful reduction in injury risk.

The flaws of this study were discussed at some length by a panel of experts in the *Journal of Bodywork and Movement Therapies* (7(2):80–96). Nevertheless, this study is not alone in finding some significant problems with generalized stretching as a mainstay of health or performance.

Even Alter (2004), who cites 2100 references in his book *The Science of Flexibility*, is hesitant to discuss the benefits of stretching due to so many contradictory pieces of research.

An important commentary to make here is that if these studies took a homogeneous sample (for example, a sample of patients with upper crossed syndrome) and asked them to perform a given stretch technique to the pectoralis minor, they would almost definitely get a statistically significant result in favor of the stretch's efficacy – at least in the short term. However, if they evaluated a heterogeneous sample, the result would be unremarkable, and if they opted to assess stretching of the middle trapezius or rhomboids in the upper crossed group they would almost definitely conclude that stretching is ineffective – as the muscle is already being held in its outer range and further stretch will disrupt the actin–myosin cross-bridges so the brain will upregulate tone to that muscle to prevent damage. Further, as is described below, there are many influences outside of biomechanical influences that may affect muscle tone.

In addition, as discussed above (see structural length versus functional tone), the homeostatic mechanisms of the body regulate the length–tension relationships of the muscles. A soleus muscle, for example, that is used for 5 hours per week to run and is stretched for three lots of 10 seconds each day, will be influenced more greatly by which of these biomechanical stressors? The answer of course is 'by the running'. In which case, the body will adaptively shorten the soleus as it will always adapt to the imposed demand by trying to enhance the efficiency of the organism. Gleim & McHugh (1997), for example, state that increased stiffness is associated with increased running and walking economy and with increased isometric and concentric force generation. Additionally, they say that muscle energetic output may be manifested most effectively by closely matching muscle stiffness to the frequency of movement in the stretch–shorten cycle. Therefore, by stretching the muscle, the efficiency of its recoil drops.

Similarly, if a muscle is utilized posturally, such as a biceps femoris compensating for poor lumbopelvic inner unit function in sacroiliac joint pain patients (Hungerford et al 2003), it doesn't matter how much that hamstring is stretched until such time as the motor control is returned to the intrinsic muscles of the trunk.

Hopefully this helps to highlight how and why stretching studies may be flawed and how, outside of the context of full biomechanical function – which includes optimal core function and optimal length–tension relationships – the general effect of stretching will always produce mixed results. To be clear, when indicated, when appropriate, stretching can be a valuable approach; however, indiscriminate stretching may be worse than useless, and may actually have a negative effect on function.

Nevertheless, stretching is an important part of maintaining function and so is discussed in greater detail below under 'Biomechanical attractors'.

Reflex profiles

Understanding the reflex profiles that patients may need to train as a component of their job or their sport is an important consideration in exercise program design.

Righting

The righting reflex is utilized when the body moves over a given surface (such as the ground).

Tilting

The tilting reflex is employed when the surface on which the body is supported moves. This is the reflex that we most commonly see engaged when a train starts to pull out of a station, or when we step onto an escalator.

The use of labile surfaces in the training environment, such as use of wobble boards, Swiss balls, disc-sits and shoes – for example, wobble shoes (Janda & Va'Vrova 2005) or the popular Masai barefoot technology shoes (MBTs) – all condition the tilting reflex.

Such conditioning has some level of application to activities of daily living, although this is limited compared to use of the righting reflex. Hence, it is important to consider use of such devices in the light of what specifically the patient is training for.

Aside from conditioning the tilting reflex, the use of labile surfaces can also help to achieve other objectives. Chek (2001b) describes the 'survival reflex' (see below) which is essentially an upregulation of neural drive to the stabilizer system as a result of being placed on a labile surface. Clinically, this technique can be used to 'fire up' a muscle that is lazy, uncon-

---

Box 9.6 Case example

A personal trainer attended for consultation who did every exercise in his training program on a Swiss ball. He squatted on the Swiss ball, lifted dumbbells on the Swiss ball, did cable-based training while kneeling or standing on the Swiss ball, as he saw this as the ultimate level of conditioning. He was consistently injuring himself when he played basketball at a semi-professional level. This was unsurprising to me as he was training himself non-specifically for his sport and was consistently conditioning his tilting reflex while neglecting his righting reflex. Since the ground rarely moves beneath your feet in a game of basketball, this was becoming detrimental to his conditioning. What this athlete needed to do was to increase exercises in his program to condition him for his sport – i.e. those that trained the righting reflex.

ditioned or inhibited. This may be another use for labile surfaces but, in general, most functional environments for activities of daily living and for sports are not labile – therefore overtraining with such methods may prove detrimental to performance.

Motor learning

Motor programs, engrams and central pattern generators

A *motor program* is defined by Schmidt & Wrisberg (2000) as 'a set of pre-structured movement commands, which define and shape the essential details of a skilled action of movement'. A generalized motor program, therefore, may incorporate a series of similar movements that have a high level of correlation and similar relative timing. For example, the back squat is similar to the front squat, which is also similar to the Jefferson squat, which is similar to the sit, which is similar to the jump. All of these would come under the generalized motor program umbrella of 'the squat pattern' (see 'Primal patterns' below).

The term *engram* can be defined as 'a set of motor commands that is prestructured at the executive level and that defines the essential details of a skilled action, analogous to a central pattern generator'.

It is the subtleties of a motor engram which mean that it is easy to locate the distance, angle and magnitude of pressure required to get your car key into the ignition of your own car, but in someone else's car, the task imposes a different level of challenge. It is also the reason that we can recognize the gait pattern of an approaching relative, long before we can recognize the face.

A central pattern generator is a centrally located control mechanism that produces mainly genetically defined, repetitive actions (Schmidt & Wrisberg 2000). Examples may include the stepping reflex of babies, the suckling reflex or prehensile (use of hand-to-mouth) feeding.

A major difference between a motor program and a central pattern generator is the anatomic region from which each is generated: the motor cortex of the brain for the former, and the brainstem or cord for the latter. The phrase 'running around like a headless chicken' is testament to the fact that gait – in chickens at least – is largely generated by a central pattern generator in the cord and not from a motor program in the (now removed) motor cortex.

Schmidt & Wrisberg (2000) explain further, when the central nervous system modifies muscle tone in response to a stimulus, what is known as the *M1 reflex* response occurs with a latency of 30 milliseconds and is generated, therefore, at the cord level. The *M2 reflex* response demonstrates a latency of 50–80 milliseconds and results from an afferent impulse generated in the muscle spindle traveling via the cord to the cerebellum and motor cortex, with a rebound efferent impulse sent back down the cord to activate the muscles. Despite cortical involvement, the M2 reflex is still considered involuntary.

Before the M3 response (true reaction time) is considered, an interim, known as the *triggered reaction*, is considered too fast to be voluntary (80–120 milliseconds) and is colloquially known as the 'wineglass effect'. This triggered reaction is most commonly initiated by cutaneous receptors and can be trained to become enhanced (Schmidt & Wrisberg 2000).

Table 9.9 Response time and the nervous system

Response type	Latency (ms)	Flexibility/ adaptability	Role of instructions	Effect of No. of choices	IU/OU response?	Consciousness/ ontogenetic level	CNS level
M1	30–50	Almost none	None	None	IU	Pre-reflexive	SC
M2	50–80	Low	Some	None?	IU	Pre-/peri-reflexive	SC/BS/(MC)
Triggered reaction	80–120	Moderate	Large	Moderate	IU + OU	Peri-/post-reflexive/ volitional	SC/BS/MC
M3	120–180	High	Very large	Large	IU + OU	Post-reflexive/ volitional	SC/BS/MC

BS, brainstem (note for this purpose, the ancient cerebellum is considered part of the brainstem); IU, inner unit; MC, motor cortex; OU, outer unit; SC, spinal cord.
Adapted from Schmidt & Wrisberg (2000).

Table 9.10 Developmental period, habitat and neuromuscular response

Developmental period	Transition to new habitat	Response dominance	Consciousness	IU/OU learning
Fetal to postnatal life	Permanent orientation: from liquid to gaseous medium; introduction of gravity; permanent orientation to perceptual information in terrestrial environment	M1, M2, [TR]	Preconscious	IU
3–7 months	Mastery of temporary orientations: postural control results in revealing new disequilibria	M1, M2, TR, [M3]	Periconscious	IU [OU]
7–15 months	Oriented locomotion: self-generated activity maps endogenous states onto action-specific information	M1, M2, TR, M3	Conscious	OU/IU

IU, inner unit; OU, outer unit; TR, triggered reaction.
Adapted from Goldfield (1995).

The M3 response is the fourth burst of EMG activity seen on testing reaction time: it is powerful, sustained and results in volitional changes – mobilization of the body.

This understanding provides important information, since it is known that the transversus abdominis and other inner unit (local stability) muscles operate in a feed-forward mechanism both to conscious movement and, more importantly, to perturbation – at least 30 milliseconds in advance of the outer unit counterparts (Richardson et al 1999). This suggests that such inner unit contraction is driven at the cord and/or brainstem level. This has implications in:

1. central sensitization at the cord (see 'Viscerosomatic reflexes' below) from any influence on the motor neuron pool:
   - viscera
   - limbic emotional
   - volitional motor
2. correlations with ontogenetic development
3. choice of rehabilitation techniques/ repercussion of volitional learning (see 'Survival reflex' below).

It has been shown that those with exceptional sporting skills are able to generate an apparent M3 response with far shorter latency than the average 120–180 milliseconds. It may be that these sports people are so rehearsed in the primary motor programs of their sport that they generate a triggered reaction that is so refined that it appears as an M3 response. As Chek (2001b) states: 'Practice does not make perfect, it is perfect practice that makes perfect.' Or put another way: 'Repetition is the mother of skill, so long as there's skill in the repetition.'

In terms of ontogenetic associations with inner unit motor control, Goldfield (1995) suggests that infants follow a course which is based upon transitions to new habitats (see 'Phylontogenetic dimensions' above for more discussion). This ontogenetic course implies that it is only at around the seventh month of postnatal life that the infant becomes oriented enough to generate action-specific movements (Goldfield 1995).

The inference is that until 7 months of age, the child is primarily reacting to their environment in an M1-, M2- and possibly triggered reaction-dominant configuration. From 7 months onwards the M3 response becomes available.

The ramifications of this ontogenetic sequence are that the learning of *cause and effect* is believed to predominate from 6 months of postnatal life onwards (Goldfield 1995). This means that pain patients are not likely to be consciously aware of inner unit function (or how to activate the inner unit) unless they are trained by a skilled practitioner. Patient-directed pain avoidance strategies are therefore only likely to target the outer unit musculature.

Lee (2003) suggests that in teaching motor relearning skills to patients, 'imagination/feeling' words should be used, rather than 'doing' commands. For example:

- *Feeling*: Imagine a laser beam between your navel and your spine, and now imagine that it is becoming charged with energy.
- *Doing*: Draw your navel towards your spine.

Because *doing* commands require volitional action – movement, they are somewhat dissociated from, and perhaps inappropriate for, retraining inner unit function. *Feeling* commands are therefore likely to be more effective, as they do not require the patient to 'move'.

Isolation vs integration

There is some debate in the literature over when, or indeed whether, to isolate individual muscle groups in rehabilitation (Comerford & Mottram 2001, Richardson et al 1999). Bobath is famously accredited with stating 'the body knows nothing of muscles, only of movements' (Edwards 2000) – and this certainly contains much merit in the field of rehabilitation. However, there are also given instances where a patient may be caught in a vicious cycle where it is initially impossible to correctly sequence the muscle contraction in a functional movement pattern (see examples below). It is in such a circumstance that isolation is fully warranted.

There are also arguments that to activate a given muscle does not necessarily mean that the targeted muscle will be activated any better in a functional environment (see examples below).

Example 1: Where isolation is useful

A patient presents with low back pain which you diagnose as sacroiliac joint (SIJ) dysfunction secondary to poor lumbopelvic motor control. We now have what might be termed a 'double whammy': the poor lumbopelvic motor control is what has likely caused the repetitive irritation at the SIJ, but now the pain is further inhibiting the muscles we need to activate in order to stabilize the segment. Since the patient is a construction worker he needs to keep working in order to pay for your treatment program, but cannot rest his back as a result. The worker needs to learn how to effectively perform a bend pattern to minimize stress on the already hypermobile joint; based on Bobath's comment, therefore, he needs to simply be taught hip–back dissociation and his lumbopelvic motor control should return.

The problem with this oversimplification is that axial load creates pain in the construction worker's SIJ, so he is unable to activate his transversus abdominis, multifidus and other inner unit muscles as he bends forwards. This means that a purely integrated movement-based approach would be completely ineffective for this worker and he would become disillusioned with the lack of results and seek a new practitioner to help him survive his environment.

Despite the shortfalls of an isolated approach, this is exactly the situation where isolation can pay dividends. As we know that the law of facilitation states that the more an impulse traverses a given neural pathway the resistance to that impulse will decrease, purely by doing isolation work we may enhance the multifidus action in more integrated movements. These muscles need to be worked, as by merely hypertrophying the multifidus and increasing tone in the transversus abdominis the construction worker will increase the stability of the SIJ. Bobath's point is that this really does not teach the construction worker how to use his body and this is where many practitioners only do half the job. The critical step that is often forgotten is to teach the patient how to sequence firing of the inner unit to provide support before they activate their outer unit musculature. This sequence can be analyzed in naturopathic terms to be dealing with causation and teaching prevention.

See below ('Ascending and descending exercises') to understand how to rehabilitate the construction worker appropriately without re-injuring him.

Example 2

Sahrmann (2005) describes a research trial in which the push-up with a plus (where movement at the top of the push-up is exaggerated to fully protract the shoulders – often prescribed to condition serratus anterior) was used to help patients with a winging scapulohumeral rhythm. Although the push-up with a plus activated and trained the serratus anterior (Ludewig et al 2004), it did not change the lack of recruitment during glenohumeral abduction – the scapulohumeral rhythm remained impaired. This occurred because simply increasing the strength of a muscle does not mean that it will be recruited in a new motor pattern or engram. The newfound strength must be consciously activated in the new motor pattern.

However, like most arguments, this one has two sides, and the answer probably lies somewhere in the middle ground. By activating a targeted muscle (in the case above, the serratus anterior), the facilitation of the efferent pathways will result in an easier (or facilitated) learning process when working on re-patterning muscle sequencing – in this scenario, in overhead work. This is a case where strengthening or facilitation on its own will not change the way the patient moves, but where it will aid the process of relearning old, lost or undeveloped motor skills.

As a practitioner, one should not forget that (as described above under 'Muscle imbalance physiology') a facilitated muscle may draw the neural drive away from an antagonistic muscle, thereby inhibiting it. In this instance, commonly the serratus anterior may be inhibited by excessive neural drive to (which

Table 9.11 Mottram/Comerford model of rehabilitation methods

Structured	Non-structured
Specific	Non-specific

Table 9.12 Examples of structure and specificity (or lack thereof) in corrective exercise prescription

Exercise example	Classification
Walking tall	Non-structured, non-specific
Walking tall, countdown timer	Structured, non-specific
Transversus activation, red dot	Non-structured, specific
Transversus activation, prone cuff	Structured, specific

can include myofascial trigger points in) the pectoralis minor.

Program design

Comerford & Mottram (2001) provide a description of differing rehabilitation approaches in Table 9.11. They observe that some patients perform better with a structured rehabilitation program, while for others this seems antagonistic to their progression. It is likely that a classic *type A personality* or a patient who exhibits dominant left-brain characteristics will perform better with a structured program, whereas those who are *type B* or have more of right-brain dominance may react better to a non-structured program. Structured program design is described in some detail below.

Examples of non-structured programs include the use of 'red dot therapy', where a red sticker is placed on a number of commonly used household or work appliances – such as the kettle, the computer, the toothbrush, the mirror, the phone. Every time the patient sees the red dot in their environment, it acts as a reminder to 'engage their transversus' or to 'enhance their postural awareness' – whatever the objective of the program is. For patients who spend a lot of time in the car or other road vehicles as part of their job, a similar strategy can be deployed where every time they spot (for example) a red car, they do a check to see if their posture is optimal, or the transversus is switched on – whatever the corrective focus is. The telephone ringing in the office or home environment can provide another unstructured cue to review posture or perform an exercise or stretch. Chek (1999a) also describes a similar approach in which a digital watch with a count-down timer is purchased and set to go off every 15 minutes. This can be a convenient alternative to a more formal structured program and, indeed, can be used in conjunction with a formal program.

A specific program of rehabilitation will target relevant muscle groups or movement patterns (for example, a prone cobra to help correct an upper crossed syndrome) whereas a non-specific program will just focus on more global goals (e.g. asking a patient with an upper crossed syndrome to walk tall, as if suspended from the crown of their head with a puppet string).

Structured program writing

Most patients, once they understand the importance of taking responsibility for their condition and prioritizing their own health, will find a structured program more motivating. There is an entire science (and art) to writing an effective corrective exercise program which is too broad to cover here, but some key general guidelines are given below.

Program design considerations

- Reps (number of repetitions of a given exercise)
- Sets (number of times you perform a given number of reps, with an interspacing rest)
- Loads (e.g. bodyweight, or a certain amount of weight of a barbell, a dumbbell, a medicine ball, etc.)
- Tempo (the amount of time under load – measured in seconds)
- Rest periods (the duration of rest between sets)
- Periodization (timetabling the program within a given time period – e.g. a week, a month, a season, etc.)
- Sequencing (the order in which the exercises should be performed – usually a safety consideration)

Depending on the adaptation targeted, based on clinical findings, different loading parameters should be applied to the patient's tissues. If it's hypertrophy that's required, then a completely different repetition (rep) range, set range, load and rest period is needed than if building endurance or power was the objective.

For example, javelin throwers (described under 'Biomechanical attractors, Chunking' section below) require the lunge, the twist and the push patterns ('chunks') to train their movement pattern. In a functional, symptom-free elite level thrower, there would be little point in training the lunge pattern for, say three sets of 20 reps at a slow tempo, as this would train predominantly the slow twitch fibers. In essence, what you would be doing is slowing down their performance speed, thereby impeding their throwing performance!

Since competitively throwing a javelin only ever entails one explosive event followed by several minutes' rest, javelin throwers need to condition themselves using power-based training variables. In other words, they would need to lunge with the maximum load they can safely train with (maintaining good form), performing four repetitions per set before fatigue, and complete between 6 and 10 sets (Poliquin 2006a).

To those inexperienced in training techniques and terminology, what this equates to is loading the athlete with a load that they can only lunge with between one and four times before they are fully fatigued – *not* using the same load that they can lunge with 20 times, but only do between one and four reps! In such an instance, the load is usually a barbell, though it could be dumbbells or other loading apparatus.

It may seem that this information is moving outside of the realm of the therapist and more into the realm of the strength and conditioning coach. However, consider the javelin thrower who is suffering with low back pain but has a major competition coming up in 3 months' time. Now we have someone who requires the skills of both a therapist and a strength and conditioning coach and, most importantly, these two professionals need to be speaking each other's language.

In this instance, the (right-handed) thrower may be experiencing pain in the right L5–S1 facet joint due the repetitive and cumulative impact through that structure from training – as the right foot is driven into the ground to generate a ground reaction force through the leg and into the spine, de-rotating the spine into left rotation and driving the upper limb girdle (including the right arm) into left axial rotation and a terminal push (throw) with the right arm. *Note*: This is the mechanism via which fast bowlers in cricket and many gymnasts develop spondylolysis and subsequent spondylolisthesis as they are trying to reclaim as much of the ground reaction force as possible to throw an object, or themselves, into the air with speed and power.

So to tell this javelin thrower to load the facet still further through power training with a barbell on the back is clearly not appropriate advice. What may be more appropriate for the thrower are the following guidelines.

Can the javelin thrower activate the deep abdominal wall and/or multifidus:

1. during a javelin throw?
   - [No – this is why there is pain]
2. in an ipsilateral loaded lunge?
   - [No – this creates too much load through the inflamed facet]
3. in a contralateral loaded lunge?
   - [No – this creates too much load through the inflamed facet]
4. in an ipsilateral unloaded lunge?
   - [No – this creates too much load through the inflamed facet]
5. in an unloaded contralateral lunge?
   - [Yes! This is the first time both multifidus and transversus appear to activate effectively in a *primal pattern* mimicking the javelin throw]
6. in an ipsilateral static lunge?
   - [No – this still seems to irritate the inflamed facet]
7. in an ipsilateral seated lunge (backside on Swiss ball)?
   - [Nearly – but not consistently]
8. in a ipsilateral seated lunge (backside on bench)?
   - [Yes!]

Thus, this athlete can activate the abdominal wall and multifidus in an unloaded contralateral lunge (i.e. on to the 'non-throwing' leg) and could activate only in a seated lunge (backside on bench) on the throwing leg. This allows us to evaluate exactly the point at which this athlete's rehabilitation program should commence – and what the next progression might be.

Ascending and descending exercises

The list above is an example of how the lunge may be *descended* from the lunge associated with a power event – the javelin throw. Any of the *primal patterns* (see below under 'Biomechanical attractors') or movement 'chunks' of a given motor skill can be either descended or ascended.

Examples of how the lunge may be ascended are as follows:

- *Loading* – as described above. Most commonly this might take the form of a barbell resting across the back. However, to ascend this further (and place more load on the thoracic erectors rather than the lumbar erectors), the barbell may be rested on the sternum. The next level of ascent might be to use dumbbells instead of a barbell – this requires control of two separate weights rather than one. Holding the chosen weight (barbell or dumbbell) in a full shoulder press position is a further level of neurological and core strength challenge. Finally, making the load asymmetrical – holding a dumbbell or, more challenging, the barbell in one hand is, again, a tougher motor challenge.

- *Dynamic loading*. To ascend the loading options described above, the client may perform a walking lunge as an ascent. A higher challenge would be to do a backward walking lunge, while a further challenge might be to perform a ballistic alternating lunge.

The range of ascents is only really limited by the imagination of the rehabilitation and movement specialist.

For the symptomatic javelin thrower, the twist and the push patterns (with appropriate descents) would also be assessed to see where the training program could begin with respect to these patterns.

As an aside, training on the side that is asymptomatic will have a training effect (predominantly neurotrophic) on the symptomatic side. This phenomenon is known as 'well-limb training'.

In addition, since the athlete requires a swift resolution to the pain, we would use other descended exercises to condition the key stabilization muscles of the lumbosacral region. For example, we may use a four-point exercise to condition the transversus, while we may use a prone or side-lying exercise to condition the multifidus.

What are we looking for?

- *Abdomen (transversus)*: Since, in the lunge and in the javelin throw in general, the trunk must rotate to generate force, we are not looking for the kind of bracing described by McGill (2002) and Siff (2003); instead we are looking for an abdominal hollowing to allow for both stability and mobility (see 'Inner unit' above). We should see a uniform hollowing throughout the abdominal wall as the athlete approaches heel strike with each step of the run up, and particularly at the strike of the right heel just before release of the javelin. A lack of hollowing, and/or hollowing of just part of the abdominal wall, is a failed assessment. With experience this can be seen at full speed –

though in the first instance video can usefully be used to watch the entire movement pattern in slow motion, repetitively, without further stressing the athlete. This information can be similarly applied to any patient in a simple walking gait analysis – a movement pattern (and therefore stressor) that is repeated 3000 times per day – even for very low activity people.

- *Back (multifidus)*: We should see minimal scoliosis, good pelvic control (i.e. no Trendelenburg[4]) and, specifically, no striations through the lumbar erector mass. Striations are a sign that the multifidus at the level of the striation is being overly recruited to try to prevent shear at that level. This is dysfunctional and a sign of segmental instability. Again this refers to all assessments – not just the lunge in the example of the javelin thrower.

Once assessment has identified the movement patterns and planes of motion in which the body needs to develop strength, a program of exercises, sequenced effectively, can be designed. Depending on the training objectives and the symptom profile of the patient, the exercise and training variables must be adjusted to meet the required objective (see Table 9.13).

If a patient were training for postural adaptation, leaving a 3-minute rest period between each set of exercises, this will allow the Type 1 postural fibers to have fully recovered well before exercise recommences. This means that the desired training effect – postural correction – is at best flawed and at worst, negated. In contrast, if an athlete is training for power with a heavy set of squats, but feels that he/she recovered from the previous set within 90 seconds, he/she may decide to commence the second set of squats at the same intensity. Unfortunately, their Type 2b fast glycolytic (explosive) muscle fibers will not recover until 3–5 minutes after the first set. This means that the Type 2a fast oxidative fibers will be recruited, with the result that it's not the explosive Type 2b fast glycolytic fibers that are being conditioned. The training in this instance would actually make the athlete

---

[4]A Trendelenburg sign indicates weakness, inhibition or paralysis of the gluteus medius of the weight-bearing leg. Typically, what is seen clinically is a drop of the opposite side of the pelvis below the horizontal (e.g. from one iliac crest to the other). In gait, a Trendelenburg sign is classically observed as a tail-wag – often volitionally accentuated in catwalk models. A compensated Trendelenburg may also occur where, rather than letting the pelvis drop, the patient leans their body (in the frontal plane) over the leg of the weak gluteus medius during weight-bearing.

Box 9.7 Testing for segmental instability

The skilled examiner may simply be able to pick out levels of segmental instabilities – most commonly as pivot points in the spine during active ranges of motion. However, commonly such segments are not easy to locate – or may not be apparent until the spine is under some level of load. The stick test allows the examiner to apply graduated load to the patient's spine and observe for dysfunction in a more controlled manner than, for example, loading the spine with a barbell. It also allows for assessment within the neutral zone, thereby minimizing risk of injury.

The stick test

Use a wooden dowel rod (or equivalent) and ask the patient to take hold of it firmly with both hands and hold it up in front of them – shoulders flexed to 90°. The patient should be stood with their back to a mirror, with the examiner looking over their shoulder to observe the response of their back in the mirror.

Explain to the patient that you are about to move the stick in various directions and that this process will start with light pressure, but the intensity of the movements will gradually increase. The objective for the patient is to not allow the stick to move.

Start by lifting up the stick in the sagittal plane (flexion-extension of the shoulder joint) and observe for striations in the patient's back. If striations are noted, the side, the spinal level, and the severity of the striation should be noted (usually with a subjective descriptor such as 'mild', 'moderate' or 'severe').

Next, try to push the patient into lateral flexion using the stick – this is testing for frontal plane stability. Again striations should be noted.

Finally, try to rotate the patient via the stick – thereby assessing transverse plane stability.

Combinations of the above motions and sudden changes in force provide a more functional assessment of the patient's ability to maintain functional stability in the lumbopelvic region.

The only difference between stick training (Fig. 9.14) and the stick test is that neither the neutralizer biofeedback device, nor any other means of feedback, would be utilized during assessment.

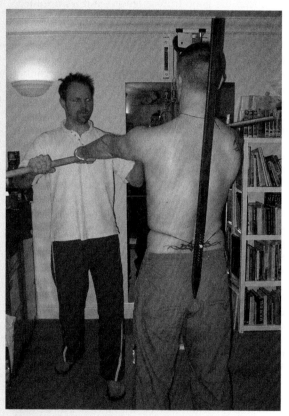

Figure 9.14 Training strength in the neutral spine position

Table 9.13 Acute exercise variables in program design

Rep range	Physiological effect	Usual set range	Usual rest period (minutes)
1–8	Power (strength) training	4–8+	3–5
8–12	Strength (hypertrophy) training	3–5	1.5–2.5
12–20	Strength-endurance	2–4	<1

Adapted from Baechle & Earle (2000), Chek (1995) and Spring et al (1991).

become slower! This is a common outcome for those who use weight training without truly understanding subtleties of the physiological adaptation they are targeting. A more common clinical example may the chronic back pain patient who needs to retrain their multifidus. Since a part of the means by which the lumbar multifidus stabilizes the lumbar spine and sacrum is through the hydraulic amplifier mechanism (Chek 2002, Lee 2004), this system requires that the multifidus has good trophic levels – if it is atrophied, the mechanism is ineffective. In this case, the multifidus first needs to be consciously activated through isolation training, and then integrated into functional loads. At this stage, loads that are designed to hypertrophy the muscle (in the 8–12 rep maximum range) must be prescribed for efficient restoration of function.

Note: Contraindications to such loading would include pain, any sign of inner unit dysfunction (such as abdominal bloating or striations at the spine), lack of proper conditioning and instructing on technique.

Tempo

A further loading parameter not discussed in Box 9.7 is 'tempo'. Tempo allows the clinician and the patient to know how much time under tension the muscle(s) is receiving. It can also be used to stress different parts of the exercise.

For example, the supine hip extension (with back on Swiss ball) exercise is particularly useful for focusing load onto the hip extensors and specifically the gluteus maximus. It is therefore an ideal exercise to help to correct a quadriceps dominant pattern, commonly associated with ACL injury and other sports injuries (Wallden 2007). It is also an excellent exercise to help correct a lower crossed syndrome, and can be used to retrain proper knee tracking (see Table 9.18). The supine hip extension exercise with the back on a Swiss ball is a descent of the squat pattern – so may also be used to help pain patients who are unable to complete a full weight-bearing squat with axial loading.

Therefore, if a patient presents with a quadriceps dominant pattern in the lunge assessment (when the knee tracks beyond the end of the foot), or poor knee tracking, yet has a layered syndrome posture, there is a conflict of interests, as one of the best exercises for correction of either of these kinematic problems is the supine hip extension, which focuses loading into the already shortened/facilitated gluteals. How can this be the case? The answer is that it is all down to the tempo of the movement, and therefore whether the targeted muscle group is being worked in its inner or its outer range – and for how long – to create adaptation.

In the example given above, the same exercise has been used to induce a different postural effect, while achieving similar performance goals. The supine hip extension with 2–2–6 tempo means that the patient is working their gluteus maximus for 10 seconds for each repetition, but for 6 seconds in its inner range and for 4 seconds in its outer range. This exercise is useful to correct a patient with a lower crossed postural pattern. The supine hip extension with the 4-4-2 tempo works the gluteus maximus for 10 seconds per repetition, yet in this instance, the muscle is being worked for 8 seconds in its outer range and only 2 seconds in its inner range. This tempo makes this version of the supine hip extension perfect for someone with a layered or sway muscle imbalance, as it trains the gluteus maximus to be strong in a lengthened position, or outer range.

Sequencing the client's rehabilitation program

Certain exercises are more demanding than others and, potentially therefore, carry a greater risk to the exerciser.

For example, if a patient with back pain were to perform a series of exercises to fatigue the abdominal wall, multifidus and gluteus medius, then is asked to squat carrying a heavy load, he/she would essentially be squatting on a 'naked' spine – as all the key stabilizers will have just been exhausted.

Equally, if a program is designed to target the (long/weak/inhibited) hip extensors of a patient with lower crossed syndrome, there is no point in doing this exercise until such time as the hip flexors have been stretched.

If the client does not stretch first, the hip extensors may only be worked in the outer range (rather than in the critical inner range where strength needs to be developed). Additionally, a facilitated psoas will reciprocally inhibit its antagonist (Korr 1978) – the gluteus maximus – and therefore compromise the neural drive to the target tissue before exercise has even commenced.

Consequently, to design a corrective program for athlete or non-athlete alike, there is a set of basic principles to be followed:

1. Stretch before strengthening (to inhibit facilitated muscles, optimize length–tension relationships and optimize axis of rotation of joint)
2. Exercise order should follow from most neurologically challenging to least neurologically challenging:

- Go from most complex (e.g. reverse standing cable woodchop) to least complex (e.g. lower Russian twist)
- Go from most loaded (e.g. heavy deadlift) to most unloaded (e.g. standing tummy vacuum)
- Go from axial loading (e.g. standing) to non-axial loading (e.g. lying)
- Go from smallest base of support (e.g. single leg squat) to largest base of support (e.g. prone transversus abdominis activation)
- From labile surfaces (e.g. Swiss ball or balance board) to non-labile surfaces (the floor)
- From uncontrolled environment (competitive sports)[5] to controlled environment (the gym)
- From dynamic to static.

For further description of these exercises, see Chek (1999b, 2003a).

Example programs (see also examples of various exercise-related interventions in relation to musculoskeletal pain in Chapter 10)

Disc pain patient[6] with upper crossed syndrome

1. Corrective stretching program:
   - McKenzie extension push-up
   - → Tape the lumbar spine into neutral lordosis
   - Foam roller longitudinal mobilization (with towel support)
   - Foam roller transverse mobilization
   - Swiss ball rectus abdominis stretch

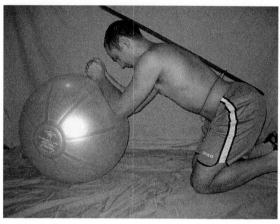

Figure 9.15 Forward ball roll exercise with biofeedback device

2. Corrective exercise program:
   - Body-weight squat (taped)
   - Forward ball roll (see Fig. 9.15)
   - Prone pelvic anterior tilt
   - Alternating superman
   - Four-point TVA

Comment: Based on the McKenzie disc derangement classification system (McKenzie 2003), a derangement 1 is described as a minor posterior displacement of the nucleus, with occasional buttock or thigh pain. There is no antalgic posture and this low-level disc derangement usually responds well to the McKenzie extension principle with corrective exercise.

Spondylolisthesis (stable, grade I) patient with lower crossed syndrome

1. Corrective stretching program:
   - Lumbar erector stretch
   - Hip flexor stretch (with gluteal activation)
   - TFL foam roller
2. Corrective exercise program:
   - Front squat
   - Supine hip extension (back on ball)
   - Horse stance vertical
   - Lower abdominal 1
   - Prone TVA activation

Comment: A spondylolisthesis is an anterior slippage of (usually) L5 on S1 – but may occur at any level of the spine. There are a number of mechanisms that may contribute to the slippage. A grade I slippage

---

[5]Many people without experience in the field of conditioning and rehabilitation believe that there is some magical danger that creeps into the equation when weights or other gym equipment, such as Swiss balls, are utilized. For example, many exercise physiology texts caution against children lifting any kind of weight until their bones have begun to fuse (usually 16 yoa+). However, this defies common sense when one considers that even during simple sprinting the child is translating up to seven times their bodyweight through one leg! Additionally, this is usually done in an unsupervised manner and most commonly in an uncontrolled environment – such as the playground – where competitors are actually trying to tackle them. Compare this with a controlled supervised environment in the gym where even lifting their own bodyweight through two legs (i.e. 14 times less load than sprinting) would be considered dangerous! This may be a case of dogmatic belief overshadowing common sense. Baechle & Earle (2000) agree that there is no lower age limit when resistance training may commence.

[6]Assuming the diagnosis is a McKenzie derangement – one (mild) disc bulge (McKenzie 2003).

indicates that the vertebra has slipped between 1 and 25% forwards. Stability of the slippage may depend on a number of factors, including, but not limited to, pain, local muscle function and dynamic imaging.

Biomechanical attractors

What is a biomechanical attractor? Well, the term *attractor* is derived from systems theory. An attractor, as described by O'Connor & McDermott (1997), is a stable, reproducible state. So, for example, the planets orbiting the sun are in an attractor state with the sun. This attractor state provides a level of stability and predictability within our macro environment – our solar system. Complex systems seem to want to revert to some kind of stable state. In chaos theory, order tends to arise from the chaos, and it is this order that is deemed a self-organizing attractor.

In the preface to their book *Signs of Life – How Complexity Pervades Biology*, Sole & Goodwin (2000) state that:

New sciences combine biology with physics in a manner that allows us to see the creative fabric of natural processes as a single dynamic unfolding. The consistent theme . . . that runs through new sciences is the understanding of biological processes in terms of complex dynamics from which emerge characteristic patterns of order.

This emergence of order from chaos eloquently describes exactly what comprises a biomechanical attractor. Goldfield's (1995) definitions of the features of an attractor (Box 9.8) will gain clarity as the discussion of biomechanical attractors unfolds below.

Box 9.8 Features of an attractor (Goldfield 1995)

1. An attractor is a region of state space (the set of all states that may be reached by a system, together with the paths for doing so) where trajectories come to rest.
2. An attractor can be a point, cycle or area of state space.
3. A physical system can have one or more attractors, and it is the number and layout of these attractors that influence the system.
4. Each attractor exerts a force on the system by means of a potential difference. The trajectory followed by the system is determined by the net sum of the forces exerted by the various attractors.
5. The configuration of attractors has a critical influence on the behavior of the system. A change in the layout of attractors leads to new competition between attractors and results in a shift to different modes.

A more human example of an attractor state might be an engram (see above for definition). For example, if an elite tennis player were to be asked to serve a tennis ball while blindfolded, they would probably have a significant success rate in: (1) hitting the ball; (2) getting it over the net; and (3) getting it to land in the service box. If a casual player were asked to perform the same task, their success would be significantly less. And if someone who has never before used a tennis racket was asked to perform the given task, the result would be almost zero serves hitting the service box. This is because the serve pattern has been so engrained in the professional tennis player that they literally can *do it with their eyes closed*. Their serving ability is so stable that even when deliberately impaired by negating them of their primary feedback tool, they are able to perform the technique with good reliability. This might be termed an *attractor state*.

Looking more to how these attractor states may have relevance to the naturopath, it must be considered how, and which, attractor states arose within the chaos of human behavior. Such attractor states will provide clues as to how the human organism has evolved to function and therefore where dysfunctional habits outside of Homo sapiens' developmental habitat may be causing biomechanical disruption. To do this requires some idea of the environment in which Homo sapiens (and his/her ancestors) developed.

Of course, knowing Homo sapiens exact developmental environment poses some level of challenge. The aquatic ape hypothesis (Attenborough 2002, Morgan 2001) is one example of how the environment may have impacted on our biomechanical evolution. Morgan's (2001) hypothesis proposes a raft of physiological rationale for how and why at some stage in our evolution we likely took to the water as our main habitat. This suggestion offers an explanation for the extraordinary leap from tetrapedalism to fully adapted, habitual bipedalism, based on the idea that our ancestors spent much of their time wading. Wading, of course, both supports some of the body weight, as well as providing resistance to the axial rotation of the body during gait – as described above under 'Phylontogenetic dimensions'.

So, what can be known for sure about the environment in which Homo sapiens' ancestors developed?

Biomechanical universality

The single biggest physical stressor on the human body is gravity. Gravity is relentless, stressing our musculoskeletal frame 24 hours a day, every day of our life (Kuchera 1997, Lee 2005).

What can be known, therefore, is that no matter where in the world our ancestors evolved, gravity was exerting itself in exactly the same way with exactly the same magnitude.[7]

Additionally, it is known that the primary surfaces from which our ancestors generated their resistance to gravity were flat or 'planar' surfaces (Cranz 2000). Humans did not evolve, for example, in a chair with lumbar support and arm rests wearing a pair of shoes with arch supports. This is why relatively narrow reference ranges in goniometric assessment of human biomechanics can be handed some level of face validity.

The following two factors:

- constant gravitational stress at 1 G (or 9.8 meters per second squared)
- resistance from planar surfaces (Cranz 2000)

provide a foundation to work with in terms of the *attractor states* that molded our biomechanical design.

Such biomechanical universality is in stark contrast to human biochemical heredity which was entirely dependent on foodstuffs available in the local environment. Of course, these factors which drive biochemical requirements are about as diverse as they could be, resulting in the well-established and very naturopathic phenomenon of biochemical individuality (Williams 1956, 1988). Hence, nutrient reference ranges have far less validity than joint range of motion reference ranges, for example.

With the combination of biomechanical universality (relatively undifferentiated physical challenges) and the organizing principle of attractor states, we are able to understand a great deal more about how the human frame was designed by nature to function. Beach (personal communication, 2003) recognized that his concept of archetypal rest postures (see below) could be classified as attractor states as they are stable states to which the human organism returns consistently after the relative chaos of daily movement. The concept of instinctive sleep postures as attractors, and primal patterns as dynamic attractors, also holds true.

Biomechanical attractors are to biomechanical health what the macronutrients are to biochemical health:

- Instinctive sleep postures   = Protein
- Archetypal rest postures   = Fats
- Primal patterns   = Carbohydrate

The correct balance of these 'staples' results in a natural homeostatic 'tuning' of the body. Just as too much carbohydrate in the biochemical environment pushes the glycemic level outside of its functional physiological range, so too much of one posture, or one exercise pattern, will push the biomechanical environment outside its functional physiological range. In biochemistry, there is insulin to compensate for this scenario; in biomechanics there are type II mechanoreceptors to compensate by inducing outer unit muscle spasm or contraction in an attempt to stabilize the area. The endpoint of this biochemical instability may be diabetes mellitus, while the endpoint of this biomechanical instability may be the laying down of osteophytes in a last ditch attempt to stabilize the unstable joint.

An imbalance or omission of one of the staples rapidly results in biomechanical imbalance and, across time, dysfunction.

Instinctive sleep postures (see in particular sections in Chapter 10 on fatigue and fibromyalgia)

Before the topics of sleep and rest postures are embraced, a key concept to acknowledge is that there is no such thing as a true position of rest. No matter what position the body is in, there is stress on certain parts more than others. In supine lying, for example, the sacrum counternutates with respect to the innominate, meaning that more stress is placed on the long dorsal sacroiliac ligament while less stress is placed on the sacrotuberous ligament (Lee 2005). Instead, a continuum from very little movement to a lot of movement is a better, more accurate way to view the body. In life, there is always movement; it's just the amplitude that varies.

Instinctive sleep postures is a concept described by Tetley (2000), a British physiotherapist, based on his observations of native cultures and ape behavior in the jungles of Uganda. Tetley suggests that sleep is nature's intrinsic manipulator, with a variety of postures helping to maintain function of a variety of joints.

Tetley (2000) identifies three primary instinctive sleep postures:

1. side-lying, with arm as pillow
2. prone with head rotation ('the lookout posture')
3. quadrupedal lying (prone with torso twist).

---

[7]It is noted that there are very slight differences in gravity based on how far the person is from the Earth's center and how much mass is underneath the individual. These differences are, however, miniscule in comparison with the influencing effects of biochemical diversity.

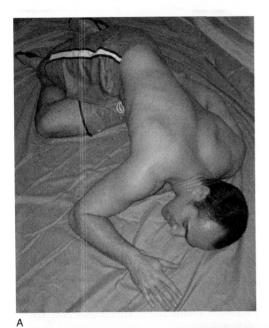

A

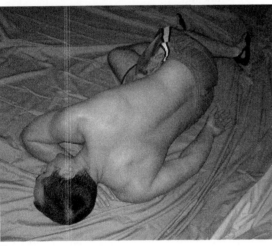

B

Figure 9.16 **A, B** Tetley's instinctive sleep postures

Tetley (2000) also describes a fully flexed kneeling posture (comparable to Sarhmann's (2002) full quadruped kneel) used by Tibetan caravaneers and sometimes called the child pose, and other rest postures such as the full squat and upright kneel.

Since around one-third of a human's life is spent sleeping, both the postures in which one sleeps and the surface on which one sleeps will, without question, impact significantly on biomechanical function. In the natural world it could be argued that sleep (and the position in which sleep occurs) is the single biggest

factor affecting the musculoskeletal system. These are true biomechanical attractor states; states that are returned to day after day and help to 're-set' biomechanical length–tension relationships.

In modern culture, significant resources are invested in finding a soft 'comfortable' bed that perhaps is 'orthopedic', with an 'orthopedic' pillow to help create a good night's sleep.

At first glance, this may seem like an excellent idea. Yet, if the major biomechanical stressors in modern society are considered, time and again the major stressor to the human frame is sitting and, specifically, Western seated posture (WSP). The topic of WSP is discussed further under the heading 'Archetypal rest postures' below but, suffice to say, the specific adaptation to the demand WSP imposes on the human frame is an upper crossed syndrome and, usually, a layered syndrome.

The relevance of the hugely prevalent upper crossed syndrome to this discussion of sleep postures is that the vast majority of patients attending a naturopathic clinic will have a forward head posture and flexed thoracic spine (specifically, the CT junction) and a flattened lumbar curve. In most cases, such patients will be unable to extend their thoracic curve fully (a functional range of motion) due to contracture of the described muscles, of the anterior longitudinal ligament and other connective tissue changes associated with fixed postural holds.

For someone with a chronic and/or fixed upper crossed syndrome to sleep supine comfortably (because they are unable to extend their CT junction) requires a pillow. *Note*: Some patients have a 'lazy' upper crossed syndrome where an upper crossed posture may simply reflect lazy postural habits, although the flexibility to be able to return to neutral has been maintained. In most patients who have had an upper crossed syndrome for a prolonged period of time (which is *most* patients), connective tissue and even bony remodeling will not allow for a reversal of pathological posture, unless significant and sustained corrective exercise, stretches and mobilizations are performed.

To sleep comfortably in a side-lying position in nature, requires a full range of flexion/abduction at the glenohumeral (GH) joint to support the head with a cushioning arm. Since to flex/abduct the arm beyond 140° requires thoracic extension (to use the arm as a pillow requires more than 140° flexion), someone with an upper crossed syndrome will either require a pillow, or will stress the anterior capsule of their GH joint or create impingement of a subacromial structure, in order to achieve this posture.

Sahrmann (2002, 2005) explains that full-range flexion or abduction of the shoulder should result in the lateral border of the scapula being pulled no more than 1 cm beyond the mid-axillary line. If the scapula does migrate further than 1 cm anterior to the mid-axillary line, this is an indication of teres major shortness or stiffness. In this example we can see that side-lying with the arm raised up as a pillow helps to maintain a functional length–tension relationship between the scapulothoracic muscles and the scapulohumeral group. This is an example of a stable state to which the body returns naturally, in order to maintain function – an *attractor state*.

Sleeping prone – something that is commonly frowned upon in 'manual therapy' groups – is something that is commonly seen in our primate cousins and in indigenous human populations (Anderson 2000, Tetley 2000). In fact, all great apes lie down to sleep and predominantly in the prone position or on their side – sleeping supine is extremely rare except in ground-nesting mountain gorillas who have little or no threat of predation (Anderson 2000). This strategy may reflect a number of benefits.

Prone

1. Decreased exposure of soft underbelly.
2. Vulnerable flexor creases are less exposed.
3. Virtually no risk of snoring when prone.
4. Rib compression may result in:
   - mobilization/synovial fluid imbibition of the costovertebral and costotransverse joints (Tetley 2000)
   - abdominal (diaphragmatic) breathing becomes a primary respiratory strategy, which, in turn, stimulates parasympathetic tone.

In addition to these benefits, one of the major threats to many ground-dwelling primates is being trampled by elephants. Having an ear to the ground may allow early detection of approaching large animals.

Side-lying

1. Flexed arms and legs result in no exposure of flexor creases:
   - minimizes exposure of superficial arteries
   - helps retain body heat
   - leaves only bony extensor surfaces (knees, elbows) exposed.
2. Virtually no risk of snoring.
3. Virtually no exposure of soft underbelly.
4. Rib compression means increased abdominal excursion during breathing and lateral breathing on the non-compressed side, which

may be used therapeutically as a mobilization technique (Lee 2003).

The first principle underlying sleep in primate groups (and any animal) is that safety from predators is paramount (Anderson 2000). Most primates sleep in elevated locations, though may sleep on the ground during daylight. The great apes differ from monkeys in that they build a nest to provide a platform in their various arboreal sleeping sites, the one exception being adult male gorillas that may sleep on the ground (Anderson 2000).

In apes, nocturnal silence is seen as an anti-predation strategy. In human groups it should be recognized that, not only is snoring the aberrant result of dysfunction in the nasopharynx – usually secondary to immune sensitization, temporomandibular joint (TMJ) dysfunction, obesity, deconditioned anterior neck musculature, or a combination thereof (Roithmann et al 2005) – it is also the best signal to any predator with a set of ears that an 'easy meal' is in the vicinity. We can deduce, therefore, that our successful ancestors – those who survived to perpetuate their genes into our current gene pool – did not have a snoring problem.

Beach (personal communication, 1994) also describes how the body and limbs in particular are designed to have enough 'give' in them, so that they can resist external compression without buckling or breaking. In supine or prone positions, for example, the arms should be able to fully abduct without any restrictive tension in the pectoral group, the latissimus dorsi or stress on the shoulder joint. This would correlate with what is known of muscle length norms (Kendall et al 1993). Similarly, the hip-knee-ankle-foot complex should be able to accept full internal or external rotation in order that, under load, the medial or lateral border of the foot (respectively) can rest against the underlying planar surface. In an *instinctive sleep posture*, therefore, the body should be resting on a firm surface with the arms in any chosen position of abduction/flexion without any level of discomfort that might prevent sleep.

If the body is unable to achieve this, it is not because the position is dysfunctional, but because the body is dysfunctional.

So the question arises, do we want to make the body comfortable within its state of dysfunction, or do we want to optimize its function? Clinically, often we have to do both, but the latter should be the foremost objective in naturopathic thinking.

With sleeping prone as an example, Neumann (2002) states that the craniocervical region of the spine should rotate approximately 90° in either direction. Sleeping prone, therefore, would equate perfectly with

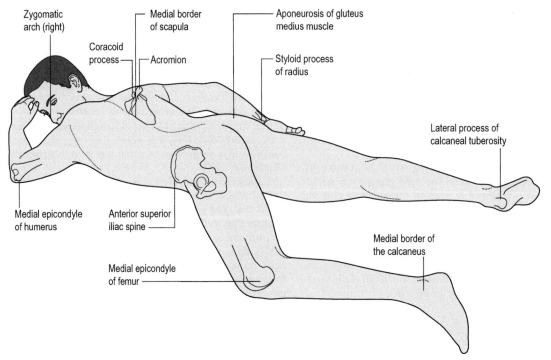

Figure 9.17 Reflexlocomotion reflex points. Redrawn from www.vojta.com. Note: The legends attaching to the figure do not necessarily identify those structures that are in touch with the floor, as discussed in the text

maintaining this full 90° range of motion, assuming that the individual hasn't gone through an extended period where pillows and soft, forgiving mattresses have allowed sleep in a non-rotated position and where range of motion has been lost.

Reflexlocomotion

Vojta (2006) takes this concept one step further by looking at how the nervous system may react to such rest postures. Vojta proposed and developed the theory that periosteal reflex points on the bony prominences of the body are stimulated by sustained bodyweight pressure.

Interstitial (type III and IV) mechanoreceptors are found in a particularly high density in the periosteum (Schleip 2003a), and respond to both rapid and slow sustained pressure changes. This, of course, implies that lying on, or sitting on, a given bony prominence will eventually result in stimulation of these periosteal receptors and motivate a change in resting posture.

Indeed, as Schleip (2003a) observes, the body's richest and largest sensory organ is not the skin, the eyes, the ears, the gustatory apparatus, the olfactory apparatus or the vestibular system, but is in fact the myofascial system.

Reflex points on the bony prominences of the medial epicondyle of the elbow, the zygomatic arch of the cheek, the anterior superior iliac spine and the medial condyle of the femur, for example, will be stimulated when the weight of the body presses against a firm planar surface (Fig. 9.17). Eventually the pain stimulus will become sufficient that the body will reflexively move. This, according to Vojta (2006), is what triggers infantile development of the reptilian crawl. The reptilian crawl is one the first examples of left–right brain integration, developing before the mammalian crawl (Goldfield 1995, Hartley 1995, Morris 1982). These and other crawl patterns are used in brain integration exercises for brain-injured patients, those with learning difficulties and those with post-traumatic vision syndrome (Wenberg & Thomas 2001).

Therefore, not only is resting in a prone position functional from a cervical range of motion, a breathing and a protection perspective but it also may help to re-pattern the brain and enhance movement coordination during sleep. That, it could be said, is an efficient system.

Morris (1982) states that there are between 40 and 70 body shifts during the average night's sleep and, since the range of adult human sleep is primarily contained within 6–9 hours, we can calculate that this equates to approximately a movement every 8–9 minutes. (This also calls into question the common assumption by many patients that they can only sleep in one position. Interestingly, many people are highly defensive about their sleep postures!)

Creep

The mechanical phenomenon in the tissues of the body known as creep, in which the connective tissues of the body will undergo plastic stretch, is an important factor in understanding the benefits and mechanisms of instinctive sleep and archetypal rest postures. Creep in the connective tissues – which would include myofascial (parallel elastic) and series elastic components – can occur in as little as 3 minutes when under load (McGill 2002). It is important to recognize that creep is both a load-dependent and time-dependent activity. The 3-minute figure presented by McGill was based on the posterior ligaments of a loaded lumbar spine, but if the load is reduced, the time taken to induce creep will extend.

Because lying down is a relatively low load activity, it is feasible and likely that creep may take a longer period which could correspond more closely with the 8- to 9-minute movement interlude described by Morris (1982) above (see 'Reflexlocomotion'). At the point at which the magnitude of afferent stimulus exceeds the threshold level at the cord, an efferent drive will occur and spontaneous movement will be generated to move the body into a new position (Slosberg 1988). This is the basis for reflexlocomotion described and utilized by Vojta and his colleagues (2006). (See Table 9.7, Definitions of tissue properties, above.)

According to Schleip (2003a), laboratory studies of force/time dependency on connective tissue creep show a high load (e.g. 60 kg) applied to the iliotibial band will result, acutely, in an approximate 18 mm (3–8%) elongation, but with tissue tearing and inflammation. With a low load, elongation will still occur, but will be less (1.5%) and will take more than an hour to achieve. Significantly, this magnitude of elongation occurs without tearing or inflammation. A further important observation is that this hour's worth of time under tension may occur across several intervals. This is congruent with the hypothesis that archetypal rest postures and instinctive sleep postures result in subtle myofascial stretch, helping to reset length–tension relationships.

Since type I mechanoreceptors are found in the superficial portions of the joint capsule they will be the first to be stimulated when the joint undergoes gradual stretch – as in the instinctive sleep postures.

Type I mechanoreceptors adapt slowly to stimulus, though they are low threshold, so when they do respond they will induce a change in firing rate to the postural system of the body (Wyke 1979). This tonic stimulation may result in changes in muscle tension but is unlikely to result in movement (as we know, postural muscles are more suited to 'holding' or compressing joints). A secondary function of the type I mechanoreceptor is to suppress pain, so this may also aid in effective sleep and/or rest.

With creep of the outer portions of the joint capsule, the type II mechanoreceptors found in the deeper layers of the capsule and articular fat pads will subsequently become stimulated (Wyke 1979). Since type II mechanoreceptors are rapidly adapting, and reflexively stimulate the phasic system, they will induce the body to move – thereby acting as a rapid response to protect the integrity of the joint. And with the tone of the postural muscles already stimulated by type I afferent drive, the equivalent of a feed-forward joint stability mechanism will be in place to allow the body to move safely during unconscious sleep.

Like the type I mechanoreceptors, type II mechanoreceptors also inhibit pain, thereby potentially aiding sleep. In general, mechanoreceptors are activated at 25% of the stimulation required to activate the nociceptors (Dvorak & Dvorak 1990). This means that well in advance of the resting individual perceiving pain (which would result in an adrenal response – antagonistic to sleep), first the postural, then the phasic system will be activated to move the joint from its potentially detrimental position of stretch.

Sleep cycles and positional changes

Interestingly, sleep is well documented to occur in several different stages, with brain-wave activity fluxing from theta-wave to delta-wave throughout the night. The non-REM portion of sleep is composed of stages 1–4 and lasts from 90 to 120 minutes, each stage lasting anywhere from 5 to 15 minutes (Hopkins 2006). Stage 5 – REM sleep – also goes through phases lasting around 10 minutes and gradually extending out until reaching durations of up to 1 hour. The entire cycle usually lasts around 100 minutes, which means that up to five cycles may be achieved during a night's sleep.

Of course, some of these stages may be of shorter duration and many patients' alarm clocks will have woken them well before they reach over 9 hours' sleep. This figure of 36 separate sleep cycles – if it were to correlate with one or two changes of sleep posture at the transition – is in close proximity to Morris's (1982) figure of 40–70 positional changes during an average night's sleep.

Table 9.14 How a hypothetical sleep pattern may look if the patient went to sleep at 10 p.m.

Time	Stage	Cumulative total of positional changes
10:00–10:15	Wake stage	1
10:15–10:30	Non-REM stage 1	2
10:30–10:45	Non-REM stage 2	3
10:45–10:50	Non-REM stage 3	4
10:50–11:05	Non-REM stage 4	5
11:05–11:15	Non-REM stage 3	6
11:15–11:20	Non-REM stage 2	7
11:30–11:40	REM (usually 90 minutes after onset of sleep)	8
11:40–12:55	Non-REM: Stage 1 (cycle stages 1-2-3-4-3-2 repeats through to . . .)	14
12:55–01:15	REM	15
1:15–02:30	Non-REM (cycle stages 1-2-3-4-3-2 repeats through to . . .)	21
02:30–03:00	REM	22
03:00–03:15	Non-REM (cycle stages 1-2-3-4-3-2 repeats through to . . .)	28
04:30–05:10	REM	29
05:10–06:25	Non-REM (cycle stages 1-2-3-4-3-2 repeats through to . . .)	35
06:25–07:25	REM	36

According to Tetley (personal communication, 2004), in some indigenous cultures – such as pygmy culture – it is forbidden to sleep off the ground, out of contact with Mother Nature. Anecdotally, many mystics and 'sensitives' also find that their sensitivities are decreased if they sleep off the ground, which may have something to do with the literal earthing effect of being in touch with the Earth, and/or may have something to do with the Earth's electromagnetic charge (Oschman 2000). Oschman (2004) has reported on studies which show that simply by earthing a person's bed to the ground their electrification decreases by 450-fold and that such earthing may help in re-regulating the 24-hour cortisol rhythm.

Further instinctive sleep postures

Another posture that may be considered an instinctive sleep posture is the *recovery position* (which effectively stretches the pectoralis minor and anterior fibers of trapezius, using pressure on the coracoid process and/or zygomatic arch as the ultimate stimulus to move; see Figs 9.16A and 9.17).

A fully supine posture may also be considered an instinctive sleep posture, though will rarely be used to sleep in the natural environment, unless there is no perceived threat. Of course, this posture is mainly recognized as being either a complete relaxation posture or a complete surrender posture.

Hence it can be concluded that, in the functional state, *pillows are props – props that propagate dysfunction.*

Similarly, a forgiving, soft mattress not only allows biomechanical dysfunction to perpetuate but also may impair the body's inbuilt postural regulation system.

This is not to suggest that everyone should sleep without pillows on a firm surface, but that everyone with a functional spine should be able to, and would probably benefit from doing so.

Archetypal rest postures

The concept of archetypal postures (rest postures) was an idea developed by Phillip Beach, a British osteopath, naturopath and acupuncturist (P Beach, personal communication 1989). Beach observed that across different cultures there were a series of postures that were adopted by all peoples throughout the world. Beach (personal communication, 2003) was the first to suggest that these postures could be viewed as 'attractor states'.

Beach identified the following archetypal postures as common to and consistent throughout all cultures across the globe (personal communication, 1989):

- the full (flat-footed) squat
- the low kneel (Fig. 9.18A)
- the high kneel
- the cross-legged (Indian sit)
- the long legged posture (Fig. 9.18B).

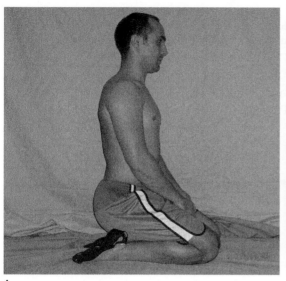 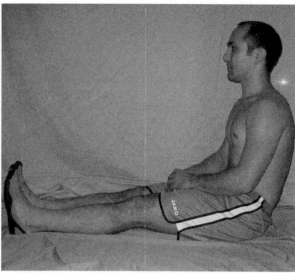

A   B

Figure 9.18 Archetypal (rest) postures: (**A**) low kneel; (**B**) long legged posture

Morris (1982) has also noted a series of rest postures adopted similar to Beach's classification, though adds the lotus position (similar to the cross-legged sit) and the squat on tiptoes (an energetically expensive version of the flat-footed squat and usually only used by those too inflexible to adopt the latter). Morris also omits the long-sit (long legged) position.

The one exception where archetypal postures are rarely utilized is in the adult population of Western culture. In Western society most adults have lost the ability to comfortably perform most, or all, of these postures, due to the fact the body adapts to its environment – its Western seated posture environment.

Western seated posture

Since, certainly from the age of 5, but commonly almost from birth, children are encouraged to adopt what we will call 'Western seated posture' (WSP) for a significant portion of their waking day, the developing body will adapt to the WSP as best it can and will gradually lose its efficacy at performing archetypal postures.

Of course, this pattern is perpetuated throughout schooling and most commonly into the workplace. In fact, the average Westerner will get up in the morning, sit down (WSP) for breakfast, jump in the car or on the train (WSP) to get into work. At work, they will typically sit all morning (WSP) until lunchtime, when they may stroll a few hundred meters (or perhaps stay sitting at their desk), before they sit (WSP) for lunch. The afternoon follows the same pattern as the morning

with sitting at work and sitting in a mode of transport to get home (WSP). They will sit down for dinner (WSP) or maybe, if they're one of the more active of the population, get down to the gym and sit (WSP) on a rowing machine, a bike or a series of weights machines. After an exhausting day of all this sitting (WSP) they will slump in the couch at home to watch the TV (WSP) before they finally head off to bed.

Hence, it would be fair to say that WSP is perhaps the most profound postural stressor on the average patient attending a naturopathic or rehabilitation-based clinic. Liebenson (2002b) explains that individuals with sedentary jobs have a higher risk of developing low back pain. Further, if in modern times the average adult sleeps less than 7 hours (Chek 2001c) and changes sleeping position around 40 times per night, this implies that, for the average naturopathic clinic's patient base, the WSP will be the most utilized posture. How to avoid this represents a challenge.

Multiple work stations

In Germany there are some businesses that have begun to incorporate multiple work stations (Cranz 2000) into the workplace. This is the most common-sense approach to minimizing cumulative micro-trauma on the musculoskeletal system for any progressive business that demands high standards for its employees and consequently high productivity.

Micropauses, or microbreaks, are also utilized to minimize the cumulative trauma of sustained posture or tasks (Liebenson 2002c). Commonly a short break of just a few seconds, moving into a different posture, or stretching out, is recommended every 20–30 minutes. However, it is likely that based on the discussion of creep above, a more regular break should be scheduled. Advice is often skewed in favor of the employer and is dependent on the mechanics of the national health care system. In New Zealand, for example, the ACC (Health Care) system will pay a certain percentage toward rehabilitation, as well as a high percentage of the patient's income (up to 80%) until they're fit to return to work. A negative outcome of this system is that it encourages malingerers. However, a benefit is that employers and the government are, in general, extremely diligent with their recommendations for micropauses, recommending them as frequently as every 3 minutes. This correlates well with what we know of connective tissue creep.

How do archetypal postures fit into this picture? Archetypal postures currently *do not* fit into this picture, and it is postulated by both Beach and Tetley that, if these more instinctive postures were commonplace in Western society, there would be a far lower incidence of musculoskeletal dysfunction and orthopedic consultation. This line of thought is supported by Cranz (2000) who suggests that chair sitting (WSP) itself causes back problems, and by Liebenson (2002b) who reports that sedentary workers have a higher incidence of disc problems than non-sedentary.

For the progressive company director, who is aware that low back pain has been the most significant cause of time off work (with work stress competing at a similar level), use of archetypal postures may provide a low-cost solution to minimize absenteeism. Archetypal workstations would likely minimize back pain, increase micropauses (thereby decreasing occupational overuse injuries) and would reduce sympathetic tone (and therefore lower stress levels) due to the stretching of large muscle groups and type II mechanoreceptors.

Akin to the dysfunctional use of painkillers, the very point of having a nervous system is not to attempt to sedate it, but to react to it. The nervous system is in place to allow the organism to respond more effectively to its environment. Modern-day ergonomics has tried to provide adaptable height chairs, adjustable lumbar supports, variable angle seats – mainly in an attempt to:

- customize the measurements of the seat to the measurements of the user, and
- minimize the pain and discomfort of sitting in one position for several hours/day by offering supports (lumbar supports, foot rests, wrist supports, head rests, etc.).

These two foci are in contradistinction to what nature has provided: a nervous system and an anthropometrically, appropriately proportioned body.

Use it or lose it

An exciting, yet patently obvious, aspect of archetypal postures is that:

- an individual's legs are anthropometrically the optimal length for the user to sit on – no customization required. For example, kneeling down, it would be extremely rare, other than through a genetic problem or surgery, to find someone whose lower leg is too short or too long for them to sit on (so their heels don't reach their buttocks)
- archetypal postures, by their nature, involve holding joint positions towards their end range, creating sustained stretch on the joint capsules. Such stretch, as described above, eventually results in cumulative afferent stimulation of the type I and II mechanoreceptors, inducing movement (a change of position) to prevent the 'user' from undergoing any cumulative trauma.

Only a small (unknown) percentage of the adult population of most Westernized societies are able to adopt archetypal postures – and usually only for a very small period of time (seconds) before becoming uncomfortable. This poses a practical problem in terms of encouraging patients to embrace this system. Simple but effective tools may be used to help patients to adopt archetypal postures that they've lost the ability to attain and/or sustain.

A comparison of proneness to osteoarthritis, between other primates and humans, identified that those joints less prone to degenerative change are those that are utilized through a similar full range of motion as other primates – such as the elbow. Joints typically used in a smaller range of motion than our primate cousins such as the hip, the knee, the shoulder and the cervical spine are more likely to develop degenerative change (Alexander 1994). Indeed, Tetley (personal communication, 2004) cites a book called *Pain, The Gift That Nobody Wants* by Brand & Yancey (1994) whose thrust is entirely congruent with this line of thought – the pain is there for a reason. Brand is an orthopedic surgeon who worked in India with those suffering from leprosy, which highlighted to him the importance of our ability to sense pain. He also observed that Indian people rarely complained of osteoarthritis in the hips. Inspired by his observation he compared radiographs of Indian and Western patients and found little difference in joint space decline. However, what struck him was the uneven wear on the hip joints of the Westerners – where degenerative change occurred primarily in the sagittal plane of the joint. Being a ball socket, the hip joint is designed to share load all around the ball – not just in one line along an anteroposterior line (Brand & Yancey 1994).

This provides an illustration of how routine use of archetypal postures, with the multiple positions that this ensures for the femoral head inside the pelvic socket, may benefit musculoskeletal health.

Research shows that 1 in 4 women, and 1 in 12 men, will suffer with osteoporosis. Of course, osteoporosis and femoral neck fracture may be associated with osteoarthritis (OA) at the hip in a reciprocal cause–effect relationship. A shocking statistic is that, from just 50 years of age onwards, according to the National Osteoporosis Foundation (2006), hip fracture results in a 24% mortality rate in the first year after the trauma.

Whilst naturopaths recognize other health and lifestyle factors contributing to hip fracture and hip OA, an attempt to address the reduced femoral neck inclination (Fig. 9.19) may not be as high on the list of therapeutic interventions. This decreased angulation is an example of the SAID principle and, more specifically, *Wolff's law* at work. However, imagine if the full squat was regularly used as an archetypal rest posture . . . how does that load the femoral neck? Interestingly, it completely reverses the loading through the

neck to help maintain an optimal angle of inclination (and therefore an optimal instantaneous axis of rotation and therefore a minimal amount of stress to the soft tissues) at the hip joint. This is a natural, inbuilt means of counteracting gravitational stress that the species, and indeed the apes, have collectively adopted.

The full squat is also very useful to support bowel function and to support the act of defecation. Tetley (personal communication, 2004) suggests that the act of defecation in the full squat position helps to balance and reset the sacroiliac joints with the concomitant contraction of the transversus abdominis. The full squat archetypal posture, the muscular action required to defecate and its suggested benefit to sacroiliac function (M Tetley, personal communication, 2004) is consistent with the work of DonTigny (1997) who recommends a variety of posterior rotation mobilizations of the innominate to return the SIJs to their self-bracing position.

Chek (2004c) also describes how the development of bipedalism and upright working postures has brought with it a digestive challenge; human beings are the only animal that needs to push fecal matter (in the 'ascending colon') uphill against gravity. Using a full squat position mechanically compresses the ascending colon (and, of course, the descending colon), aiding peristalsis in the former and stimulating urgency to evacuate (secondary to stimulation of

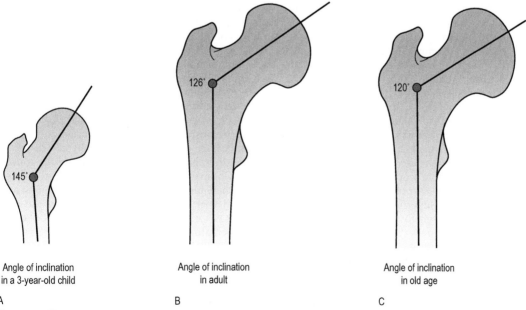

Angle of inclination in a 3-year-old child

Angle of inclination in adult

Angle of inclination in old age

A   B   C

Figure 9.19 Progressive decrease in angulation of femoral neck across time. Reproduced with permission from Platzer et al (2000)

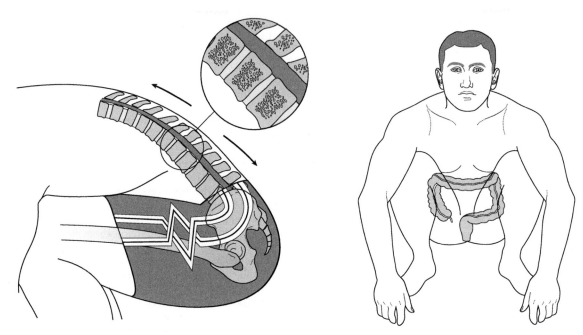

Figure 9.20 In the full squat, compression of the thighs against the body wall results in lift through the lumbar discs and compression of the terminal GI tract, which aids healthy bowel motion, particularly in the ascending colon. Redrawn from an image kindly provided by Paul Chek

colonic stretch receptors) in the latter. Additionally, the full squat assists decompression of the lumbar spine by creating lift through pressure of the thighs against the trunk (see Fig. 9.20).

Table 9.15 outlines some of the characteristics of the various archetypal rest postures and how they may facilitate stretching, compression and function of different bodily processes.

The full quadruped position is rarely used by adults, though by babies it is commonly used as a sleeping position. This is why it is more colloquially known as the 'child pose'. Tetley (2000) observes that this posture is commonly utilized by Tibetan caravaneers as a sleep posture – meaning that only bone is in contact with the ground – all significant muscle mass is kept clear of the frozen ground. It is also an excellent position for assessment and for treatment of various joint pathologies as described by Shirley Sahrmann (2002), so is therefore worthy of mention.

Interestingly, the Ruffini corpuscles (a type II mechanoreceptor found more superficially than the Pacini type IIs) are particularly sensitive to tangential forces and as a result of such forces create an inhibition of sympathetic activity. This, of course, would be exactly what one would want after a hunt, after a fight, after being chased – and, most importantly, when resting.

Such inhibition of sympathetic activity would also make these postures ideal positions to eat in and to encourage the body to make its diurnal switch from sympathetic dominance towards parasympathetic dominance by nightfall.

Archetypal postures and tissue repair

It is thought that fibroblasts and fibroclasts are responsive to piezoelectric charges which are generated by external pressure. This process is commonly discussed in terms of scar tissue formation (Croft 1995) and the laying down of a functional scar with collagen deposition along the lines of stress (Lederman 1997). Instinctive and archetypal rest postures would aid in tissue healing through this mechanism. Additionally, an increase in static pressure on muscles tends to lower arterial blood pressure (Schleip 2003a). Each of the archetypal postures results in compression through weight-bearing on different tissues, thereby distributing the therapeutic effect across multiple muscle groups. Compression with or without traction through muscles may also induce a 'wringing effect'. Just as if presented with a sodden rag doll, turning the neck fully so it is 'wrung' will squeeze the fluid out of the microvasculature, enhancing venous return. So sleeping prone with the neck fully rotated in one direction may support removal of waste metabolites from the neck's daily battle with gravity.

Schleip (2003b) explains that static stretching is likely to inhibit capillary blood flow in the targeted tissues, which, he suggests, may inhibit tissue repair. However,

Table 9.15 Archetypal postures, their features and associated human behaviors

Archetypal posture	Descriptors	Behavior
Squat	**Feature**: Soleus stretch/colon compression	**Bowel/bladder evacuation**
Stretches	Soleus/vasti/gluteus maximus/lumbar and thoracic erectors/ Achilles + patella tendons	
Compresses (tangential force)	Gastrocnemius/soleus/hamstrings/ascending + descending colon/disc	
Decompresses	Femoral neck/facets (lumbar)/prostate/genitalia	
Works	Tibialis anterior	
Base of support	Feet (plantar aspect)	
Long sit	**Feature**: (Lower) Hamstring stretch	**Eating** (legs provide natural collection tray)
Stretches	Hamstrings/gluteus maximus/knee ligaments dural stretch	
Compresses (tangential force)	(Disc) Prostate	
Decompresses	(Facet)/Knee joint (although lock home)	
Works	Psoas/internal oblique	
Base of support	Ischial tuberosities/legs	
Kneel	**Feature**: Lumbar spine neutral	**Prayer**: Christian/Catholic
Stretches	Tibialis anterior/vasti/(gluteus maximus)/patella tendon/ anterior knee capsule + anterior talocrural capsule	
Compresses (tangential force)	Gastrocnemius/soleus/hamstrings/lateral compartment of shin	
Decompresses	Posterior annulus/posterior ligamentous system/thoracolumbar fascia/prostate/genitalia	
Works	Lumbar erectors/obliques	
Base of support	Lateral aspect of shin/dorsum of foot	
High kneel	**Feature**: Plantar fascia/toe flexors, lordosis	**Prayer**: Christian/Catholic
Stretches	Toe flexors/plantar fascia/Achilles tendon/patella tendon/ anterior knee capsule, etc.	
Compresses (tangential force)	Myofascial trigger points/hamstrings/soleus/gastrocnemius/ pre- + postpatella bursae	
Decompresses	Posterior annulus/posterior ligamentous/prostate/genitalia	
Works	Lumbar erectors/obliques	
Base of support	Toes + knees	

Continued

Table 9.15 Archetypal postures, their features and associated human behaviors continued

Archetypal posture	Descriptors	Behavior
Side kneel	**Feature**: Corrects/compounds scoliosis, frontal plane	**???**
Stretches	Ipsilateral internal rotators, quadratus lumborum, lumbar factors/contralateral external rotators/dorsiflexors	
Compresses (tangential force)	Ipsilateral gluteus maximus/contralateral lateral annulus + facet	
Decompresses	Ipsilateral lateral aspect of annulus + facet	
Works	Contralateral quadratus lumborum and obliques	
Base of support	Ipsilateral shin/foot/hand – thorn in foot, tetrapod vs biped loading	
Indian sit	**Feature**: Stretches adductors (facilitated)/aerial/ability to remove thorns ± tend to soles	**Prayer/meditation:** Hindu/Buddhist
Stretches	Adductors/internal rotators, including piriformis/upper hamstrings/anterior hip capsule	
Compresses (tangential force)	Ischial tuberosities/prostate	
Decompresses	Knee/lateral subtalar joint	
Works	Lumbar erectors/(? psoas)	
Base of support	Ischial tuberosities/lateral knee	

Table 9.16 Full quadruped posture, feature and associated human behavior

Archetypal posture	Descriptors	Behavior
Full quadruped	**Feature**: Transversus + serratus anterior activation/maximal motion coupling through body's joints	**Prayer**: Muslim
Stretches	Vasti/tibialis anterior/dorsiflexion/gluteus maximus/posterior hip capsule/lumbar erectors/latissimus anterior	
Compresses (tangential force)	(Pre- + postpatella bursae)/anterior annulus/calves/hamstrings/quadriceps	
Decompresses	Facets/posterior annulus	
Works	Transversus/serratus anterior	
Base of support	Hands, knees, dorsum of foot	

on the contrary, Knobloch et al (2007), studying the pathophysiology of Achilles tendinopathy, found perfusion in the microcirculation of the tendon to be significantly elevated in symptomatic when compared with non-symptomatic tendons. Alfredson & Ohberg (2002) suggest that this may be due to a process of neovascularization and they have demonstrated that using sclerosing techniques on the neovessels results in effective treatment of Achilles tendinopathy. Further, Alfredson & Lorentzon (2000) showed that an eccentric contraction of the triceps surae promotes an ischemic environment within the tendon, explaining the dramatic success of their eccentric training protocol for presurgical cases of Achilles tendinopathy.

Therefore, far from Schleip's (2003b) suggestion that inhibition of capillary blood flow may be counterproductive to healing, it may in fact facilitate healing or even prevent tendinopathy. The high kneel and full squat would be particularly effective for inducing ischemia in the Achilles tendon and all of the archetypal postures (high/low/side-kneel, cross-legged sitting, full squat, quadruped) – bar the long sit – would be effective for inducing ischemia in the patella tendon.

Archetypal postures and movement

Because each of the archetypal rest postures induces stretch to a number of different tissues, each posture will become uncomfortable after a given period of time (between 3 and 15 minutes) as the tissues start to undergo creep. This results in the inclination to move, which is a functional thing to do. Far from discomfort being the *problem* with archetypal rest postures, it is the *solution* to avoiding musculoskeletal damage and dysfunction.

Many therapists suggest to their patients that sitting with the legs crossed is not good for the health of the back. Snijders et al (1997) assessed the activation of different trunk muscles during Western seated posture and found that leg crossing permitted decreased muscular action and therefore stabilization could be achieved more efficiently by putting stretch through the passive subsystem (sacrotuberous ligament and thoracolumbar fascia). Sitting with the legs crossed can therefore be classified as a functional response to aid stabilization of the back. Thus, as argued by Vleeming (2003), it is sitting that is dysfunctional – not leg crossing!

Archetypal postures and lordosis

The astute observer may note that all of the archetypal postures, bar the kneeling postures, result in some degree of posterior tilt of the pelvis and a propensity to lumbar flexion. Surely this just would add to the known problem with WSP creating disc injury (Liebenson 2002b).

Figure 9.20 above explains one reason why a full squat may not be as detrimental to the lumbar disc as it may first appear, but it should also be borne in mind that the significant use of walking in developmental times means that the spine would constantly have undergone compressive (axial flexion) loads with each heel strike and weight-bearing phase of gait. In a functional spine, with functional anteroposterior spinal curvatures, this will result in increased load of the spinal curves, increasing lordotic load (or sagittal extension). A set of rest postures biased somewhat towards flexion and therefore a reduction of lordotic curve may have provided optimal rebalancing.

For the modern environment, it may be that a slight bias toward rest postures enhancing lumbar extension may be more beneficial for the hypothetical 'average' person. There are devices that have been developed to counteract the flexion bias of modern lifestyles such as the prone prop – though many will naturally adopt a similar posture to read or watch television.

Other postures that may be considered archetypal rest postures include supine lying (as described under instinctive sleep postures), side-lying with head propped, or lying prone with upper body propped on elbows.

The first of these postures has a number of benefits described above (see 'Instinctive sleep postures'), the second has fewer biomechanical benefits as it works against the strong drive of the righting reflex of the optic, otic and occlusal planes, as well as stressing the tissues of the cervical spine – although Butler (1994) has pointed out that this posture makes for an effective ulnar nerve mobilization (or ULTT3 in the language of neurodynamics). The last of these three postures is almost the perfect antidote to the flat-backed posture and high disc injury incidence associated with WSP (McKenzie 2003). In fact, the prone propped position is commonly used by manual therapists in rehabilitation of disc pain patients (posterior annular bulges).

Perhaps one of the most exciting aspects of archetypal postures is the fact that there is little doubt these postures were inextricably a part of how Homo sapiens 'got here' on their 4+ million year evolutionary journey.

Moreover, returning to the idea that stretching to warm up for a sport or prevent an injury simply has no foundation in nature, equally unnatural is sitting in one single posture for 8 or more hours per day. Observation of any animal – even a domesticated animal – reveals that there is movement even when at rest. It is almost without question, therefore, as proposed by Tetley and Beach, that these postures are designed to hone and refine the body's myofascial length–tension relationships (though there are probably numerous other benefits), thereby maintaining an optimal instantaneous axis of rotation at the joints (see Fig. 9.7 above). And what's even better, is that using archetypal postures costs nothing and can be easily incorporated into patients' daily lives with a little improvisation.

The slow protracted style stretching found in archetypal postures is comparable with so-called 'developmental' stretching described in sports and exercise science (Alter 2004). Rather than discussing the optimal duration to stretch, it should be apparent by now that the optimal stretch time – particularly in the context of archetypal rest and instinctive sleep postures – is the length of time it is comfortable to hold it. When the discomfort becomes sufficient for the subject to want to move, *then* is the time to move. This is utilization of the nervous system in the role for which it was designed. It is suggested that such developmental stretching stimulates the Golgi receptors (type III mechanoreceptors) that lie in series, with fascial fibers influencing alpha motor neurons to downregulate their drive – thereby relaxing the tone in the phasic system (Schleip 2003c).

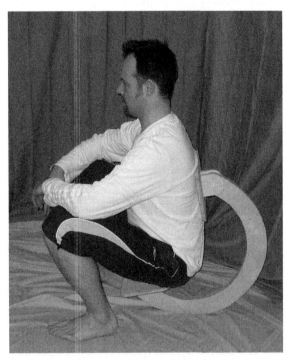

Figure 9.21 Illustration of a patient improvising to create a comfortable environment for the squat archetypal posture

Primal patterns

In studies of different cultures that exhibit longevity, many disparate health and lifestyle factors appear to support their health successes. A moderate to high level of daily activity is one of several common links between such cultures (Buettner 2005). Of these daily activities, whether involving walking to collect water, working in the fields, or hunting and gathering, all will incorporate multiple aspects of the primal patterns.

Primal patterns is a concept developed by Paul Chek (personal communication, 1993) based on kinesiological studies and a comprehensive foundation of motor learning. Chek describes seven different primal patterns, the last being gait with the three subgroups of walking, jogging and running, each with their own motor program (P Chek, personal communication, 1993, Chek 2000a).

These primal patterns are as follows:

1. The squat
2. The bend
3. The lunge
4. The twist
5. The push
6. The pull
7. Gait
   - Walk
   - Jog
   - Run.

Primal patterns are used in exercise kinesiology to understand more about how an athlete moves within their environment – whether that environment is competitive or not.

In terms of the primal patterns as biomechanical attractors, it is reasonable to suggest that gait could be termed a primary dynamic attractor with the other six patterns as secondary dynamic attractors. The rationale for this is that gait was utilized for many hours each day in the nomadic ancestral environment, whereas powerful lunging, twisting, pushing, pulling, squatting or bending would likely have only been used for a matter of seconds or minutes per day –

Table 9.17 Neuromuscular/articular interactions

Motor neuron	Muscles	System	Conscious	Stimulation from ligamentous or capsular stretch	Brain
Gamma motor neuron	Inner unit	Tonic	Unconscious	Powerful	Ancient cerebellum
Alpha motor neuron	Outer unit	Phasic	Volitional	Weak	Neocortex

albeit regularly enough to define them as attractor states. However, see stressor model (Fig. 9.22) below.

The squat

The squat pattern as a primal pattern should be differentiated from the squat used as an archetypal (rest) posture. As a primal pattern, the squat is primarily used for lifting, for sitting and for jumping and, as such, is commonly only utilized to a depth where the thighs reach parallel to the ground. In archetypal postures, the squat is a rest posture and a defecation posture, hence is usually 'full' in nature with the back of the thighs in contact with the calves and the front of the thighs in full contact with the abdominal wall.

The squat is an important movement skill allowing the arms to reach down close to the ground to lift low-level objects and to share the load of those objects through the large muscle groups of the quadriceps, the hamstrings, the gluteals and the lumbar erectors.

If, during the squat, the load is between the legs (known as a Jefferson squat), or resting on the sternum (a front squat), this tends to focus the load more into the thoracic extensors and the lower scapula stabilizer (lower trapezius in particular) – as the load is trying to collapse the shoulder girdle anteriorly. If the load is behind the legs (a hack squat) or resting atop of the shoulders and cervicothoracic region of the spine, this tends to stress the lumbar erectors more – as now the load is trying to pull the body posteriorly and so to compensate the trunk must be inclined forwards somewhat.

An understanding of these simple principles and the wherewithal to select the most 'specific' loading parameter to the patient's sport or activity of daily living – as well as their muscle imbalance pattern – makes for a more effective exercise prescription.

The squat primarily works the deep longitudinal system and the posterior oblique sling (see sling systems above).

The bend

The bend pattern is an important movement skill and brings with it much controversy. There are two schools of thought with regard to the bend pattern, mainly

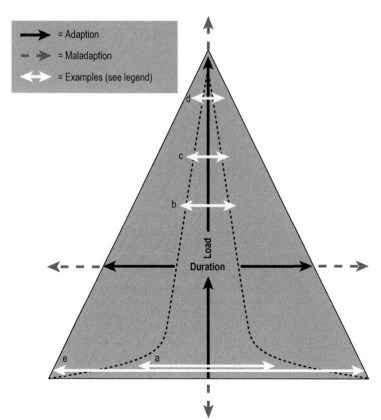

Figure 9.22 Stressor model. The higher the load, the less duration is required to create an adaptation. However, if the duration is too long or the load is too high, maladaption will occur (i.e. tissue failure). Examples are given: (a) doing a corrective exercise to train the stability muscles for only 2 minutes' duration means the white line does not move outside of the black dotted line, so that little or no adaption will take place. A postural exercise must have a minimum of 3–5 minutes of time under tension to have a training effect on the type 1 muscle fibers. Example (b): a strength endurance stimulus must last for a shorter duration than the pure endurance training, and the load will be higher. This will result in adaption of primarily type IIa fibers in the muscle. Example (c): strength conditioning requires shorter duration than strength–endurance, with higher loads. Example (d): power conditioning requires extremely short duration, explosive exercise, with even higher loads. Example (e): a very low load activity such as sitting may be carried out for such a long duration that it exceeds the body's adaptive capacity and results in breakdown (see Chapter 2 for more on adaptation)

contested between Gracovetsky (1988) and McGill (2002).

Gracovetsky's approach maintains that a functional spine should, and must, use the posterior ligamentous system to lift a heavy load. This approach is based on the study of Olympic power lifters who, Gracovetsky calculated, could not possibly lift the loads they were lifting with their lumbar erectors alone; they needed to use their hip extensors (hamstrings and gluteal group) via their thoracolumbar fascia to lift through the spine and into the arms.

However, McGill (2002) recommends an attempt to maintain a neutral spinal position when lifting heavy loads. This results in a more equal load distribution through the three-column system of the spine (the disc and bilateral facets). Liebenson supports McGill's contention, as does Chek.

Chek (2002) provides a useful and rational clinical insight into these two philosophies. If the lift starts from a neutral spinal position (while flexed at the hips – 'the hip hinge') the lumbar spine and lumbar erectors are already engaged in their inner range. To lift a very heavy load from this position may result in some lumbar flexion (as maintained by Gracovetsky), but at least if the start is from the neutral position weight-bearing is equally distributed between disc and the two facets (the tripod mechanism of the spine), the nucleus is centralized within the disc, and if the spine migrates forwards into flexion to allow for tensioning of the posterior ligamentous system, at least the lumbar erectors are now working eccentrically. In eccentric contraction muscles are approximately 1.2 times stronger (Bompa 1999). Additionally, if you're able to breathe while lifting the load, this implies that the load is not heavy enough to warrant a neutral spine and, assuming no back pain or disc injury indicators, the ligamentous strategy is both functional and safe. Another way of assessing whether the load is safe to lift with a flexed spine is the number of repetitions you could perform without fatigue; if it is 20 or more reps it is again considered safe. It should, however, be borne in mind that connective tissue creep is both time and load dependent. Therefore, if someone lifts a 5 kg load across 4 seconds 100 times without time for the tissues to regain their form, it would be the equivalent of lifting 1 kg across 1 second 4000 times, or 50 kg across 10 seconds, just once.

The bend is a similar movement pattern to the squat and is sometimes (mistakenly) performed with an identical kinesiological profile. Since the bend pattern is most commonly trained using a deadlift (see Fig. 9.22), confusion arises because the deadlift is also used as an explosive Olympic lift. Naturally, when people want to learn how to do something properly they watch 'the experts' and then copy them. An Olympic lifter will typically use a squat pattern to lift the bar from the ground to help share the load across more working joints and muscle groups.

However, the bend pattern is a necessary skill for many people in their activities of daily living where a squat is impractical. Take, for example, a new mother who has to spend a significant portion of time changing her new baby's nappy (diaper), dressing and undressing the baby, bathing the baby and putting the baby into and out of its cot. In each of these situations, it is unlikely that she will be able to squat to put the baby down – as there is a side to a cot, many changing tables are solid or have storage underneath, dressing the baby is often done on a changing table or on a bed with a solid side, bathing the baby also means reaching over the lip of the bath with little scope to bend the knees.

With all that relaxin in her system and an abdominal wall that has undergone a significant laying down of sarcomeres during pregnancy (i.e. it is not in its optimal length–tension relationship) and a pelvic floor that may have been recently traumatized, this means that the new mother had better know how to bend with a competent level of skill.

The bend pattern then, is also sometimes known as the hip hinge (Liebenson 2003) and requires good hip–back dissociation skills – especially in those who are injured or deconditioned. The primary muscle groups involved in power generation are the hamstrings, the gluteals (to a lesser extent) and the erector spinae. The quadriceps are far less actively involved in the bend pattern as the knee should not flex more than around 20° and should remain relatively static compared to the pattern in the squat (Hodges 1999).

The bend primarily works the deep longitudinal system and the posterior oblique system bilaterally (hamstrings, gluteus maximus and latissimus dorsi being prime movers in lifting).

The lunge

The lunge pattern is most commonly utilized in sports and can be viewed as a descent of the running gait pattern. However, it should be recognized that in running gait, two feet are never on the ground at the same time, whereas when changing direction in sports (or historically, in hunting/escaping predators) the lunge is utilized – usually accompanied by a twist. The lunge is also used to reach for distant objects (such as in racket sports) and may be utilized to step over ground-lying obstacles, such as fallen trees, pot-holes or streams.

In terms of carry-over, the lunge is primarily useful for change of direction – for example, in planting and cutting sports – where the foot must plant into the ground to cut and change direction. For this, the multidirectional lunge is an excellent conditioning exercise. In more day-to-day situations, climbing stairs is a modified lunge pattern, while raking the lawn, sweeping the driveway, vacuuming the house or stepping over a puddle may all utilize the lunge pattern. The lunge may also be used to lift heavy objects from a low level, but with the drawback that it creates significant shear at the pelvis, and commonly requires significant activation of the frontal plane musculature (such as quadratus lumborum and gluteus medius) for successful execution. As such, those with sacroiliac joint problems should avoid the lunge pattern in the acute phase and should only proceed with caution at the subacute phase.

The lunge primarily works the lateral system and the deep longitudinal system (see sling systems above). Due to the loading on the lateral system, the lunge will often highlight the Trendelenburg and compensated Trendelenburg patterns.

The twist

The twist pattern is essential to most powerful movement patterns, including gait. In almost any explosive situation in sports (which of course are metaphoric of predation and prey circumstances in evolution), sprinting, punching, kicking and throwing all involve explosive rotation of the trunk – the twist pattern. In the home the twist pattern may be used to turn to reach something from a cupboard, or to lift a small child onto a bed or cot, for example. Turning to reverse the car also – if done properly – should incorporate a full twist through the length of the spine – not just the neck. The twist pattern primarily conditions the obliques, as well as the anterior and posterior oblique slings. If a lateral shift is incorporated into the pattern, as is commonly the case, the twist will also work the lateral system (see slings systems above; see also discussion on abdominal wall function above).

Clinically, the twist may be assessed through use of a cable pulley system, or through the *stick test* described above (see Fig. 9.14). The twist particularly highlights motor control deficits in the transverse plane. If a deficit is located, motor control must be reestablished – commonly through descending the exercise to one in which motor control is restored. This may involve completely removing the axial load through the spine.

The push

The push pattern commonly incorporates a twist as a component, though it may also be executed in isolation. In most functional environments the twist and the push will couple to create a powerful punching or

throwing action; however, in the therapeutic environment, it is sometimes useful to train movement patterns in isolation or to train isometric (static) trunk stability while dynamically moving a limb. This would be referred to as shoulder–trunk dissociation. The push is effective for training the anterior oblique sling. In daily living the push is most often utilized to push ourselves up out of bed, off the ground or out of a chair, to open heavy doors, or perhaps to get a car rolling for a bump-start.

Pushing may be achieved in the closed chain, such as a push-up, or in the open chain, such as a bench press or a cable push. The versatility of performing a push pattern using a cable allows for multiple movement patterns and therefore retraining of motor patterns as well as strength and conditioning. For example, Sahrmann's (2005) assertion that strengthening the serratus anterior will not change the functional pathomechanics of the glenohumeral joint may be countered under the tutelage of a skilled practitioner, by training activation of serratus anterior through utilizing a push pattern 'with a plus' through multiple angles. This will enhance serratus activation and sequencing in functional movement patterns, as well as increasing drive to the muscle through neural pathway facilitation.

The pull

As with the push pattern, the pull pattern also typically incorporates a twist as a component, though it may be executed in isolation. Again, this may be used therapeutically to isolate an area for strength development before integrating the strength into a functional movement pattern. However, it is also very useful for assessment of the patient (see below). The pull pattern is particularly effective for conditioning the posterior oblique sling.

From a survival point of view, pulling was essential for climbing and for dragging food or logs back to the home base. In today's modern world, it is probably most commonly utilized for raking the lawn, pulling out weeds, moving furniture or pulling open a door. The pull may be assessed in the closed chain, such as the pull-up, or in the open chain, such as a latissimus dorsi pull-down or a standing cable pull.

Clinically, the pull is particularly useful for assessing how the patient transfers load between their legs, trunk and arms and how they integrate their shoulder musculature. For example, are they arm dominant (don't use their trunk at all), do they hitch their shoulder (scapula elevators may be facilitated), do they recruit their scapulohumeral or their scapulospinal muscles equally, or is one group dominant over the other?

Gait

Gait has been correctly described by Chek (2000a) as a primal pattern. Indeed, it is likely to be, by far, the most primal movement pattern when viewed through the lens of biomechanical attractors.

Gait can be divided into three major subgroups based on motor learning:

- The walk
- The jog
- The run.

Gait in the guise of walking and jogging is classically recognized as 'cardiovascular training' despite the fact that so-called 'anaerobic training', such as lifting weights or sprint training, is also a significant cardiovascular training tool, as the cardiovascular system works to repay the accumulated oxygen debt. Gait can be used successfully to train each of the major energy systems of the body (aerobic, fast oxidative and fast glycolytic).

Walking

Human walking is a unique biomechanical phenomenon. It has been said that 'man stands alone because man alone stands' (Morris 1982).

Lovejoy is renowned as one of the world's leading experts on the evolution of human gait (Goldfield 1995). Lovejoy & Latimer (1997) emphasize the development of the lumbar lordosis as one of the key anatomic changes allowing efficient bipedal gait. The importance of lordosis in gait is also expounded by Gracovetsky (1997, 2001) who explains that the kinetic energy of the ground reaction force is captured as potential energy in both the annulus of the disc and the collagen of the facet joints. If the lumbar spine loses its lordosis, increased energy will be focused into the disc and, across time, will increase wear and tear to the disc complex. Considering it is estimated that humans will have in excess of 10 million footfalls across their lifespans (Morris 1982) and that, each time they do so, between three and seven times their body weight returns through their body mechanics, this is some significant cumulative load, which may struggle to survive even a subtle shift of weight-bearing towards the disc.

Walking results in a low y-axis sine wave, meaning that there is relatively little compressive impact through the spine when walking. Sprinting is similar to walking in terms of axial load, whereas jogging is far higher impact with a far higher sine wave. This pattern is paralleled by horses' gait (walk = walk, jog = trot, run = canter, sprint = gallop), which is partly why horse riding is so therapeutic for helping children with motor learning deficits, providing an affer-

ent stimulus almost identical to that if the child was ambulating themselves.

This sine wave differential is why it has been clinically noted that when the patient complains of low back pain while jogging but not during sprinting or walking, this is almost pathognomonic of compressive spinal injury, and usually a disc injury (Cowie 1999).

As Lederman (1997) and Stone (1999) have discussed, pumping of synovial joints – as occurs in repetitive passive mobilization techniques – stimulates the synovial membranes to produce synovial fluid, thereby increasing hydrostatic pressure in the joints and preventing wear and tear to the joint cartilages and to the spinal discs. The same process occurs as a 'natural oiling mechanism' when the joint is mobilized actively through repetitive motions – such as gait. Of course, the efficacy of this system only holds true if the patient is appropriately hydrated; it is likely that under states of chronic dehydration, fluids will be redirected to more vital processes, such as digestion and blood pressure regulation (Batmanghelidj 2001).

Liebenson (2004) states that slow walking with little arm swing is associated with increased static loads through the spine and is not recommended for those with back pain. This information would correlate with Van Emmerick et al's (1999) work showing that a walking pace below 0.75 meters per second (which is an extremely slow ambling pace) is associated with a lack of interlimb coupling (where opposing upper and lower limbs 'couple' in their motion). Applied anatomy reveals that it is this coupled motion that utilizes the 'smart spring' mechanism (Chek 2001b, 2001d) or the posterior oblique and anterior oblique muscle slings. This provides a clear explanation for why strolling around the shops for an afternoon, where the total distance traveled may be only 2–3 km, is far more tiring on the body than taking a 7–8 km walk with free-swinging arms in the countryside.

Such countryside walking is, developmentally, what our biomechanics have adapted to over thousands of millennia. This evolutionary inheritance has been shown to:

- reduce blood pressure
- enhance balance
- increase mobility
- reduce varicose veins and deep vein thrombosis
- decrease fatigue (Vines 2005)

and these benefits are enhanced if the walking is completed barefoot.

It is worthy of note that the two things that are most likely to quieten a distressed newborn is being carried

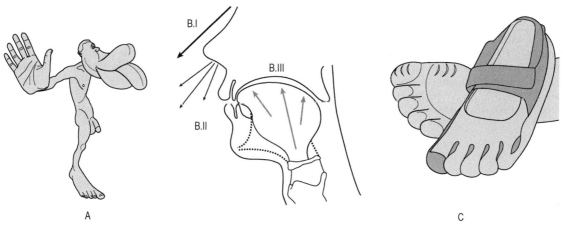

Figure 9.23 **A** Homunculus. **B** Tongue position and nasal breathing. **B.I**: line of vision when walking barefoot. The downward gaze results in activation of the deep cervical flexors – thereby supporting stabilization of the neck. **B.II**: air passing out through the nose as a result of (**B.III**) the tongue being held in its physiological rest position against the roof of the mouth. This positioning of the tongue also serves to create stability through the supra- and infrahyoid muscle groups of the neck. **C** 'Fivefingers' shoes for barefoot walking

close to the body and walked, or to be breast-fed. Because survival in the wild would have required a high level of stealth (Grimes 2002), keeping a newborn contented would have been a tribal priority and walking was, no doubt, a key daily routine.

Both feeding and being walked involve close physical contact, usually with a parent, but the latter also involves motion. There is undoubtedly a comforting effect of being held close and of being rocked in a gait-like motion (as the child would have been in the womb), but there is also the added benefit that such movement inevitably acts as an afferent stimulus to the child's nervous system, laying down the foundations of central pattern generators at the cord level. A lack of movement at this early stage of life – such as the child only ever being put in a pram – may result in later developmental and movement skill difficulties. In pygmy culture, the child barely ever loses its skin–skin contact with its mother across its first year of life.

Jogging

Jogging is the second gait pattern. It has a different motor engram from walking and sprinting. The most obvious discriminating factors are that in walking gait one foot is always on the ground, in running gait there is always a period of time (flight phase) when there are no feet on the ground. Sprinting is delineated from jogging in that it is explosive and therefore not sustainable for bursts of longer than 8 seconds.

Jogging efficiency (and gait efficiency in general) has been shown to be maximized by running barefoot. Of course, in many terrains – particularly man-made terrains, but also parks and trails where people may have dropped litter – barefoot running may be ill advised. There are, however, certain commercial options open to runners who would like the benefits of running barefoot, without the dangers. Benefits of barefoot running include:

- earthing effect to the ground – decreasing electrification of body (Oschman 2004)
- lower prevalence of acute injuries of the ankle
- lower incidence of chronic injuries of lower leg
- increased running efficiency (decreased oxygen consumption by ~4%) (Warburton 2001).

The peripheral sensorium is significant – one need only look at the classic homunculus to see how much afferent information is received from the foot complex. Larkins (2004) claims that 70% of the terminal nervous system is housed in the hands and feet.

Any gait pattern carried out barefoot brings with it the need to scan both the immediate and the upcoming terrain. This requires activation of both the superior oblique extrinsic ocular muscles and, secondary to the oculocervical reflex (Lewit 1999), the deep cervical flexors of the neck and supra/infrahyoid group. As such, for the infrahyoid group to efficiently lever the head into an effective barefoot running posture the suprahyoid group must be in their physiological rest position (Caine 2004, Rocabado & Iglarsh 1990), co-contraction of the styloglossus and hyoglossus being particularly important to achieve stability.

The implications of this are that any kind of barefoot gait is beneficial in terms of central nervous system activation, venous return, injury reduction and in driving optimal tongue position and therefore optimal breathing patterns. Douillard (2001) has researched the effects of nose breathing (an inescapable consequence of having the tongue in its physiological rest position) on trained aerobic athletes, and has found it to consistently improve their times and other measurable parameters, such as their VO$_2$max.

Running

Running is a more explosive gait action – commonly anaerobic, utilized in short bursts (ATP-CP system) – and is only sustainable at top sprint speed for periods of about 8 seconds (Telle 1994). Indeed, it is generally the rule that the most elite 100-meter sprinters in the world are those that decelerate slower than the others toward the end of the race – as opposed to the appearance that they continue to accelerate.

However, running may also utilize fast oxidative, or fully aerobic (slow twitch) fibers. According to Attenborough (2003), the 'persistence hunt' is the most ancient of hunting techniques. This method of hunting involves picking out the (usually largest) male stag of a herd and chasing it and tracking it during the middle of the day. This latter fact is of great significance as:

- humans have a cooling system of sweat glands covering their naked skin which other large mammals do not
- humans walk upright, minimizing their exposure to the overhead midday sun
- humans use a series of energy-conserving sling systems to effect a more efficient gait than tetrapods
- humans have the ability to carry water with them which an animal does not
- the risk of attracting attention from feline predators is at a minimum during the middle hours of the day since they are primarily nocturnal hunters.

Hence, it is suggested that the ability to run is a significant part of our genetic heritage. It is an interesting aside that Beach (personal communication, 2003) states that there is no way that an animal as feeble as Homo sapiens could have traversed every ecosystem of the planet without help from our canine cousins. It is believed that ancestral dogs would have been attracted to the warmth of hominid fires (Koyonagi 2006) when they came on the scene some 230 000 to 1.5 million years ago, depending on which evidence you accept as definitive (Nicholson 1998). Anthropologist Dr Colin Groves now suggests that the human–dog relationship could be almost as old as modern man himself. Basing his hypothesis on a recent DNA research project, Dr Groves uses the results to support his statement that: 'Humans domesticated dogs and dogs domesticated humans' (Koyonagi 2006). It may be no coincidence then that dogs, like humans, also pack hunt, and also run down their prey through endurance or persistence hunting. It may be a truism therefore, that dogs really are man's best friend. Did you ever wonder why dogs get so excited at the idea of going out for a 'walk' with their owner?

Running (as mentioned above under 'Gait'), particularly at high (sprint) speeds, creates a lower axial load through the spine than jogging. It is also, of course, faster than walking or jogging and therefore inherently more stable. Additionally, since sprinting is maximal, there is increased neural drive to the active subsystem, meaning that the spine is under less risk of injury from instability in sprinting than it is in jogging, for example.

Gait as a biomechanical attractor

Gait, in general, can be viewed as a repetitive mobilization of all the joints of the human body. Importantly, the sacroiliac joints, which are the point of summation of ground reaction and descending inertial forces during gait, are mobilized into posterior rotation during the weight-bearing phase of gait via the deep longitudinal sling mechanism. Since heelstrike – and therefore greatest kinetic loading – occurs when the innominate is in its most posteriorly rotated position, it is plausible that the cumulative effect of multiple heel-strikes is a relative posterior mobilization of the innominate, suggested by some authors to be a prerequisite for good sacroiliac joint function (DonTigny 1997). Maintaining the sacroiliac joint in its optimal position is critical to avoid the slackening of the iliolumbar ligament which occurs when the innominate rotates anteriorly and the subsequent compromise of the passive subsystem of the L5–S1 motion segment.

Gait-based activities may also play an important role in normalization of blood sugar regulation, energy levels and mood (see below). This last point may be coupled with the fact that most gait-based activities are outdoor activities and therefore expose the participant to sunlight, which will contribute to rebalancing of disrupted circadian cycles and boost immunity. Due to the rhythmical nature of gait, and particularly if completed while nose breathing, it will result in a meditative state and a mental calming effect.

Biomechanical attractor summary

It is proposed that *archetypal rest* and *instinctive sleep postures* are a homeostatic mechanism to maintain appropriate myofascial length, reduce hypertonus and aid sleep and repair through inhibition of sympathetic activity, supporting digestive function, maintaining joint range of motion, allowing optimal recovery of tendons after activity and helping to repattern the brain through unconscious rehearsal of reptilian crawl patterns.

Primal patterns have a more dominant role in fashioning muscle tone, maintaining joint health through synovial function, supporting visceral health through compression–relaxation cycles, and supporting cardiovascular health through use.

Assessment using primal pattern analysis

The primal patterns may be used to evaluate 'chunks' of the patient's motor skill and programming. If a basketball player, for example, kinesiologically tests well in the lunge pattern, but demonstrates poor motor skill or movement sequencing in the squat pattern, we know which part of his game is most likely deficient – his jump shots and rebounds.

Chunking

Take, for example, the javelin thrower. To throw a javelin efficiently requires a combination of the primal patterns 'lunge', 'twist' and 'push'. A deficiency in any of these patterns, or getting these patterns in the wrong order, will be significantly detrimental to the performance outcome. Hence, in training for the event of javelin, it would be wise to incorporate these three movement patterns into the conditioning program. To train a javelin thrower mainly with squats and standing cable pulls is not likely to enhance their performance (see periodization below for further discussion).

For the javelin thrower therefore, the lunge, the twist and the push can each be considered a 'chunk' of the motor skill required to throw for performance.

For the mum who is a part-time office worker, the lunge, the pull and the push are less likely to be useful movement patterns in which she should become adept. For her, it is far more important to be successful in her environment, to be good at the squat pattern, the twist and the bend pattern. Squatting with optimal form is the start point for good seated posture. If, as for most office workers, the squat pattern is faulty, the office worker will 'hit' the seat with a posteriorly tilted pelvis and a flexed lumbar spine. This starts office workers in an inappropriate and detrimental spinal posture before they even begin their multiple hours at their desk (see 'Neutral spine philosophy' above). The ability to be able to bend with appropriate and effective biomechanics is a critical skill for a parent who has to pick up the children and lift other loads as a component of activities of daily living.

It is a common clinical observation that a patient may be able to properly stabilize and generate power in four or five of these primal patterns, but in the sixth is totally unable to activate their transversus abdominis, for example. This gives us a window into: (1) which movements are likely to have caused the symptoms; and (2) which movement pattern needs to be descended and retrained to prevent future injury.

A study was conducted by researchers in Florida (McCullough et al 2005) to assess the effects of primal pattern training on functional mobility in an elderly population. The purpose of the study was to establish the validity and reliability of using primal movements as an alternative assessment tool for functional mobility in the elderly. Thirty subjects were evaluated with an average age of 81.6 (22 females and 8 males). Tools utilized by physical therapists to assess function, including the Timed Up and Go (TUG), have been shown to be valid and reliable for measuring function, balance and risk of falls in the elderly. A statistically significant correlation between the primal movement functional assessment tool and the TUG suggests that the primal movement grading criteria is a valid tool to assess functional mobility in the community-dwelling senior adult. The inter-rater reliability findings demonstrate that the primal movement functional assessment tool is a reliable tool for assessing functional mobility in the elderly. These findings cannot be assumed to apply to all senior citizens since this was a small group of subjects chosen from a sample of convenience. There was also an unequal distribution of male and female subjects, all of whom regularly participated in a weekly exercise program provided at the retirement community center. Participation in an ongoing exercise program may have conditioned these subjects so that they were more physically fit than the general senior adult population. These findings support the use of primal movements in physical therapy assessment of functional disability in the elderly as well as showing promise for use in physical therapy interventions and as a predictor of falls in the community-dwelling elderly population. Further investigation is warranted to determine the efficacy of primal movements as a functional assessment tool.

To assess for function and/or dysfunction in any of the primal patterns, including gait, there are several simple key assessments to look out for, and which are applicable as foundation observations in any given movement pattern. These key assessment features are summarized in Table 9.18.

It is noted that handedness, footedness or 'laterality' patterns contribute to postural imbalances – particularly in the frontal plane. However, in the context of gravitational strain pathophysiology, and the known

Table 9.18 Key assessment features

Body part	Functional	Dysfunctional
Hallux	In axial alignment with 1st metatarsal, 65° extension when loaded	*Commonly*: Hallux valgus, hallus rigidus (inability to extend great toe of weight-bearing foot to 65°)
Foot	Good arches, lateral malleolus in line with lateral border of foot	*Commonly*: Pes planus, pronation at subtalar joint, Achilles valgus *Sometimes:* Pes cavus, supination at subtalar joint (commonly on short leg as functional compensation)
Knee	Center of patella in alignment with 2nd toe Static load Dynamic load	*Commonly*: • Static: Medial rotation of patella in relation to 2nd toe • Dynamic: Exaggerated medial rotation of patella, commonly with poor control *Rarely*: Lateral rotation of patella relative to 2nd toe
Hip	Controls femur (therefore as above), and in closed chain hitches pelvis in frontal plane	*Commonly*: Trendelenburg or compensated Trendelenburg at hip, poor control of medial rotation
Sacroiliac joint	Innominate posteriorly rotates on sacrum at heel strike, anteriorly rotates on sacrum at toe-off.	Restriction in either direction → restricted step length, or early shift to opposite foot In squat, bend → shift to opposite foot
Lumbar spine	30–35° lumbar curve No frontal plane curvature No hip-back dissociation in lifting Ability to adopt hip-back dissociation on demand	*Commonly*: Flattened lumbar curve, slight 'functional' scoliosis. Striations observed under dynamic load – especially in frontal and transverse plane, e.g. twist pattern *Sometimes*: Hyperlordotic curve, significant 'functional' scoliosis or 'structural' scoliosis
Thoracic spine	30–35° thoracic curve No frontal plane curvature Ability to fully extend (reverse) thoracic curve Ability to maintain neutral curve under load	*Commonly*: Increased thoracic curve – especially at C-T junction – with increased (dropped) 1st rib angle – rib cage held in exhalation *Sometimes*: Flattened portion of thoracic spine, very restricted ± fused zone
Cervical spine	30–35° cervical curve No frontal plane curvature No forward head posture (zygomatic arch directly above sternal notch)	*Commonly*: Forward head posture, head tilt ± rotation *Rarely*: Flattened lordosis, military posture
Upper limb posture	Balanced claviculoscapular complex in frontal plane One-third of humeral head anterior to acromion	*Commonly*: Protraction, shoulder hitching (especially under load) *Sometimes*: Winging, other movement impairment syndromes
Abdominal wall	Observable pre-contraction of transversus abdominis (hollowing) just prior to gross body motion, including heel strike, initial swing Good e-concentric contraction of transversus during quiet breathing	*Commonly*: No observable pre-contraction, no contraction, no lower abdominal contraction. Bracing or flaccidity of transversus during quiet breathing – especially standing *Sometimes*: No upper abdominal contraction

neurological manifestation of joint capsule stress on tonic postural control, such imbalance can never be viewed as 'functional' (see 'Biomechanical attractors' above). Instead, laterality patterns are a dysfunctional result of imbalanced use and therefore a consequence that must be corrected for if the patient is to biomechanically optimize (or 'survive') their environment. This can be easily and successfully achieved with a properly designed corrective exercise program.

Barriers to rehabilitation success

There are two major barriers to rehabilitation success: time and physiological load.

Many patients are already overcommitted with their time before they come in to see us – and commonly this is a component of the symptom etiology. In addition, many patients attending naturopathic clinics do so because they are in pain – not because they want to improve function. This means that a part, or parts, of their body have reached the point where the rate of cumulative stress has outpaced their rate of healing. To add extra load to such a system through corrective exercise may further compromise an already compromised system.

Time

In this day and age, many patients attend health clinics with pain conditions or health complaints that are largely caused by a sedentary lifestyle and the inability to express a perceived stress, such as a deadline or monthly target, with physical reaction, such as running or fighting. Making time for exercise and stretching is a major challenge for many patients. As most therapists know, the best motivator for exercise is symptoms. As soon as the patient is symptom-free, they most commonly 'forget' to do their stretches or exercises, until something else goes wrong some months down the line.

This, in part, can be attributed to the fact that we are probably not designed to 'stretch' for stretching's sake (see 'Biomechanical attractors, Archetypal rest postures' above). Neither are we designed to exercise for exercise's sake (see functional exercise above).

Historically, exercise has had a significant purpose, namely survival. This 'survival' is metaphorically played out by many a sports person and is exactly why people will usually work themselves several times harder chasing after (hunting) a ball, than they will running on a static treadmill in front of a wall, for example.

Studies have shown that working a longer day does not always pay dividends in terms of productivity.

The volume of work completed by workers doing a 12-hour day is equivalent to the volume completed by workers doing an 8-hour day (Pheasant 1991). While the critic may question how motivated the workers were, this study does demonstrate that there is a likely benefit in terms of productivity by 'framing' work duration with strict start–finish boundaries – which may include scheduling some form of exercise program at 5 p.m. or before work starts at 9 a.m.

The whole concept of biomechanical attractors – and in particular instinctive sleep postures and archetypal rest postures – suggests that, if such postures were utilized in the work or home environment, corrective stretching may not be needed at all. This would mean that the precious commodity of time is not spent on mundane stretch programs and could actually form an intrinsic part of the work and home environment.

Strides in this direction have been achieved in some workplaces in Germany (Cranz 2000) where floor-based, seated and standing workstations are utilized. It is the floor-based workstation that specifically offers its own secondary range of working postures – the archetypal postures. As has been discussed above, it is not that sitting should be made more comfortable – quite the opposite. The discomfort experienced with sitting is the body's natural mechanism to move to a new working (or resting) position. To ignore this warning system is akin to taking a painkiller in order to play sport. To try to 'cushion' or dampen this system (as is the objective of most modern ergonomics approaches) is the equivalent of bandaging an ankle in order to play sport. The problem is being acknowledged, but not really addressed. With the rapid evolution of the communications age, with connectivity and wireless gadgetry, multiple workstations are becoming more of a workable reality.

By the same token, utilizing primal patterns, in particular the gait patterns, health of most synovial joints can be maintained, ranges of motion, proprioception, coordination and many of the body's natural pumping and pressure-regulated mechanisms can be preserved (see 'Primal patterns' above).

Physiological load

Physiological load refers to the cumulative total of stressors on the individual's system. This is sometimes referred to as adaptive load. Such physiological load results in increased adrenal stress and commonly reaches a point where adding further load to the figurative 'camel's back' is literally enough to break it.

Exercise as a stressor

Before advising patients to exercise, in whatever form that may take, it is important to recognize that most patients attending a clinic will be attending not because they are well and just want to improve, but because they have musculoskeletal pain and are usually under the influence of multiple visceral, hormonal or limbic-emotional stressors.

It is not unusual, for example, for patients to attend only after 'saving up' an impressive list of symptoms and with pain that has become chronic. Anyone who has chronic pain has a corresponding limbic-emotional load – as pain is stressful and disrupts function. Accompanying will commonly be a number of hormonal stressors and/or imbalances – as pain results in adrenal release (and eventually fatigue). As a result, the patient will most likely have visceral symptoms – as adrenaline shuts down digestive and assimilative processes, sending the body into a catabolic state.

To further load such a patient with a complex exercise program may be exactly the *wrong* thing to do. The concept of adaptational overload – where all forms of therapy, including exercise prescription, are seen as additional stressors – is discussed in Chapter 2, as well as in Chapter 10.

It is important to recognize that the bulk of available literature on training and adaptation to training is taken from young elite sportsmen and women who:

- have higher levels of growth hormone than your average middle-aged patient
- have a greater training age[8] than the average patient
- may be eating more healthily than the average patient
- have a greater genetic propensity for adaptation (hence the reason they are elite athletes).

Physics of exercise (after Bentov 1978)

For many highly driven, type A personality achievers, the idea of relaxation or early nights is completely foreign to them. To many, the way that they relax is by going for a run, playing a game of squash, or doing an 'adrenaline sport' such as rock-climbing, parachute jumps or bungee jumping. However, this simply overlays a high amplitude stress with a second high amplitude stressor. In physics this may be seen to result in an apparent decreased stress level, but the underlying dysfunction has not been effectively dealt with.

---

[8]Training age equates to the number of years that the patient has been training with that methodology. A soccer player, for example, may have 'soccer age' of 20 years, but may have only just started training his lunge pattern with a barbell for one season – therefore his training age for lunging with a barbell is 1.

> **Box 9.9 Assessing physiological load**
>
> Assess yourself: how many indicators do you recognize from the lists below? As a loose rule, the more symptoms from these lists you experience, the higher your physiological load.
>
> 1. Sympathetic indicators:
>   - Poor digestion/↓ salivation
>   - Constipation
>   - Anxiety
>   - ↑ Respiratory/heart rate
>   - Poor sleep quality
>   - Night sweats
>   - Orgasm/genital inhibition
>   - Waking unrested
>   - Nervousness
>   - Jittery
>   - ↑ Muscle tension
>   - ↑ Inflammatory conditions
>   - ↑ Susceptibility to infection
>   - Sensitive to bright lights
> 2. Parasympathetic indicators:
>   - Strong or excessive digestion
>   - Hyperactive bowel; colicky
>   - Incontinence
>   - Orthostatic failure upon rising
>   - ↓ Respiratory rate
>   - Poor sleep quality; *hibernation*
>   - ↑ Mucus secretions
>   - Nervousness; depression; somnolence
>   - Hands warm and dry
>   - ↑ Gag reflex
>   - ↑ WBC count and more allergies
>
> *Note*: Most people who test as being parasympathetic dominant are not dominant in that system because they are exceedingly laid back (though that can occasionally happen!), but instead their sympathetic drive is so exhausted, they have drifted into increased parasympathetic tone (Wolcott & Fahey 2000). This is commonly a sign of significant adrenal fatigue (Wilson 2004).

Stress and breath

Stressors come in many guises: from work stress to relationship stress, financial stress to postural stress, chemical stress to electromagnetic stress. All of these stressors will result in an elevated respiratory rate and, potentially, a subsequent breathing pattern disorder. Such breathing pattern disorders may have a profound effect on the physiology of the body (Chaitow 2004). Respiratory influences on health are discussed more fully in Chapter 10. Refer also to Figure 2.7 in Chapter 2 for a summary of the effects of breathing pattern disorders.

Reflexively mouth breathing and accessory breathing are associated, while nose breathing and diaphragmatic breathing are associated (Chek 1994).

As Douillard (2001) explains, nasal breathing allows the turbinates in the nose to literally turbine the air in the nasopharynx, firstly cleaning particulate matter via the air in the mucous membranes and cilia and, secondly, warming the air so that it will pass deep into the lower lobes of the lungs. In the lower lobes there is a greater preponderance of parasympathetic afferent receptors, while reciprocally in the upper lobes there are more sympathetic afferent receptors. When mouth breathing, cold unfiltered air enters the lungs and will only service the upper lobes (Douillard 2001), presumably due to bronchoconstriction. The deeper, longer inhalation with nose breathing (and, incidentally, humans are the only animal in which obligate nose breathing is no longer 'obligatory') allows for greater stretching of the alveoli, which results in increased production of endogenous nitric oxide. Nitric oxide is a potent sympathetic inhibitor (as well as a stimulator of immune function) – so this is a secondary way that deep breathing will decrease sympathetic and reciprocally increase parasympathetic tone (Douillard 2001).

Consequently, we can see that the physiology of the body can be utilized within breath-based disciplines to switch the patient from a sympathetically charged state to a parasympathetic state. Since parasympathetic stimulation is associated with rest, digestion, tissue repair and anabolic processes, most patients benefit from parasympathetic-enhancing exercises.

Additionally, Douillard (2001) has shown that by manipulating the respiratory environment to breathe using the nasal airway only, helps to enhance performance by keeping the athlete relaxed and focused. Indeed, maintaining a higher level of parasympathetic activity during running and other sports performance makes good sense, when one considers that many sports involve right-brained creative expression as much – if not more – than left-brained logical, strategic expression. It is being in the right brain that is equated with being 'in the zone'. Too much mouth breathing stimulates sympathetic activity and therefore left brain function, meaning that 'thinking outside the box' becomes a challenge (Chek 2006). This may pose a real problem for anyone requiring a creative capacity in their work or home life. Table 9.19 demonstrates some of the benefits to all naturopathic patients from nasal breathing.

Neck stability is also optimal when the tongue is in its physiological rest position (Chek 1994, Rocabado

Table 9.19 Benefits of nasal breathing

Mouth breathing	Nose breathing
Accessory breathing	Diaphragmatic breathing
↓ Nitric oxide	↑ Nitric oxide
Sympathetic stimulation	Parasympathetic stimulation
Air cold	Air warm
Air unfiltered	Air filtered
↓ Neck stability • Tongue on floor of mouth	↑ Neck stability • Tongue in physiological rest position
↑ Left brain activity	↑ Right brain activity
Fight, flight, fright, tight	Rest, digest, decongest, tension-less
Catabolic	Anabolic
Compromised visceral health	Facilitated visceral health
Compromised venous/lymphatic return	Facilitated venous/lymphatic return

& Iglarsh 1990) and nullifies any ability to breathe through the mouth – assuming the tongue posture is correct (Caine 2004). This results in the myriad benefits described in Table 9.19 and is likely to be further facilitated by running barefoot, as this means significant attention must be paid to the upcoming ground beneath the feet. Such attention with the eyes results in facilitation of the deep cervical flexors via the oculocervical reflex (Lewit 1999). For further discussion of barefoot running, see 'Primal patterns, Gait', above.

Muscular system as expression of psychological state

Since the muscles are an innervated continuation of nervous system expression, Keleman (1989) suggests that the muscles may be seen as 'fat nerves'. This is consistent with Schleip's (2003a) observation that the myofascial system provides more afferent feedback to the central nervous system than any of the special senses. As well as their afferent feedback, they are also commonly facilitated (as in muscle imbalance physiology) – an efferent phenomenon. This understanding is important both from a treatment viewpoint and to understand the biography that may be affecting the biology.

Box 9.10 The breath and chi connection: Water...

Water may well be the connection between breath and chi (or prana). Water is one of the most diamagnetic substances known to science, while oxygen is one of the most paramagnetic substances. Just like an electrical circuit, the polar opposite properties of water and oxygen results in work potential, or energy production, when they meet in an 'earthed' human being.

It is well established that, historically, towns and cities have typically grown up around rivers and streams. In the West, such water supplies were most commonly sanitized through distillation. In the East, water supplies were most commonly sanitized through boiling the water and adding leaves with high antioxidant levels. This is the root of the well-established fact that many people of Eastern origin convert alcohol to acetaldehyde more rapidly, resulting in earlier intoxication.* This is a reflection of adaptation to the specific demands of the biochemical environment and is a classic example of metabolic typing, or biochemical individuality in action.

It is interesting to note that many natural health authorities suggest that because Western social drinks (alcohols, black tea, coffee, cola) are diuretics, most Westerners are chronically dehydrated (McKone 1996),

while a common observation of Westerners made by Traditional Chinese Medicine is that they are often yin (water) deficient.

If we place on this foundation the fact that all of the traditional breath-based disciplines (e.g. yoga, meditation, tai chi, Xi gong) developed not in the West, but in the East, the average chronically dehydrated Westerner attending a tai chi class may come away unmoved by their experience. However, a well-hydrated, open-minded Westerner is likely to actually perceive the benefit of the cultivation of chi as a result of the interaction between increased oxygen and well-hydrated cellular machinery (for further discussion of cellular hydration see 'Hydration' section below).

- *Paramagnetism* is the tendency of the atomic magnetic dipoles, due to quantum-mechanical spin as well as electron orbital angular momentum, to align with an external magnetic field. Paramagnetic materials attract and repel like normal magnets when subject to a magnetic field.
- *Diamagnetism* is a form of magnetism that is only exhibited in the presence of an external magnetic field. It is the result of changes in the orbital motion of electrons due to the external magnetic field.

*Such individuals have the genetic alleles alcohol dehydrogenase 2 and dehydrogenase 3. Though to some this may seem a disadvantage, it also means that people with this profile have very low risk of alcoholism.

Janda (1994), for example, discusses the fact that some muscles in the neck, the levator scapulae in particular, may be used to literally 'dump' excessive neural drive from the limbic-emotional system. This enhanced neural drive to the levator and other postural muscles results in the hunched, red-light or upper crossed posture we are all familiar with in stressed states (whether they be emotional, physical, thermal, etc.) (Hanna 1988).

Because the body is a closed system, neural energy generated from nervous system activation – whether it be through chronic pain or acute emotional situations – will result in peripheralization of that neural drive, usually down those pathways that are most facilitated. The common outcome of this is tension in the tonic muscle system and relative inhibition in the phasic muscle system, though there are exceptions (see Table 9.6 for explanation of tonic and phasic muscle characteristics).

The multifidus, transversus and other deep stabilizer muscles have a lower threshold to stimulus (Sahrmann 2002) and therefore are the first muscles to be affected by aberrant neural events at the cord level. Hence, visceral dysfunction or any limbic-emotional

crisis may affect the firing of the deep, local stabilizer system. Since the system is tonic, we might expect that it would become facilitated and tight (as does the pectoralis minor or the levator scapulae), but this depends on the nature of the stimulus and whether that stimulus arrives at the cord via the alpha-afferent or the beta-afferent system. The former (low threshold system) may acutely alter postural reflexes, such as the guarding associated with peritonitis, but the latter system is more associated with activity-dependent plasticity, has greater convergence with the somatic B-afferent nerves and is sensitized by repetitive stimuli from the viscera or limbic systems.

In addition, the Arndt–Schultz law states that a low stimulus will upregulate, while a high stimulus will inhibit physiological processes, so the response of the motor nerve at any given level will depend entirely upon the cumulative inputs into its motor neuron pool from elsewhere.

The notion of the musculoskeletal system as a dampener for aberrant energies from the organ systems, from emotional input or from pain generators is consistent with Traditional Chinese Medicine's meridian theory and with Ayurveda's chakra principles.

Psychology of corrective exercise

Many patients have a faulty rehabilitation model – looking externally, or outside of themselves for someone to fix the problem. While a trained clinician may be better able to understand a patient's symptom profile, it is critical in rehabilitation to both teach patients about their condition as well as to offer advice and coaching as to how to make better choices, whether this involves exercise, nutrition or other lifestyle choices.

In his article 'Motivating Pain Patients', Liebenson (1999) has described some of the following concepts for working with patients. While this kind of approach is most commonly considered applicable to chronic pain patients, it should be equally applicable to acute and all pain patients – particularly bearing in mind that 85% of patients presenting for orthopedic consultation have an unknown causative onset of their pain. This, of course, suggests that the problem is one of cumulative microtrauma based on dysfunctional biomechanical, biochemical or emotional patterns. The list in Box 9.11 is adapted from Liebenson (1999) and should be considered when designing a corrective exercise program for *any* patient:

Movement approaches and mood

Depressive symptomatology is more prevalent among sedentary than physically active individuals (Berlin et al 2006). According to Weinberg & Gould (1999), mental health problems account for 30% of total duration of hospitalization in the USA and about 10% of medical costs – ranking them third as a cause of disability. See topic of depression in relation to exercise influences in Chapter 10.

The effects of exercise on anxiety and depression can be defined as either acute or chronic. The acute effects of exercise on mood tend to focus on state anxiety. The vast majority of research into the effects of exercise on psychological well-being has been conducted using aerobic exercise. Nevertheless, activities such as weight or strength training, yoga, and other 'non-aerobic' exercises have produced positive effects on psychological health (Weinberg & Gould 1999).

Higher levels of physical activity in depressed patients have been shown to be associated with less concurrent depression, even after controlling for gender, age, medical problems and negative life events (Harris et al 2006). Physical activity counteracted the effects of medical conditions and negative life events on depression.

Exercise has been shown to have an irrefutable benefit in helping to optimize mood – both in those who are non-symptomatic and in those with clinically defined depressive episodes (Warburton et al 2006).

Box 9.11 Designing a corrective exercise program

1. Treat 'activity intolerances' rather than pain
2. Set goals (e.g. to be able to play a full round of golf by . . .; to be able to walk to the shops by . . .)
3. Bear in mind socioeconomic effects of pain:
   - Job performance
   - Sports performance
   - Ability to engage in hobbies
4. Bear in mind sexual activity being affected by pain:
   - Does the pain affect libido?
   - Does pain inhibit performance?
   - Feelings of inadequacy or inability to provide
     - effects on relationship
5. Any other lifestyle changes or compromises due to the pain
6. Distinguish between hurt and harm:
   - Pain during an exercise
   - Pain during a stretch
   - Pain after an exercise
     - delayed onset muscle soreness (DOMS)
   - Treatment reaction
7. Manage your patient properly by offering comprehensive information
8. Flare-ups are not failures to manage the pain, but *education* as to how to better manage the pain in future
9. Focus your patient on function rather than pain
10. In order to do this, firstly provide education about the dysfunction, and explain how it arose out of a deviation from normal function
11. Do not over-focus on dysfunction – also explain which areas are functioning well
12. Progress should be monitored every 2–4 weeks to give patients accurate feedback of their changes/improvements
13. Assess using pain provocation tests/quantifiable testing to demonstrate gains

---

How this occurs probably involves many mechanisms, including the fact that exercise is commonly performed in an outdoor environment which allows exposure to sunlight, known to have antidepressant effects and to help to re-regulate circadian rhythms. The exercise itself may also help to re-regulate a disrupted circadian rhythm, thereby aiding sleep and psychogenic restoration. If the circadian rhythm is disrupted, this alone may be a major cause of depression (Spiegel et al 2003). Other benefits of exercise on mood will be due to the ability of exercise to exert a regulatory effect on blood sugar stability – also commonly indicated in episodes of depression (Chek 2003, Holford 1997, 1999, McTaggart 2003). Exercise is also known to increase opiate-like endorphin production in the brain, and may contribute to a natural high from exercise – alongside the possibility of a feel-good factor from knowing that time has been used constructively and to move towards a positive goal.

Similar to antidepressants, exercise has been hypothesized to increase the synthesis of new neurons in the adult brain. Studies on rats reveal a two- to threefold increase in hippocampal neurogenesis with regular access to a running wheel when compared with control animals (Ernst et al 2006). Recent rat studies also show that exercise (in this instance swimming) enhances short-term memory (Alaei et al 2008).

In one study (Berlin et al 2006), 40 regular exercisers were deliberately deprived of exercise across just 2 weeks and assessed using multiple profiles and testing procedures to measure fatigue and somatic depressive symptoms. Both fatigue and depressive symptoms emerged after just 1 week of exercise withdrawal ($p = 0.05$) and subsequently predicted the development of cognitive-affective depressive symptoms at 2 weeks ($p = 0.046$). Exercise withdrawal also resulted in increased negative mood ($p \leq 0.01$), and this increase was correlated with decreases in fitness level ($p = 0.03$). Depressed mood and fatigue are commonly observed in individuals deprived of usual exercise activities, and the increase in fatigue may be partially mediated by reduced fitness levels. For the naturopath, these findings may highlight the importance of recognizing patient mood changes in response to short-term exercise withdrawal following events such as injuries and recovery from medical procedures that do not require full bed rest. This is of particular psychosocial importance for those whose careers, identities or social activities are built around a given sport or activity (see Liebenson's recommendations in Box 9.11 above).

Physical activity is associated with reduced concurrent depression. In addition, it appears that physical activity may be especially helpful in the context of medical problems and major life stressors. Clinically, encouraging depressed patients to engage in physical activity is likely to have potential benefits with few obvious risks – particularly if the guidelines contained within this chapter are followed. Use of exercise to offer similar benefits to the use of antidepressants is of great excitement to the practitioner of natural medicine – offering both fewer side-effects and many additional benefits compared with taking an antidepressant medication.

There is irrefutable evidence of the effectiveness of regular physical activity in the primary and secondary prevention of several chronic diseases (e.g. cardiovascular disease, diabetes, cancer, hypertension, obesity, depression and osteoporosis). Some of this evidence is described in Chapter 10. Governmental physical activity guidelines are variable but commonly fall within the approximate range of 20–30 minutes' duration of >60% of maximal heart rate three to five times per week (Weinberg & Gould 1999). Such guidelines are sufficient to elicit health benefits, especially in previously sedentary people.[9] Commonly, those unaccustomed to exercise use their lack of exercise history as an excuse for not taking on the advice of the clinician to do an exercise program; however, the less conditioned they are, the greater the benefits they will receive (Warburton et al 2006).

Many people who suffer with depression are focused on one or multiple earlier life experiences (such as a bereavement, a divorce, or a time(s) they have felt cheated). Alternatively, such individuals may be focused on a kind of hopelessness about the future and how certain past (or anticipated future) events may impact the potential for future happiness. This means that the focus and energy is not invested in the present but in past events that cannot be changed or future events that may never happen (Tolle 2001). When a negative mental state exists, this compounds and reinforces the pain felt or anticipated. Active engagement in exercise encourages the participant into the present, into the now, potentially decreasing pain, increasing endorphins, and enhancing self-image and self-esteem (see Box 9.12).

Exercise and body composition ratios

While effective motor control and sequencing is far more important to biomechanical function than body fat levels, it is a general trend that if body fat is high, muscle activation and sequencing may be compromised. This can be attributed to a number of physiological cascades – such as the ingestion of allergenic foods resulting in weight gain (Deitsch & Rivera 2002) and concomitantly disrupting activation of the abdominal wall musculature (see 'Viscerosomatic reflexes' below). Similarly, excess bodyweight has an inverse relationship to high physical activity and high performance. Therefore, typically those who have a poor lean body mass ratio will tend to be inactive or sedentary and therefore their underlying neuromuscular function is more likely to be deconditioned. Likewise, those whose nervous system development is poor and/or their inherent biomotor abilities are poor, will tend not to gravitate toward sports, which

---

[9]However, see below as to why these guidelines may fail to help those with excess weight or obesity problems.

Box 9.12 Positive effects of exercise on mood

- Beneficial in mood regulation for both depressed and non-depressed groups
- Re-regulation of circadian rhythms
- Stabilization of glycemic control
- Increased release of endorphins (Weinberg & Gould 1999)
- Potential exposure to sunlight
- Potential social effects of exercise (Weinberg & Gould 1999)
- Feel-good factor of constructive intervention (Weinberg & Gould 1999)
- Synthesis of new hippocampal neurons (Ernst et al 2006)
- Greater effects in sedentary people
- Encourages participant to be 'present'
- Empowerment (Weinberg & Gould 1999)
- Minimal negative side-effects
- Multiple positive side-effects (including decreased risk of cardiovascular disease, diabetes, cancer, hypertension, obesity, osteoporosis and others) (Baechle & Earle 2000, Weinberg & Gould 1999)

---

otherwise may have helped them to overcome their relative physical insufficiencies. For these and other reasons, a poor lean body mass ratio is commonly associated with defective motor control and sequencing.

Since body fat typically tends to deposit in different parts of the body depending on the endocrine dominance (Wolcott & Fahey 2000), it is not possible to generalize and say that all body fat tends to deposit in the abdominal region – as this simply is not the case. However, when adipose tissue does accumulate in the abdominal cavity, this can pose a problem for low back stabilization, since it tends to distend the abdominal wall and promote visceroptosis, which in itself can increase mechanical loading in the back.

Additionally, body fat in excess of the desirable social level is both detrimental physically for health, increasing the risk of a number of significant diseases, and psychologically very damaging for vast swathes of the population.

Hence, there is both good and bad news for those with weight issues. Firstly, the bad news is that excess weight is a health issue which requires addressing just as any other issue for optimal health and therefore for optimal expression of self. Unfortunately, there is much written about weight loss in the popular press – and even taught on professional training courses – which is simply not true. This is part of the reason that

there are so many diet books, exercise fads and miracle cures which only serve to eventually disappoint.

The good news it that with some applied physiology, it certainly is possible to effectively lose weight, but it does require a high level of commitment and persistence – which commonly means a prerequisite of support from friends and family and may well require an additional psychological/emotional support, such as hypnosis, neurolinguistic programming, emotional freedom technique or similar approaches.

Of course, obesity or weight gain should not be seen as a symptom of eating too much food (for which the cure would be to eat less food), but moreover it should be recognized as a symptom of one or more dysfunctional patterns in the sufferer's life. Often combined in the mix are poor food choices, emotional comfort eating, and disappointment with the lack of results from starvation protocols resulting in binge eating. One viewpoint is that being overweight is a sign of metabolic imbalance, just like any other health complaint such as dry skin, allergies, chronic fatigue, etc. When the body chemistry normalizes, weight tends to seek its natural, normal, genetically programmed 'set point'. Balancing body chemistry, improving metabolic efficiency and building good health, rather than attempting to force weight loss, is critical (Wolcott 2006).

Most so-called 'weight loss programs' result in a loss of water or muscle weight, neither of which is desirable. Loss of muscle is particularly unfortunate, as it is actually muscle tissue that is responsible for burning stored fat for energy. Losing muscle means losing the very means whereby you can lose weight effectively. In addition, dieting by cutting calories results in blood sugar fluxes which, in turn, increase the production of lipogenic enzymes and a greater propensity to store energy as fat.

Forcing the body to lose weight without correcting the underlying cause is similar to taking an antihistamine to stop sneezing during hay fever season. Sneezing is not the problem – it is an expression of the problem. When antihistamines are stopped, the sneezing resumes because the cause was not addressed by the antihistamine. Similarly, when the forced weight loss regime is discontinued, excess weight returns, and often with the unhappy new quality of being increasingly difficult to drop with each successive attempt.

Furthermore, since muscle weighs more than fat, should you lose fat while adding lean muscle, your scales would indicate you're gaining – not losing – weight, so weighing scales are not the best monitor of positive changes (Wolcott 2006).

Eating appropriate foods to satisfy your cellular machinery is the realm of metabolic typing and beyond the confines of this chapter. Nevertheless, this approach to weight loss through optimizing your nutritional intake is really without challenge as the best nutritional approach to weight management.

Exercise for weight management

Surprisingly for most, the exercise protocols that are most effective for weight management are commonly far more conducive to the sufferer's life than one might think.

Really there are two ways to effectively lose weight and they are at either end of the exercise spectrum:

- very low intensity, long duration exercise
- very high intensity, short duration exercise.

Method 1

Very low intensity (<50% VO_2max) (Shephard & Astrand 1992) exercise may include walking or gentle cycling sustained for a period in excess of 90 minutes. The use of glycogen for energy production is predominant for the first 30 minutes of exercise (Parker 1998) and by 90 minutes glycogen is all but exhausted (Shephard & Astrand 1992). This is known as 'hitting the wall'. Thereafter, fats become the primary substrate for energy production, and exercise – even at low intensity – becomes a significant challenge. Commencing exercise at a low intensity means that the body will switch to a combination of glycolysis and lipoxidation at an earlier juncture in the exercise session and therefore exercise is sustainable for longer and more fat is burned. This is particularly effective if done first thing in the morning before the night's fast is broken – as the body is already in a lipoxidative state (Shephard & Astrand 1992). If the exerciser starts at a higher pace (>50% max), they will not even begin burning any fat until at least 30 minutes into the exercise program (Parker 1998).

It should come as no surprise that few gym-users exercise on any one machine for longer than 30 minutes as, firstly, their nervous system gets very sedated on static machines so motivation is naturally very difficult to muster and, secondly, most gyms have a policy that you're not allowed to use any given machine for longer than 20 or 30 minutes! This means that weight loss on the cardiovascular machines at the gym is extremely difficult to achieve physiologically and psychologically.

The non-exerciser is caught in a negative spiral where a lack of aerobic conditioning means greater dependence on glycogen to supply energy to the working muscles. With the introduction of exercise, cellular oxidative efficiency improves, so fat is recruited as an energy substrate earlier and earlier in the exercise session. For example, one study showed that the gastrocnemius muscle is seven times more effective at burning fat after marathon training than before (Costill 1979). Of course, the great motivation for the aspiring athlete – whether the goal is to be able to comfortably go for a countryside hike, or to be able to run ultralong distance marathons – is that as soon as they break their previous non-athletic habit, they are in an upward spiral – with each exercise session helping them burn fat earlier in their session, and more efficiently.

The benefit of a low-intensity form of weight loss is that many who need to lose weight dislike the idea of the gym environment, and many spend much of their week indoors, sat-down and overcommitted timewise. To use this form of exercise as a way to 'wind down' and stimulate the parasympathetic nervous system, perhaps on a mid-week day if possible, and once or twice more at the weekend, serves a double benefit.

Method 2

Very high intensity, circuit-based, multijoint training. This approach typically involves lifting loads and/or doing bodyweight exercise, so the exerciser needs to have a minimum of good core function before applying this method (Shephard & Astrand 1992). The exerciser should perform a circuit of between four and six exercises that are at an intensity of 70%.[10] The circuit should be completed without a break moving from one station to the next. At the end of one circuit, the exerciser is allowed up to 1 minute's break, but no more. The circuit should then be repeated a further two or three times (between three and four circuits in total). This approach results in an increased metabolic rate for between 24 and 48 hours after exercising due to a surge in growth hormone as a result of the lactate levels in the blood (Chek 2004d, Poliquin 2006b). This serves to both repair the tissues and to therefore increase metabolically hungry lean muscle mass – meaning the participant burns more calories, even when at rest.

A great benefit of this approach to losing weight is that, for the busy businessman or mother of three

---

[10]An intensity of 70% refers to the percentage of the one-rep maximum lift the exerciser can perform. For example, if the exerciser can lift only 100 kg for one repetition in the squat pattern, then they should be performing this routine (orthopedic concerns cleared) with 70 kg on the bar. How can one calculate their 70% value? There are a number of ways, but the easiest way is to calculate the load that the individual can only lift four times before fatiguing. This load is equivalent to 90% of their 'one rep max'. By dividing this figure by 9, then multiplying the result by 7, the 70% intensity can be calculated. Of course, this form of training may be contraindicated for the pain patient and those with stability issues.

children, this workout can be done in between 20 and 30 minutes from start to finish, yet has fat-burning benefits for a significant period afterward. Across time, this second method will also increase the lean muscle mass, which elevates the basal metabolic rate, meaning that more calories are burned per day, just from being alive – quite aside from further exercise interventions.

Periodizing exercise for weight loss

Some experts in the field of weight loss suggest that combining the two styles of training above within the same session or week is not as effective as persisting with one for a longer period of time (say, 3 weeks) then persisting with the other for a similar period. This is termed 'zigzagging' where the former method works primarily through stimulating catabolic processes, while the latter method stimulates anabolic processes. Switching from a catabolic method to an anabolic method in any one week means that the body doesn't know whether it's coming or going. To take full advantage of either environment (catabolic or anabolic), it is suggested, requires a minimum of 2–3 weeks on each program, with each cycle being repeated across a series of months.

The author suggests that, as a general rule, any conditioning program should either be adapted or completely changed every 6 weeks or less in order to change the stimulus on the body and thereby take advantage of the body's relative inefficiency in the new movement pattern or exercise. If change is not introduced, the body will firstly become increasingly efficient at that movement pattern – and therefore will not burn so many calories – and secondly will be left prone to 'staleness', pattern overload injuries or cumulative trauma disorders.

Other more complex and customized means of losing weight are available through effective evaluation of various physiological factors, such as adrenal function and lactate threshold (J Alexander, C Maund, founders of 'Endurance training for athletes', CHEK Studio, San Diego, personal communication, 2006).

Rehabilitation/movement re-education approaches

Functional training and functional movement patterns

We have discussed functional movement patterns above under the section 'Biomechanical attractors, Primal patterns'. A broad definition of a functional exercise may be 'an exercise which achieves the goal for which it is designed'.

Such a definition is inclusive, inasmuch as an isolation or intramuscular stimulating exercise, such as a machine bench press, may be entirely functional for a bodybuilder trying to achieve hypertrophy, or for an injured patient who needs to rehearse motor control of a given muscle. However, for most sportspeople and for return to full function, intermuscular training is critical and, in general, far more important to optimize performance and decrease injury risk.

More specifically, a functional exercise in terms of activities of daily living and sports is one in which the exercise demonstrates:

1. a comparable reflex profile to stated objective
2. maintenance of center of gravity over base of support:
   - static stability
   - dynamic stability
3. generalized motor program compatibility
4. open/closed chain compatibility
5. relevant biomotor abilities
6. isolation to integration (Chek 2000a).

Examples have been cited in the text as to where many popular exercises have very little functional carry-over to the environment in which the patient lives. Functional carry-over, based on the factors listed above, has to be a primary consideration in the design of any corrective exercise program.

Ascending and descending activities of daily living and sports specific movement patterns

The concept of primal patterns helps the clinician to understand where the patient needs proficiency and movement skill in relation to their activities of daily living and their sports.

An office worker, for example, is in a very static posture for prolonged periods of the day and will need good antigravity muscle endurance. Hence, a corrective exercise that would be ideal for the office worker would be the prone cobra – sometimes referred to as a dorsal raise (see below under 'Examples of big bang exercises'). They would also need to be able to squat with good form to get in and out of their chair with good form.

Descending

An inability to squat may result in the individual 'falling into' and 'hauling themselves out of' their chair. If they are unable to squat due to a strength deficit in, for example, their hip extensor group, descending the squat pattern to a supine hip extension exercise (see Tempo, Example Programs) is an appropriate way to target an appropriate load to the target muscles in a similar movement pattern with a similar reflex profile but less loaded spine.

Ascending

If, after work, this same office worker would normally go to basketball practice, then being able to ascend the squat pattern to a power-oriented jump is a biomotor requirement. If they're unable to do this successfully and safely in the closed environment, they're unlikely to be able to do it successfully or safely in the open environment of competition. Training with heavily loaded squats (1–8 reps, depending on training experience and stability), or with depth squats or more plyometric-based training, is important to prevent injury and optimize performance.

Dynamic versus static stability

Above we have discussed how important it is for the therapist to evaluate the body in both a static assessment in the clinic and in a more dynamic environment – ideally also in the clinic, but possibly in the gym or in the sporting arena.

It is true to say that many sportspeople – and especially those that are commonly injured – reach a point during performance where they surpass their stabilization threshold. In fact, many of these sportspeople go from having one muscle imbalance when standing in the clinic room (e.g. a layered syndrome) to entirely the opposite muscle imbalance (e.g. a lower crossed syndrome) when in the dynamic environment. Also, commonly when under load, the body will migrate to its position of strength – which for most people is the position they spend most of their day in – an upper crossed syndrome. This is what is consistently observed when people lift loads that are too heavy for them, such as when moving a heavy piece of furniture – they most commonly round into an upper crossed syndrome as this is the position in which they are strongest.

Concept of 'big bang' exercises

A big bang exercise is one which works multiple muscles and/or joints, usually in multiple planes of motion and/or has multiple benefits to the user. Therefore it has the characteristic of being extremely efficient in terms of time management and goal attainment.

Examples of big bang stretches (Alexander 2001, Chek 2001b)

90–90 stretch

The 90–90 stretch is considered a big bang stretch as it stretches both the internal rotators of the hip and an external rotator of the hip (piriformis). It also stretches the upper hamstrings and works to facilitate (activate) the lumbar erectors while teaching hip–back dissociation.

Foam roller longitudinal

The foam roller longitudinal is a big bang mobilization as it focuses gravitational force into the thoracic spine to help reverse the thoracic curve, as well as allowing the (usually protracted) shoulders to retract, thereby effectively creating a myofascial stretch on the pectoralis minor. The foam roller can also be placed in such a way as to exert pressure into the suboccipital region, like a therapist performing a suboccipital inhibition. The user can also rotate their trunk on the foam roller from side to side to add a new dimension to the stretch and pump the facet joints without axial load. This adds a balance challenge and, based on the work of Haynes (2003), is likely to result in activation of lumbar multifidus and other deep, intrinsic spinal muscles.

Swiss ball rectus abdominis

The Swiss ball rectus abdominis stretch doubles as a thoracic spine extension mobilization. It can also be modified to target a specific anterior oblique sling by activating one arm and leaving the other rested, or can simply be used to help inhibit external oblique dominance by activating both arms together. Of course, in raising the arms above the head we are putting a stretch into the pectoralis major in particular. This oft-tight muscle can also benefit from this stretch.

Examples of big bang exercises (Alexander 2001, Chek 2001b)

Lower abdominal exercises

Lower abdominal exercises, such as those described by Sahrmann (2002) and Chek (1999b, 2001b), which utilize the legs to focus load on the lower abdominal wall, may be seen as big bang exercises, though they are mainly corrective and not very functional. For example, Chek's 'lower abdominal 2' (2001b), Sahrmann's 'lower abdominal progression – hip and knee flexion with alternate foot unsupported' (2002) and Liebenson's 'dead bug' exercise (2004) involve an alternating extension of the knee and hip (from a fully flexed position) to place load on the abdominal wall. The big bang nature of this exercise includes the following factors:

1. Motor sequencing (inner unit before outer unit contraction)

2. Motor control:
   - transversus must overcome force from rectus abdominis to prevent stomach from 'bulging' and inducing a flexor moment into the lumbar spine
   - a pressure biofeedback unit may be placed under the apex of the lumbar curve (deep to umbilicus) to allow the patient to hone control of the lumbar curve and maintain a neutral spine during loading (see 'Neutral spine philosophy' above for further discussion)
3. Alternating gait-like pattern
4. Asymmetrical load puts emphasis through anterior oblique sling:
   - may be used to bias conditioning through the weaker sling.

Prone cobra

The prone cobra (sometimes called the 'dorsal raise') is an excellent exercise to correct an upper crossed syndrome and may also be discriminatively utilized to correct imbalances at the pelvis. Again, this exercise could not be described as highly functional, but is an excellent corrective exercise. The prone cobra works the following muscle groups:

1. Primary muscle groups worked:
   - thoracic erectors
   - scapula retractors
   - scapula depressors
   - GH external rotators
   - deep cervical flexors
   - long cervical extensors
2. Secondary muscle groups worked:
   - lumbar erectors – including multifidus (for those with a flat lumbar curve)
   - gluteus maximus (for those with lower crossed syndrome).

The prone cobra may also be performed on the Swiss ball, which results in the following changes:

- Decreased leverage on erectors of back
- Increased neurological demand (mainly righting reflex)
- Works hamstrings in lengthened position, if feet are supported by wall – meaning an excellent exercise for correcting a sway posture or layered syndrome (see 'Muscle imbalance physiology' section above)
- Can work in front of the mid-frontal plane.

Due to this last point, the prone cobra from the floor may be the best method of correcting length–tension imbalances in the spinal erector muscles associated with decreased lumbar lordosis and/or increased thoracic kyphosis.

Horse stance vertical

The horse stance vertical is a four-point exercise, which means that there are no exteroceptive stimuli to the outer layers of the abdominal wall facilitating their contraction. This means that it is easier to perform a relatively isolated contraction of the transversus abdominis, before moving the limb girdles – which invokes action of outer unit musculature.

To perform this exercise with correct posture means the spine should be maintained in its neutral position throughout the exercise. To aid this, a wooden dowel rod can be placed longitudinally down the spine to help both the practitioner and the patient to observe for/feel for spinal position. There should be three points of contact with the dowel rod – the sacrum, the mid-thoracic spine and the occiput.

The exercise itself should be preceded by a transversus abdominis contraction (to train optimal motor sequencing) and then the opposing hand and knee should be lifted upward, almost enough to take them off the ground, yet still maintaining a very subtle contact with the ground.

This contact with the ground minimizes the tendency for the patient to shift their weight onto their leg and away from their arm. The subtlety of the movement and the axial torque it induces mean that the intrinsic muscles of the spine will be activated. To maintain a neutral spinal posture and to prevent the stick from rolling off the body, the anterior oblique sling must activate, the rectus abdominis and the lumbar erector spinae must co-contract, the posterior fibers of gluteus medius must activate, and the rotator cuff muscles and serratus anterior, in particular, must all work.

Horse stance vertical primarily works the following muscle groups:

- Anterior oblique sling
- Deep lumbar multifidus (and rotatores)
- Intrinsic muscles of the hip (including gluteus medius)
- Rotator cuff at shoulder (including serratus anterior)
- Deep cervical flexors
- Long cervical extensor (short cervical extensors in lengthened position).

Supine lateral ball roll

The supine lateral ball roll is regarded as a big bang exercise due to the fact that it works the exerciser in all three planes of motion. The hip extension required to keep the body and legs parallel to the ground is the sagittal component, while the lateral movement on the ball is the frontal component and in moving laterally results in a transverse plane torque through the trunk.

The primary muscle groups that resist the torque through the trunk are the anterior and posterior oblique slings. For this reason, the supine lateral ball roll is excellent for rehabilitation of sacroiliac joint instability as a mid/late phase corrective exercise, and due to it working the scapula retractors and gluteal muscles may be useful for correcting both upper and lower crossed syndromes, respectively.

Front squat

The front squat is the same movement pattern as the squat described above under 'Primal patterns', or that is commonly seen in the gym environment where a barbell is placed across the shoulders. However, the difference with the front squat is that the load (whether it be a bar, a dumbbell or a medicine ball) is place atop the chest. This means that the front squat has greater carry-over to most activities of daily living and, because the load is placed on the front (anterosuperior aspect) of the rib cage, it is the muscles on the back (posteroinferior aspect) of the rib cage that have to do most of the work. As such, the front squat works the lower trapezius and the lower thoracic extensors, meaning it is an excellent exercise for correcting an upper crossed syndrome in a functional movement pattern.

The front squat is important to help retrain the sitting pattern, the jumping pattern and lifting technique. It works primarily the lower trapezius, thoracic extensors, gluteus maximus, hamstrings and quadriceps, though also active are all trunk stabilizers, hip–knee stabilizers, soleus and intrinsic muscles of the feet.

Performing a squat wearing a flat shoe, or barefoot, allows for better proprioceptive development, which is important for sporting carry-over.

Standing cable pull

The standing cable pull is an integrated exercise useful for correction of an upper crossed syndrome due to the way it works the scapula retractors, the rhomboids and middle trapezius. Force is primarily generated from the posterior and anterior oblique slings. Due to the fact that this exercise is normally done at a fast to explosive pace, it may be useful as an active mobilization of the thoracic spine.

Because this is a standing exercise, the righting reflex is activated and has a significant carry-over to activities of daily living and to sports.

Big bang benefits

A great benefit of a big bang exercise is that the patient receives multiple gains in one effort. This means that not only is the exercise prescription more efficient but also, because the clinician recognizes that this single exercise is helping the patient on multiple levels, the belief that they can help the patient is enhanced and this enhances the patient's belief in the process. Though it may not be the first thing considered when prescribing an exercise, the placebo effect is nevertheless as present with an exercise as it is with a pill. If the practitioner is convinced that a given exercise will benefit the patient through advanced biomechanical understanding, this will be conveyed to the patient.

For example, comparing the front squat (a big bang exercise) with a crunch from the floor, the conviction in recommending the crunch from the floor would be based on 'it's useful to help you get up off the floor'. Other than that, it has practically no functional carry-over for the patient and commonly compounds muscle imbalances already present including rectus abdominis dominance (since there is little requirement to stabilize when lying on the floor). On the other hand, the list of benefits of the front squat described above speaks for itself and allows the practitioner to confidently relay (verbally and non-verbally) the expected benefit to the patient.

Swiss ball training

The Swiss ball (also known as physio ball, gym ball or stability ball) is perhaps one of the most useful and versatile training devices available to the rehabilitation specialist. Developed by Casani in the 1960s in Italy, the Swiss ball was mistakenly given its geographically incorrect name by American physical therapists who observed their use by clinicians in Switzerland (Chek 1996). In its early days, the Swiss ball was used primarily to rehabilitate those with neural deficits – such as victims of polio. It was also employed by Bobath in her work to help rehabilitate neurologically damaged patients. However, it was only really popularized as a piece of gym equipment in the early 1990s by exercise specialist Paul Chek. Since his pioneering work to explain the benefits of the Swiss ball over the very non-functional machine-based culture in most commercial gyms, the Swiss ball has been increasingly utilized in gyms and in the rehabilitation setting.

What can the Swiss ball be used for?

Many people make the assumption that, because the Swiss ball is a labile surface, the person using it has to activate their stabilizer system to stay balanced on it (in whatever context). However, this is not strictly true. In a gym full of Swiss balls, assuming there's no wind in the room and the floor is flat, the balls will sit still quite happily and exhibit good stability – in fact they would probably sit there for many, many years without becoming unstable. It is what's put on the Swiss ball that is unstable . . . the patient!

Because, for most, use of the Swiss ball is a new movement skill, it can pose something of a challenge on its first few uses. However, anyone without a significant balance problem should adjust to Swiss ball use very quickly and, if they don't, it's all the more evidence that they need to work at it (see discussion below regarding base of support and neurological demand).

Stretching on the Swiss ball

There is some evidence to suggest that use of the Swiss ball for stretching or for corrective exercises facilitates the higher centers involved in regulation of length–tension relationships, particularly the cerebellum. This facilitation may result in a regulation of length–tension relationships – and therefore joint mechanics – more rapidly than static stretching alone (Chek 1996b).

The number of stretches and exercises that can be performed on the Swiss ball is only bound by the imagination (and probably the knowledge) of the user, so the key thing to address is the core principles for Swiss ball use:

1. Initially, most Swiss ball exercises are best completed in the neutral spine posture. This ensures development of strength in the neutral position and means that stresses through the weight-bearing tissues are equally dispersed (see 'Neutral spine philosophy' above).
2. The smaller the base of support, the more neurologically demanding the exercise.
3. The more planes of motion worked through, the more neurologically demanding the exercise (see 'Supine lateral ball roll' above).
4. The transversus should activate when on the Swiss ball; if it fails to do so, the exercise is too advanced for the user.

(See other considerations under the key assessment features outlined in Table 9.18.)

Neural drive/survival reflex

Chek (1996, 2000b, 2001b, 2004e) has described what he terms a survival reflex where the body will reflexively recruit all the muscles it can to avoid an actual, or perceived, catastrophic event. Certainly these observations seem to have good founding, both in the clinical environment and in the neurophysiological literature. For example, Davidoff (1992) explains that the capacity of the segmental myotatic reflex system to compensate for changing loads is only modest. What the Swiss ball does not tend to do is to place the body under significant load (as would occur in some sports or in weightlifting). Davidoff goes on to say that reflexive adjustments at the segmental level may be effective at compensating for perturbation when the errors of position are small and the stretch is rapid (Chek 2000b). This is exactly what we tend to find with Swiss ball use – a small rapid need to correct the posture.

Nitz & Peck (1986) also observe that a characteristic of the deeper, inner unit muscles is that they have an increased concentration of spindle cells, making them particularly important for (and reactive to) stability challenges. As Panjabi et al (1989) discuss, the typically shorter length of the inner unit muscles and their lower threshold to stimulus allow them to react more quickly; hence their response to anything that induces a stability challenge, such as a Swiss ball, wobble board or balance shoes.

Additionally, Janda (personal communication, 1999) comments that a classic way of combating low back pain utilized by the Native Americans was to run in dried-out river beds. Presumably, those of you who have tried to run on the soft sand of a beach will recognize that this probably posed something of a perturbation and/or balance challenge to help reactivate their inner unit.

In contrast, Hides et al (1996) showed that, even 1 year after resolution of low back pain, the lumbar multifidus had not recovered its normal function. They proposed that this may be a mechanism for the onset of chronic back pain. What Hides et al's research implies is that if someone has a pain problem, they cannot properly recover from it unless they see a trained therapist to teach them to consciously activate multifidus/transversus abdominis and other inner unit muscles. However, this may be a somewhat simplified view.

Indeed, the implication would be that prior to Hides et al's research in 1996 – which would include the whole of human evolution – a single bout of low back pain or a back injury would result in compromised inner unit function and therefore presumably compromised ability to move to hunt or to evade predators. In short, the prognosis after even one bout of back pain wouldn't be too good. In their paper, Hides et al do not state how many of their experimental subjects were actively engaged in sports, how many were entirely sedentary – or any shade in between. In a meta-analysis of the high-quality literature available on core rehabilitation in 1998, the author concluded that, since there are so many potential methodological flaws with most exercise prescriptions at that time, it would seem that the best way to effectively rehabilitate function of the core musculature would be to play sports that involved multiple movement patterns.

Since then, knowledge has moved on, and effective core activation can be progressed from floor-based to Swiss ball-based to standing functional exercises, as described throughout this chapter. But to play interactive sports is still a very reasonable piece of advice for core conditioning – assuming that the patient is able to activate their deep stability system when they play their sport. The primal pattern system of assessment described above can be utilized to see if, when and in which movement patterns (motor chunks) the patient is able to activate their core.

This conclusion seemed to coincide somewhat with the concept of the 'survival reflex' and with the nature of existence in the great outdoors. There is little doubt that in running as fast as your body will take you to climb the nearest tree – even perhaps then swinging through the vines to escape a big cat – would be enough to activate both Chek's 'survival reflex' and the perturbations described by Davidoff, and to show some parallels to Liebenson's river-bed running.

Parasympathetic enhancement exercises

Parasympathetic activity is exactly what most pain patients are missing and is commonly a large factor in why rehabilitation may be impeded or arrested. Chronic pain cycles can include a multiplicity of phenomena, but a classic example might be as follows: A pain patient's sleep quality is disrupted because of their pain. They wake feeling tired, so take stimulants throughout the day to keep them alert – this tips their physiology into a sympathetic state and therefore they are catabolic. Their blood sugar fluxes up and down because of the lack of sleep, the stimulant consumption and the pain, so they crave sweet foods – requiring 'sugar fixes' to keep them going. The sensibility of their food choices dwindles, so the availability of nutritional factors for repair becomes limited. They can't wind down in the evening because stimulants such as caffeine have a half-life of 6 or more hours. So they go to bed 'tired, but wired' and are unable to get to sleep. The cycle perpetuates, and all the time they remain catabolic.

This is an example of a patient who would simply 'break down' further if put onto a sympathetic-stimulating corrective exercise program. They first need to address their autonomic imbalance, through parasympathetic work and addressing fundamental lifestyle factors, and then – and only then – should the introduction of sympathetic-stimulating exercise be considered.

Many classical books on Ayurveda, Traditional Chinese Medicine and polarity approaches to rehabilitation have documented many different exercises to support function of a given chakra, element or energy center.

The basis of these exercises is to generate an electromagnetic charge (via gentle muscle contraction) in the region of the targeted energy center of the body. Such a generation of charge – which physicists would view as an action potential on an EMG – would be viewed as the cultivation of chi, or prana, in Eastern disciplines. The production of such energy in these disciplines is believed to have an adaptogenic effect – in the same way that ginseng biochemically is an adaptogen – either upregulating depleted energy when fatigued, or downregulating nervous energy when stressed, as required by the body. In this way, chi, prana or the naturopathic 'vital force' is seen as an intelligent, organizing energy. Normally, exercises designed to cultivate these energies are combined with breath work, visualization and positive affirmations to increase the effect in the intended geographical zone. (For further discussion of breath, see Box 9.10 above.)

One of the prime objectives of parasympathetic stimulation is to avoid any increase in the resting respiratory rate. An increase in breathing rate is a direct indication that the sympathetic nervous system is coming into ascendancy and the exercise is no longer therefore serving its purpose.

Certain exercise categories naturally fill the criterion of 'parasympathetic stimulating'. Traditionally, tai chi, Xi gong, Hatha yoga and meditation in their various forms fit the description best, but there are many other disciplines or activities that stimulate a parasympathetic response – though they are idiosyncratic, of course, based on taste and enjoyment. Examples may include, but are not limited to:

- candle-lit dinner
- bath/jacuzzi
- sauna/steam room
- massage
- reading poetry
- creative writing
- visualization techniques
- chanting/drumming

- singing
- painting/drawing/doodling.

Classical movement and rehabilitation approaches

The purpose of the preceding pages has been to provide a larger contextual framework within which to place the following disciplines. Each of these disciplines has undoubtedly expanded the horizons of how the body may be moved and re-educated, yet all too often they are embraced more as belief systems, rather than tools.

Far from being an encyclopedic regurgitation of the various rehabilitation and movement re-education approaches, hopefully this chapter has provided the reader with a wider appreciation of the benefits and limitations of these and other disciplines.

Alexander technique (see also Alexander technique in Chapter 7, particularly Fig. 7.17)

Underlying premise

The work is based on the premise that our coordination is the deepest and truest expression of who we are, and that, to redirect our energy towards our aspirations, requires a deep and profound knowledge of how we are coordinating ourselves as we do that.

Key principles

The primary object of attention is towards what Alexander called our 'primary control', which can be understood as being how our head movements are affecting the rest of our coordination. Alexander discovered that our head movements govern vertebral coordination, which in turn governs the quality of all our movements.

The second object of our attention is remembering that this is a perfect mechanism – therefore our sole intention is to become aware of how we interfere with its usage, and in turn give up this interference, which then results in free and flexible movement.

The third object of our attention is to realize that if we are successful in the first two, the result will be an entirely new experience not in keeping with anything we have experienced before. We therefore resist trying to be 'right' based on our old idea of 'right' and enjoy the new experiences we are having.

Aston patterning

Underlying premise

The premise is that the environment should be adapted to the human body, not the other way around. It includes perceptions about our body's natural form and function, our processes of learning and self-expression, and our interaction with the physical properties of the planet and our environment. Key to the paradigm is the recognition that the human body is an asymmetrical structure, that its motion and form take on three-dimensional asymmetrical spiral patterns and that each human body is unique.

Key principles

The underlying principle of Aston movement is that each individual body is unique, three-dimensional and subtly asymmetrical, and thus movement naturally forms ascending and descending spirals. There are no straight lines in the body.

True balance and ease come from learning about and cooperating with our natural structures rather than imposing through effort a linear and strict unnatural symmetry. Aston movement allows for individuality. So each body will interpret an exercise in its own unique way. Traditional forms of exercise may try to fit your body into a position, whereas the Aston method aims to fit the exercise to match you – a simple but key difference.

Dr Rolf asked Aston to develop a movement education counterpart to Rolfing, with the aim of helping clients to preserve the changes achieved in the structural integration bodywork. Dr Rolf enrolled Aston in the next Rolf training program in 1968. Aston developed and taught the movement education curriculum from 1971 to 1977.

The Aston-Paradigm® is the empirically based philosophy that emerged from Aston's observations of the movement of energy as it manifests in all human activity. This new paradigm recognizes that nature's asymmetrical three-dimensional spiral can negotiate between seemingly conflicting forces, thereby evoking a dynamic movement. Its perspective can be applied to psychological processes such as teaching and learning, to interpersonal dynamics and to the physical actions that constitute any human task.

When applied to human biomechanics, Aston-Mechanics® shows how, when the body is appropriately aligned, this negotiation through the spiral can be used to dynamically transmit the force of gravity and its complement, ground reaction force. The principles of Aston-Mechanics can be applied to any system of human movement, such as yoga or Pilates training, to any sport, or to playing a musical instrument, as a way of more accurately addressing each individual's limitations and possibilities.

Aston-Patterning®, the integrated system of techniques based on the Aston-Paradigm, includes bodywork, movement education, fitness training and ergonomic applications. In the Aston problem-solving approach, there is no 'ideal body type' to achieve or conform to; the uniqueness of each individual is honored and respected. The practitioner and the client work together in a gentle, precise and powerful way to unravel the layers of history stored in the tissue. Visible changes in alignment and movement patterns accompany the relief felt as the person is guided to discover and redefines his or her natural sense of what feels 'right'.

Brain Gym

Underlying premise

This program is distinctive because it addresses the physical (rather than mental) components of learning. It builds on what the learner already knows and does well; it meets the learner just as he or she is, without any judgment of capabilities; and it teaches the student key elements of learning theory that he or she will be able to apply. Brain Gym is based on the premise that all learning begins with movement, also supporting the idea that any learning challenges can be overcome by finding the right movements to subsequently create new pathways in the brain.

Key principles

- *Laterality* is the ability to coordinate one side of the brain with the other, especially in the visual, auditory and kinesthetic midfield, the area where the two sides overlap. This skill is fundamental to the ability to read, write and communicate. It is also essential for fluid whole-body movement, and for the ability to move and think at the same time.
- *Focus* is the ability to coordinate the back and front areas of the brain. It is related to comprehension, the ability to find meaning, and to the ability to experience details within their context. People without this basic skill are said to have attention disorders and difficulty in comprehending. At a deeper level, focus allows us to interpret a particular moment or experience in the greater context of our lives or to see ourselves as unique individuals within the larger framework of our society.
- *Centering* is the ability to coordinate the top and bottom areas of the brain. This skill is related to organization, grounding, feeling and expressing one's emotions, a sense of personal space, and responding rationally rather than reacting from emotional overlay.

The Brain Gym movements interconnect the brain in these dimensions, allowing us to easily learn through all the senses, to remember what we learn, and to participate more fully in the events of our lives. We are able to learn with less stress, and to express our creativity using more of our mental and physical potential. The movements also assist in clearing emotional stress that can affect us both mentally and physically.

Reported benefits include improvements in such areas as vision, listening, learning, memory, self-expression, and coordination in children and adults. Teachers typically report improvements in attitude, attention, discipline, behavior, and test and homework performance for all participants in the classroom.

Breathing rehabilitation methods (see Chapters 2, 4, 6 (Box 6.45) and 10 for additional notes on aspects of breathing dysfunction)

Underlying premise

- Establish a functional breathing pattern and rate utilizing primary muscles of respiration.

Key principles

- Facilitate use of diaphragmatic breathing through tongue in physiological rest position, and through nasal breathing (see Table 9.19 above).
- Optimal rate of breathing through guided imagery, music, environmental manipulation.
- Multiple factors may be etiological, individually or together, in breathing pattern disorders, including psychological, allergic and nutritional factors.
- Biomechanical influences on breathing pattern may receive special attention, based on the principle that structure and function are so closely inter-related.
- Various disciplines already focus on breathing as a key component of their practice. These may include the Buteyko method, yoga-based therapies, voice training, Xi gong, Traditional Chinese Medicine and even running performance (Douillard 2001).

Core stability training

Underlying premise

- Establish function of the key core muscles for stabilization, for motor control and for performance.
- Movement emanates from the core (Gracovetsky 1988).

- The deep core muscles fire in a feed-forward mechanism – ahead of the more superficial mobilizer muscles (Richardson et al 1999).

Key principles

- Pre-contraction of the inner unit muscles before activating outer unit muscles results in minimal trauma to the passive subsystem of the spine and as a result optimal force generation.
- Conditioning the core muscles and establishing correct sequencing minimizes stress on the spinal and peripheral joints.

Feldenkrais

Underlying premise

- Russian-born Israeli educator Moshe Feldenkrais based the Feldenkrais method on the importance of awareness in human functioning.
- Re-establishment of proprioceptive awareness and movement skill.

Key principles

- Rolling motions mimic the very first movements attempted in ontogenetic development.
- Feldenkrais consists of two branches: Awareness Through Movement® and Functional Integration.
- Feldenkrais believed awareness had to be experienced, not taught verbally. To that end, participants accomplish movements and postures they thought unattainable, producing greater vitality.
- Functional integration involves treating the nervous system primarily through the skeletal structure, by using hands-on, painless manipulation.

Pilates

See Chapter 8 for brief notes on Pilates.

Underlying premise

- Developed by Joseph Pilates as 'active rest' for elite ballet dancers in New York City.
- Works the core muscles with fine control and attention to breathing.

Key principles

- Mainly floor-based or fixed axis machine-based exercise.

- Significant use of core muscles.
- Commonly class-based, though can be one-to-one instruction.
- Has been popularized over recent years, with many hybrid versions appearing and differing standards of knowledge and/or clinical application.

Tai chi

Underlying premise

- Tai chi chuan is an internal Chinese martial art. There are different styles of tai chi, although most agree they are all based on the system originally taught by the Chen family to the Yang family starting in 1820.
- It is often promoted and practiced as a martial arts therapy for the purposes of health and longevity, sometimes even to the point of being taught exclusively as an exercise technique ignoring martial applications entirely (some recent medical studies support its effectiveness).
- Tai chi chuan is considered a 'soft' style martial art, an art applied with as much deep relaxation or 'softness' in the musculature as possible, to distinguish its theory and application from that of the hard martial art styles which use a degree of tension in the muscles.
- Development and integration of inner calm and inner strength with outer strength and control.

Key principles

- Traditional tai chi training is intended to teach awareness of one's own balance and what affects it, awareness of the same in others, an appreciation of the practical value in one's ability to moderate extremes of behavior and attitude at both mental and physical levels, and how this applies to effective self-defense principles.
- Tai chi is considered a soft martial art, and there are many other soft martial arts that have not been described here. This omission is not to negate their value as therapeutic modalities, but to recognize the common thread of most martial arts, i.e. to develop their devotees physically, mentally, emotionally and spiritually.

Trager

Additional discussion of Trager work is found in Chapter 7.

Underlying premise

- A bodywork therapy developed by American medical practitioner Dr Milton Trager in the 1920s.
- Trager work makes extensive use of touch contact, and encourages the patient to experience the 'freeing up' of different parts of the body.

Key principles

- The technique consists of simple exercises called mentastics and deep, non-intrusive, hands-on work.
- The idea is to use motion in the muscles and joints to produce positive sensory feelings which are then fed back into the central nervous system.
- The result is a feeling of lightness, freedom and flexibility. Treatments vary with the individual.

Voice work

Underlying premise

- The voice is our primary means of expression, and, as such, is important for the expression of emotion that may otherwise be suppressed, and for communication and performance.

Key principles

- A combination of posture, breathing work (of which diaphragmatic control is a large part), tongue position and use of vowel sounds allows the constrictors of the pharynx to function optimally and to produce a confident and pleasing resonance.
- Awareness of TMJ function and head posture is particularly important and will be screened to ensure there are no compromises on the voice.
- Voice work raises the confidence and competence of the patient in expressing themselves, thereby enhancing self-esteem and effective communication and expression of ideas.

Xi gong

Underlying premise

- There are in excess of 100 different styles of Xi gong, which can be roughly divided into two categories: the first is Taoist/Buddhist Mi-Tzong (Secret Religion). These methods concentrate on the effort of opening up the channel (meridian) system of the human body. The second category is the Buddhist Zen's way of 'quiet sitting with an empty mind' or Taoist 'Tai Xi'.
- These methods belong to the basic training of the 'Ru Ding', using the methods of accounting the breath, thinking as a special object to gradually eliminate the unconscious random thoughts and reach the state of an empty mind.

Key principles

- The objective of Xi gong is to build qi (also referred to as and pronounced as 'chi') through use of slow rhythmical movement, breath work, attention and intention.
- One biological basis for generating qi is the enhancement of alpha brain waves. This may be the Xi gong practitioner connecting with the Earth's natural Schumann resonance – as described by Oschman (2000).

Yoga

Additional information on yoga research results is given in Chapter 10.

Underlying premise

- Yoga first arose more than 3000 years ago in what we now call India. The word 'yoga' comes from the Sanskrit word *yuj*, which means 'to bind, join, attach, yoke'.
- *Yuj* also means 'union, to direct and concentrate one's attention on, to use and apply'.
- Yoga requires concentrating on your mind and body to bind yourself to God. It's about disciplining yourself to balance your mind, soul and emotions, so that you can connect with your individual spirit (your 'jivatma'), which is, in turn, part of the Supreme Universal Spirit ('Paramatma' or God).

Key principles

There are many different styles of yoga. The term 'yoga' can refer to any of the following:

- Karma yoga – focuses on giving of oneself without expecting any reward
- Jnana yoga – a philosophical approach to unveiling the illusions of the world
- Bhakti yoga – channeling emotional energy into one's spiritual practice
- Raja yoga – focuses on concentration and mind control.

Hatha yoga

Hatha yoga, the physical practice, is a form of raja yoga.

There many forms of Hatha yoga. Current popular styles include (but are not limited to):

- Hatha yoga – a gentle style of yoga. Use of the term 'hatha' is debatable, some believing the term should only be used to refer to the general idea for all physical yogas, while others use it colloquially to refer to the gentler style. In Hatha yoga, the focus is on long stretches and flexibility, with slow, deep breathing (yogic breathing is known as 'pranayama'). This can be very soothing for the mind – it is a parasympathetic-stimulating style of yoga.
- Kundalini yoga, which works on the premise that the body has eight 'chakras' and, through use of 'breath of fire' (rapid breathing), one can heat up the body from the bottom up, eventually 'raising kundalini' to achieve a feeling of high enlightenment.
- Power yoga, which is also known by the Sanskrit term Vinyasa yoga (a 'vinyasa' is a series of rapid movements which warm up the body all over). This is a very active form of yoga, in which a person moves quickly through the poses (called 'asanas'), not holding them as long as in other styles. This is more of a sympathetic-stimulating style of yoga.

Nutritional considerations in rehabilitation

Although nutrition is technically outside of the remits of this chapter, there are two major and important considerations:

1. eating appropriate macronutrient ratios
2. avoiding intestinal irritants.

A third consideration is hydration, which is a prerequisite for good digestion and will be discussed separately below.

Eating appropriate macronutrient ratios

Barry Sears popularized the idea of eating appropriately portioned macronutrient ratios in his highly acclaimed book *The Zone Diet* (1999). However, Sears did not incorporate a model of biochemical individuality (see 'Biomechanical universality' above). Wolcott is considered by many as the forerunner in the field of biochemical individuality or metabolic typing (Chaitow 2002, Wharton 2001). Wolcott's extremely naturopathic book *The Metabolic Typing Diet* (Wolcott & Fahey 2000) and his global network of advisers employ a hierarchical system incorporating all of the major forms of metabolic typing in a prioritized order.

To eat the appropriate macronutrient proportions based on your unique biochemical heritage is a pseudo-scientific, commonsense way of answering the question 'How can I achieve optimal health through nutrition?' without using a double-blind randomized controlled trial on a heterogeneous population (which therefore has no individual specificity). The answer is to look at how we got here – the single biggest experiment in history. What did our ancestors eat? How did they survive in a harsh, competitive environment? How were they selected out by nature? In what environment and with what foodstuffs were they selected out?

These are fundamentally the questions metabolic typing goes a long way toward answering, with excellent clinical results.

Avoiding intestinal irritants

Foods that irritate the digestive system are many. In fact, most foods will irritate the digestive system if eaten in enough quantity as the food in question will always technically be 'non-self' and will eventually spark an immune response resulting in stimulation of ubiquitous mast cells, setting off a cascade of biochemical events leading to inflammation of the digestive tract – see Chek (2003) for further detail.

Such inflammation, if sustained, will create intestinal permeability and sensitize the immune system further. Sensitization of the immune system will, in itself, have a negative impact on the systemic response to inflammatory and repair processes, thereby having a direct impact on rehabilitation.

It is a congruent observation to note that the primary food sensitivities in the Far East are to rice and soya, whereas in the West the primary food sensitivities are to gluten and/or gliadin from all grains (except corn, rice, buckwheat and millet), or to the lactose or casein in dairy (Shils et al 1994). This, then, is a reflection of quantity of consumption – in tandem with the given qualities of the foods in question. The simple interpretation – and reality of the situation – is that the more any one foodstuff is consumed, the more likely your immune system is to respond to it, as described above.

Viscerosomatic reflexes

The net result of cumulative inflammation is repetitive stimulation of the afferent nerves returning to the spinal cord from the digestive tract. As Willard (1997, 2001, 2002) states, the B-afferent visceral nerves specifically are sensitive to repetitive stimuli. This means that they are able to set up a zone of sensitization in the spinal cord at the level of the spinal cord to which they return. This sensitization may travel up to five levels above and below the primary segment affected, though the stimulus will always be greatest at the segmental level of the returning afferent nerve (see Box 9.13).

The various characteristics of the B-afferent system mean it is ideally suited to respond to recurrent stimulation from irritating foodstuffs, from dysbiotic conditions (parasite, candida, other yeasts, amoeba and others), or from alcohol or many medical drugs. A large number of pharmaceutical agents – and NSAIDs in particular – are renowned for causing gastrointestinal (GI) inflammation as a side-effect. In nature, of course, foods are cycled seasonally and geographically – as we know the larger part of the development era that shaped Homo sapiens was nomadic (see 'Primal patterns, Walking' above).

The response of B-afferent stimulation may be manifold. B-afferent nerves have the greatest preponderance in the GI tract, and also have the most neural convergence with other visceral and somatic nerves. They are known to be involved in the inflammatory and general adaptive response, and when activated exhibit plasticity – in other words they may actually change and maintain a new firing rate or level of excitability after the initial stimulus has gone. Often this facilitation of the intrinsic spinal cord circuitry may be maintained for several days after the irritation in the gut has subsided.

A further common clinical source of viscerosomatic reflex is the uterus. The effects of the menstrual cycle on core stability have been studied by Nella (2005). Nella assessed 18 healthy asymptomatic female undergraduate osteopathic students for motor control of their lower abdominal wall using a pressure biofeedback unit. Measurements were taken over the 4 weekly phases of one menstrual cycle. Women were divided into two groups of nine subjects each according to oral contraceptive pill (OCP) status.

Results: A one-way repeated measures ANOVA revealed a statistically significant difference in core stability success rates between weeks ($p < 0.0001$) regardless of OCP status. A post-hoc test revealed that success rate during menstruation was significantly less than other weeks ($p < 0.001$).

Actual results were as outlined in Table 9.20, measured in percentage achieving successful control.

The conclusion of the study was that, regardless of OCP status, lumbopelvic motor control was reduced during menstruation. It was suggested that nociceptive input from the uterus or uterine tubes, which share the same nerve roots as transversus abdominis, may result in increased afferent drive and later the outflow to the muscles, causing them to undergo 'reflex inhibition' resulting in spinal instability.

What is the significance of such visceral sensitization at the cord level?

The significance is that those muscles of the inner unit, whose predominant function is stabilization of joints, have a low threshold to stimulus. This means that any

---

Box 9.13 Characteristics of B-afferent visceral fibers (after Willard 2001)

1. Small fiber system/unmyelinated and myelinated
2. Sensitive to repetitive stimuli
3. Most neural convergence between visceral and somatic B-afferents
4. Nociception and general adaptive response
5. Activity-dependent plasticity
6. Once initiated, intrinsic spinal cord circuitry maintains facilitation.
7. Secrete neuropeptides when activated:
   - substance P
   - somatostatin
   - vasoactive intestinal polypeptide
   - neurokinin A
8. Higher preponderance than A-afferent fibers

Table 9.20 Study results assessing lumbopelvic motor control during different stages of the menstrual cycle

	Preovulation	Ovulation	Postovulation	Menstruation
Exercise 1L	99 ± 2	98 ± 3	96 ± 9	68 ± 22
Exercise 1R	99 ± 5	96 ± 11	97 ± 7	57 ± 21
Exercise 2L	98 ± 5	98 ± 7	95 ± 10	59 ± 20
Exercise 2R	99 ± 2	98 ± 7	98 ± 6	60 ± 20

aberrant stimulus in the spinal cord circuitry is likely to first affect the inner unit muscles.

Why don't patients' transversus abdominis or multifidus muscles 'spasm'?

The most likely explanation is that, in the early stages of facilitation, it may well be that the lumbar multifidus and transversus abdominis have upregulated tone, but since they are well equipped to work for prolonged periods, it is unlikely that the patient would notice any adverse effects of this increased tone. In fact, they may feel even better than normal. However, when the stimulus reaches a given level, in accordance with the Arndt–Schultz law: 'A high stimulus inhibits physiological processes, and a low stimulus facilitates physiological processes.' Therefore, in the example of the multifidus or transversus, these low threshold muscles will be the first to become inhibited.

Inhibition is described by Richardson et al (1999) as the most likely explanation for their findings where they identified that within 2 weeks of the onset of low back pain, the lumbar multifidus may shrink to 69% (±8%) of its original size when viewed on magnetic resonance imaging. This shrinkage cannot be explained by atrophy within such a short time-frame. The only explanation could be a decreased neural drive and therefore decreased tone resulting in decreased cross-sectional area. This correlates with clinical findings of apparent lack of firing of the muscle, combined with the fact that the muscle may begin to fire when the neural drive is enhanced through perturbation or 'survival reflex' stimulation (see above).

As we know, anatomically the spinal level of innervation of the GI tract corresponds very closely with the innervation of the key stability muscles of the lumbopelvic region.

Hydration

Not only is hydration critical for its well-documented role in performance but also it is essential for tissue repair, for loading of the tissues and for chi-based (parasympathetic-enhancing) exercise.

Tissue repair

Hydration at the cellular level helps to maintain cell volume and is critical for tissue repair. As Waldegger et al (1997) state, the paramount importance of cell volume for the regulation of cell function, including protein metabolism, is well recognized. Cell shrinkage, as a result of dehydration, stimulates proteolysis and inhibits protein synthesis. This is corroborated by Ritz et al (2003) who state that protein metabolism is probably regulated by cellular hydration in humans. In a state of dehydration the body will compensate by borrowing water from its stores – 66% from the intracellular reservoir, 26% from extracellular sources and about 8% from the blood volume (Batmanghelidj 2001). Quite aside from musculoskeletal dysfunction, a decrease in cell volume correlates with catabolic states in a variety of diseases (Haussinger et al 1993). Peripheral tone is increased to compensate for decreased blood volume, thereby slowing the rate of injury healing in the extremities (Batmanghelidj 2001.

Hydration at the cellular level also affects cell adhesion properties and so may be an important determinant in clotting and other tissue repair mechanisms.

Tissue loading

It is well documented that the weight-bearing joints of the body operate on a hydrostatic pressure mechanism whereby the loads involved in static and dynamic posture are transduced through the joint (or disc) fluid through to the next structure up the kinetic chain. If we took as an example the knee when jumping, we would see that up to nine times bodyweight is directed from the ground reaction force upward through the tibia into the knee joint where the tibial cartilage will direct that force into the synovial fluid, and the synovial fluid will translate the force into the femoral cartilage and into the femur. This force then passes in a similar way through the hip and sacroiliac joints into the spine where it will sequentially derotate the facets and discs, storing potential energy in each of the facet cartilages and annuli. This stored energy is converted to kinetic energy at the next step (Gracovetsky 1988, 1997, 2001, 2003). This a mechanical component of the interlimb coupling observed in humans whenever their gait speed exceeds 0.75 meters/second (Van Emmerick et al 1999).

A dehydrated body will draw fluids from relatively non-vital reserves (joints and discs) in order to maintain vital functions such as digestion, respiration and blood pressure regulation (Batmanghelidj 2001). The medium/long-term consequence of this is early degenerative change in the discs or in the articular cartilage of the usually non-touching joint surfaces.

Chi cultivation

Due to the subtle quantum properties of water and oxygen, when the two combine it is theorized that work potential is realized and energy is harvested. This has been termed 'chi' in Chinese philosophy, 'qi' in Japanese philosophy, 'prana' in Hindu philosophy, and 'life-force' or 'vitality' in naturopathic philosophy (see Box 9.10 above for further discussion).

Model of dimensional mastery

Hopefully the model of dimensional mastery will put any corrective program that is designed for the patient into a relevant context. The patient should not be left at the level of the amoeba (transversus abdominis activation with a pressure biofeedback cuff), nor should they be started at the level of primate (unloaded transverse plane) if they are not even functioning well at the fish level (frontal plane)!

This chapter has, in some detail, discussed the dimensions through to the 4th dimension of time. However, it would be remiss to not consider where this model may lead if followed to its logical conclusion – which is the 5th dimension – or the spiritual realm.

Though spirituality is, for some, contentious, there are no known cultures in the world that do not have some form of spiritual belief system – a framework within which to place their unanswerable questions and to gain a true sense of purpose (Hick 1999).

Such pursuit of answers to the challenges faced in life can not only stimulate hope but also act as a catalyst to think: How can I learn from this problem? What can I do to remedy or to 'flow with' this problem?

In this way, even the most calamitous of events can be seen from a symbolic, a meaningful or purposeful perspective, which in itself is health promoting. To quell the concerns a Newtonian scientist might have at this thought, it is known from pharmaceutical production, from cognitive behavioral psychology and from neurophysiology, amongst others, that the overriding influence on the motor neuron pool is the limbic-emotional system (Davidoff 1992, Willard 1997)

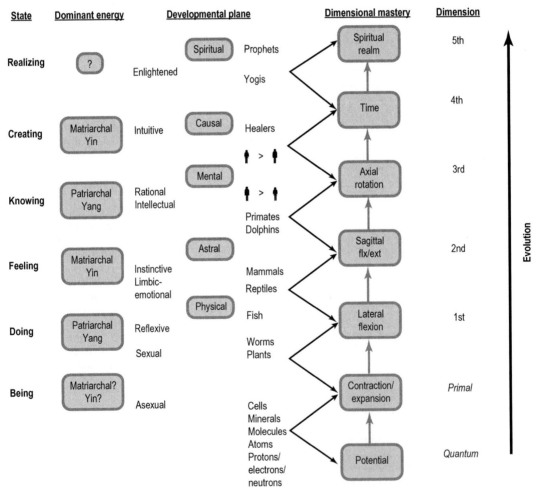

Figure 9.24 Dimensional mastery model. flx/ext, flexion-extension

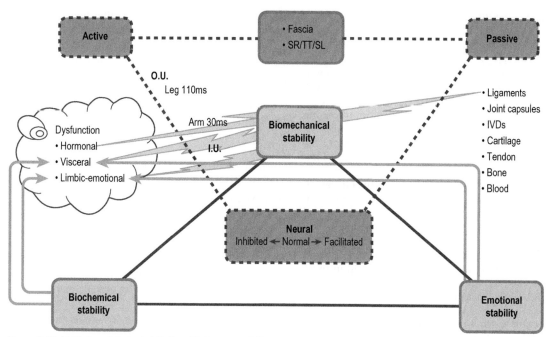

Figure 9.25 Unified model of rehabilitation. I.U., inner unit; IVDs, intervertebral discs; O.U., outer unit; SL, sarcolemma; SR, sarcoplasmic reticulum; TT, t-tubule

and therefore what that person believes. With this in mind, there is no way that spirituality, psychology, limbic-emotional, visceral and many other factors can be ignored in the study of rehabilitation, as exemplified by the naturopathic triad, the model of dimensional mastery (Fig. 9.24) and the unified model of rehabilitation above (Fig. 9.25).

The unified model of rehabilitation

To review the chapter and to summarize it down into a synoptic diagram, it can be seen that rehabilitation and movement re-education techniques may be approached from multiple dimensions – and may incorporate physical, mental, emotional and spiritual modalities.

It is hoped that this holistic view of movement rehabilitation has added competent, qualified and, most importantly, clinically useful observations to the current knowledge-base in this field. Not all that has been discussed has been tested in randomized, controlled, double-blind trials, but then we know that reductionist research methodologies investigating the parts – for all of their value – simply cannot effectively add up to the function of the whole organism we have presenting in practice. For this a combination of physiology, anthropology, neurology, clinical observation

and the current randomized controlled trial knowledge-base provides a balanced path forward. In some instances, quantitative research will never find statistical significance in a concept we know physiologically to be true. In such cases a statistically meaningful result could be chased for a matter of years – with the only true result being disappointment, while in the meantime many thousands of people could have been helped if what is known through other means were applied.

In general, if the body is under stress or in pain (whether the source is biochemical, physical, limbic-emotional or spiritual) there is increased cortisol secretion. Perpetuation of this situation brings with it a detrimental impact on the ability to repair tissues (Wilson 2004). Additionally, if the pain associated with this stressor is sustained it may inhibit the inner unit musculature associated with the stressed area (Richardson et al 1999). This compromises biomechanical stability and sets up a positive feedback cycle of further wear and tear (stress), resulting in decreased active subsystem control due to pain inhibition. Ultimately, the passive subsystem tends to take the brunt of the neural and active subsystem's incompetence.

If there is a problem with emotional stability this, too, adds to the cortisol drive inhibiting tissue repair in the longer term. Another common cause of emotional instability in women is premenstrual syndrome. Premenstrual syndrome is hypothesized to be associated with the biochemical instability 'estrogen-dominance' (Heitz et al 1999). Increased estrogen levels have been suggested to compromise ligamentous function (Faryniarz et al 2006, Heitz et al 1999, Wojtys et al 2002) by binding with the estrogenic receptors in these connective tissues, thereby compromising the passive system and increasing the risk of injury. In the same patient, the visceral afferent drive from the uterus will be increased secondary to uterine inflammation and/or pain (Nella 2005). Since the uterus also reflexes to the thoracolumbar cord, like the GI tract, it has the propensity to inhibit the inner unit of the lumbopelvic region, adding to the relative instability and injury risk (see 'Viscerosomatic reflexes' above).

If the body is eating the wrong macronutrient ratios it will become hormonally challenged and will result in decreased ability to repair tissues. If, within these macronutrients, there are any foodstuffs that irritate the digestive tract (or there is another pharmaceutical or dysbiotic stressor in the gut tube), the inner unit muscles will be the first to become compromised due to their low threshold to stimulus. This knocks out the active subsystem and biomechanical stability becomes compromised. Examples of how this model may be applied to ensure optimal biomechanical stability are endless, but the point of the exercise is to illustrate that without consideration of this unified model, clinical success will not be close to realizing its potential.

The unified model of rehabilitation (Fig. 9.25) combines some of what is known about biochemical influence on the stability of the body, with some of what is known about limbic-emotional factors and demonstrates that, without integration, the clinician can only expect disintegration.

References

Adams M, Bogduk N, Burton K, Donan P 2002 The biomechanics of back pain. Churchill Livingstone, Edinburgh

Ahlberg P 2001 The missing link. Horizons – BBC Science and Nature. 1 February 2001. BBC 2

Alaei HA, Moloudi RA, Sarkaki AR 2008 Effects of treadmill running on mid-term memory and swim speed in the rat with Morris water maze test. Journal of Bodywork and Movement Therapies (in press)

Alexander C 1994 Utilization of joint movement range in arboreal primates compared with human subjects: an evolutionary frame for primary osteoarthritis. Annals of Rheumatic Diseases 52:720–725

Alexander J 2001 CHEK Level I certification. Intensive 9 day training course. Harbour Club, London

Alfredson H, Lorentzon R 2000 Chronic Achilles tendinosis: recommendations for treatment and prevention. Sports Medicine 29(2):135–146

Alfredson H, Ohberg L 2002 Ultrasound guided sclerosis of neovessels in painful chronic Achilles tendinosis: pilot study of a new treatment. British Journal of Sports Medicine 36(3):173–175; discussion 176–177

Allen RE 1990 The concise Oxford dictionary of current English. Oxford University Press, Oxford

Alter M 2004 Science of flexibility, 3rd edn. Human Kinetics, Champaign, IL

Anderson J 2000 Sleep related behavioural adaptations in free-ranging anthropoid primates. Sleep Medicine Reviews 4(4):355–373

Astrand PO, Rodahl K, Dahl H, Stromme S 2003 Textbook of work physiology, 4th edn. Human Kinetics, Champaign, IL, p 1–7

Attenborough D 2002 The life of mammals. BBC Books, London

Attenborough D 2003 The life of mammals, DVD series. BBC Productions, London

Backster C 2003 Tapping into the etheric field. In: Primary perception: biocommunication with plants, living foods, and human cells. White Rose Millennium Press, Anza, CA, p 75–76

Baechle T, Earle R 2000 Essentials of strength training and conditioning, 2nd edn. Human Kinetics, Champaign, IL

Barnes M 1997 The basic science of myofascial release: morphologic change in connective tissue. Journal of Bodywork and Movement Therapies 1(4):231–238

Batmanghelidj F 2001 Your body's many cries for water. Tagman, London

Bentov I 1978 Stalking the wild pendulum – on the mechanics of consciousness. Bantam Books, New York

Berlin AA, Kop WJ, Deuster PA 2006 Depressive mood symptoms and fatigue after exercise withdrawal: the potential role of decreased fitness. Psychosomatic Medicine 68(2):224–230

Berrill N 1954 Sex and the nature of things. Gollancz, London, p 149

Bogduk N 1997 Clinical anatomy of the lumbar spine and sacrum. Churchill Livingstone, Edinburgh, p 81–85, 117–118

Bompa T 1999 Periodization training for sports. Human Kinetics, Champaign, IL

Boos N, Rieder R, Schade V et al 1995 Volvo Award in clinical sciences. The diagnostic accuracy of magnetic resonance imaging, work perception, and psychosocial factors in identifying symptomatic disc herniations. Spine 20(24):2613–2625

Bradley D, Chaitow L, Gilbert C 2002 Multidisciplinary approaches to breathing pattern disorders. Churchill Livingstone, Edinburgh

Bradley N 2001 Age-related changes and condition-dependent modifications in distribution of limb movements during embryonic motility. Journal of Neurophysiology 86(4):1511–1522

Brand P, Yancey P 1994 Pain, the gift that nobody wants. HarperCollins, New York

Brennan B 1988 Hands of light: a guide to healing through the human energy field. Bantam Books, New York

Brostoff J, Gamlin L 1998 The complete guide to food allergy and intolerance. Bloomsbury, London

Bryson B 2003 A short history of nearly everything. Doubleday, London

Buettner D 2005 The secrets of long life. National Geographic Magazine, November

Bullock-Saxton J, Murphy D, Norris C, Richardson C, Tunnell P 2000 The muscle designation debate: the experts respond. Journal of Bodywork and Movement Therapies 4(4):225–241

Butler D 1994 Mobilisation of the nervous system. Churchill Livingstone, Edinburgh

Caine A 2004 Voicegym book. The Voice and Body Centre, Southampton

Chaitow L 2001 Muscle energy techniques, 2nd edn. Churchill Livingstone, Edinburgh

Chaitow L 2002 Individuality. Journal of Bodywork and Movement Therapies 6(3):141–142

Chaitow L 2004 Breathing pattern disorders, motor control and low back pain. Journal of Osteopathic Medicine 7(1):33–40

Chek P 1994 Posture and craniofacial pain. In: Curl DD (ed) Chiropractic approach to head pain. Williams & Wilkins, Baltimore, p 121–162

Chek P 1995 Program design – choosing reps, sets, load, tempo and rest periods. Correspondence course. CHEK Institute, San Diego, CA

Chek P 1996 Swiss ball training. Correspondence course manual. CHEK Institute, San Diego, CA

Chek P 1999a Advanced program design. Correspondence course. CHEK Institute, San Diego, CA

Chek P 1999b The golf biomechanics manual. CHEK Institute, Vista, San Diego, CA

Chek P 2000a Movement that matters. CHEK Institute, Vista, San Diego, CA

Chek P 2000b How to activate 'survival reflexes' for improved strength. Online. Available: www.dragondoor.com/articler/mode3/231/

Chek P 2001a Flatten your abs forever. Video. Producer: CHEK Institute, Vista, San Diego, CA

Chek P 2001b Scientific core conditioning. 2 day seminar. Maidenhead, UK. Organizer: www.paulchekseminarsuk.com

Chek P 2001c Nutrition and lifestyle coach certification course. Brighton, UK. Organizer: www.paulchekseminarsuk.com

Chek P 2001d The outer unit. Online. Available: www.coachr.org/outer.htm, and www.ptonthenet.com/displayarticle.aspx?ArticleID = 102

Chek P 2002 Scientific back training. 2 day seminar, Brighton, UK. Organizer: www.paulchekseminarsuk.com

Chek P 2003 How to eat, move and be healthy. CHEK Institute, San Diego, CA

Chek P 2004a Breathing squats, spinal position and chi flow. CHEK Forum, 29 January 2004. http://health.groups.yahoo.com/group/chekforum/message/1313

Chek P 2004b Balance training for the elderly. Online. Available: www.mercola.com/2005/apr/9/balance_training.htm

Chek P 2004c Fear the squat no more! Parts I and II. Online. Available: www.mercola.com/2004/jul/28/fear_the_squat.htm

Chek P 2004d How to get off your fat and get the fat off! Online. Available: www.mercola.com/2004/nov/13/get_off_fat2.htm

Chek P 2004e How to activate 'survival reflexes' for improved strength and function. Online. Available: www.mercola.com/2004/jun/19/survival_reflexes.htm

Chek P 2006 Nutrition and lifestyle coaching – level III training. Copenhagen, Denmark. Organizer: www.alun.dk

Comerford M, Mottram S 2001 Functional stability retraining: principles and strategies for managing mechanical dysfunction. Manual Therapy 6(1):3–14

Cordain L 2002 The Paleo diet. Wiley, New York, p 32–57

Costill D 1979 A scientific approach to distance running. Tafnews Press, Los Altos, CA, p 60

Cowie C 1999 The female triad. Osteopathic Sports Care Association 2nd Annual Conference, Leighton Buzzard, Bedfordshire

Cranz G 2000 The Alexander technique in the world of design: posture and the common chair. Journal of Bodywork and Movement Therapies 4(2):90–99

Cresswell A, Grundstrom H, Thorstensson A 1992 Observations on intra-abdominal pressure and patterns of abdominal intra-muscular activity in man. Acta Physiologica Scandinavica 144:409–418

Critchley D 1990 Butterworth's medical dictionary. Butterworths, London

Croft A 1995 Management of soft tissue injuries. In: Foreman SM, Croft AC (eds) Whiplash injuries: the cervical acceleration/deceleration syndrome, 2nd edn. Williams & Wilkins, Baltimore

Davidoff R 1992 Skeletal muscle tone and the misunderstood stretch reflex. Neurology 42:951–963

De Waal F, Lanting F 1997 Bonobo: the forgotten ape. University of California Press, Berkeley, CA

Deitsch R, Rivera R 2002 Your hidden food allergies are making you fat. Random House, New York

Diepersloot J 1997 Warriors of stillness. Center for Healing and the Arts, Walnut Creek, CA

DonTigny R 1997 Mechanics and treatment of the sacroiliac joint. In: Vleeming A, Mooney V, Dorman T, Snijders C, Stoeckart R (eds) Movement, stability and low back pain – the essential role of the pelvis. Churchill Livingstone, New York, p 461–476

Douillard J 2001 Body, mind, and sport, Three Rivers Press, New York, p 147–168

Drews U 1995 Color atlas of embryology. Thieme, New York

Dvorak J, Dvorak V 1990 Manual medicine: diagnostics. Thieme, Stuttgart, p 35–45

Edwards S 2000 Neurological physiotherapy – a problem-solving approach. Churchill Livingstone, Edinburgh, p 6–7

Elias J, Faust A, Chu YH, Chao E, Cosgarea A 2003 The soleus muscle acts as an antagonist for the anterior cruciate ligament – an in vitro experimental study. American Journal of Sports Medicine 31(2):241–246

Ernst C, Olson AK, Pinel JP, Lam RW, Christie BR 2006 Antidepressant effects of exercise: evidence for an adult-neurogenesis hypothesis? Journal of Psychiatry and Neuroscience 31(2):84–92

Erwin D, Valentine J, Jablonski D 1997 The origin of animal body plans. American Scientist 85:126–137

Faryniarz DA, Bhargava M, Lajam C, Attia ET, Hannafin JA 2006 Quantitation of estrogen receptors and relaxin binding in human anterior cruciate ligament fibroblasts. In Vitro Cellular and Developmental Biology, Animal 42(7):176–181

Gerber R 2000 Vibrational medicine for the 21st century. Piatkus, London

Gilbert C 1998 Breathing: an essential component of bodywork. Journal of Bodywork and Movement Therapies 2(2):64–65

Gleim G, McHugh M 1997 Flexibility and its effects on sports injury and performance. Sports Medicine 24(5):289–299

Glenister T 1958 A correlation of the normal and abnormal development of the penile urethra and of the infra-umbilical abdominal wall. British Journal of Urology 30:117–126

Goldfield E 1995 Emergent forms: origins and early development of human action and perception. Oxford University Press, Oxford

Gracovetsky S 1988 The spinal engine. Springer, Vienna

Gracovetsky S 1997 Linking the spinal engine with the legs: a theory of human gait. In: Vleeming A, Mooney V, Dorman T, Snijders C, Stoeckart R (eds) Movement, stability and low back pain – the essential role of the pelvis. Churchill Livingstone, New York, p 243–252

Gracovetsky S 2001 Analysis and interpretation of gait in relation to lumbopelvic function. In: Proceedings of the 4th Interdisciplinary World Congress on Low Back and Pelvic Pain, Montreal

Gracovetsky S 2003 The story of the vertebrate spine. Evening lecture. Royal Geographical Society, London. Organizer: www.chekclinic.com

Gracovetsky S 2004 Stability or controlled instability? 1 day workshop, London. Organizer: www.chekclinic.com

Grimes K 2002 Hunted! New Scientist 2338:34–36

Hanna T 1988 Somatics – reawakening the mind's control of movement, flexibility and health. Perseus Books, Cambridge, MA, p 49–59

Harris AH, Cronkite R, Moos R 2006 Physical activity, exercise coping, and depression in a 10-year cohort study of depressed patients. Journal of Affective Disorders 93:79–85

Hartley L 1995 Wisdom of the body moving. North Atlantic Books, Berkeley, CA

Hartman LS 1997 Handbook of osteopathic technique, 3rd edn. Chapman & Hall, London

Haussinger D, Roth E, Lang F, Gerok W 1993 Cellular hydration state: an important determinant of protein catabolism in health and disease. Lancet 341(8856):1330–1332

Hawker G, Wright J, Coyte P et al 2000 Differences between men and women in the rate of use of hip and knee arthroplasty. New England Journal of Medicine 342(14):1016–1022

Haynes W 2003 Rolling exercises designed to train the deep spinal muscles. Journal of Bodywork and Movement Therapies 7(3):153–164

Haywood K, Getchell N 2005 Life span motor development, 4th edn. Human Kinetics, Champaign, IL

Heglund N, Schepens B 2003 Ontogeny recapitulates phylogeny? Locomotion in children and other primitive hominids. In: Bels VL, Gasc J-P, Casinos A (eds) Vertebrate biomechanics and evolution. BIOS Scientific, Oxford

Heitz NA, Eisenman PA, Beck CL, Walker JA 1999 Hormonal changes throughout the menstrual cycle and increased anterior cruciate ligament laxity in females. Journal of Athletic Training 34(2):144–149

Herbert R, Gabriel M 2002 Effects of stretching before and after exercising on muscle soreness and risk of injury: systematic review. British Medical Journal 325:468

Hick 1999 The fifth dimersion: an exploration of the spiritual realm. One World, Oxford

Hides J, Carolyn A, Richardson C, Jull G 1996 Multifidus muscle recovery is not automatic after resolution of acute, first episode low back pain. Spine 21:2763–2769

Hodges P 1999 Is there a role for transversus abdominis in lumbo-pelvic stability? Manual Therapy 4(2):74–86

Hodges P, Heijnen I, Gandevia SC 2001 Postural activity of the diaphragm is reduced in humans when respiratory demand increases. Journal of Physiology 537(3):999–1008

Holford P 1997 The optimum nutrition bible. Piatkus, London

Holford P 1999 100% Health. Piatkus, London

Hopkins H 2006 Sleep stages. Alegent Health, Sleep, and Breathing Disorder Laboratory, Omaha, NE. Online. Available: www.sleepdisorderchannel.net/stages/

Hungerford B, Gilleard W, Hodges P 2003 Evidence of altered lumbopelvic muscle recruitment in the presence of sacroiliac joint pain. Spine 28(14):1593–1600

Hunter G 2005 Hamstring strain in professional football. Football Association Medical Society Non-League Conference, Lilleshall, UK, October 2005

Ingber D 1999 How cells (might) sense microgravity FASEB Journal 13:S3–S15

Janda V 1968 Postural and phasic muscles in the pathogenesis of low back pain. Proceedings of the XIth Congress of the ISRD, Dublin, p 553–554

Janda V 1978 Muscles, central nervous motor regulation and back problems. In: Korr M (ed) Neurobiologic mechanisms in manipulative therapy. Plenum Press, New York, p 27–41

Janda V 1983 On the concept of postural muscles and posture in man. Australian Journal of Physiotherapy 29:83–84

Janda V 1994 Muscles and motor control in cervicogenic disorders: assessment and management. In: Grant R (ed) Physical therapy of the cervical and thoracic spine. Churchill Livingstone, New York

Janda V, Va'Vrova M 2005 Sensory motor stimulation. In: Liebenson C (ed) Rehabilitation of the spine – a practitioner's manual. Lippincott Williams & Wilkins, Philadelphia, p 319–328

Kapandji I 1974 The physiology of the joints, vol 3: the trunk and the vertebral column. Churchill Livingstone, Edinburgh, p 20–21

Kapandji I 2003 Fuzzy biomechanics. 1 day workshop, London. Organizer: British School of Osteopathy

Kardong K 2002 Vertebrates. McGraw-Hill, New York

Keleman S 1989 Emotional anatomy. Center Press, Berkeley, CA, p 90

Kendall F, McCreary E, Provance P 1993 Muscles, testing and function. Williams & Wilkins, Baltimore

Kent G, Carr R 2001 Comparative anatomy of the vertebrates, 9th edn. McGraw-Hill, Dubuque

Knobloch K, Schreibmueller L, Kraemer R et al 2007 Eccentric training and an Achilles wrap reduce Achilles tendon capillary blood flow and capillary venous filling pressures and increase tendon oxygen saturation in insertional and midportion tendinopathy: a randomized trial. American Journal of Sports Medicine 35:673

Korr I 1978 Neurobiologic mechanisms in manipulative therapy. Plenum Press, New York

Koyonagi M 2006 Evolution of dogs. Online. Available: www.suite101.com/article.cfm/about_dogs/12072

Kuchera M 1997 Treatment of gravitational strain pathophysiology. In: Vleeming A, Mooney V, Dorman T, Snijders C, Stoeckart R (eds) Movement, stability and low back pain – the essential role of the pelvis. Churchill Livingstone, New York, p 477–499

Kuno M 1984 A hypothesis for neutral control for the speed of muscle contraction in the mammal. Advanced Biophysics 17:69–95

Lardner R 2001 Stretch and flexibility: its importance in rehabilitation. Journal of Bodywork and Movement Therapies 5(4):254–263

Larkins P (ed) 2004 Run faster, easier and injury free – your bare feet are key. Running Fitness September:32–34

Larsen W 1998 Essentials of human embryology. Churchill Livingstone, Edinburgh

Lederman E 1997 Fundamentals of manual therapy. Churchill Livingstone, Edinburgh, p 105

Lee D 2003 The integrated approach to the thorax. 2 day course, London. Organizer: www.physiouk.co.uk

Lee D 2004 The pelvic girdle, 3rd edn. Churchill Livingstone, Edinburgh

Lee D 2005 Recent advances in the assessment of the lumbopelvis. Evening lecture, British College of Osteopathic Medicine, London

Lewit K 1999 Manipulative therapy in rehabilitation of the locomotor system, 3rd edn. Butterworth-Heinemann, Oxford

Leys S, Eerkes-Medrano D 2006 Feeding in a calcareous sponge: particle uptake by pseudopodia. Biological Bulletin 2(11):157–171

Liebenson C 1999 Motivating pain patients. Journal of Bodywork and Movement Therapies 3(3):143–146

Liebenson C 2002a Functional exercises. Journal of Bodywork and Movement Therapies 6(2):108–113

Liebenson C 2002b Are prolonged sitting postures bad for the back? Journal of Bodywork and Movement Therapies 6(3):151–153

Liebenson C 2002c Taking micro pauses: patient's information for self-help procedures. Journal of Bodywork and Movement Therapies 6(3):154–155

Liebenson C 2003 Activity modification advice: Part 1 – the hip hinge. Journal of Bodywork and Movement Therapies 7(3):148–152

Liebenson C 2004 Spinal stabilization – an update. Part 3. Journal of Bodywork and Movement Therapies 8(4):286–287

Lorenz B, Bohnensack R, Gamulin V, Steffen R, Muller WE 1996 Regulation of motility of cells from marine sponges by calcium ions. Cellular Signalling 8(7):517–524

Lovejoy C 1988 Evolution of human walking. Scientific American 259(5):118–125

Lovejoy C 2005 The natural history of human gait and posture. Part 1: Spine and pelvis. Gait and Posture 21:95–112

Lovejoy O, Latimer B 1997 Evolutionary aspects of the human lumbosacral spine and their bearing on the function of the lumbar intervertebral and sacroiliac joints. In: Vleeming A, Mooney V, Dorman T, Snijders C, Stoeckart R (eds) Movement, stability and low back pain – the essential role of the pelvis. Churchill Livingstone, New York

Lovejoy C, McCollum M, Reno P, Rosenman B 2003 Developmental biology and human evolution. Annual Reviews of Anthropology 32:85–109

Ludewig P, Hoff M, Osowski E, Meschke S, Rundquist P 2004 Relative balance of serratus anterior and upper trapezius muscle activity during push-up exercise. American Journal of Sports Medicine 32(2):484–493

McCullough L, Litwin B, O'Conner K, Weiser E 2005 A randomized trial of primal movements to assess functional mobility in the elderly adult. Journal of the American Physical Therapy Association. Online. Available: www.apta.org/AM/abstracts/pt2005/abstractsPt.cfm?pubNo = PO-RR-36-TH

McGill S 2002 Low back disorders: evidence based prevention and rehabilitation. Human Kinetics, Champaign, IL

McKenzie R 2003 The lumbar spine: mechanical diagnosis and therapy. Spinal Publications, Waikanae, NZ

McKone WL 1996 Osteopathic athletic health care: principles and practice. Chapman & Hall, London

McTaggart L 2003 The field: the quest for the secret force of the universe. HarperCollins, London

Morgan E 2001 The aquatic ape hypothesis. Souvenir Press, London

Morris D 1982 Man watching: a field guide to human behaviour. Grafton Books, London

Morris D 1985 Body watching: a field guide to human species. Grafton Books, London

Murray M, Pizzorno J 2000 Encyclopaedia of natural medicine. Little, Brown, Boston

National Osteoporosis Foundation 2006 Information available at: www.nof.org/osteoporosis/diseasefacts.htm

Nella C 2005 The effects of the menstrual cycle on core stability. British College of Osteopathic Medicine BSc (Hons) Thesis, University of Westminster, London

Neumann D 2002 Kinesiology of the musculoskeletal system. Mosby, St Louis

Newman Turner R 1990 Naturopathic medicine. Thorsons, Wellingborough, p 26

Nicholson W 1998 Fire and cooking in human evolution, rates of genetic adaptation to change, hunter-gatherers, and diseases in the wild. Online. Available: www.beyondveg.com

Nitz A, Peck D 1986 Comparison of muscle spindle concentrations in large and small human epaxial muscles acting in parallel combinations. American Surgeon 52(5):273–277

O'Connor J, McDermott I 1997 The art of systems thinking. Thorsons, Wellingborough

O'Rahilly R, Müller F 2003 Human embryology and teratology. Wiley-Liss, New York

O'Reilly J, Ritter D, Carrier D 1997 Hydrostatic locomotion in a limbless tetrapod. Nature 386:269–272

Oschman J 2000 Energy medicine. Churchill Livingstone, Edinburgh

Oschman J 2004 Our place in nature: reconnecting with the Earth for better sleep. Journal of Alternative and Complementary Medicine 10(5):735–736

Oxford Park Academy 2006 Sponges – phylum porifera. Oxford Park Academy, Overland Park, Kansas. Online. Available: www.geocities.com/sciencejanetc/7th_8th_grade/animal_kingdom/sponges.html

Panjabi M, Abumi K, Duranceau J, Oxland T 1989 Spinal stability and intersegmental muscle forces. A biomechanical model. Spine 14(2):194–200

Parker J 1998 Heart monitor training, 2nd edn. Cedarwinds Publishing, Tallahassee, FL, p 63–64

Pheasant S 1991 Ergonomics, work and health. Palgrave Macmillan, Basingstoke, p 161–163

Platzer W, Kahle W, Frotscher M 2000 Color atlas and textbook of human anatomy: locomotor system (Flexibook), 4th edn. Thieme, Stuttgart

Poliquin C 2006a Modern trends in strength training. Poliquin Performance Center, East Greenwich, RI

Poliquin C 2006b The German body comp program. Poliquin Performance Center, East Greenwich, RI

Proctor B 2003 The freedom series – CD Home Learning Series. Online. Available: www.bobproctor.com

Radinski L 1987 The evolution of vertebrate design. University of Chicago Press, Chicago

Raff R 1996 The shape of life – genes, development, and the evolution of animal form. University of Chicago Press, Chicago

Richardson C, Jull G, Hodge P, Hides J 1999 Therapeutic exercise for spinal segmental stabilization. Churchill Livingstone, Edinburgh

Ritz P, Salle A, Simard G et al 2003 Effects of changes in water compartments on physiology and metabolism. European Journal of Clinical Nutrition 57(Suppl 2): S2–S5

Rizk N 1980 A new description of the anterior abdominal wall in man and mammals. Journal of Anatomy 131(3):373–385

Robinson G 2006 Plant cell cytoskeleton. Online. Available: http://sun.menloschool.org/~birchler/cells/plants/cytoskeleton

Rocabado M, Iglarsh Z 1990 Musculoskeletal approach to maxillofacial pain. Lippincott Williams & Wilkins, Philadelphia

Roithmann R, Demeneghi P, Faggiano R, Cury A 2005 Effects of posture change on nasal patency. Revista Brasileira de Otorrinolaringologia (English ed.) 71(4):478–484

Sahrmann S 2002 Diagnosis and treatment of movement impairment syndromes. Mosby, St Louis, p 23–27

Sahrmann S 2005 Diagnosis and treatment of movement impairment syndromes – the upper extremity. 2 day workshop, Manchester, UK. Organizer: www.physiouk.co.uk

Sale D 1988 Neural adaptation to resistance training. Medicine and Science in Sports and Exercise 20(5 Suppl):S135–145

Schaefer R 1987 Clinical biomechanics, musculoskeletal actions and reactions. Williams & Wilkins, Baltimore

Schleip R 2003a Fascial plasticity – a new neurobiological explanation. Part 1. Journal of Bodywork and Movement Therapies 7(1):11–19

Schleip R 2003b The stretching debate. Journal of Bodywork and Movement Therapies 7(2):104–116

Schleip R 2003c Fascial plasticity – a new neurobiological explanation. Part 2. Journal of Bodywork and Movement Therapies 7(2):104–116

Schmidt R, Wrisberg C 2000 Motor learning and performance. Human Kinetics, Champaign, IL

Sears B 1999 The zone diet. Thorsons, London

Shephard R, Astrand P 1992 Endurance in sport. Blackwell Scientific, London, p 127–130

Shils M, Olsen J, Shike M 1994 Modern nutrition in health and disease. Lea & Febiger, Philadelphia

Siff M 2003 Transversus abdominis revisited. Online. Available: www.ptonthenet.com/displayarticle. aspx?ArticleID = 1929

Slosberg M 1988 Effects of altered afferent articular input on sensation, proprioception, muscle tone and sympathetic reflex responses. Journal of Manipulative and Physiological Therapeutics 11(5):400–408

Snijders C, Vleeming A, Stoeckart R, Mens J, Kleinrensink G 1997 Biomechanics of the interface between spine and pelvis in different postures in movement stability and low back pain. In: Vleeming A, Mooney V, Dorman T, Snijders C, Stoeckart R (eds) Movement, stability and low back pain – the essential role of the pelvis. Churchill Livingstone, New York, p 103–114

Sole R, Goodwin B 2000 Signs of life – how complexity pervades biology. Basic Books, New York, p ix–11

Spiegel K, Leproult R, Van Cauter E 2003 Impact of sleep debt on physiological rhythms. Revue Neurologique (Paris) 159(11 Suppl):6S11–20

Spring H, Illi U, Kunz H-R et al 1991 Stretching and strengthening exercises. Thieme, Stuttgart

Stokes B 2002 Amazing babies: essential movement for your baby in the first year. Move Alive Media, Inc. Online. Available: www.amazingbabies.com

Stone C 1999 Science in the art of osteopathy. Stanley Thornes, Cheltenham

Telle J 1994 Beyond 2001 the next real step: new approaches to scientific training for the advanced body builder. Edict, Denver, CO, p 216–217

Tetley M 2000 Instinctive sleeping and resting posture: an anthropological and zoological approach to treatment of low back and joint pain. British Medical Journal 321:1616–1618

Tolle E 2001 The power of now. Hodder & Stoughton, London

Tracy B 1997 The luck factor. Nightingale Conant, Niles, IL

Van Emmerick R, Wagenaar R, Van Wegen E 1999 Interlimb coupling patterns in human locomotion: are we bipeds or quadrupeds? Annals of the New York Academy of Sciences 860:539–542

Vaughn B 2003 The stretching debate. Journal of Bodywork and Movement Therapies 7(2):80–96

Verma K 1999 Ethics and aesthetics. Eubios Journal of Asian and International Bioethics 9:12–13

Vines G 2005 Put a wild wobble in your walk. New Scientist 2531:51

Vleeming A 2003 Movement, stability and low back pain. One day workshop, Birkbeck College, London. Organizer: www.physiouk.co.uk

Vleeming A, Snijders C, Stoeckart R, Mens J 1997 The role of the sacroiliac joints in coupling between spine, pelvis, legs and arms. In: Vleeming A, Mooney V, Dorman T, Snijders C, Stoeckart R (eds) Movement, stability and low back pain – the essential role of the pelvis. Churchill Livingstone, New York, p 53–71

Vojta 2006 What is reflexlocomotion and how does it work? Online. Available: www.vojta.com/cgi-local/ivg_eng.cgi

Waldegger S, Busch GL, Kaba NK et al 1997 Effect of cellular hydration on protein metabolism. Mineral and Electrolyte Metabolism 23(3–6):201–205

Wallden M 2008 The hamstring syndrome. Part 1. Journal of Bodywork and Movement Therapies (in press)

Wallden M, Patel A 2008 A caveat to the feed-forward mechanism of the transversus abdominis? Spine (in press)

Warburton DE, Nicol CW, Bredin SS 2006 Health benefits of physical activity: the evidence. Canadian Medical Association Journal 174(6):801–809

Warburton M 2001 Barefoot running. Sportscience 5(3). Sportsci.org/jour/0103/mw.htm,2001

Weinberg R, Gould D 1999 Foundations of sport and exercise psychology, 2nd edn. Human Kinetics, Champaign, IL, p 355

Wenberg S, Thomas J 2001 Post traumatic vision syndrome and the locomotor system: Part 1. Journal of Bodywork and Movement Therapies 4:4

Wharton C 2001 Metabolic man – ten thousand years from Eden. WinMark Publishing, Orlando, FL

Willard F 1996a Somatic dysfunction generated by visceral problems. The feedback loop. AAO Convocation video, American Academy of Osteopathy, Indianapolis, IN

Willard F 1996b Somatic dysfunction generated by joint surface irritation. AAO Convocation video, American Academy of Osteopathy, Indianapolis, IN

Willard F 1996c Somatic dysfunction generated by nerve root irritation. AAO Convocation video, American Academy of Osteopathy, Indianapolis, IN

Willard F 1997 The autonomic nervous system. In: Ward R (ed) Foundations for osteopathic medicine. Williams & Wilkins, Baltimore

Willard F 2001 Somatovisceral interactions at the spinal cord level. Course Notes, British College of Naturopathy and Osteopathy, London

Willard F 2002 Viscerosomatic and somatovisceral integration. Course Notes, British College of Osteopathic Medicine, London

Willard F, Mokler D, Morgane P 1997 Neuroendocrine-immune system and homeostasis. In: Ward R (ed) Foundations for osteopathic medicine. Williams & Wilkins, Baltimore

Williams P 1995 Skeletal muscle – non-myofibrillar structures of the sarcoplasm. In: Gray's anatomy, 38th edn. Churchill Livingstone, Edinburgh, p 739–764

Williams P, Goldspink G 1973 The effect of immobilization on the longitudinal growth of striated muscle fibers. Journal of Anatomy 116:45–55

Williams P, Goldspink G 1978 Changes in sarcomere length and physiological properties in immobilized muscle. Journal of Anatomy 127:459–468

Williams R 1956 Biochemical individuality. Keats Publishing, New Canaan, CT

Williams R 1988 Biochemical individuality, 2nd edn. McGraw-Hill Contemporary, New York

Wilson J 2004 Adrenal fatigue – the 21st century stress syndrome. Smart Publications, Petaluma, CA

Wojtys E, Huston L, Boynton M, Spindler K, Lindenfeld T 2002 The effect of the menstrual cycle on anterior cruciate ligament injuries in women as determined by hormone levels. American Journal of Sports Medicine 30(2):182–188

Wolcott W 2006 Excellence in health. Online. Available: www.healthexcel.com

Wolcott W, Fahey T 2000 The metabolic typing diet. Doubleday, London

Wyke B 1979 Neurological mechanisms in the experience of pain. Acupuncture and Electro-therapeutic Research 4:27–35

10

Leon Chaitow ND DO

With contributions from:

Hal Brown ND DC

Nick Buratovich ND

Brian Isbell PhD ND DO

Lisa Maeckel MA CHT

Dean E. Neary Jr ND

David Russ DC

Roger Newman Turner ND DO

Naturopathic Physical Medicine Approaches to General Health Enhancement and Specific Conditions

In this chapter research studies (commonly osteo-pathic and/or chiropractic) relating to a selection of named conditions are discussed. However, this should not be taken to mean that the treatment methods being reviewed are necessarily recommended for use in a naturopathic setting. The objective of their inclusion in the chapter is to offer a sense of the scope and potential influence on health, deriving from physical medicine interventions, rather than creating a veritable cookbook of therapeutic choices.

Some of the manual methods that are described – both specific and general – appear to be effective in assisting homeostatic regulation of physiological functions (Hoag 1977, Kuchera & Kuchera 1991). However, the authors wish to be clear from the outset that the citations offered do not provide conclusive evidence of efficacy, only that the data strongly suggest the usefulness of the modalities and methods, when applied in a wide range of pathological or dysfunctional settings, whether the condition can be specifically diagnosed or not.

General approaches (as discussed particularly in Chapters 7 and 8, and historically in Chapter 3) have been demonstrated to benefit patients with a variety of named conditions or syndromes (see evidence/citations in Chapters 3, 7 and 8, and in this chapter).

By extrapolating such evidence, there emerge *general constitutional guidelines* regarding useful therapeutic physical medicine approaches that may variously improve immune function, lymphatic drainage and circulation, encourage a more balanced autonomic function, and assist respiration and elimination, as well as modulating pain, while enhancing other physiological functions.

In this way, a generic, rather than specific, model of naturopathic care is provided, in which manual and/or hydrotherapeutic and/or electrotherapeutic interventions (where appropriate), synchronous with biochemical and/or psychosocial interventions (also where appropriate), are selected in order to encourage self-regulation.

Thus, in naturopathic terms, they are seen to be influencing or stimulating the *vis medicatrix naturae* to operate more efficiently – as in the examples of shorter duration hospital stays reported on in Chapter 7 (and in this chapter).

In this way naturopathic principles can be seen to have been translated into practical clinical approaches.

Integrated, not isolated, interventions

It is self-evident that when treating general health problems manual methods should seldom be applied in isolation, but should rather be offered alongside attention to the individual's specific biomechanical, biochemical and/or psychosocial/emotional needs.

Even when treating apparently localized biomechanical/musculoskeletal conditions – such as painful tenosynovitis affecting the elbow, for example – naturopathic physical medicine requires attention to the context out of which this problem has evolved, calling for an integrated approach.

The individual's history, posture and current activities, as well as biochemical and psychological status, may all have an influence of what appears to be a localized inflammatory process, accompanied by pain, edema and restricted movement.

The local condition would clearly receive attention – possibly involving variations on the theme of hydrotherapy, electrotherapy, soft tissue or joint manipulation, acupuncture, etc. In addition, nutritional, botanical and/or homeopathic strategies that encourage self-regulatory functions might usefully be prescribed – as appropriate in any given situation. Additionally, stress coping and other strategies could be advised to avoid behavioral changes. This combination of inputs, to an apparently localized condition, would be an ideal naturopathic response.

As mentioned, one focus of this chapter is towards identifying practical, evidence-informed, physical medicine clinical approaches to named conditions or syndromes, deriving from the osteopathic, chiropractic, physical therapy, massage, hydrotherapy and more general therapeutic literature, in the hope that this will encourage their use as part of comprehensive naturopathic care, that also includes nutritional, psychological, botanical and other modalities. These associated complementary modalities and methods are, however, not detailed.

Apart from specific physical medicine approaches, general mobilization protocols, incorporating both osseous and soft tissue manipulation, are recommended. These commonly have no specific objective in mind, but possess the potential to offer multiple, health-enhancing benefits.

Generalized naturopathic physical medicine methods are discussed in Chapter 3, as well as in Chapter 8, and below.

General approaches – and the lack of evidence from purely 'naturopathic' sources

Along with the use of specific therapeutic interventions, as indicated by evidence (see this chapter as well as Chapters 7 and 9), naturopathic practitioners are strongly urged to incorporate aspects of general osteopathic or general naturopathic approaches, or general therapeutic massage as described in Chapter 7, in care of patients – *whatever their health problems may be*.

The question may legitimately be asked as to why, in this chapter (and others), does the supporting evidence for, say, manipulation and other physical medicine modalities not derive directly from naturopathic research?

When research evidence was being evaluated and collected for this book, searches of major data banks such as Medline, ScienceDirect and Scopus resulted in the accumulation of some 700 studies in which the key words *naturopathy* or *naturopathic* appeared in the titles or abstracts.

Of these studies, apart from a handful in which hydrotherapy was identified, and one in which massage was mentioned, *none* described any aspect of physical medicine, or any of the modalities discussed in Chapter 7. The almost exclusive focus was on the biochemical aspect of patient care – nutritional, botanical medicine and homeopathy.

The massage paper mentioned above described the work of the German physician Georg Groddeck (1866–1934) who pioneered a combination of psychotherapy and massage techniques in the treatment of very ill patients, whose illnesses he considered to be psychosomatic in origin. Groddeck's approach, over 100 years ago, showed 'the importance of a combination of psychosomatic medicine and naturopathy for contemporary medicine' (Häfner 2005).

The data search results relating to naturopathy demonstrated clearly that physical medicine strategies are almost totally ignored when it comes to research into, or reviews of, naturopathic medicine. There is therefore no evidence to present, from such sources, in this chapter.

However, there is an abundance of evidence deriving from osteopathic, chiropractic, physical therapy, massage and yoga sources, for example, of methods that *do* form part of naturopathic training and practice, and these are therefore the sources that have been used in this chapter to validate naturopathic physical medicine's employment of the variety of modalities, listed below, in care of patients with a variety of named conditions and pathologies.

Before evaluating the evidence for the use of physical medicine modalities in health care, it is appropriate to briefly offer an overview of what naturopathic physicians or practitioners are taught during their training, in the arena of physical medicine, and what aspects of these methods they use in practice.

What is taught to NDs, and what is currently practiced, in naturopathic care of patients?

The notes below summarize aspects of naturopathic physical medicine training in Canada, USA, Australia and the UK, as well as key points taken from a 2006 survey of naturopathic doctors in Canada relating to their use of physical medicine (Verhoef et al 2006). A perspective is also offered regarding German naturopathic medicine.

Additional information derives from an analysis of insurance statistics involving some 600 000 enrollees from western Washington State in 2002 (Lafferty et al 2006), as well as from a 2004 Australian survey of naturopathic and (Western) herbal medicine practitioners (Bensoussana et al 2004).

Before evaluating aspects of the results of these surveys, and details of ND training, a widely accepted definition of naturopathic physical medicine should be restated.

Naturopathic physical medicine (and manipulative therapy) defined

In Chapter 1 (Box 1.5) extracts were given from the *Position Paper on Naturopathic Manipulative Therapy*, published by the American Association of Naturopathic Physicians (AANP) (Buratovich et al 2006).

This is an important document, with elements of its content worthy of repeating, in order to emphasize the unique nature of naturopathic physical medicine, in which practitioners with a wide range of integrated manual and physical skills are seen to be capable of treating not only musculoskeletal dysfunction but also broader health issues, as well as aiming to 'optimize the structure and function of healthy individuals'.

An abbreviated version states (for fuller extract see Box 1.5, Chapter 1):

- Naturopathic physicians use appropriate diagnostic and imaging methods with physical medicine modalities and procedures as part of an integrated approach to the diagnosis and treatment of the full spectrum of health disorders . . . including but not limited to the musculoskeletal/postural, nervous, circulatory, respiratory, metabolic, psychosocial, and bioenergetic systems.
- Naturopathic physical medicine (NPM) is the therapeutic use . . . of the physical agents of air, water, heat, cold, sound, light and the physical modalities/procedures including but not limited to hydrotherapy, electrotherapy, diathermy, ultrasound, ultraviolet, infrared and

low level laser light, therapeutic exercise, naturopathic manipulative treatment and the use of needling and injection therapies, including dry needling, regenerative injection therapy (prolotherapy), mesotherapy, neural therapy and myofascial trigger point therapy.

- Naturopathic manipulative treatment (NMT) is treatment by manual and other mechanical means of all body tissues and structures . . . [involving] the use of oscillation, thrust, and sustained tension including but not limited to high and low velocity techniques, high and low amplitude techniques, traction, mobilization through physiologic and extra-physiologic ranges of motion, including passive intrinsic mobility of all body joints, and repositioning of displaced body tissues and organs.

- Naturopathic medical education includes . . . courses devoted specifically to NPM and NMT and integrated with other courses and clinical experience and prepares NDs to competently perform NPM and NMT, to recognize the limits of their skills, understand the risks, contraindications and limitations of the modality and to refer patients to specialists when appropriate.

Generalist or specialist?

It is important to remember that naturopaths are trained to be generalists, to ensure that after qualifying as physicians (in the USA and Canada) or practitioners (with a Bachelor's degree, in the UK and Australia), they are competent health care providers, capable of integrating the many naturopathic modalities proficiently – including physical medicine, homeopathy, nutritional medicine, botanical medicine, counseling and health psychology, as well as other naturopathic modalities such as acupuncture.

At graduation many NDs already have specialist qualifications – for example, in chiropractic, osteopathy or physical therapy. And many ND graduates, subsequent to graduation, choose to go on to a second phase of professional training in order to achieve a full discipline level of skill, a specialization, to add to their generalized naturopathic skill competence.

The primary naturopathic training therefore aims to produce competent generalists, and this should be kept in mind when evaluating the details of training discussed below.

Canadian survey evidence (Verhoef et al 2006)

A useful survey of naturopathic medicine in Canada offers insights into the range of physical medicine modalities used by naturopathic physicians and practitioners in North America.

The survey points out that:

*Naturopathic practitioners are trained in a variety of complementary/alternative medicine (CAM) therapies, such as botanical medicine, homeopathy, traditional Chinese medicine (including acupuncture), nutrition, and **some forms of manipulation**. Strong emphasis is placed on lifestyle counselling. [Emphasis added]*

The survey notes that there are variations in emphasis, as well as content, within North American (Canada and USA) naturopathic training:

Canadian trained NDs were significantly more likely [than US trained graduates] to have received training in acupuncture, electro-acupuncture, iridology and magnetic therapy, but less likely to have received training in biofeedback, colon therapy, hypnosis, natural childbirth, polarity therapy, reflexology and yoga.

When asked about the degree of thoroughness with which training had been offered, in particular physical medicine modalities, the 300+ responders to the survey made the observations outlined in Table 10.1.

Canadian-trained NDs (and American-trained NDs working in Canada) would, on the basis of this survey, appear to have received what they consider to be a sound training in manipulation (HVLA, mobilization and soft tissue methods), hydrotherapy and massage, but not in some of the other modalities listed (such as yoga and polarity therapy).

How does this perception translate into application?

What aspects of naturopathic physical medicine, that lie within their scope of practice, do naturopathic physicians working in Canada actually apply, and what health problems are their patients consulting them about?

- The naturopathic practitioners in the survey estimated that the majority of their patients were female (73.8%), and that on average they saw mostly patients between the ages of 36 and 64 (45.8%), followed by patients between the ages of 18 and 35 (24.5%).

- The most important reasons for consultation were gastrointestinal complaints (72%), followed by women's health issues such as premenstrual symptoms and menopause (66%), fatigue (65.3%), allergies (56.7%), musculoskeletal conditions (43.3%) and psychiatric conditions such as anxiety and depression (34.6%).

Table 10.1 Perceived physical medicine coverage of topics in colleges of naturopathic medicine[a]

Topic	Adequate/ thorough (%)	Limited (%)	Not covered (%)	Total number
Naturopathic manipulation[b]	89.0	9.2	1.7	292
Hydrotherapy	83.8	14.2	2.0	296
Massage	78.8	15.1	6.2	292
Lymphatic drainage	21.5	47.4	31.1	293
Acupressure	16.4	36.6	46.9	292
Craniosacral therapy	9.2	27.3	63.5	293
Yoga	4.8	19.1	76.1	293
Polarity therapy	3.4	12.4	84.1	290
Alexander technique	2.7	10.0	87.3	291

[a] Responders to the survey were trained in both Canadian and US colleges. Most received their ND degree from the Canadian College of Naturopathic Medicine (Toronto, 65.9%), followed by the US National College of Naturopathic Medicine (Portland, Oregon, 17.1%).
[b] Manipulation, as taught in naturopathic schools, colleges and universities, includes HVLA, mobilization and soft tissue methods. The term 'naturopathic manipulation' (which may include HVLA thrust-type methods) is used deliberately to distinguish it from chiropractic manipulation which almost always incorporates HVLA methods.

Clearly these percentages suggest that many patients consulting NDs have multiple symptoms.

Note: As indicated by the research data provided later in this chapter, there is strong evidence that there is the potential for physical medicine methods to be able to offer significant assistance in restoration of health *in all of these conditions*.

Practitioners in the survey were asked to indicate whether they provide physical medicine modalities for more than half of their patients, for less than half of their patients, or never (see Table 10.2).

The evidence therefore is that, despite very high scores on perceived quality of training, neither massage nor manipulation is offered to almost 50% of patients seen by naturopathic practitioners in Canada.

The breadth of naturopathic training makes this finding relatively unsurprising. Not all NDs will utilize all the modalities and methods they are taught, any more than all MDs use all that they are taught.

Licensing (USA, Canada) demands the ability to demonstrate competence in the core elements of naturopathic practice, including physical medicine; however, this does not guarantee that any particular aspect of the training will be utilized extensively, or at all. For example, all NDs are trained in botanical and homeopathic methods of treatment, though not all will choose to use these approaches.

For many NDs the manual/physical aspect of their work is of less interest than focus on normalizing the biochemistry of their patients, by means of lifestyle modification and use of nutritional and botanical substances, in order to enhance self-regulation.

Because NDs are trained as generalists, not specialists, particular therapeutic preferences are likely to emerge during training and when in practice. For these reasons, although the majority of respondents in this survey considered that the training in, say, manipulation was 'adequate/thorough', the individual choice may still be made to place therapeutic emphasis elsewhere.

It is unsurprising that modalities such as lymphatic drainage and acupressure are offered to fewer than 50% of patients, since these modalities were reported either to have been taught poorly, or not to have been taught at all, by the majority of responders to the survey.

Washington State survey evidence (Lafferty et al 2006)

Washington State mandates that all commercial health insurance companies cover the services of all categories of licensed health care provider – including naturopathic medicine (as well as acupuncturists, massage therapists and chiropractors).

Table 10.2 Types of modalities provided by the naturopathic practitioners in the survey

	More than 50% (%)	Less than 50% (%)	Never (%)	Total number
Naturopathic manipulation[a]	40.8	15.8	43.4	292
Hydrotherapy	65.2	10.8	24.0	296
Massage	47.8	7.0	45.3	287
Lymphatic drainage	42.5	4.8	52.7	292
Acupressure	37.3	5.6	57.0	268
Craniosacral therapy	35.3	4.6	60.1	283
Yoga	32.1	3.1	64.8	287
Polarity therapy	4.2	0.3	95.5	286
Alexander technique	2.3	0.0	97.5	284

[a] The HVLA aspects of naturopathic manipulation equate fairly closely with chiropractic manipulation, since the majority of tutors of these methods in naturopathic colleges have a chiropractic background. However, as mentioned earlier, naturopathic manipulation is more likely to also involve soft tissue manipulation and mobilization strategies than would be utilized by most chiropractors. See Box 1.5, Chapter 1, for a description of naturopathic manipulation.

When attempting to tease out how many of the 600 000 individuals covered by these schemes consulted specific CAM and mainstream professions, the statistics are sometimes blurred. This is because some insurance companies conflate naturopaths, acupuncturists and massage therapists into one category ('NAM'). Other insurance companies list the numbers of individuals consulting each of these provider groups specifically – acupuncture, naturopathy, etc.

Amidst the wide range of statistical data, a recent survey reveals the following number of visits in 2002, to different categories of CAM health care providers, in western Washington State. Among more than 600 000 enrollees, 13.7% made CAM claims, including:

- acupuncture 52 542 (1.3%)
- naturopathy 41 106 (1%)
- massage 116 543 (3%)
- NAM (made up of naturopathy, acupuncture and massage) 210 191 (5.3%).

In this same period there were 3 246 793 (82.4%) visits to conventional providers (MDs, DOs, PTs, etc.).

The percentages of major diagnostic categories assigned to those attending naturopathic physicians were (with the percentages of these diagnoses ascribed to patients attending conventional medical practitioners in brackets):

- Musculoskeletal   30.7% (21%)
- Cardiovascular   8.1% (9%)
- Female reproductive   18.2% (8.6%)
- Neurological (e.g. headache) 13.2% (5.2%)
- Gastrointestinal/hepatic   12.2% (4.2%)

Note: The conditions selected for this list, from the data in the report, are those where strong evidence exists for benefit deriving from receipt of application of physical medicine modalities – as detailed later in this chapter.

Comparison of ND practice in two US states (Connecticut and Washington)

A random survey of approximately 200 licensed naturopathic practitioners, conducted in Connecticut and Washington State, produced useful information regarding the type of conditions treated (over 70% chronic or chronic flare-up), the gender (75% female), the age groups (60% between 35 and 64) and the therapeutic modalities employed (see Table 10.3).

Boon et al (2004), who conducted the surveys, note that:

The only physical therapies that are part of the naturopathic scope of practice used in more than 5% of the visits were naturopathic manipulation, physiotherapy (Washington only), and hydrotherapy (Washington only).

Table 10.3 Comparison of ND practice in Connecticut and Washington State

	Connecticut (*n* = 631 visits) (%)	Washington (*n* = 1186 visits) (%)
Naturopathic therapeutics		
Botanical medicine	51	43
Vitamins	41	43
Minerals	35	39
Homeopathy	29	19
Acupuncture	14	4
Allergy treatment	11	13
Glandular therapies	4	13
Physical therapies		
Naturopathic manipulation	8	15
Physiotherapy	1	13
Hydrotherapy	4	10
Ultrasound	2	9
Mechanotherapy	2	7
Counseling/education		
Therapeutic diet	26	36
Self-care education	17	23
Exercise therapy	9	12
Mental health	4	6

Table 10.4 Practice time estimated by naturopaths devoted to modalities/disciplines

Modality	Practice time (%)
Herbal medicine	43.7 ± 25.6
Homeopathy	24.6 ± 23.8
Nutritional medicine	42.5 ± 25.7
Massage and tactile therapies	31.0 ± 24.1
Other (including iridology and aromatherapy)	36.0 ± 27.0

The figures in Table 10.3 highlight a large discrepancy between use of naturopathic physical medicine modalities in the two states surveyed, despite over 95% of practitioners, in both states, graduating from the same two training establishments (Bastyr University, Seattle, and National College of Naturopathic Medicine, Portland, Oregon).

Australian survey evidence

A comprehensive survey involving 795 respondents was conducted in Australia in order to 'map the practice of naturopathy and Western herbal medicine, in particular the characteristics of its workforce' (Bensoussana et al 2004).

Of the 795 participants, 604 (76%) identified naturopathy as a practice descriptor, while 489 (61.5%) also described themselves as herbalists, 208 (26.2%) as homeopaths, 315 (39.6%) as nutritionists and 277 (34.8%) as massage therapists.

Clearly many practitioners identified more than one title to describe their clinical practices, which is perfectly understandable considering the eclectic nature of modalities employed in naturopathy.

The survey notes that: 'The practices of herbal medicine and naturopathy make up a sizeable component of the Australian healthcare sector, with approximately 1.9 million consultations annually.'

The principal findings regarding practice time devoted to different modalities by naturopathic practitioners – expressed as a mean percentage (with standard deviation) – are outlined in Table 10.4.

Sixty-two per cent report that they perform physical examination assessments including auscultation and palpation.

The survey results suggest that up to one-third of practice time in Australian naturopathic care involves aspects of physical medicine.

German naturopathic medicine

There are two distinct 'grades' of naturopathic practice in Germany: physicians (MDs) who train additionally in naturopathy (or other CAM disciplines) and 'Heilpraktikers' (health practitioners), who are not physicians, but whose practice is regulated by the state.

The number of Heilpraktikers increased from 9000 in the year 1993 to nearly 20 000 in 2004 (Joos et al 2006).

In 2004 the German Federal Medical Chamber documented:

- 15 970 MDs with an additional qualification in chiropractic

- 5538 MDs with an additional qualification in homeopathy
- 13 502 MDs with an additional qualification in naturopathy – equal to 18.5% of physicians working in the ambulatory (non-hospital) sector (Haltenhof et al 1995).

German naturopathic practice

In 2004, Hartel & Volger published a national representative sample showing that:

> ... *herbal medicine, exercise therapy and hydrotherapy are the most frequently used CAM methods – all of which belong to the so-called classic naturopathy, also known as kneippism from its originator Sebastian Kneipp (1821–97). Besides the classic naturopathic methods homeopathy, manual therapy and acupuncture are commonly used CAM therapies in Germany.*

Comment: It is not clear to what degree Heilpraktikers utilize physical medicine.

Additionally, the data showing that many MDs practice chiropractic and many practice naturopathy do not indicate how much overlap there is between these physicians, i.e. how many have trained in both disciplines.

What is clear is that physical medicine (manual therapy and hydrotherapy), as well as exercise prescription, forms an integral part of naturopathic care in Germany.

How adequate, overall, is naturopathic physical medicine training?

Data are provided below of ND training hours in physical medicine during ND studies, with reference to Canada, Australia, the USA and the UK.

Canadian ND physical medicine training (Ritter 2005)

Curricula

Although both adequately meet the minimum requirements, the two Canadian Colleges, *Canadian College of Naturopathic Medicine* (CCNM), Toronto, Ontario, and *Boucher Institute of Naturopathic Medicine* (BINM), New Westminster, BC, have dissimilar requirements as to hours spent in the physical medicine training that they offer.

Both CCNM and BINM have very similar hours in regard to Basic Science Prerequisites (126 hours) and Clinical and Diagnostic Foundations (138 hours). These hours are devoted to topics such as Anatomy

---

Box 10.1 Manual skills training at CCNM and BINM

CCNM manual skills training (based on course outline 2003)

1. Soft tissue manipulation	39 hours	
• Palpation		
• Manual therapy		
2. Naturopathic manipulation I	45 hours	
• Spine and extremities		
3. Naturopathic manipulation II	<u>84 hours</u>:	168 hours
• Spine and extremities		
Prerequisite (264 hours) plus skills training	**=**	**432 hours**

BINM manual skills training (based on course outline 2004/5)

• Myofascial manipulation	156 hours	
• Additional (to prerequisite) orthopedic testing	20 hours	
• HVLA spinal manipulation	156 hours	
• Master class spinal manipulation	<u>12 hours</u>:	344 hours
Prerequisite (264 hours) plus skills training	**=**	**608 hours**

Note: These Canadian figures do not include hydrotherapy training.

---

and Physiology, Symptomatology, Diagnosis and Differential Diagnosis, History and Interviewing Process, and Orthopedic Physical Assessment (including radiology) – a total of 264 prerequisite hours.

However, subsequent to meeting prerequisite requirements, manual skills training is not the same in these two Canadian ND training establishments (Box 10.1).

US ND physical medicine training[1]

The figures listed below represent averages of what was being taught in relation to physical medicine, and for how long, at two leading American colleges of naturopathic medicine, after the year 2000.

The total number of hours, over the duration of the courses, devoted to physical medicine study, was between 224 and 240 for lab and between 55 and 60 for lectures, representing slightly less than

---

[1]Personal communications from present or former Chairs of Physical Medicine Departments.

10% of the total curriculum time of ND training in the USA.

- Palpation – 36 lab hours (none at some colleges)
- Hydrotherapy – 18 lab/10 lecture hours
- Orthopedic diagnosis – 36 lab hours
- Physiotherapy – 36 lab hours, comprising electrical, sound, light, heat, cold, laser and mechanical therapeutics
- Manipulative therapies – 90 lab/36 lecture hours.

It is important to note that, in addition, ND students are exposed to lectures on anatomy, physiology, rheumatology and other topics that overlap with the topics listed above, as well as supervised clinical activities, some of which inevitably involve physical medicine modalities.

Australian ND physical medicine training[2]

The information offered regarding Australian ND training relates to the year 2006 and to the Bachelor of Naturopathy degree course taught at Southern Cross University.

Compulsory

- One semester Tactile Therapies 1 = 30 hours of lectures, 40 hours of practical (relaxation and lymphatic massage).
- Clinical practicum = 24 hours in internal university supervised physical medicine clinic, plus 24 hours external placement – therapeutic massage in hospital placements (palliative care, rehabilitation, medical, aged care).
- Naturopathic Clinic in final year – estimated 80 hours of physical medicine on basis of patient requirements.

Total core hours = 198 (in the context of a 2420 hour degree course, this equals 8%).

Physical medicine is regarded as a minor modality in the four-modality course, with Herbal medicine and Nutritional medicine receiving the major focus (see summary below).

Elective

Approximately 50% of students take electives units – Tactile Therapies 2 and 3.

---

[2]Details supplied by Paul Orrock ND DO, Senior Lecturer and Director of Clinical Education, Southern Cross University, New South Wales, Australia.

Each elective unit comprises 15 hours of lectures, 35 hours of practical and 24 hours of clinical practicum.

The units cover advanced therapeutics, hydrotherapy, systemic considerations, myofascial techniques, pain management and exercise prescription.

If both electives are taken, the total physical medicine hours = 346, i.e. 14% of the 2420 hour course.

None of the hours specified above includes topics such anatomy, physiology or pathology, which are taught separately.

In terms of modality training, the majors (nutrition, herbal medicine) each comprise 300 contact hours and approximately 200 hours in clinical practicum – about 20% of the curriculum for each topic.

Australian ND course as a whole, in summary

- Sciences — 20% of curriculum face-to-face hours
- Medical studies — 10%
- Naturopathy studies — 15% plus clinical practicum integration (600 hours total)
- Herbal medicine — 20%
- Nutritional medicine — 20%
- Tactile therapies — 8–14% (see above – based on compulsory + electives)
- Homeopathy — 4–12%

The percentage of Australian naturopathic training that involves physical medicine, based on this example (between 8 and 14%), is therefore not very different from the approximately 10% of curriculum time in North American training.

UK ND physical medicine training
(University of Westminster, London)

Brian Isbell PhD ND DO

Since September 1996, when the Complementary Therapies degree of the BSc Honours scheme was first offered, naturopathy has been an option available for students to study. The naturopathy content has been steadily developed so that in 2004 a pathway of naturopathy modules, within the Complementary Therapies degree, was accredited by the General Council and Register of Naturopaths (GCRN). Due to the continuing development of the naturopathy theme and the popularity of the pathway of modules it was decided to validate a named course in naturopathy with its first intake in September 2006. The BSc (Hons) Health Sciences: Naturopathy is accredited by the GCRN.

The course as a whole, in summary, contains the following components:

- Sciences   15%
- Medical studies   5%
- Naturopathy studies   20%
- Naturopathic physical medicine   20%
- Nutritional medicine   10%
- Herbal medicine   5%
- Homeopathy   5%
- Practitioner development skills   10%
- Research skills/project   10%

The total number of taught hours (not including clinic) over the duration of the course, devoted to physical medicine, is 135 for practical/laboratory work and 100 for lectures. These hours represent approximately 20% of the total taught curriculum time of 1200 hours of the BSc (Hons) Health Sciences: Naturopathy course. Students are expected to complete 2400 hours of self-directed study and practice.

In addition, during the course, students have to complete 400 hours of supervised clinical experience in the University of Westminster's Polyclinic, approximately 50% of which is likely to involve the application of physical medicine techniques. Students may also study up to two additional optional modules that would represent another 100 hours of tuition, of which 75% would be practical and 25% lecture.

The 235 hours devoted to physical medicine are allocated as follows:

- Palpation   40 lab/20 lecture
- Hydrotherapy   25 lab/25 lecture
- Orthopedic diagnosis   10 lab/10 lecture
- Physiotherapy   15 lab/15 lecture
- Exercise therapies   5 lab
- Manipulative therapies   40 lab/30 lecture
  (not HVLA)

The above physical medicine topics are consolidated by practice within the clinic, with additional workshops being organized where necessary. In addition, students are able to attend a 1-week residential hydrotherapy course in Germany.

A summary of ND physical medicine training in Australia, Canada, the USA and the UK is outlined in Table 10.5.

Note: While the course hour figures shown in Table 10.5 are not directly comparable because of factors such as the inclusion in some of hydrotherapy, and

Table 10.5 Summary of ND physical medicine training in Australia, Canada, USA, UK

Country	Possible NPM hours	% of curriculum
Australia	198 to 346 (if electives taken)	8–14
Canada	168 or 344	8–14
USA	300	<10
UK	235 + ~200 supervised clinical + optional 100	20

not in others, a broad conclusion can be drawn, i.e. that the hours devoted to physical medicine – on some courses more than others – involve a relatively low level in the hierarchy of importance in curricula of naturopathic training, compared with nutritional and botanical subjects.

This in no way implies inadequate training, only that the structural, biomechanical, physical aspects of the human condition appear to be seen as relatively less important than the biochemical dimensions by the administrators of some naturopathic training institutions.

Should HVLA be employed by naturopaths?

In a recent submission to the British Columbian Minister of Health, to justify the use of HVLA manipulation, in response to chiropractors arguing for an exclusive right to manipulation, and exclusion of NDs from this right (Ritter 2005), the following observations were made:

*In Canadian Naturopathic Colleges the student will receive between 432 and 608 hours of training for spinal manipulation in basic science prerequisites, clinical and diagnostic foundations and manual skills. Within the manual skills 156 hours will be devoted to palpation and hands-on therapy and **168 hours specifically to the safe and effective application of high velocity, low amplitude spinal manipulations**. In addition the student clinician must demonstrate proficiency of spinal manipulation under supervision in order to meet competency standards and successfully complete clinic.*

The right of naturopathic physicians to continue to utilize HVLA manipulation has been affirmed in British Columbia. This issue remains current in other Provinces and in the USA, where chiropractic lobbyists periodically attempt to restrict the rights of other professions in this regard.

Comment:

The evidence from the survey quoted, and the scheduled course times quoted, suggest that physical medicine methods, in the context of naturopathic training, should be allocated greater curriculum time.

This might help to ensure that physical medicine modalities would be more widely utilized within naturopathic practice, to the benefit of patients.

However, even if training hours remain unchanged, the evidence suggests that ND graduates achieve a competency to deliver the range of modalities their generalized practices require.

Are other physical medicine providers offering naturopathic care?

In order to establish trends in chiropractic care, data were obtained from a total of 7651 patients of 161 chiropractors, in 110 practices, in 32 states in the USA, as well as two Canadian provinces; data from two Australian practices were also included (Hawk et al 2001).

- Non-musculoskeletal complaints (frequently ones with complex or poorly understood etiologies that are not well managed under standard medical care) accounted for 10.3% of the chief complaints reported by these DCs.
- Chiropractic practices with the highest proportion of patients with non-musculoskeletal chief complaints (>17%) were less likely to accept insurance, and more likely to be in locations with populations greater than 100 000.
- The most common chiropractic manipulation techniques were used less frequently by DCs who identify part of their practice as 'naturopathic', while more non-adjustment procedures were employed, especially diet/nutrition counseling, nutritional supplementation, herbal preparations, naturopathy and homeopathy.

Quite what 'naturopathy' represents, when detached from diet, use of HVLA manipulation, nutritional supplementation, herbal treatment and homeopathy, is not easy to establish from this study. However, what is clear is that a fairly high proportion (a little under 20%) of chiropractors regularly utilize non-adjustment methods, including what they perceive to be 'naturopathy'.

With a huge chiropractic population – over 50 000 in the USA alone – this percentage (20%) represents a far greater number of chiropractors practicing what they term 'naturopathy' in North America than the entire world population of naturopathic physicians and practitioners.

The organizational role of the musculoskeletal system

It is worth reflecting on a profound truism that is often lost in the minutiae of analyzing the multiple influences on health, that the musculoskeletal system (constituting as it does over 60% of the human body) can be conceived as an active and organized organ, and not just for its movement functions.

Thorpe (1971) has expressed this succinctly:

*[The musculoskeletal system] takes an **active** part in the interplay between the person, his internal functions, his environment, and the other biological entities contacted, both hostile and friendly.*

Korr (1970) has memorably labeled the musculoskeletal system as the 'primary machinery of life', for it is the musculoskeletal system (not our digestive or our immune, or other systems) that is the largest energy consumer in the body. It allows us to perform tasks, play games and musical instruments, make love, give treatment, paint, dance, run and jump, and, in a multitude of other ways, engage in life.

Korr stated that the parts of the body act together 'to transmit and modify force and motion through which man acts out his life'. This coordinated integration takes place under the control of the central nervous system as it responds to a huge amount of sensory input from both the internal and the external environment.

Thorpe (paraphrased) outlines the multiple functions of the musculoskeletal system as:

1. organizing posture
2. providing the basis for function and motion
3. operating as a major sensor of the external environment and the internal milieu
4. acting as a transducer in response to stimuli, with biochemical and neurological effects and influences
5. acting to increase (facilitate or increase gain of) neurological responses
6. acting as an inhibitor to decrease (dampen or block) neurological responses
7. producing, storing and utilizing energy

8. organizing the multiple roles of connective tissue and fascia.

It would be reasonable to add to this list that the musculoskeletal system provides a framework within which circulatory and neural functions, as well as the organ systems, operate. In other words, providing a structure through which the functions of multiple systems and organs can be expressed.

It is with these multiple, over-arching influences in mind, and the potential effects – for good or ill – that these have on the economy and function of the whole person, that general approaches to manual therapy are suggested.

The evidence for general (constitutional) physical medicine approaches

Massage

Field and colleagues (2005) have demonstrated an almost universal benefit deriving from massage therapy. They have reviewed studies on depression (including depression related to sexual abuse and eating disorders), pain syndrome studies, research on autoimmune conditions, immune system studies (including HIV and breast cancer), and studies on the reduction of stress at work, the stress of aging and pregnancy stress.

- In studies in which cortisol was assayed in relation to massage, either in saliva or in urine, significant decreases were noted in cortisol levels (averaging decreases of 31%).
- In studies in which the activating neurotransmitters (serotonin and dopamine) were assayed in urine, an average increase of 28% was noted for serotonin, and an average increase of 31% was noted for dopamine, following massage.

These studies, when considered together, demonstrate the stress-alleviating effects (decreased cortisol) and the activating effects (increased serotonin and dopamine) of massage therapy in relation to a variety of medical conditions and stressful experiences.

Exercise

Exercise – carefully selected to match the needs of the individual, and sufficiently non-arduous (or actually pleasant) to ensure a reasonable chance of compliance – has been shown to offer widespread benefits in cases as divergent as metabolic syndrome-related disorders (insulin resistance, type 2 diabetes, dyslipidemia, hypertension, obesity), heart and pulmonary diseases (chronic obstructive pulmonary disease, coronary heart disease, chronic heart failure, intermittent claudication), muscle, bone and joint diseases (osteoarthritis, rheumatoid arthritis, osteoporosis, fibromyalgia, chronic fatigue syndrome) and cancer, depression, asthma and type 1 diabetes (Pedersen & Saltin 2006).

Integrated manual methods

Non-specific physical medicine approaches (as outlined in Chapter 8 – for example, OMT and GNTT) are in accord with the roots of naturopathy. Kirchfield & Boyle (1994) note that both Lindlahr and Lust employed combinations of physical exercise, massage, osteopathy and chiropractic.

Discussing 'women's suffering' in his classic text *Philosophy of Natural Therapeutics*, Lindlahr (republished 1988) states:

While studying Nature Cure in Europe . . . I learned that correction of spinal and pelvic lesions and consequent removal of pressure and irritation of nerves, the cure of chronic constipation and malnutrition by pure food diet and hydrotherapy, the strengthening of pelvic nerves and muscles by active and passive movements and exercises were sufficient to correct local symptoms in a natural manner.

In Chapters 3 and 8 the naturopathic 'general tonic treatment' is noted as being well established by the 1920s. See later in this chapter, under the subheading 'Fatigue, including chronic fatigue syndrome', for evidence offered of benefit deriving from a variety of integrated non-specific osteopathic and soft tissue mobilization methods (Perrin et al 1998, 2007).

To help in summarizing the positive effects of physical medicine on general health and specific pathologies, named conditions have been considered and evidence offered of benefits deriving from application of a wide range of physical medicine methods.

In order to do this, searches have been made of all the major data banks seeking research evidence. Not all studies located have been reported, as this would have been unproductive in terms of the mass of information. Instead, a selective gathering of data has been exercised, accompanied by an attempt at identification of the physiological mechanisms involved.

Before considering specific conditions, a review of the effects of manual/physical medicine approaches on biological processes are discussed below. This evidence should be seen alongside that offered in Chapters 7 and 8 in particular, where specific tissue, as well as neurological, lymphatic and psychophysiological, influences were reviewed.

The physiology of physical (manual) medicine

A variety of general physiological (biological) effects that relate to self-regulatory processes have been shown to result from aspects of physical medicine treatment.

A number of these have been summarized by Khalsa et al (2006):

> There is increasing evidence that manual therapies may trigger a cascade of cellular, biomechanical, neural, and/or extracellular events as the body adapts to the external stress. Collectively, reports of animal studies (Boal & Gillette 2004, Pickar & Wheeler 2001), case studies (Dishman et al 2005, Mohammadian et al 2004) and numerous clinical trials of chiropractic and physical therapy (Buchmann et al 2005, Childs et al 2004, Hoiriis et al 2004) suggest that spinal manipulation can alter the activity of nearby mechanically sensitive neurons (Bolton 2000, Pickar 2002), including those that function proprioceptively (which sense body position and muscle movements) and, that these changes can in turn lead to responses by the central and autonomic nervous systems (Boal & Gillette 2004). These responses may, in turn, lead to observed changes in circulating levels of various neuropeptides and regulatory proteins. Whether this cascade is responsible for the reported clinical efficacy of manipulation for back and neck pain, for example, is unknown.
>
> Studies of massage-like stimulation of animals indicate that such treatment can stimulate pain-modulating systems working through the action of endogenous opioids (Lund et al 2002). Massage-induced cardiovascular changes in animals have also been observed, and found to be related to the action of the hormone oxytocin, at the level of the midbrain (Kurosawa et al 1995, Lund et al 2002, Wikstrom et al 2003). However, although these preliminary studies are promising and suggest several hypotheses, the exact mechanisms of action for any treatment effects attributable to manual therapies are currently unknown.

Changes in autonomic nervous system (ANS) activity have been offered as one explanation for some of the remote effects of manual therapies, including spinal manipulation (Gosling et al 2005). For example, it has previously been demonstrated that manual interventions applied to the cervical spine can elicit a rapid hypoalgesic effect at the elbow (Vicenzino et al 1996), can alter beta-endorphin and pain levels (Vernon et al 1986), modify distal skin temperature (Harris & Wagnon 1987, Sterling et al 2001, Vicenzino et al 1998a,b), alter pupil diameter (Briggs & Boone 1988), blood pressure (Crawford et al 1986, Knutson 2001) and other measures of cardiopulmonary function, such as respiratory rate and heart rate (Driscoll & Hall 2000, McGuiness et al 1997, Vicenzino et al 1998a).

Such effects are not confined to manipulation of the cervical spine. For example, one study demonstrated that spinal manipulation, outside the region of the sympathetic outflow in the lumbar spine, resulted in an increase in cutaneous blood flow in the lower limbs, bilaterally (Karason & Drysdale 2003).

The long-disputed concept that spinal restrictions ('subluxations' in chiropractic terminology; 'somatic dysfunction' or 'osteopathic lesion' or 'facilitated segment' in osteopathic terminology) can directly influence visceral function appears to be resolving, with support emerging from neuroscience research involving both animal (Budgell et al 1997, 1998, Sato & Swenson 1984) and human (Budgell & Sato 1996, Budgell et al 1995, Fujimoto et al 1999) studies, that at least partially validate what has been held to be clinically obvious to the osteopathic and chiropractic professions for well over a century.

Neuroscience research now appears to support a neurophysiological rationale for the concept that aberrant stimulation of spinal or paraspinal structures may lead to segmentally organized reflex responses of the autonomic nervous system, which in turn may influence visceral function (Budgell 2000).

Clearly far more research is needed; however, there is now sufficient validation to be certain that somatic modulation may occur following the application of physical/manual medicine methods and modalities, well beyond those involving purely muscle and joint problems.

Immune and healing responses

It is a truism to state that all treatment demands adaptational responses from the body/mind complex. 'Treatment' therefore fits the definition of 'stress'. Whether treatment involves manipulation, exercise or a physiotherapeutic model – including hydrotherapy and electrotherapy – a physiological adaptive response is being called for. If these (or other) short-term therapeutic stressors do not overwhelm the adaptive capacity of the individual, it appears that the provoked responses are likely to be beneficial.

Dhabhar & Viswanathan (2005) have shown that an 'acute' response to psychological stress has largely beneficial effects, as compared with chronic, repetitive, long-term stress-related adaptations:

Acute stress may selectively mobilize specific leukocyte subpopulations into sites of surgery, wounding, or immune activation. Such a stress-induced increase in leukocyte trafficking may be an important mechanism by which acute stressors alter the course of different (innate versus adaptive, early versus late, or acute versus chronic) immune responses.

Khalsa et al (2006) expand on these findings by stating:

Emotions were identified as potential causes of disease some 2600 years ago, and psychoneuroimmunology is an attempt to apply principles and techniques of modern science to the age-old question of emotion-caused disease. Acute stress lasts minutes to hours; chronic stress lasts weeks to months, disturbing the diurnal rhythm. Acute stress – brief and with normal circadian rhythm – is an adaptive response that prompts increased leukocyte mobilization and protective immune response. Chronic stress or distress – prolonged and repeated – incites dysregulated immune responses and decreased leukocyte mobilization and protective immune response.

The research of Dhabhar & Viswanathan (2005) has helped to identify some of the processes involved, and has shown the potential for both positive and negative effects to derive from what can be termed therapeutically focused stress:

Stress-induced increases in leukocyte trafficking may enhance immuno-protection during surgery, vaccination, or infection, but may also exacerbate immuno-pathology during inflammatory (cardiovascular disease, gingivitis) or autoimmune (psoriasis, arthritis, and multiple sclerosis) diseases.

Naturopathic physical medicine should be practiced with consideration that therapeutically applied stress demands may produce self-regulating changes of this sort.

Stress and adaptation-related issues are discussed more fully in Chapter 2, which looks at general and local adaptation processes as described by Selye (1971, 1976).

Defining and redefining 'stress'

Stress and adaptation issues are discussed at length in Chapter 2.

In relation to the research of Dhabhar & Viswanathan discussed above, it may be useful to briefly re-evaluate current (and historical) meanings of this much abused term.

Romero (2004) explains that the term 'stress' is extremely difficult to define. Historically, 'stress' has been used to refer to several different concepts, including:

- the noxious stimuli that an individual is exposed to
- the physiological and behavioral coping responses to those stimuli, and
- the overstimulation ('stress overload') of the coping responses that results in disease.

The word 'stressor' is used to refer to a noxious stimulus, and 'stress response' refers to the suite of physiological and behavioral coping mechanisms. 'Chronic stress' relates to long-term overstimulation of coping responses.

Acute stressors last a short period of time, such as predator attacks; however, if they persist they become chronic stressors, e.g. long-term subordination, famine, etc.

McEwen & Wingfield (2003), adapting Selye's (1946) concepts, proposed a change in nomenclature. They introduced three new concepts:

- 'allostasis', the maintenance of homeostasis through change
- 'allostatic load', the measure of how hard an individual must work (e.g. energy requirements) to accomplish a normal life-history task (e.g. breeding)
- 'allostatic overload', the state in which energy requirements exceed the capacity of the animal to replace that energy from environmental resources.

They propose that 'stress' only be used to refer to stimuli that require an emergency energetic response. This provides a way to determine the impact of stress. If the stimulus pushes the animal/individual into allostatic overload, physiological and/or behavioral changes will be required to survive. If allostatic overload is not reached, however, coping will be adequate.

From a naturopathic perspective these terms and stages can be seen to clearly equate with the evolution of dysfunction and ultimately ill-health – with symptoms emerging as signs of the physiological or pathological changes underway.

Application of any form of treatment (manipulation, change of diet, exercise regime, acupuncture needling, medication, etc.) can be seen to be acting in the mode of a stressor, demanding a response.

If the stressor matches the ability of the organism to respond appropriately (i.e. does not overwhelm it), the adaptation response is likely to be beneficial, as in the example provided by Dhabhar & Viswanathan in relation to psychological stress.

Biomechanical influences on the pathophysiology of pain

In relation to the most common of all presenting symptoms, pain, Khalsa et al (2006) observe:

Several generalized pain syndromes (e.g. fibromyalgia, irritable bowel syndrome, temporomandibular syndrome, etc.) exhibit commonalities, which are more significant than their differences. They are highly dependent on sex hormones, predominantly seen after puberty, and effects are driven by stress and a variety of inputs. Sensory motor integration is important in such syndromes, and manual therapies may affect those systems.

Amongst the most common uses of manual manipulation therapy has been the treatment of pain, which markedly influences the magnitude of some of the components of inflammatory responses, and which induces a feedback control of plasma extravasation and neutrophil function. This feedback control itself is powerfully modulated by vagal afferent activity, and both the function of the primary afferent nociceptor and the modulation of inflammatory hyperalgesia by vagal afferent activity, have been shown to be highly sexually dimorphic (Levine et al 2006). Gender differences in nociception do not reflect the use of generally different mechanisms; instead, a common set of signaling pathways may be modulated by hormones (Hucho et al 2006) and/or emotion.

Rhudy & Williams (2005) propose that *emotion influences pain* through a valence-by-arousal interaction. Specifically, negatively valenced (pleasant–unpleasant) emotions can enhance or inhibit pain, depending on the level of arousal (calm–excited) that accompanies the emotion (i.e. how intensely the negative emotion is experienced). Pain is enhanced with negative emotions that range from low to moderate arousal, but it is inhibited at higher arousal levels (Fig. 10.1). Alternatively, positive emotions always inhibit pain,

as long as minimal arousal is obtained. Moreover, evidence suggests that highly arousing positive emotions (i.e. orgasmic bliss) profoundly attenuate pain.

Working from this model, these researchers propose that gender differences in the experience of pain may arise from differences in the experience and processing of emotion that, in turn, differentially alters the processing of pain. Specifically, the defensive system may be more attuned to threatening stimuli in women. As a result, women are more reactive to unpleasant stimuli than men.

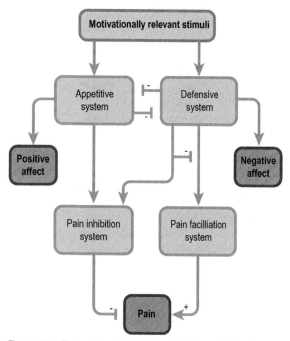

Figure 10.1 The relationship between affective motivational systems and pain modulation. Reproduced with permission from Rhudy & Williams (2005)

Box 10.2 Managing the patient in pain

David Russ DC

Note: The information in this section does not constitute training in counseling or psychotherapy. Patients with mental illness, cognitive or personality disorders can benefit from physical medicine, but they should also have appropriate psychological or psychiatric care.

Patients in pain have cognitive and emotional reactions that may color their perception of their condition. Emotional pain is as real – and as painful – as a torn muscle, arthritic joint or compressed nerve.

Acknowledgement and understanding of this allows the practitioner to more effectively treat the whole patient and the whole condition (DiMatteo et al 1986, Kim et al 2004, Squier 1990).

Practitioners can gain insight into the mental/ emotional component of a condition simply by listening to the patient (Reynolds & Scott 1999). Once a patient's psychological state has been observed and hopefully identified, practitioners can adopt simple tactics to help patients feel better emotionally.

Continued

Box 10.2 Managing the patient in pain continued

There are three predominant emotions which accompany physical pain: sadness, anxiety (Hagen et al 2006) and anger (Mollet & Harrison 2006). Each of these is discussed along with ways of identifying and considering them as part of the patient's overall condition.

Grief

Patients may feel grief or sadness because they have lost something as the result of their condition. This is especially true with cases of chronic pain, in relation to which patients may express sadness by talking about what they have had to give up.

- 'I can't dance any more.'
- 'Ever since my injury I haven't been able to carry my daughter.'
- 'I have lost the feeling in my feet.'
- 'I have had to spend thousands of dollars in tests and treatment.'

Non-verbal behaviors which may indicate sadness include:

- sighing
- crying
- monotone voice, lack of facial expression
- holding back tears
- lips or voice trembling.

These statements and behaviors may reflect that the patient feels that something has been lost and that grief over that loss is being experienced. The grieving patient may cry during the consultation as what has happened is recounted.

When patients express grief about a condition, a possible course of action is to simply acknowledge or name the grief.

- You've had to give up dancing. You must really miss that.
- You really wanted to run that marathon this year.
- You want to be able to pick up your daughter again.

These statements affirm to the individual that what has been said has been heard and understood (Reynolds & Scott 1999). Sometimes this simple response can be very touching, and may provoke the onset of crying.

The patient should be allowed to cry and/or to express the sadness being experienced. Waiting patiently, without judgment, shows compassion and understanding. Most daily social interactions do not allow room for grieving and sadness, so it can be powerful simply to allow the patient to express

this difficult and painful emotion (Reynolds & Scott 1999).

Usually a few minutes of crying, silence or talking will remove significant stress from the patient's mind, and although still grieving, the patient will be more present, allowing the interview or treatment to continue.

When patients have cried during the initial interview, or during treatment, it is appropriate to be gentle and deliberate with manual therapy. Patients feel vulnerable at such times, and pressure which may otherwise have been well tolerated may feel too deep. Consider making the treatment session gentle, and spending some time simply encouraging the patient to breathe more slowly.

If the patient cannot stop crying it is best to stop treatment, allowing a quiet, safe period, while a friend or family member is contacted to accompany them home, or to see a practitioner with appropriate training in mental health issues.

Anger and frustration

Anger and frustration are components of the grieving process (Dunne 2004). Patients experiencing these emotions in relation to their condition – and what they have lost – may appear irritable, negative or grumpy. Similar statements may be made to those expressed by the grieving patient, but the demeanor will be different. Rather than crying, some of the following behaviors may be noted:

- Clenched fists or jaw
- Shaking the head (as in saying 'no') as the condition is discussed
- Brow furrowed or frowning
- Speaking with a loud voice.

In the author's experience, angry patients tend to go off at tangents, often displaying frustration or negativity regarding other areas of their life apart from health issues – for example, work, relationships, money or politics.

A useful course of action in such a case would be to avoid being 'drawn in' by the negativity or irritability. It is important to understand that a patient in pain may well wish to have a more positive outlook but might feel unable to do so. Being complicit with the expressed criticisms of the world affirms this pessimism, which is unhelpful. Neither is it helpful to try to talk the patient out of being angry or frustrated since such emotions are valid and significant current components of their condition. Caring for this aspect of the individual's health is as important as caring for the hurt shoulder or hip.

It is also appropriate to feed back to the patient what you are observing:

Box 10.2 Managing the patient in pain continued

- You seem frustrated.
- You seem to be having a hard time with your boss/spouse/friend.
- You really have gone through a lot, and it seems like you could use a rest from it all.

Making these 'mirroring' statements *with the same care and compassion that you show for their physical malady* will often create an immediate connection. The patient might lower the defensive irritability shield, and express the grief or sadness that underlies this, relieving some of the physical and emotional tension.

Patients in a state of anger or frustration usually appreciate physical medicine modalities that promote relaxation, such as heat and gentle massage. It is appropriate to use such modalities (unless otherwise contraindicated) to help a patient relax. This relaxation should create greater receptivity in the patient and make further treatment easier and more effective.

Fear and anxiety

Patients are often anxious about their condition and the pain which accompanies it. This is especially true of those who do not know what is wrong, what kind of treatment they need, and how long they can expect to be in pain. In other words, the patient reacts with anxiety to the *uncertainty* that comes with pain and injury. Sometimes patients are anxious simply being in a practitioner's office, even if not particularly anxious about their condition.

There are some common non-verbal clues that may indicate that a patient is anxious or afraid:

- Nail biting or hand wringing
- Shifting in their chair
- Hurried speech, which sometimes results in interrupting, stuttering and stumbling over words
- Voice shaking
- Very close observation of the practitioner and the surroundings
- Modified breathing pattern, sighing, 'air hunger', increased swallowing rate.

Patients may also identify their anxiety verbally:

- 'I'm really worried about this.'
- 'My mother had arthritis and I'm afraid that's what I have, too.'
- 'I'm scared because I can't afford to miss any more work. I might lose my job.'

It is tempting for the practitioner to make unfounded or overly optimistic statements to assuage a patient's fears. This should be avoided:

- 'You'll be just fine soon.'
- 'I'm sure you don't have arthritis.'
- 'You'll be back to work in no time. Don't worry.'

A more positive approach may be to offer information regarding whatever facts are available regarding their condition, along with a straightforward opinion and assurance that the condition will be investigated until it is identified and treated appropriately. Explain the diagnosis/assessment results, the treatment plan and the prognosis. Offer a degree of control by appropriately involving the individual in the decision-making about their care.

The practitioner's demeanor and behavior are powerful cues to the patient. The following behaviors may help a patient feel less anxious:

- Sitting up straight, attentive, and using appropriate eye contact will assure the patient that they are recognized and heard.
- Speaking in a calm, clear, soft voice.
- A relaxed posture, smooth efficient movement, and the appropriate use of humor exhibits confidence.
- Soliciting and directly answering questions offers assurance that questions and concerns will be addressed appropriately.
- Acknowledging that a particular question, or a certain aspect of a patient's health, would be better addressed by another practitioner, assures the patient that the practitioner is aware of their own limitations.
- Collaboratively develop a treatment plan that is outlined to, and discussed with, the patient (see below).

Anxious patients appreciate extra explanation of treatments, and a gentle approach, at least at first. In this author's experience, gentle treatment modalities (e.g. positional release technique) are particularly appropriate for anxious patients.

Usually, patients will feel less anxious as they are offered more information and gain greater confidence in the practitioner. Signs that a patient's fear is decreasing include:

- eyes relaxed and closed during treatment
- easy laughter and relaxed smiling
- smooth, slow breathing and relaxed sighing
- voice softens
- patient stops paying close attention to the practitioner's every move.

Box 10.3 The therapeutic plan

In formulating a treatment plan in relation to a painful condition, objectives are essential – for example, functional improvement, reduction in pain, enhanced mobility, etc.

The means whereby objectives are achieved may vary, but until there is a review and possible revision, the objective(s) should remain unchanged. This may sound obvious but it lies at the heart of the process of creating a plan of action.

Before considering objectives a sifting process is useful, in which the patient and the condition are evaluated in relation to the following types of query:

- Is this a pain-related condition that is likely to improve/resolve on its own?
- If it is, therapeutic intervention should be refined to avoid inhibition of the natural processes of recovery. An example might be a strained joint, which in time will recover unaided. Intervention might be focused on ensuring sound muscle balance and joint mobility, possibly including normalization of localized soft tissue fibrosis.
- Or is this a condition that might improve on its own, but that is more likely to remain a background problem unless suitable treatment is offered? In such a case a plan of action, with clear objectives and regular review of progress, is appropriate. Self-help rehabilitation strategies and re-education of use patterns (posture, breathing, etc.) might be appropriate.
- Is this a problem that is unlikely to improve, that is more likely to deteriorate (involving degenerative arthritic changes for example) but which has the potential to be eased symptomatically and/or functionally? In such a case therapeutic objectives need to take account of the likely progression of the condition, with palliative and self-help interventions designed to retard degeneration and to encourage better adaptation. 'Progress', in some instances of chronic pain and dysfunction, is measured not by improvement, but by the slowing of the seemingly inevitable process of degeneration.
- Is this a condition which has almost no chance of either improvement or possibly of even slowing the degenerative processes? In such cases palliation is an approriate objective, to ease discomfort and to make the process of decline as comfortable as possible.

All these objectives may be of value to the patient. Likelihood that improvement is not possible should not mean that the patient should not be helped to cope better with the inevitable decline.

In designing a treatment plan the following general questions might usefully be considered:

- What is it that needs to be achieved (reduction/removal of a particular pain; restoration of movement to a restricted joint; improved function, etc.)?
- What are the best ways available of achieving those ends (which techniques, modalities and strategies are most likely to help in reaching the objectives)?
- Am I capable of delivering these methods/techniques, or would referral be more appropriate?
- How long is it likely to take before progress is noted (taking account of the acuteness/chronicity of the problem, exacerbating features, and the condition of the patient)?
- Are there things the patient could be doing to assist in the process (home stretching, hydrotherapy, change in diet, relaxation procedures, etc.)?

After an appropriate period of time, depending on the nature of the condition and the patient, progress should be reviewed:

- Have the original objectives been partly or wholly achieved?
- If not, are there other ways of trying to achieve them?
- Or, are there other/new objectives?
- How can these best be achieved?

The treatment plan needs to take account of the patient's ability to respond, which depends largely on the patient's vitality levels. Kappler (1996) summarizes this need by saying:

The dose of treatment is limited by the patient's ability to respond to the treatment. The practitioner may want to do more and go faster; however the patient's body must make the necessary changes toward health and recovery.

The old adage, 'less is more', is an important lesson which most practitioners learn by experience, often after discovering that because a particular approach worked well, doing more of the same often did not.

These thoughts highlight a truth which can never be emphasized too strongly, particularly in a naturopathic context, that the body alone houses the prerogative for recovery. Healing and recovery are achieved via the expression of self-healing potentials inherent in the mind–body complex. Treatment is a catalyst that should encourage that self-healing process, by removing factors that may be retarding progress, or by improving functional abilities.

Biomechanical influences on pain

Khalsa (2004) has offered a summary of the biomechanical influences on pain:

Mammals in general, and humans in particular, have evolved a highly sophisticated system of pain perception, which is characterized in humans by complementary but distinct neural processing of the intensity and location of a noxious stimulus, and a motivational/emotional or affective response to the stimulus. The peripheral and central neurons that comprise this system, which has been called the 'neuromatrix', dynamically (temporally) respond and adapt to noxious biomechanical stimuli. However, phenotypic variability of the neuromatrix can be large, which can result in a host of musculoskeletal conditions that are characterized by altered pain perception, which can and often does alter the course of the condition. This neural plasticity has been well recognized in the central nervous system, but it has only more recently become known that peripheral nociceptors also adapt to their altered extracellular matrix environment.

Pain perception in humans is a highly complex system that integrates noxious stimuli from the tissues, with the overall status (physical, emotional, and mental) of the individual. Unlike the five primary senses, pain is strongly influenced by positive and negative feedback systems within the brain, spinal cord, and the primary nociceptor. Nonetheless, within the pain perceptive system, there is a sensory/discriminant component for which the intensity of an acute noxious stimulus is essentially proportional to the perceived pain. As we continue to better understand the complexity of this system, we will be better able to create treatments to prevent and treat patients suffering from pain.

Note: Due to its complexity there is no exploration in depth of the topic of pain in this text; however, the topic of naturopathic care of pain, including painful musculoskeletal conditions, is evaluated later in this chapter.

Naturopathic physical medicine leans heavily on the research that has provided an evidence base for the methods long employed in the osteopathic, chiropractic, physical therapy and massage professions. By incorporating what has been validated in these settings, together with naturopathy's own unique perspective, naturopathic practitioners can be seen to have a wide range of safe tools, modalities, methods and approaches, on which to draw.

The body is self-regulating. The opportunity to normalize dysfunction or disease resides as an innate ability that may be retarded by biomechanical imbalances and restrictions.

In Chapter 2 evidence was offered as to the inability of cells to metabolize normally when distorted, where structure was shown clearly to govern function. This consideration – together with the mountain of evidence that shows that circulatory, immune, neurological, eliminative and other functions, as well as the individual's psychosocial balance, are all capable of being beneficially influenced by manual and movement methods of treatment – should be a major part of all clinical decision-making.

The evidence for their safe employment, in a variety of conditions, is outlined below.

Self-regulation and manual methods

Before considering the evidence for physical medicine treatment, involving the listed range of conditions, it is useful to reproduce (see Box 10.4) the list of conditions previously shown in Chapter 7 of the evidence that exists of beneficial results deriving from osteopathic or chiropractic manipulation.

Box 10.5 lists a variety of conditions where evidence shows clear benefit deriving from application of massage. This list is also to be found in Chapter 7 under the subheading 'Massage'.

Box 10.6 lists a number of the validated benefits of yogic practice.

It is important that naturopaths remind themselves of the potential value of such approaches, particularly when the lure of biochemical interventions seems to dominate clinical decision-making.

Placebo power

It would be short-sighted in a text on naturopathic physical medicine to ignore discussion of the role of placebo in healing. Since naturopathy stands on a platform of enhancement of self-regulation, it makes sense to acknowledge that self-regulation may be triggered, encouraged or enhanced by suggestion that affects the individual's mind positively, if this removes obstacles to homeostatic function.

Along with safe therapeutic measures, the time and effort taken by any practitioner seriously delving into an individual's problems and needs is itself a force for good in health promotion, whether this is labeled as placebo or as merely offering a 'sense of support'.

Powerful evidence suggests that if someone believes a form of treatment (any form of treatment) will relieve pain, it will do so far more effectively than if the belief is that the treatment cannot help. In trials involving over 1000 people suffering from chronic pain, dummy medication reduced the levels of the pain by at least 50% of that achieved by *any* form of pain-killing drug, including aspirin and morphine.

The researchers Melzack & Wall (1989) explain:

Box 10.4 Partial list of conditions where there exists evidence of benefit deriving from osteopathic or chiropractic manipulation

- ADHD (Giesen et al 1989, Upledger 1978)
- Asthma (pediatric) (Bachman & Lantz 1991, Guiney et al 2005)
- Asthma (adult) (Rowane & Rowane 1999)
- Cardiac arrhythmia (Jarmel et al 1995)
- Duodenal ulceration (Pikalov & Kharin 1994)
- Dysmenorrhea (Boesler et al 1993, Hondras et al 1999)
- Enuresis (Gemmell & Jacobson 1989)
- Fibromyalgia (Gamber et al 2002)
- Headache (Mootz et al 1994)
- Hypertension (Johnston & Kelso 1995, Yates et al 1988)
- Infantile colic (Klougart & Nilsson 1989, Tanaka et al 1998)
- Multiple sclerosis (enhancing exercise effects) (Yates et al 2002)
- Otitis media (Fallon 1997, Vallone & Fallon 1997)
- Parkinson's disease (enhanced gait) (Wells et al 1999)
- Pneumonia (decreased antibiotic usage, shorter hospital stay) (Noll et al 2000)
- Premenstrual syndrome (Walsh & Polus 1998)
- Prenatal care (improved outcomes for labor and delivery) (King et al 2003)
- Pyloric stenosis (Fallon & Lok 1994)
- Visual acuity enhancement (Kessinger & Boneva 1998)

Naturopathic perspective

Manipulation can mean anything from light stretching of the skin to high velocity, low amplitude manipulation of an osseous articulation (HVLA 'adjustment'), with a huge range of variables in between. Triano (2001) has observed that:

There are currently over 90 different named systems of manual procedures. The problem is that there is no current triage system available that predicts which patient has the greater likelihood of benefiting from manual treatment or the procedure type.

It is a virtual certainty that in treatment of patients with the variety of conditions listed above, the treatments used would have had an equally wide range. Selection of what is appropriate in any given setting relates to tailoring the forms of manipulative interventions to the patient's characteristics and needs, so that the adaptive responses that follow improve functionality. This makes appropriate use of 'manipulation' an ideal naturopathic modality (the right method, involving the right degree of force, at the right time, for the right patient, or area). It also requires that those using manipulation have competence in safe application of as wide a range of complementary and alternative techniques and modalities as possible.

This shows clearly that the psychological context – particularly the physician's and patient's expectations – contains powerful therapeutic value in its own right, in addition to the effect of the drug [or any other form of treatment] itself.

Placebo facts

- Placebos are far more effective against severe pain than mild pain.
- Placebos are more effective in people who are severely anxious and stressed than in people who are not, suggesting that the 'anti-anxiety' effect of placebos accounts for at least part of the reason for their usefulness.
- Placebos work best against headache-type pain (over 50% effectiveness).
- In about a third of all people, most pains are relieved by placebo.
- A placebo works more effectively if injected, rather than if taken by mouth.
- Placebos work more powerfully if accompanied by the suggestion that they are indeed powerful and that they will rapidly produce results.
- Placebos which are in capsule or tablet form work better if two are taken rather than one.
- Large capsules work as placebos more effectively than do small ones.
- Red placebos are most effective of all in helping pain problems.
- Green placebos help anxiety best.
- Blue placebos are the most sedative and calming.
- Yellow placebos are best for depression and pink are the most stimulating.

Box 10.5 Massage influences

Following courses of massage:

- aggressive youngsters were less aggressive (Diego et al 2002)
- agitated physical behavior in Alzheimer patients was reduced (but not verbal aggression) (Rowe & Alfred 1999)
- peptic ulcer symptoms improved (Aksenova et al 1999, Bei 1993)
- symptoms of anxiety were significantly reduced (Shulman & Jones 1996)
- pain reduction and improved functionality were evident in patients with rheumatoid arthritis (Field & Hernandez-Reif 1997)
- there was significantly enhanced forced expiratory flow in asthmatics (Field et al 1997a)
- stereotypical behavior was reduced in autistics, and there was more socializing and fewer sleep problems (Escalona et al 2001)
- breast cancer patients demonstrated reduced anxiety, reduced depression, increased urinary dopamine, serotonin values, increased natural killer cell numbers and lymphocytes (Hernandez-Reif et al 2004)
- bulimia patients reported immediate reductions in anxiety and depression (Field et al 1998)
- there was a reduction of arm pain and discomfort following lymph node dissection in patients with breast cancer (Forchuk & Baruth 2004)
- massage treatment of trigger points reduced blood pressure significantly (systolic and diastolic) and decreased heart rate, as well as resulting in improvement in emotional state and muscle tension (Delaney et al 2002)
- chronic fatigue syndrome patients reported reduced depression and somatic symptoms, as well as improved sleep (Field et al 1997b)
- people with constipation had more normal bowel function and reduced incidence of soiling (Bishop et al 2003)
- compliance with insulin and food regulation improved and glucose levels decreased from 159 mg/dL to within normal range in diabetics over a 30-day period (Field et al 1997c)
- there was immediate decreased anxiety and depressed mood, long-term increased sleep hours

and decreased sleep movements in fibromyalgia patients; substance P levels dropped as did pain ratings (Field et al 2002)

- HIV patients had enhanced immune system cytotoxic capacity (Ironson et al 1996)
- diastolic pressure reduced significantly in hypertensives (Hernandez-Reif et al 2000a)
- mood improved as did white blood cell and neutrophil counts in leukemic patients (Field et al 2001)
- numerous studies as well as systematic review show benefit greater than acupuncture and self-care in cases of low back pain (Ernst 1999)
- multiple sclerosis patients demonstrated reduced anxiety and depression, improved self-esteem and social functioning (Hernandez-Reif et al 1998)
- numerous studies show enhanced tolerance to pain, raised pain threshold and improved function in a variety of settings, including chronic and postoperative pain (Walach et al 2003)
- Parkinson's disease patients showed improved daily living activities, less disturbed sleep (Hernandez-Reif et al 2002).

Note: The forms of massage utilized in these examples are almost certainly not standardized in all the examples; however, in many it was. Nor is it certain that the benefits noted derived from massage alone, as in some of the studies cited combinations of modalities, including massage, were employed.

Naturopathic perspective

Massage can be deep or superficial, slow or rapid, general or localized, brief or lengthy, heavy or light, and can involve a range of different mechanical influences ('load'; see discussion on massage in Chapter 7). Therefore no two massage sessions are ever quite the same, and if tailored to meet the perceived needs of the individual, appear to be capable of enhancing self-regulatory functions, as well as removing/reducing obstacles to recovery via improved circulatory, neurological, lymphatic or other functions. Massage is therefore an ideal modality for use in naturopathic settings, involving almost all forms of ill-health or dysfunction.

- Placebos have been shown to be effective in a wide variety of conditions including anorexia, depression, skin diseases, diarrhea and palpitation.
- Placebo effects do not only occur when taking something by mouth or injection – any form of

treatment from manipulation to acupuncture to surgery carries with it a degree of placebo effect.

Recognition of the placebo effect allows us to realize the importance of the power of suggestion on all of

Box 10.6 Yoga influences

Yogic approaches have been reported (Goyeche & Ikemi 1977, Singh 2006) to have been successfully used in the management of:

- anxiety (Selvamurthy 1994)
- bronchial asthma (Faling 1986, Manocha et al 2002)
- cardiovascular disease (Harinath et al 2004) related to diabetes (Malhotra et al 2002, Singh et al 2004)
- chronic sinusitis (Telles et al 1994)
- depression (Khumar et al 1993, Pilkington et al 2005)
- epilepsy (Ramaratnam & Sridharan 2000)
- headache (Latha & Kaliappan 1992)
- hypertension (Patel & North 1975)
- insomnia (in cancer patients) (Cohen et al 2004)
- irritable bowel syndrome and gastritis (Taneja et al 2004)
- low back pain (Galantino et al 2004)
- menstrual disorders (Chen 2005, Sridevi & Krishna-Rao 1996)
- multiple sclerosis (Oken et al 2004)
- peptic ulcer (Bhole 1983)
- stress-related symptoms in epilepsy (Panjwani et al 1995).

Naturopathic perspective

There are probably as many variations of yoga as there are varieties of manipulation and massage approaches (see yoga discussion in Chapter 7). What is common to all of them is that they require individual attention and effort to achieving an aspect of the required discipline, whether meditation, breathing function, a specific posture or even a modification of diet. What makes yoga an intrinsically naturopathic approach to health is the fact that the ultimate benefit of its use derives from enhanced self-regulatory functions.

us, with some people being more influenced than others. It is essential that we should not think that because a placebo 'works' in an individual that the person is not genuinely suffering, or that the reported relief is false (Millenson 1995). A person's attitudes and emotions can be seen to be powerful aids (or hindrances) to recovery. Feelings of hope and expectation of improvement, coupled with a relationship with caring helpers, professional or otherwise, assist in recovery and coping.

An example of placebo potency is exemplified by a study by Price et al (2007) associated with brain activity and irritable bowel syndrome. They note that:

*Previous experiments found that placebos produced small decreases in neural activity of pain-related areas of the brain, yet decreases were only statistically significant after termination of stimuli and in proximity to when subjects rated them. These changes could reflect report bias rather than analgesia. This functional magnetic resonance imaging (fMRI) study examined whether placebo analgesia is accompanied by reductions in neural activity in pain-related areas of the brain, during the time of stimulation. Brain activity of irritable bowel syndrome patients was measured in response to rectal distension by a balloon barostat. **Large reductions in pain and in brain activation within pain-related regions (thalamus, somatosensory cortices, insula, and anterior cingulate cortex) occurred during the placebo condition.** Results indicate that decreases in activity were related to placebo suggestion, and a second factor (habituation/attention/conditioning). Although many factors influence placebo analgesia, it is accompanied by reduction in pain processing within the brain in clinically relevant conditions. [Emphasis added]*

Appropriate treatment, together with education, patient focus and a strong suggestion – for example, that self-regulation will assist recovery if appropriate lifestyle modifications are undertaken, and if posture and exercise are attended to – may assist not only in practical ways but also via the placebo effect.

Conclusion: All the evidence suggests that the placebo effect is a reliable ally of naturopathic care.

Further reading

1. Peters D 2001 Understanding the placebo effect in complementary medicine: theory, practice and research. Churchill Livingstone, Edinburgh

Naturopathic physical medicine approaches to specific and general conditions

The following is an alphabetical list of specific and general conditions in which use of physical medicine methods have been described in this chapter:

1. Anxiety, panic attacks and phobic behavior
2. Asthma
3. Breathing pattern disorders (BPD) – see Box 10.7
4. Cardiovascular disease
5. Depression
6. Fatigue (CFS)
7. Fibromyalgia syndrome (FMS)

Box 10.7 Breathing pattern disorders (e.g. hyperventilation) and medically unexplained symptoms

Almost all the physical medicine methods outlined above as being appropriate for treatment of asthma (and anxiety) are appropriate in treatment of people with breathing pattern disorders.

Acute episodes of hyperventilation represent only approximately 1% of all cases, far outnumbered by chronic patterns (Nixon 1989).

Chronic hyperventilation leads to hypocapnia (reduced levels of carbon dioxide) and can present with a myriad of respiratory, cardiac (De Guire et al 1992), neurological or gastrointestinal symptoms, without any clinically apparent overbreathing by the patient (Pryor & Prasad 2002a). In the United States as many as 10% of patients in a general internal medicine practice are reported to have hyperventilation syndrome as their primary diagnosis (Beales & Dolton 2000).

Studies show that, relative to men, women have a higher rate of respiration and a greater tendency to respiratory alkalosis, which is exaggerated during the luteal (progesterone) phase of the menstrual cycle (Lum 1987).

Hyperventilation syndrome and breathing pattern disorders are therefore female dominated, with a female : male ratio ranging from 2 : 1 to 7 : 1. Women may be more at risk because of hormonal influences, since progesterone stimulates respiration, and in the luteal (postovulation/premenstrual) phase, CO_2 levels drop, on average, by 25%. Additional stress can subsequently 'increase ventilation at a time when carbon dioxide levels are already low' (Damas-Mora et al 1980).

Beales & Dolton (2000) have summarized the problems of managing patients with multiple vague symptoms where there is no obvious organic cause:

Katon and Walker (1998) estimate that 14 common physical symptoms are responsible for almost half of all primary care visits. Yet over a one-year period, only about 10%–15% of these symptoms are found to be caused by an organic illness. **Abdominal pain, chest pain, headache, and back pain** are *commonly found to be medically unexplained. Primary care physicians find patients with medically unexplained symptoms frustrating, and these patients tend to be frequent attenders, who account for a disproportionate amount of healthcare resources. Consequently, they are also common among frequent attenders in secondary care where they present in most specialties. Reid et al (2001) examined the records of the 361 patients who attended outpatients most frequently (i.e. the top 5%). In 208 of the 971 consultation episodes, after full investigation, their symptoms were medically unexplained.*

It is suggested that the respiratory status of such patients might prove illuminating.

Reducing levels of apprehension, anxiety and fear may be seen to have the potential for allowing a variety of features, including motor control, to improve.

Breathing retraining is one way of achieving this objective. There is good evidence that breathing rehabilitation is a useful method for achieving reduced anxiety/panic levels and for improving postural control and somatic complaints, such as low back pain (Aust & Fischer 1997, Han et al 1996).

Hyperventilation can usually be corrected by breathing retraining.

Lum (1984) reported on a study in which more than 1000 anxious and phobic patients were treated using breathing retraining, physical therapy and relaxation. Symptoms were usually abolished in 1–6 months, with some younger patients requiring only a few weeks. At 12 months, 75% were free of all symptoms and 20% had only mild symptoms; however, about one patient in 20 had 'intractable symptoms'.

8. Gynecological disorders and menstrual irregularities
9. Headache (and migraine)
10. Hypertension
11. The hospitalized patient (and postoperative care)
12. Infection including respiratory tract infections (including pneumonia)
13. Irritable bowel conditions
14. Insomnia
15. Interstitial cystitis and chronic pelvic pain
16. Pain – musculoskeletal and other.

Anxiety, panic attacks and phobic behavior

Anxiety can be seen to be a normal response to anxiety-provoking events (Angst & Volrath 1991). It would be bizarre, to say the least, if anxiety was not the response to a life-threatening situation. As with so many 'normal' life responses, anxiety only becomes a problem if it is excessive, prolonged and/or inappropriate. There are undoubtedly biochemical features associated with severe anxiety (Coplan et al 1998), which is more generally considered to be an emotional/psychological disturbance.

There also exists a clear biomechanical/functional aspect in which respiratory function can be shown to have a direct impact on both the causes and the control of anxiety states (Asmundson & Stein 1994) and the common repercussion – panic attacks (Breier et al 1986).

Hyperventilation and anxiety symptoms

If severe anxiety is prolonged, there is an almost predictable progression as anxiety translates into panic, and all too frequently phobic behavior. A common thread in this progression is hyperventilation and an imbalance in CO_2 levels (Caldirola et al 1997).

Dratcu (2000) has noted:

Provocation of panic experimentally has indicated that several biological mechanisms may be involved in the onset of panic symptoms. Evidence from provocation studies using lactate, but particularly carbon dioxide (CO_2) mixtures, suggests that panic patients may have hypersensitive CO_2 chemoreceptors. Klein (1993) proposed that this may be due to a dysfunctional brain's 'suffocation alarm' and that panic patients hyperventilate to keep pCO_2 low.

He continues:

Studies of panic patients in the non-panic state have shown EEG abnormalities in this patient group, as well as abnormalities in cerebral blood flow and cerebral glucose metabolism. These abnormalities can be interpreted as signs of cerebral hypoxia that may have resulted from previous hyperventilation.

What appears to happen is that habitual patterns of breathing are adopted to maintain low CO_2 levels, with anxiety-provoking consequences. This process is more prevalent in women than in men (Loeppky et al 2001).

Low CO_2 levels equate with respiratory alkalosis and a wide range of changes apart from inducement of heightened anxiety, including smooth muscle constriction affecting blood vessel (Castro et al 2000) and gut diameter, with consequences on oxygen delivery, cardiovascular and bowel function (Ford et al 1995).

As Foster et al (2001) explain:

Respiratory alkalosis is an extremely common and complicated problem affecting virtually every organ system in the body [producing as it does] multiple metabolic abnormalities, from changes in potassium, phosphate, and calcium, to the development of a mild lactic acidosis. Hyperventilation syndrome is a common etiology of respiratory alkalosis.

There are, in addition, negative effects on balance (Balaban & Thayer 2001), motor control (Van Dieën et al 2003), pain thresholds (Rhudy & Meagher 2000) and autonomic imbalance characterized by sympathetic arousal (Dempsey et al 2002). Lum (1994) reports:

During moderate hyperventilation, loss of CO_2 ions from neurons stimulates neuronal activity, causing increased sensory and motor discharges, muscular tension and spasm, speeding of spinal reflexes, heightened perception (photophobia, hyperacusis) and other sensory disturbances. More profound hypocapnia, however, increasingly depresses activity. This parallels the clinical state: initial alertness with increased activity, progressing, through decreased alertness, to stupor and coma.

Hypoglycemia as an aggravating factor

These changes are exacerbated if there are simultaneous hypoglycemic episodes, and are particularly severe in deconditioned individuals whose metabolism relies excessively on anaerobic glycolysis, since lactate, a by-product of this, stimulates the respiratory rate even further. Hyperventilation is also more common during the postovulation phase of the menstrual cycle as progesterone is a respiratory accelerator (Damas-Mora et al 1980).

Blood sugar level is 'clinically a most important non-ventilatory factor. When blood glucose is below the middle of the normal range (i.e. below 4.4 mmol/L) the effects of overbreathing are progressively enhanced' (Brostoff 1992).

Effects of bicarbonate loss

The process of respiratory alkalosis triggers a homeostatic rebalancing via the kidneys, leading to excretion of bicarbonate which can result in marked calcium and magnesium imbalances. Hyperventilation decreases $PaCO_2$ (hypocapnia) and starts the acid–base changes that end as respiratory alkalosis. These changes in $PaCO_2$ produce secondary changes in plasma bicarbonate concentration. In chronic hypocapnia changes in plasma bicarbonate occur as a result of adjustments in renal mechanisms that are attempting to restore homeostatic balance (Madias & Adrogue 2003).

With symptoms ranging from insomnia to headaches, irritable bowel syndrome, chronic fatigue, menstrual irregularities (Loeppky et al 2001), musculoskeletal pain, loss of balance, cognitive difficulties ('foggy brain'), anxiety, panic attacks and phobic behavior, it is difficult to imagine the individual being anything other than anxious.

Breathing retraining (see below) has as one of its aims the objective of raising the threshold of tolerance for CO_2, and so allowing a slower breathing rate to be well tolerated (Jennett 1994).

Rehabilitation strategies

Strategies that can help to normalize such a cascade of health problems have been shown in many studies to require (for optimum results) a combination of breathing retraining and physical medicine interventions that focus attention on the thoracic cage, diaphragm and accessory respiratory muscles (Lum 1994).

Reducing levels of apprehension, anxiety and fear may be seen to have the potential for encouraging improvement in breathing patterns and all the negative symptoms that flow from these.

There is also good evidence that breathing rehabilitation is a useful method for achieving reduced anxiety/panic levels and for improving postural control (Aust & Fischer 1997) and somatic complaints, such as low back pain (Mehling & Hamel 2005), and conditions such as chronic fatigue (Nixon & Andrews 1996).

Anxiety studies

1. *Breathing rehabilitation and anxiety states*: In one study (Lum 1987) more than 1000 anxious and phobic patients were treated using a combination of breathing retraining, physical therapy and relaxation. Symptoms were usually abolished in 1–6 months, with some younger patients requiring only a few weeks. At 12 months, 75% were free of all symptoms, 20% had only mild symptoms and about one patient in 20 had intractable symptoms.

2. *Breathing retraining and anxiety disorders*: In another study (Han et al 1996) the effects of breathing retraining were evaluated in patients with hyperventilation syndrome in which most of the patients met the criteria for an anxiety disorder. The diagnosis was based on the presence of several stress-related complaints, reproduced by voluntary hyperventilation, patients with organic diseases having been excluded. Therapy was conducted in the following sequence:
   - Brief, voluntary hyperventilation to reproduce the complaints in daily life
   - Reattribution of the cause of the symptoms to hyperventilation
   - Explaining the rationale of therapy – reduction of hyperventilation by acquiring an abdominal breathing pattern, with slowing down of expiration
   - Breathing retraining for 2–3 months by a physical therapist. After breathing therapy, the sum scores of the Nijmegen questionnaire were markedly reduced. A canonical correlation analysis relating the changes of the various complaints to the modifications of breathing variables showed that the improvement of the complaints was correlated mainly with the slowing down of breathing frequency.

3. *Mothers massaging babies reduces anxiety*: Anxiety levels and depressed mood were significantly reduced in mothers when they learned to give their babies regular preterm infant massage (Feijó et al 2006).

Nijmegen questionnaire (see Fig. 10.2)

The Nijmegen questionnaire provides a non-invasive test of high sensitivity (up to 91%) and specificity (up to 95%) (Vansteenkiste et al 1991). This easily administered, internationally validated diagnostic questionnaire is the simplest, kindest and to date most accurate indicator of acute and chronic hyperventilation (Van Dixhoorn & Duivenvoorden 1985).

The questionnaire enquires as to the following symptoms, and their intensity: constriction in the chest, shortness of breath, accelerated or deepened breathing, inability to breathe deeply, feeling tense, tightness around the mouth, stiffness in the fingers or arms, cold hands or feet, tingling fingers, bloated abdominal sensation, dizzy spells, blurred vision, feeling of confusion or losing touch with the environment.

Physical medicine therapeutic measures for symptoms linked to anxiety states

- *Physical medicine approaches aimed at normalization of breathing pattern disorders include selective use of many of the modalities discussed in Chapter 7: massage, myofascial release, muscle energy techniques, positional release techniques, mobilization, HVLA manipulation, rib raising directed at short, tight, restricted thoracic cage and accessory respiratory muscles.*

- *Massage in particular, and to some extent reflexology, have been shown in studies to offer anti-anxiety effects (commonly involving reduced cortisol levels as a measure of a calming effect) (Field et al 2005).*

- *These manual methods should be combined with appropriate breathing exercises (see Further reading suggestions below).*

- *When such methods are combined with use of biofeedback from a capnograph, linked to a computer monitor, results are commonly more rapid.*

	Never 0	Rare 1	Sometimes 2	Often 3	Very often 4
Chest pain					
Feeling tense					
Blurred vision					
Dizzy spells					
Feeling confused					
Faster or deeper breathing					
Short of breath					
Tight feelings in chest					
Bloated feeling in stomach					
Tingling fingers					
Unable to breathe deeply					
Stiff fingers or arms					
Tight feelings round mouth					
Cold hands or feet					
Palpitations					
Feelings of anxiety					

Total: /64*

* Nijmegen. Patients mark with a tick how often they suffer from the symptoms listed. A score above 23/64 is diagnostic of hyperventilation syndrome.

Figure 10.2 Nijmegen questionnaire. Reproduced with permission from Chaitow et al (2002)

- *Psychotherapy, counseling and stress management can also usefully be combined with the biomechanical focus, when appropriate.*
- *Nutritional strategies require attention to maintenance of a stable blood-sugar status, as well as to replenishment of potentially unbalanced nutrients such as calcium, magnesium and potassium.*
- *Hydrotherapeutic and electrotherapeutic measures may be helpful in easing anxiety.*

Asthma

Lum (1996) points out that there are many people with breathing pattern disorders such as hyperventilation who have been labeled as asthmatics:

Thirty percent of cases of asthma are known to be induced by emotion or exercise, and many symptoms are common to hyperventilation and to asthma: intermittent, labored breathing; relief from bronchodilators (transient in hyperventilation); exercise; cough; fear, anxiety and panic. It is thus a matter of individual preference whether the clinician calls such cases asthma or hyperventilation. The distinction is important. Treatment of hyperventilation

cures the patient. The asthmatic is condemned to a life of medication.

Concepts and methods as outlined in the previous section on anxiety, insofar as they relate to respiratory function, can therefore be applied in full to patients with asthma, as well as to individuals whose breathing patterns are less than normal but whose level of respiratory dysfunction does not justify a diagnosis of hyperventilation or asthma.

Assessment by means of a capnograph reading of less than 30 mmHg, of end-tidal CO_2 (ETCO$_2$), is diagnostic of hyperventilation, as (with over 90% certainty) is a score of 23 or more (out of 64) using the Nijmegen questionnaire, as discussed earlier in this chapter.

What is increasingly evident is that many individuals, intermittently or constantly, have breathing patterns that, while not 'qualifying' for a hyperventilation diagnosis, are heading in that direction.

If breathing patterns were routinely evaluated (the Nijmegen questionnaire takes no more than a minute or two to complete), such individuals could be recognized and helped towards normality by simple means (Aust & Fischer 1997, Han et al 1996, Mehling & Hamel 2005).

Systematic review of manual therapy and asthma

A Cochrane systematic review (Hondras et al 2005) has been conducted to evaluate the evidence for the effects of manual therapies (such as massage, chiropractic, physiotherapy) for treatment of patients with bronchial asthma. The conclusion was that there is insufficient evidence to support, or refute, the use of manual therapies for patients with asthma, and that there is a need to conduct adequately sized randomized controlled trials that examine the effects of manual therapies on clinically relevant outcomes.

Studies that support the use of manual methods in treatment of asthmatics (alongside the nutritional, botanical, pharmacological and other strategies that may assist self-regulation to operate more efficiently) include the following:

- *Soft tissue manipulation and asthma*: Studies have demonstrated that soft tissue manipulation can improve movement of the chest, increase the flow of air, and generally ease the symptoms of chronic asthma (Bockenhauer et al 2002, Rowane & Rowane 1999). Soft tissue manipulation (deep massage-type and stretching techniques, often based on osteopathic methods) can significantly relax the respiratory muscles and mobilize the spine and ribs. Many osteopaths and chiropractors, as well as those physiotherapists who are trained in manual methods (and some licensed massage therapists), use these methods.
- *Upper thoracic manipulation and asthma*: Specific manipulative attention to the upper thoracic spine (to the first four or five vertebrae just below the neck) and to the first joint of the neck (occipitoatlantal joint) can influence the activity of the vagal nerve, relax the diaphragm, and help to ease asthma symptoms. When the sympathetic nervous system is in an 'alarm' phase (as it is likely to be when someone is stressed or anxious), breathing becomes more rapid, and shallower, and asthma symptoms increase. The vagal nerve controls the parasympathetic nerve supply to the diaphragm (among other things) and stimulation of this nerve, by careful manipulation of the area, has been shown to help normalize the excessive degree of sympathetic activity that accompanies asthma (Szentivaneji & Goldman 1997).
- *Breathing exercise and asthma*: Pursed-lip and anti-arousal, yoga-type diaphragmatic breathing exercises have been shown to be very effective in improving the mechanics and efficiency of breathing in asthmatics (Faling 1986, Tisp et al 1986). The instructions involve focus on breathing in through the nose (slowly if possible) and then exhaling slowly (taking 4–6 seconds) through pursed lips ('kiss position', as though blowing a balloon). This is repeated for several minutes. The benefits include slowing the breathing rate, increased amount of air movement through the lungs ('tidal air'), so improving oxygen supplies to the blood and producing an anti-arousal effect (Cappo & Holmes 1984).

- *Buteyko breathing and asthma*: The Russian Buteyko rehabilitation method uses exercises that include variations of controlled breathing, including pursed-lip breathing. A specific tactic is use of a 'control' pause. Daily practice of this is recommended in which the breath is slowly exhaled, and then held out for as long as is comfortable, followed by breathing shallowly (i.e. the holding of the breath is not followed by a deep breath). This is thought to encourage a build-up of CO_2, which relaxes the smooth muscles around the lungs, easing the breathing afterwards. An Australian study of this method, involving 39 patients, resulted in reduced steroid medication usage and significantly improved breathing function in asthma patients (Bowler et al 1998).

- *Chiropractic and asthma*: There have been a number of positive studies showing benefit in asthma of chiropractic attention. For example, 3 months of chiropractic manipulation (involving 20 treatments sessions) was shown to reduce the symptoms of persistent childhood asthma, with benefits still present a year after treatment ceased (Bronfort et al 2001). Nevertheless, there seems to be a consensus that although quality of life and bronchodilator use have been demonstrated, there is currently not sufficient evidence to support the use of chiropractic as a primary treatment for asthma (Balon & Mior 2004). However, there is some evidence suggesting that chiropractic care, in conjunction with standard medical treatment, may be of value (Gibbs 2005). The author notes:

  Three cases of asthma where patients, being treated by conventional pharmacological means, had chiropractic manipulation administered to the upper thoracic spine twice a week for a period of 6 weeks. Objective measurements were collected using a peak flow meter and subjective data using an asthma specific questionnaire. All three cases resulted in increased subjective and objective parameters and suggest the need for larger studies with appropriate methodology.

- *Hydrotherapy and asthma*: The effect on 25 patients with bronchial asthma (10 male, 15 female, mean age 60 years) of complex spa therapy (swimming training in a hot spring pool + fango (seaweed mud) therapy + inhalation of iodine salt solution) was evaluated. Physical symptoms and respiratory system function improved significantly after spa therapy. The results also suggested that complex spa therapy improves psychological factors in patients with bronchial asthma (Yokota et al 1997).

- The improvement of ventilatory function by spa therapy was examined in 37 patients with steroid-dependent intractable asthma (SDIA) in relation to clinical asthma types. All subjects had been on long-term corticosteroid therapy before spa therapy. Spa therapy was found to improve the values of ventilatory parameters. The results show that spa therapy improves the condition of small airways disorder in patients with SDIA (Tanizak et al 1993).

Exercise, asthma and the menstrual cycle

In the previous section on anxiety it was noted that progesterone is a respiratory accelerator, making the postovulation (pre-period) segments of the cycle a time when symptoms emerging from breathing pattern disorders (or asthma) were most likely to be exacerbated. Stanford et al (2006), in a study evaluating the effects of these cyclical phases on female athletes, have confirmed this connection. This study investigated the relationship between menstrual cycle phase and exercise-induced bronchoconstriction (EIB) in female athletes with mild atopic asthma. Seven subjects with regular 28-day menstrual cycles were exercised to volitional exhaustion on day 5 (mid-follicular, FOL) and day 21 (mid-luteal, LUT) of their menstrual cycle. Pulmonary function tests were conducted pre- and post-exercise. The maximal percentage decline in post-exercise forced expiratory volume in 1 second (FEV_1) and forced expiratory flow from 25 to 75% of forced vital capacity (FEF 25–75%) was significantly greater ($p < 0.05$) on day 21 (mid-LUT phase) when salivary progesterone concentration was highest, compared to day 5 (mid-FOL phase) when salivary progesterone concentration was lowest. The deterioration in the severity of EIB during the mid-LUT phase was accompanied by worsening asthma symptoms and increased bronchodilator use. This study demonstrates that menstrual cycle phase is an impor-

tant determinant of the severity of EIB in female athletes with mild atopic asthma.

Naturopathic clinicians should be aware of this influence when prescribing exercise and when informing asthmatic female patients of times when particular attention to breathing retraining should be considered.

Exercise and asthma

Exercise-induced asthma is a well-known phenomenon (Caffarelli et al 2005) that can lead to an avoidance of active exercising. Instead of this course of (in)action, education should be offered as to the value of submaximal exercise.

- *Physical exercise and asthma*: A Cochrane systematic review (Ram et al 2005) has found that, in people with asthma, physical training can improve cardiopulmonary fitness without changing lung function. It is not known whether improved fitness is translated into improved quality of life. It is important to know that physical training does not have an adverse effect on lung function and wheeze in patients with asthma. Therefore, there is no reason why patients with asthma should not participate in regular physical activity.

- *Submaximal exercise and asthma*: To investigate the effects of regular submaximal exercise on quality of life in children with asthma, exercise capacity and pulmonary function of 62 children with mild/moderate asthma were evaluated. The children were randomly allocated into exercise and control groups. The exercise group underwent a moderately intensive basketball training program for 8 weeks. A home respiratory exercise program was advised to both groups. The Pediatric Asthma Quality of Life Questionnaire (PAQLQ) was used for the evaluation of activity limitation, symptoms and emotional functions. Exercise capacity was evaluated through the physical work capacity (PWC 170 test) on a cycle ergometer and 6-minute walk test. Spirometric tests were also performed and medication and symptom scores were recorded. Results showed that although PAQLQ scores improved in both groups, the improvement in the exercise group was significantly higher. The exercise group performed better in the PWC 170 and 6-minute walk tests, whereas no improvement was detected in the control group at the end of the trial. Medication scores improved in both groups, but symptom scores improved only in the exercise group. No significant changes were detected in pulmonary function in either group, except for peak expiratory flow values in the exercise group (Basaran et al 2006).

- *Physical activities of daily life and asthma*: Adults with asthma who had derived benefits from a 10-week exercise program were evaluated 3 years later to see whether continued adherence to exercising, or not, had impacted on their condition. All 21 participants were found to be physically active in daily life, less limited by their disease, and better able to control their asthma, irrespective of whether they were adherent with exercise recommendations or not. The study findings suggest that physical activities in daily life are sufficient to maintain a good physical condition (Emtner & Hedin 2005).

Yoga and asthma

- *Yoga breathing and asthma*: Over 100 asthma patients were taught basic yoga breathing (similar to the pursed-lip methods described above). The results showed a reduction in use of drugs and improved breathing function, which was still apparent 4 years after the study (Nagarathna & Nagendra 1985).
- *Sahaja yoga and asthma*: A randomized controlled trial has shown that the practice of Sahaja yoga does have limited beneficial effects on some objective and subjective measures of the impact of moderate to severe asthma (Manocha et al 2002).
- *Diet therapy, yoga and asthma*: 37 asthmatic patients (19 men, 18 women) were involved in a study in which yoga therapy was combined with 'a non-pharmacological approach of naturopathy' (ingredients/modalities not specified apart from 'diet therapy' and 'nature cure treatment'). The various parameters, including lung function test, were measured on admission and once a week. Results showed significant improvement in PEFR, VC, FVC, FEV_1, FEV/FEC %, MVV, ESR and absolute eosinophil count. The patients reported a feeling of well-being, freshness and comfortable breathing (Sathyaprabha et al 2001).

Physical medicine therapeutic measures for asthma

- *Soft tissue and joint manipulation, particularly involving the diaphragm and upper thoracic region, offers benefits to asthmatics.*

- *Breathing rehabilitation methods, including yoga breathing techniques, enhance respiratory function for people with asthma.*
- *Regular submaximal exercise improves quality of life and respiratory function for people with asthma.*
- *Spa treatment improves objective and subjective criteria in asthmatic patients.*

Cardiovascular disease

Manipulation and cardiovascular health

Segmental spinal changes and heart disease

Beal (1983) has noted that it is almost always possible to predict that cardiovascular disease is present (or is likely to develop) when two or more segments of the spine in the region of T2, T3 and T4 display tense, rigid, 'board-like' characteristics on palpation, especially if these tissues do not respond to normal efforts to reduce their hypertonicity. (See Box 6.38, in Chapter 6, for Beal's palpation method for identification of facilitated segments.)

Burns (1943) has also explained this phenomenon as resulting from afferent stimuli, arising from dysfunction of a visceral nature. The reflex is initiated by afferent impulses arising from visceral receptors, which are transmitted to the dorsal horn of the spinal cord, where they synapse with interconnecting neurons. The stimuli are then conveyed to sympathetic and motor efferents, resulting in changes in the somatic tissues, such as skeletal muscle, skin and blood vessels.

Abnormal stimulation of the visceral efferent neurons may result in hyperesthesia of the skin, and associated vasomotor, pilomotor and sudomotor changes. Similar stimuli of the ventral horn cells may result in reflex rigidity of the somatic musculature. Pain may accompany such changes.

The degree of stimulus required, in any given case, to produce such changes will differ, because factors such as prior sensitization of the particular segment, as well as the response of higher centers, will differ from person to person.

Korr (1976) and Lewit (1999) suggest that, in many cases, viscerosomatic reflex activity may be noted before any symptoms of visceral change are evident, and that this phenomenon is therefore of potential diagnostic and prognostic value.

The first signs of viscerosomatic reflexive influences are vasomotor reactions (increased skin temperature), sudomotor (increased moisture of the skin) and skin textural changes (e.g. thickening), increased subcutaneous fluid and increased contraction of muscle. There is value in using light skin palpation for identification of areas of facilitation as discussed in Chapter 6.

These signs disappear if the visceral cause improves. When such changes become chronic, however, trophic alterations are noted, with increased thickening of the skin and subcutaneous tissue, and localized muscular contraction. Deep musculature may become hard, tense and hypersensitive. This may result in deep splinting contractions, involving two or more segments of the spine, with associated restriction of spinal motion. The costotransverse articulations may be significantly involved in such changes. Such changes would be readily identifiable using neuromuscular assessment palpation as described in Chapter 5.

More on the facilitated segment

Patterns of somatic response will be found to differ from person to person, and to be unique, in terms of location, the number of segments involved, and whether or not the pattern is unilateral or bilateral. The degree of intensity will also differ, and is related to the degree of acuteness of the visceral condition (Hix 1976).

An understanding of the nature of facilitated spinal segments in relation to visceral pathology may explain why appropriate treatment of spinal joints of the neck and upper back can influence, and at times can assist in normalizing, irregular heart rhythms (Jarmel et al 1995).

Jarmel (1989) explains that:

Disturbances in sympathetic and parasympathetic regulation of the heart are associated with increased vulnerability to sudden cardiac death. Destabilizing neural input to the vagus and cardiac sympathetic nerves may originate from mechanically irritated intervertebral joints. Asymptomatic spinal joint dysfunction can affect the autonomic nervous system and may activate potent somato-cardiac reflexes. Aberrant neural impulses from vertebral dysfunction may adversely affect the electrical stability of the heart and increase susceptibility to ventricular fibrillation. Correcting the spinal joint dysfunction which activates these articulovisceral reflexes may have beneficial effects in decreasing vulnerability to sudden cardiac death.

Congestive heart failure

Structural changes and cardiovascular disease

Stiles (1977) observes, in relation to individuals with congestive heart failure, that once the condition has been stabilized, physical evaluation and treatment should focus on the rib cage to ensure optimal diaphragmatic function, as well as the region of ribs 1, 2 and 3, where the thoracic duct joins the internal jugular and subclavian veins. The upper thoracic spine should also receive particular attention, as restrictions of these segments can affect the sympathetic ganglia (Korr et al 1970).

Stiles writes (addressing his own profession):

The osteopathic physician must try to restore normal physiologic motion in the upper thoracic and lower cervical areas, since these are the sites of origin of the sympathetic innervation supplying the coronary vessels. Also, somatic dysfunction of this area can, by affecting the sympathetic ganglia, affect the sympathetic motor supply to the cardiac plexus. This in turn can contribute to changes in cardiac rate. . . . Since the parasympathetic supply to the cardiac plexus is via the vagus, somatic dysfunction in this area, from the atlanto-occipital area, through the cervical region, and into the upper dorsal junction, can have adverse effects on vagal innervation and thus on myocardial rate and rhythm.

Another reason for uneven heart rhythm can be the activity of trigger points in the muscles between the 5th and 6th ribs, a little to the right side of the sternum (in the intercostal or pectoral muscle fibers) (Simons et al 1999a).

Pseudo-angina (functional cardiac symptoms)

As far back as 1948, mainstream medical journals were reporting the phenomenon of pseudo-coronaries and pseudo-angina (Davis 1948). These were episodes of angina where the symptoms did not derive from the cardiovascular system, but were musculoskeletal in origin.

- *Hyperventilation and pseudo-angina*: Angina-like symptoms can also occur in people without coronary artery disease as a result of constriction of the blood vessels, caused by excessive exhalation of carbon dioxide, during unbalanced breathing episodes. Such stress-induced changes can occur during hyperventilation, which frequently have nothing to do with true heart disease. One study suggests *up to 90%* of non-cardiac chest pain can be brought on by hyperventilation syndrome and other breathing pattern disorders (De Guire et al 1992). It is therefore important that chest pain associated with breathing pattern disorders such as hyperventilation are investigated, so that heart disease can be excluded as a diagnosis, and breathing rehabilitation started (see below and discussion of breathing pattern disorders in Chapter 1).

- *Syndrome X*: A condition known as syndrome X (not to be confused with metabolic syndrome, also referred to as syndrome X) refers to those people with a history of angina, whose symptoms can be provoked by an exercise test (chest pain comes on within 6 minutes or less) but who have normal cardiac arteries. Respiratory imbalances may be a key element in such conditions. This is much more common in women than in men (Kumar & Clark 1998, Nakao et al 1997).

- *Spinal restrictions and angina symptoms*: Spinal restrictions and disc degeneration can also cause symptoms identical to angina, without any cardiac involvement at all. One series of 164 such cases of pseudo-angina were reported, with all patients experiencing angina symptoms as well as neck pain, headaches and arm pain. In about a quarter spinal surgery was required, but the majority were successfully treated using methods such as intermittent traction, the wearing of hard collars, stretching of neck muscles and use of anti-inflammatory medication (Jacobs 1990).

- *Lower cervical dysfunction and pseudo-angina*: In another study, seven cases of pseudo-angina were reported, involving typical angina symptoms together with nausea and shortness of breath. In all the patients the lower cervical region was found to be involved (C5/6). Angina symptoms were relieved in five cases, either by surgery to remove damaged discs (three patients) or by use of soft collars (two patients) (Booth & Rothman 1976).

- *T4 syndrome*: The thoracic spine can also be a major source of pseudo-angina. Swedish research, involving nearly 1000 patients admitted to a hospital coronary unit, showed that pseudo-angina resulting from thoracic spinal dysfunction (described as 'T4 syndrome') was the third most common diagnosis after coronary thrombosis and true angina pectoris (Bechgaard 1981).

- *Manipulation and pseudo-angina*: Treatment of the spinal causes, by manipulation, has been shown to relieve such 'angina' symptoms, often in as little as one treatment, with no return of symptoms for up to 10 years (Hamberg & Lindahl 1981).

- *Trigger points and pseudo-angina*: Many cases of pseudo-angina have been reported resulting from trigger points in the pectoral muscles but also in various shoulder and neck muscles. Trigger points are local, irritable, sensitive (to pressure) areas in muscles that usually cause pain or discomfort, not only where they are situated but also in target areas some distance away (Epstein & Gerber 1979).

- *Lidocaine injections, manual therapy and pseudo-angina*: In one report, symptoms of angina-like pain together with palpitations and shortness of breath were reported to clear up following treatment of trigger points by lidocaine injections, as well as massage, hydrotherapy (hot packs, ice packs, whirlpool) and muscle stretching (Pellegrino 1990).

- *Costovertebral joints and pseudo-angina*: Studies by Erwin et al (2000) and Wyke (1975) have also identified the costovertebral joints as a source of back pain and/or pseudo-angina, which may be ameliorated by spinal manipulation. These joints have the requisite innervation for pain production in a similar manner to other joints of the spinal column.

Massage and cardiovascular health

In Chapter 7 the virtually universal usefulness of massage therapy was highlighted. Studies show that massage treatment of trigger points reduces blood pressure significantly (systolic and diastolic) and decreases heart rate, as well as improving the emotional state and muscle tension (Delaney et al 2002). Diastolic blood pressure has been shown to reduce significantly in hypertensive individuals following massage (Hernandez-Reif et al 2000a).

Although much of the evidence of benefit of physical medicine methods in treatment of cardiovascular disease and dysfunction is anecdotal, support also comes from studies that suggest positive general cardiovascular benefits (McGuiness et al 1997), sometimes relating to single case studies, from which extrapolation to a wider application would be speculative (Driscoll & Hall 2000), or which show positive benefits in measures such as heart rate variability (Zhang et al 2006).

General and (where appropriate) specific manipulative and soft tissue methods, in cases of patients with cardiovascular disease, are shown to be of potential value in naturopathic care, particularly where attention is given to contextual issues such as lifestyle, exercise, nutrition and stress management.

Hydrotherapy and cardiovascular health

Treatment of cardiovascular disease and dysfunction by means of hydrotherapy/balneotherapy has a long tradition.

Kneipp (1979; first published in 1893) described his treatment of a young man with 'head and heart complaints' as follows:

Every morning the young gentleman walked for half an hour in the wet dewy grass, and daily stood in the water up to the pit of his stomach, with a lavation of the upper body . . . later on, by way of strengthening, he received frequent upper affusions daily, one or two, in alternation with semi-baths. Head and heart complaints soon vanished with the gradual increase of his general strength.

Over 100 years later researchers in Germany evaluated Kneipp's empirical approach. They explain:

In central-European physical therapy, warm-water baths and sauna are commonly supplemented by repeated cold water stimuli with peripheral cold water immersions and cold water pourings (hydrotherapy according to Kneipp) (Bühring 1988). Serial hydrotherapeutic cold- and warm-water applications are also used as a supportive treatment for patients with coronary artery disease and patients with CHF in cardiological rehabilitative facilities. The beneficial effects of hydrotherapy in patients with chronic heart failure (CHF), hypertension, and coronary artery disease have been described in some empirical and observational reports (Brüggemann 1986, Gutenbrunner & Ruppel 1992). However, its efficacy has never been tested in controlled trials. The current study was designed to test whether a specific and intensive home-based hydrotherapeutic treatment program, consisting of a structured combination of warm and cold thermal applications, can induce improvements in exercise performance, quality of life (QOL), and heart-failure–related symptoms in patients with mild CHF.

The home-based hydrotherapy is described as follows:

Patients were advised to practice warm and cold applications at least three times a day to a total maximum of 30 minutes daily. Warm thermal applications consisted of peripheral warm water baths (arm baths, foot baths) with incremental temperature (maximum 40°C) and warm sheet packs. For cold applications, short-term arm or foot baths and peripheral water pourings with a water temperature below 18°C were taught. Patients were instructed to apply the hydrotherapeutic applications long enough to induce a postprocedural reactive feeling of warmth with respective mild redness of the treated skin area, but no longer than 15 minutes for baths and 5 minutes for cold pourings.

After the 6-week study the researchers noted:

Our findings imply that an appropriately performed home-based hydrotherapeutic program may provide a

practical, salutary, nonpharmacological therapy for patients with CHF without the need for expensive rehabilitation facilities. Furthermore, this therapy approach may be applicable in patients who are unable to participate in exercise training. We conclude that a simple, home-based, hydrotherapeutic program is feasible and effective in improving symptoms, QOL, and hemodynamics of patients with non-severe CHF. Further studies are needed to investigate the effects of hydrotherapy in patients with larger populations and more severe heart failure, and to clarify the mechanisms behind this non-pharmacological therapy approach.

More recently, scientific studies have revealed more about the value of different forms of hydrotherapy in treatment of cardiovascular disease:

- *Hemodynamic effects of training in warm water*: Low workload exercises for mobility, strength and cardiovascular fitness, when immersed (standing) in warm (33–34°C) water, induces beneficial hemodynamic effects in patients with chronic heart failure. There were no signs of adverse reactions. The findings indicate that an increased venous return is balanced by a reduction of heart rate and a probable decrease in afterload, promoting an increase in left ventricular output. These positive hemodynamic effects of short-term immersion support previous evidence of positive effects during training in warm water (Cider et al 2006). This evidence is supported by other studies (Gabrielsen et al 2000, Meyer 2001).
- *Balneotherapy and the heart*: Balneotherapy involving sulfur baths has been shown Leibetseder et al 2004) to beneficially modify plasma homocysteine, long associated with cardiovascular disease (McCully 1969).

Exercise and cardiovascular health

- *Walking and the heart*: Treadmill exercise test data have confirmed that heart rate recovery is a marker of physical fitness and exercise capacity, that abnormal heart rate recovery is a strong predictor of mortality in both asymptomatic individuals (Cole et al 1999, 2000, Messinger-Rapport et al 2003) and cardiac patients (Nishime et al 2000, Shetler et al 2001) and that exercise training improves heart rate recovery in cardiac patients (Tiukinoy et al 2003). The 6-minute walk test has a range of applications in characterizing exercise response in both cardiac and non-cardiac patients. It has also been proposed as a valid measure of functional capacity after a cardiac rehabilitation program (Wright et al 2001).

- *Exercise and the heart*: Because the ultimate goal of any prophylactic measure in myocardial pathophysiological conditions is the restoration of full contractile function, it is logical to use contractile pump function as the primary dependent measure in the study of myocardial response. A considerable number of research studies have demonstrated that exercise attenuated the significant impairments in left ventricular developed pressure (LVDP), maximum rate of left ventricular pressure development and decline (±dP/dt), systolic and diastolic pressure, coronary flow, cardiac output and work, induced by several cardiotoxic and pathological stressors (Ascensão et al 2007, Hamilton et al 2001).

- *Muscle strengthening exercise and coronary heart disease*: A number of studies have demonstrated beneficial effects from muscle strengthening exercises in healthy persons including: increased endurance, bone density, metabolic rate; improved sleep; reduced depression; decreased body fat; improved digestion; prevention of falls and frailty and diabetes mellitus. It is still not clear which exercise is best for prevention of heart disease, but it is now clear that regular exercise is preventive. In a recent study (Tanasescu et al 2002), running, weight training and rowing were all protective against coronary artery disease.

- *Graduated exercise and cardiovascular function*: Although there is some disagreement regarding different effects of exercise on cardiovascular function in males and females (Paroo et al 2002, Xi 2002), a graduated and prescribed exercise program based on research evidence of benefit in cardiovascular rehabilitation should be introduced (BACR 2000).

Tai chi cardiovascular effects, compared with walking

It may be of interest that when brisk walking exercise was compared with tai chi, the latter produced the better outcomes.

Tai chi chuan more effective than brisk walking for fitness

A study by Audette et al (2006) compared the effects of a short style of tai chi chuan (TCC), versus a brisk walking training program on aerobic capacity, heart rate variability (HRV), strength, flexibility, balance, psychological status and quality of life in elderly women. Outcomes measured before and after training included estimated VO$_2$max, spectral analysis of HRV (high-frequency, low-frequency power as well as high- and low-frequency power in normalized units) as a measure of autonomic control of the heart, isometric knee extension and handgrip muscle strength, single-leg stance time, the State Trait Anxiety Inventory (STAI), Profile of Mood States (POMS) and Short Form-36 (SF-36) questionnaires.

The conclusion was that a short style of TCC was an effective way of improving many fitness measures (including cardiovascular) in elderly women over a 3-month period. TCC was also found to be significantly better than brisk walking in enhancing certain measures of fitness including lower extremity strength, balance and flexibility.

Breathing rehabilitation (including yoga) and cardiovascular health

There are several ways in which a habitual upper chest breathing pattern, that automatically involves excessive carbon dioxide exhalation and increased alkalinity of the bloodstream (Foster et al 2001), can disrupt the normal oxygen supply to the heart, at times causing abnormal rhythmic behavior or worse:

1. The smooth muscles that surround the blood vessels constrict, reducing blood supply to the heart muscles and vessels, resulting in acute episodes such as coronary artery spasm (Nakao et al 1997).
2. The red blood cells release the oxygen they should be delivering to the heart muscles less efficiently (Bohr effect), provoking angina-like symptoms (Pryor & Prasad 2002b).
3. The sympathetic nervous system becomes stimulated, unbalancing heart rhythms.

An upper chest breathing pattern also creates a great deal of additional work for particular muscles, including those that may house trigger points involved in heart arrhythmia, the intercostals and pectorals. Trigger points often develop in overused muscle tissues, especially if they are relatively oxygen starved (ischemic), as they would be when there is an upper chest breathing pattern (Simons et al 1999a).

Breathing retraining (yogic-type patterns) can help to restore normal nerve and oxygen supply to the heart, easing disturbances such as palpitations (Han et al 1996) (see 'Anxiety' and 'Asthma' sections for more on breathing).

Yoga (pranayama) and the heart

Breathing is proposed as having a beneficial effect on cardiovascular function. Pranayamic breathing, defined as a manipulation of breath movement, has been shown to contribute to a physiological response characterized by the presence of decreased oxygen consumption, decreased heart rate and decreased blood pressure, as well as increased theta wave amplitude in EEG recordings, increased parasympathetic activity, accompanied by the experience of alertness and reinvigoration (Harinath et al 2004, Malhotra et al 2002, Pal & Velkumary 2004, Singh et al 2004).

Mechanisms

The mechanisms as to how pranayamic breathing interacts with the nervous system affecting metabolism and autonomic functions are not yet fully understood.

It is hypothesized (Edrya et al 2006) that voluntary slow deep breathing functionally resets the autonomic nervous system through stretch-induced inhibitory signals and hyperpolarization currents propagated through both neural and non-neural tissue which synchronizes neural elements in the heart, lungs, limbic system and cortex. During inspiration, stretching of lung tissue produces inhibitory signals by action of slowly adapting stretch receptors (SARs) and hyperpolarization current, by action of fibroblasts. Both inhibitory impulses and hyperpolarization current are known to synchronize neural elements, leading to the modulation of the nervous system and decreased metabolic activity indicative of the parasympathetic state. It is proposed that pranayama's (breathing pattern) physiological mechanism acts through both cellular and systems levels, involving both neural and non-neural elements. This theoretical description illustrates a common physiological mechanism underlying pranayama and may explain the role of the respiratory and cardiovascular systems in modulation of the autonomic nervous system.

From a naturopathic perspective it would seem to be irrelevant whether Western or Eastern models of breathing retraining are incorporated into therapy, as long as this vital function is addressed.

Physical medicine therapeutic measures for cardiovascular disease

- *Manipulation, mobilization and soft tissue treatment of the upper thoracic spine can positively influence cardiovascular function.*
- *Manual treatment of the rib cage, with specific attention to ribs 1, 2 and 3 and the upper thoracic spine, is potentially helpful in cases of congestive heart failure.*
- *Pseudo-angina symptoms may be eased by appropriate manual treatment of cervical and upper thoracic vertebrae, the costovertebral joints or trigger points in key local muscles (e.g. pectoralis major).*
- *Massage can frequently balance both systolic and diastolic blood pressure irregularities, and helps to induce a more normal cardiac rhythm.*
- *Various forms of hydrotherapy, including balneotherapy, have been shown to be helpful in treatment of a variety of cardiovascular conditions.*
- *Graduated and regular exercise (e.g. 6-minute walk test) and/or muscle strengthening exercises offer cardiovascular benefit in prevention as well as rehabilitation.*
- *Tai chi is a useful means of achieving cardiovascular benefits in a stress-free environment.*
- *Breathing exercises, including pranayama yoga, are helpful in cardiovascular conditions.*

Depression

Manipulation and depression

- *Depression retards benefits of physical treatment methods*: While anxiety had little or no effect on outcomes, coexisting depression has been shown to significantly reduce the likelihood of success of treatment of chronic resistant musculoskeletal pain, involving a multidisciplinary treatment program incorporating myofascial technique physical therapy, clinical psychophysiology (biofeedback, counseling), medications and trigger point injections (Sorrell et al 2003).
- *BEST chiropractic and depression in chronic pain patients*: While there is little evidence that depression can be successfully treated using manipulative methods alone, a subtle form of chiropractic known as bio-energetic synchronization technique (BEST) has demonstrated such an effect in treatment of chronic pain conditions (Rupert et al 2005). Twenty-four adult patients with chronic pain-related conditions that had failed to respond to previous chiropractic care were recruited. The patients were given baseline assessments including pain visual analog scale, Profile of Mood States, and the Global Well-being Scale. The 5-week treatment program consisted of an initial 3-day session with BEST therapy, followed by a single treatment session for the following 4 weeks. Patients were re-evaluated at the end of the 3-day session and at weekly intervals throughout the course of care. Global Well-being Scale scores significantly improved

at the end of the 3-day session ($p > 0.05$) but not subsequently. The Profile of Mood States reflected favorable changes in all areas. Significant improvement in vigor ($p > 0.003$) and fatigue ($p > 0.006$) existed at the end of 5 weeks ($p < 0.01$). The reduction of pain was significant at both the end of the 3-day session and at follow-up ($p = 0.0003$). *A statistically significant decrease in depression* ($p = 0.004$) *was noted after 3 days, and a substantial although not significant* ($p = 0.06$) *decrease in depression existed at the end of 1 month.*

Mobilization and depression

There are also encouraging results from some studies that point to the value of mobilization methods in patients whose depression is reactive – for example, in people suffering from phobic conditions and panic attacks.

Osteopathic manipulative therapy, depression and panic disorder

Michaud (2004) tested the proposal that an osteopathic approach could be seen as an alternative treatment to the two types of presently proposed therapies, alone or combined (pharmacological, psychological). It is observed that panic disorder (PD) is a mental health problem that takes too long to detect, tending to become chronic and lessening the quality of life. The experimental design involved a clinical study involving nine subjects suffering from PD with agoraphobia who did not take any prescribed medication for PD during the study, nor were they treated by a psychologist, in order to isolate the effect of the osteopathic treatment. Evaluation of the quality of life was made by six standard questionnaires used in psychological evaluation in research for PD in pretreatment and post-treatment.

- *Step 1*: Pretreatment evaluation (1st week): (a) PRIME-MD questionnaire to verify the diagnosis; (b) psychological evaluation with the six questionnaires; (c) osteopathic evaluation.
- *Step 2*: Osteopathic therapy: four sessions of osteopathic treatment according to protocol (around 1 hour each).
- *Step 3*: Post-treatment evaluation (13th week): re-evaluating the subjects with the same psychological questionnaires as in step 1.
- *Step 4*: Follow-up 3 years later: using the same psychological questionnaires in order to verify if the acquired conditions have maintained or disappeared. *Results*: First, the results that were

obtained show a significant improvement in the quality of life with regard to factors of *depression*, fear, anxiety, physical sensations and panic attack. Secondly, these acquired conditions were maintained or improved after 3 years.

Massage and depression

There a large number of studies supporting the value of massage in treatment of depression.

- *Slow-stroke massage and depression*: A randomized cross-over trial (Müller-Oerlinghausen et al 2004) evaluated the benefits of 'slow-stroke' massage in treatment of 32 depressed patients (24 women, 8 men; average 48 years). The trial involved three massage sessions at set times and sessions in two control groups of relaxation and perception, lasting for 60 minutes, 2–3 days apart. Under the control conditions there was no touching. The effects of depression-specific variables were measured by both the patients' own assessment and that of an independent observer. *Results*: Under conditions of both massage and control, comparison of before and after effects, there was not only a mood-enhancing effect but also some very marked changes in almost all criteria. The benefits of massage compared with control treatment were confirmed by both female and male patients. *Conclusion*: Slow-stroke massage is suitable for adjuvant acute treatment of patients with depression, and should be available in both hospital and general practice settings.
- *Massage and depression during pregnancy*: Eighty-four depressed pregnant women were recruited during the second trimester of pregnancy and randomly assigned to a massage therapy group, a progressive muscle relaxation group or a control group that received standard prenatal care alone (Field et al 2004). These groups were compared to each other and to a non-depressed group at the end of pregnancy. The massage therapy group participants received two 20-minute therapy sessions (by their significant others) each week for 16 weeks of pregnancy, starting during the second trimester. The relaxation group provided themselves with progressive muscle relaxation sessions on the same time schedule. Immediately after the massage therapy sessions, on the first and last days of the 16-week period, the women reported lower levels of anxiety and depressed mood and less leg

and back pain. By the end of the study the massage group had higher dopamine and serotonin levels and lower levels of cortisol and norepinephrine. It is suggested that these changes may have contributed to the reduced fetal activity, and the better neonatal outcome, for the massage group (i.e. lesser incidence of prematurity and low birth weight). The data suggest that depressed pregnant women and their offspring can benefit from massage therapy.

- *Massage and biochemical markers affecting both depression and anxiety*: Biochemical markers of these conditions have been shown to significantly change following massage. Field et al (2005) report that in studies in which cortisol was assayed either in saliva or in urine, significant decreases were noted in cortisol levels (averaging decreases of 31%). In studies in which the activating neurotransmitters (serotonin and dopamine) were assayed in urine, an average increase of 28% was noted for serotonin, and an average increase of 31% was noted for dopamine. These studies combined demonstrate the stress-alleviating effects (decreased cortisol) and the activating effects (increased serotonin and dopamine) of massage therapy on a variety of medical conditions and stressful experiences.

In these representative studies, as well as in hundreds of others, massage has been shown to be a valuable adjunct to patient care in cases of depression. Naturopathic care of individuals with depression should clearly consider incorporating massage as part of the therapeutic plan.

Exercise and depression

- *Physical activity and depression*: A 10-year study by Harris et al (2006) examined associations between physical activity, exercise coping and depression in a sample of initially depressed patients. These patients ($n = 424$) completed measures of physical activity, exercise coping, depression, and other demographic and psychosocial constructs at baseline, 1 year, 4 years and 10 years. The results showed that more physical activity was associated with less concurrent depression, even after controlling for gender, age, medical problems and negative life events. Physical activity counteracted the effects of medical conditions and negative life events on depression. It appears that physical activity may be especially helpful in the context of depression associated with medical

problems and major life stressors. Clinically, encouraging depressed patients to engage in physical activity is likely to have potential benefits with few obvious risks.

- *Ballroom dancing and depression*: Ballroom dancing as a form of exercise has been studied in relation to geriatric depression (Haboush et al 2006). Twenty depressed, community-dwelling older adults (average age = 69) completed a pilot study of ballroom dance lessons as a treatment for geriatric depression. Participants were randomly assigned to either an immediate or delayed treatment condition. All participants received eight ballroom dance lessons from a selection of six dances (foxtrot, waltz, rumba, swing, cha-cha and tango) from the National Dance Council of America's syllabus. There was some support for self-efficacy and hopelessness as outcome predictors. Participant feedback indicated the dance lessons were enjoyable and well-received.

- *Exercise and mental well-being*: Associations between exercise and mental well-being have been well documented. A meta-analysis of 11 treatment outcome studies of individuals with depression yielded a very large combined effect size for the advantage of exercise over control conditions: $g = 1.39$ (95% CI: 0.89–1.88), corresponding to a $d = 1.42$ (95% CI: 0.92–1.93) (Stathopoulou et al 2006).

Based on these findings naturopaths are strongly encouraged to consider the role of exercise interventions in care of depressed patients.

Hydrotherapy and depression

There is a modest degree of support for the value of spa therapy (thermal, flotation, chemical) in treatment of moderate depression; however, since the majority of spas do not accept individuals with serious behavioral problems or those who are at risk of suicide, this form of therapeutic intervention offers only limited evidence of value in such conditions (Dubois 1973, Dubois & Arnaud 1983, Guillard 1990).

Flotation tank treatment and depression

Restricted environmental stimulation technique (REST) using a flotation tank has been shown to reduce anxiety and depression in patients with chronic pain (Kjellgren et al 2001). Treatment comprised a procedure in which the individual was immersed in a tank filled with water of an extremely high salt concentration. Thirty-seven patients (14 men and 23 women) suffering from chronic pain participated in the study. They were randomly assigned to either a control group (17 participants) or an experimental group (20 participants). The experimental group received nine flotation-REST treatments over a 3-week period. The results indicated that the most severe perceived pain intensity was significantly reduced, whereas low perceived pain intensity was not influenced. Flotation-REST treatment elevated the participants' optimism and reduced the degree of anxiety or depression, and improved the sleep pattern.

While the foundational treatment for depression is likely to call for attention to psychosocial issues, as well as biochemical nutrition, etc., factors, the evidence offered suggests that additional benefit is available via use of exercise, massage and other manual methods, and possibly hydrotherapy.

Physical medicine therapeutic measures for depression

- *Manipulation, mobilization and particularly massage have all been shown to offer significant benefit for people with depressive illness.*
- *Major antidepressive benefits derive from all forms of exercise (walking, ballroom dancing).*
- *Spa treatment appears to offer benefit for some people with depression.*

Fatigue, including chronic fatigue syndrome (see also instinctive sleep postures in Chapter 9)

Apart from pain, fatigue is one of the most widespread of symptoms (Lane et al 1990), ranging from mild to extreme, intermittent and fluctuating to constant, physical to mental ('brain fog', depression), primary (chronic fatigue syndrome) or secondary to a host of influences, seasonal, toxic, deficiencies, cyclical, justifiable or just plain mysterious. Clearly, with etiologies that range from endocrine to nutritional, psychological to physiological and/or pathological, there are no magic bullets for remedying fatigue, any more than there are for pain.

What underlying failure of adaptation, inability of coping systems and/or excessive demands of a physical or psychological nature, or just plain breakdown of normal functions such as energy (ATP) production, are involved, determines what therapeutic measures should be recommended. Causes, as with most health problems, usually lie in a combination of the three major influences: biochemical, psychosocial or biomechanical. Self-regulating processes that are overwhelmed or underfunctioning need to be identified and offered assistance towards recovery, by means of removal of identifiable causes, together with enhancement of function.

Compression and manipulation for fatigue associated with fibromyalgia

Patients with diagnosed fibromyalgia received 30 chiropractic treatments that combined ischemic compression applied to trigger/tender points for 10 seconds at a time, as well as spinal manipulation, in order to evaluate the effects on the intensity of pain, sleep disturbance and fatigue (Hains & Hains 2000). Between 15 and 30 treatments were administered over a 30-day period. After 30 days there was an average lessening of 77.2% (standard deviation, SD = 12.3%) in pain intensity and an improvement of 63.5% (SD = 31.6%) in sleep quality and 74.8% (SD = 23.1%) in fatigue. The improvement in the three outcome measures was maintained after 1 month without treatment.

Low force (BEST) chiropractic and fatigue

In their 2005 study, Rupert et al state:

The treatment approach involves extensive education related to nutrition, diet, and lifestyle modification. BEST also emphasizes the patient's responsibility for their own health and attempts to motivate and empower them to be more responsible for their own lives. The nutritional education consisted of encouraging patients to increase vegetable consumption and reduce dietary animal protein. Supplementation consisted of ground barley plant tablets, a digestive enzyme, and trace minerals.

Treatment involves the patient lying on a treatment table where muscle strength tests are performed with the patient in both the prone and supine positions. These tests commonly involve strength assessment of the arm or leg. During the test, while in the supine position, the patient is asked to think about the chief complaint, or the major stress in their life. This process is believed to determine if there is an emotional component involved. The treating doctor then places the patient prone and uses leg-length assessment in an attempt to evaluate 'balance'. This is believed to be a method of assessing the balance of the autonomic nervous system. If the treating practitioner finds leg-length variations other than anatomical variations that would suggest autonomic imbalance, then a treatment is administered. This consists of the placing of one hand on the back of the skull of the prone patient, and the other on the sacrum. Light pressure is then applied to these 2 regions. The pressure is described as a form

---

Box 10.8 Osteopathic management of chronic fatigue syndrome

Roger Newman Turner ND DO BAc

A disturbance of sympathetic nervous function has been hypothesized as a significant factor in the etiology of chronic fatigue syndrome (CFS) by Perrin (1993). He draws a correlation between the incidence of chronic back pain and the later onset of CFS (myalgic encephalomyelitis).

In a later paper, Perrin was able to demonstrate a significant reduction in a number of measures of CFS severity following a course of osteopathic treatment (Perrin et al 1998). A clinical trial assessed 58 people with confirmed CFS. They were divided into two groups – a patient group ($n = 34$) and a control group ($n = 24$). Only those in the patient group were given osteopathic treatment whilst the control group did not receive any manual treatment. They were, however, allowed to receive any other treatment available for this condition.

The treatment of each CFS patient consisted of the following procedures:

- Soft tissue massage of paravertebral muscles, trapezii, levator scapulae, rhomboids and respiratory accessory muscles
- High- and low-velocity manipulation of the thoracic and upper lumbar spinal segments
- Gentle articulation of thoracic and upper lumbar spine and ribs

- Functional techniques to suboccipital region and sacrum
- Stimulation of craniosacral rhythm by functional cranial techniques
- Effleurage to aid drainage of thoracic and cervical lymphatic vessels
- Exercises to improve mobility of thoracic spine and physical coordination
- Contrast bathing (warm and cold compresses) to tender areas of their backs.

Treatment continued for 12 months during which both groups underwent continual assessment. Two types of measurement were used: the first consisted of objective measurements of the physical condition of the leg muscles and mobility of the thoracic spine using biomechanical tools; the second involved asking the subjects to complete questionnaires about their symptoms.

On the qualitative assessments made after 1 year, the patient group showed an improvement of 40% ($p < 0.0005$) as against a 1% worsening of symptoms for the control group. Objective measurements of knee extensor muscle fatigability also revealed significant improvement in the treatment group. This was achieved solely through the protocol described above, without direct treatment of the quadriceps or lower limbs.

Note: It may be useful to compare the osteopathic protocol described for treatment of CFS with the general osteopathic (and naturopathic) physical medicine approaches discussed in Chapter 8.

---

of light touch with about the same amount of pressure that could be placed on the eye without pain.

After the use of the BEST treatment approach involving 24 chronic failed chiropractic patients, significant improvement was noted in the level of pain, improved vigor, fatigue and an improved sense of well-being. These results were obtained despite both the long-standing nature of the symptoms and failure to respond to previous chiropractic care.

Graduated exercise and chronic fatigue syndrome

Chronic fatigue syndrome (CFS) appears to be a heterogeneous disorder when it comes to both clinical presentation and possible patho-etiology; however, there are patients at one end of the spectrum who fit with the commonly quoted psychiatric model of inactivity and depression, leading to abnormal illness beliefs and/or behavior, while at the other end there are those in whom there is evidence of neuromuscular pathology and no psychiatric comorbidity (Lane 2000). Clinical approaches should clearly take account of such variables.

While some studies have demonstrated that graded exercise regimes can markedly benefit patients with CFS (Bazelmans et al 2001), others have shown that caution should be applied in prescribing exercise protocols to CFS patients, as overambitious exercise can precipitate a significant and sustained period of relapse (Lapp 1997).

In terms of percentage of successful outcomes of graded exercise applied in chronic fatigue settings, White & Naish (2001) observe that:

Graded exercise therapy is a clinically useful treatment for chronic fatigue syndrome in about half of the patients referred, but a significant minority fail to complete their treatment successfully.

Gradual increases in physical and mental activity are suggested, a process commonly known as pacing. This needs to take into account the considerable fluctuations in symptom severity that occur in CFS. Pacing involves appropriate periods of rest and relaxation. In the largest support group questionnaire 1949 respondents found pacing helpful, 201 reported no change, and 30 stated they were made worse. These results indicate that pacing is a highly acceptable and effective approach to activity management in CFS (Shepherd 2001).

Exercise and yoga for fatigue deriving from neurological disease

Fatigue is one of the most common causes of disability in patients with neurological disease such as multiple sclerosis, with peripheral and central mechanisms often coexisting. Studies have demonstrated benefit with therapeutic exercise and yoga, although the mechanisms of action are poorly understood and may not be specific (Berger & Owen 1988, Oken et al 2004, Petajan et al 1996).

Multidimensional physical medicine approach (including exercise, massage and relaxation) and fatigue (and other symptoms) related to cancer and chemotherapy

The results of a study by Andersen et al (2006) indicate that 6 weeks of a multidimensional exercise (structured physical activity, relaxation, body-awareness techniques and massage intervention) for cancer patients with or without disease, and who are undergoing chemotherapy, can lead to a reduction in symptoms and side-effects. As such, the total burden of pain, including myalgia, arthralgia, paresthesia and other pain, was reduced significantly ($p = 0.046$).

The researchers divided fatigue into different categories:

- *Physical fatigue*: The sense of fatigue that follows physical exercise and other forms of physical activities, characterized by, for example, relaxed sense and energy.
- *Treatment-related fatigue*: This sense of fatigue can be related to the chemotherapy (and perhaps radiation therapy) and may be characterized by influenza-like symptoms unrelieved by rest or sleep.
- *Mental fatigue*: The sense of being unconcentrated and lacking energy to carry out any activities.

The following reflect the symptom score changes over a 6-week period of this combined treatment:

- Physical fatigue: dropped from 0.95 to 0.74
- Treatment-related fatigue: from 0.83 to 0.55
- Mental fatigue: from 0.75 to 0.57
- Other pain: from 0.53 to 0.39
- Paresthesia: from 0.53 to 0.43
- Lack of appetite: from 0.43 to 0.34
- Constipation: from 0.40 to 0.24
- Myalgia: from 0.36 to 0.17
- Arthralgia: from 0.31 to 0.29
- Diarrhea: from 0.17 to 0.06.

From the first to the last week the myalgia scores ($p = 0.013$) and other pain scores ($p = 0.041$) significantly changed. None of the other changes reached statistical significance at the 95% level. The score for vomiting was unchanged (from 0.04 to 0.04) and nausea increased from 0.22 to 0.24.

Massage and acupressure and fatigue related to end-stage renal disease (ESRD) (Cho & Tsay 2004)

A study was conducted to evaluate whether depressed and fatigued patients with ESRD might benefit from acupressure. Patients were divided into two groups, with the experimental group receiving acupressure with massage, while having hemodialysis treatment. The control group received routine care. Of those receiving acupressure, the treatment consisted of a 12-minute massage, three times per week, for 4 weeks. Findings were that those individuals in the treatment group had significantly decreased depression scores (10.1 vs 13.0) and fatigue scores (3.4 vs 5.1).

Physical medicine therapeutic measures for fatigue

- *Light forms of manipulation (e.g. BEST) as well as compression techniques have been shown to relieve fatigue for some patients.*
- *Carefully graduated exercise protocols offer benefit to most chronic fatigue patients.*
- *Patients with neurologically derived fatigue have benefited from yoga and general exercise measures.*
- *Fatigued individuals suffering from cancer, and the effects of chemotherapy, have benefited from multidimensional exercise protocols incorporating physical activity, relaxation, massage and body awareness techniques.*

Note: The pain experienced by many patients with CFS is discussed under the subheading 'Pain' later in this chapter.

Fibromyalgia syndrome (see instinctive sleep postures in Chapter 9; see also page 46 for more details of fibromyalgia syndrome (FMS)

In a major survey, 63% of patients with rheumatological disorders other than fibromyalgia syndrome (FMS) and 91% of those with FMS currently use some form of CAM (Pioro-Boisset et al 1996) compared with 42% of the general population (Eisenberg et al 1998).

Note: A number of studies relating to the pain experienced in fibromyalgia are discussed later in this chapter under the subheading 'Pain'.

Manipulation and FMS

In a review of chiropractic efficacy in treatment of FMS, Blunt and colleagues (1997) suggest that chiropractic manipulation should be associated with additional potentially useful adjunctive methods, including soft tissue massage and 'spray and stretch'. To what extent, in any given case, the soft tissue approaches alone might be responsible for the resulting benefits is open to debate.

Various mechanisms could be involved. Pain inhibition may be achieved as a result of:

- increased spinal mobility following manipulation that tends to decrease central transmission of pain from adjacent structures (Gatterman et al 1990)
- release of endogenous opioids following manipulation (Irving 1981)
- modification of pressure pain thresholds of cervical paraspinal musculature increasing following manipulation
- paraspinal muscles relaxing due to stretching of apophyseal joint capsules during manipulation, reflexively inhibiting motor neuron pools which may be facilitated and therefore responsible for increased tone. Intrafusal fibers are also stretched during manipulation, helping restore balanced afferent/efferent impulses in the proprioceptive system of the joint and local musculature (Shambaugh 1987)
- articular adhesions being reduced or broken in chronic cases (Kirkaldy-Willis et al 1984)
- increased range of motion (Lewit 1985).

Chiropractic and FMS

A combination of chiropractic manipulative treatment and applied local pressure (ischemic compression) was assessed for efficacy in a group of 15 women (mean age 51.1) by Hains & Hains (2000). The women received 30 treatments, two or three times weekly. The treatment consisted of:

- ischemic compression applied to previously identified (by palpation) tender points. The pressure was applied for 10 seconds, and was sufficient to reach the patient's pain tolerance level. The technique was repeated at each session until the tender points failed to cause pain with the application of 4 kg (8.8 lb) of pressure.
- manipulation of the upper thoracic and cervical region using rotational and high velocity thrust techniques to areas judged to be restricted in mobility ('decrease in the quality of segmental motion') and increased tenderness.

Of the 15 women, nine (60%) reported at least 50% improvement in pain intensity (77% improvement), fatigue levels (63.5% improvement) and sleep quality (74.8% improvement). These improvements were reported after both 15 and 30 treatments and were sustained for at least 1 month following the end of the treatment.

Among those who did not report benefit after 30 treatments it was observed that there had been a less than 35% improvement by the end of 15 treatments, and that this: 'suggests that a minimum 35% improvement in pain intensity must be observed after 15 treatments or it may no longer be appropriate to pursue this form of treatment'.

Comment: In this small study, benefit for the majority of patients was achieved, suggesting possible benefits for some FMS patients where combined ischemic pressure (trigger point deactivation) and mobilization is offered. However, this does not clarify whether the ischemic pressure, which calmed the trigger points, would have, on its own, achieved similar results.

Symptomatic relief from chiropractic

It is reported that 46% of patients with FMS receiving chiropractic attention report symptom relief (Wolfe 1986).

To date there have been no large controlled trials to validate benefit following the use of chiropractic in treatment of FMS; however, what evidence there is suggests possible value, particularly when combined with other manual approaches (Holdcraft et al 2003).

Soft tissue treatment, manipulation, education and FMS

In a pilot study (a randomized cross-over trial), a group of Canadian chiropractors (Blunt et al 1997) selected 21 rheumatology patients with FMS, aged between 25 and 70 years. Ten patients received treatment between three and five times per week for 4 weeks. During this time the remainder (the controls) received no treatment, but received it in the following 4-week period (only nine were involved by this stage, as two patients had dropped out). Treatment consisted of:

- soft tissue massage using a counterirritant cream
- soft tissue stretching with and without fluoromethane as a chilling agent (used especially in early stages and on the scalene muscles)
- spinal manipulation (minimal amplitude, low velocity) applied to joints with a 'hard' end-feel
- education, involving provision of information of aggravating factors, sleep habits, body mechanics, understanding the etiology of FMS.

The study confirms the benefit in pain modulation and functional status in FMS patients of carefully applied manipulative methods incorporating both osseous and soft tissue methods. Studies which compare joint manipulation with soft tissue approaches would help to clarify their relative benefits. There is no evidence that the underlying condition is assisted by these methods, although they clearly have an important role to play in management.

Osteopathic manipulative treatment (OMT) and FMS

- *OMT and FMS*: Doctors at Chicago College of Osteopathic Medicine measured the effects of OMT (including strain/counterstrain and muscle energy technique; see Chapter 7 for more detail) on the intensity of pain felt in the diagnostic tender points in 18 patients who met all the criteria for FMS (Stoltz 1993). Each had six visits/treatments and it was found over a 1-year period that 12 of the patients responded well in that their tender points became less sensitive (14% reduction in intensity as against a 34% increase in the six patients who did not respond well). Most of the patients – the responders and the non-responders to OMT – showed (using thermographic imaging) that their tender points were more symmetrically spread after the course than before. Activities of daily living

were significantly improved, and general pain symptoms decreased overall.

- *OMT, self-care or moist heat, and FMS*: Doctors at Texas College of Osteopathic Medicine selected three groups of FMS patients, one of which received OMT, another had OMT plus self-teaching (learning about the condition and self-help measures) and a third group received only moist-heat treatment. The group with the least reported pain after 6 months of care was that receiving OMT, although some benefit was noted in the self-teaching group (Jiminez et al 1993).
- *Medication and OMT*: Another group of doctors from Texas College of Osteopathic Medicine tested the difference in results involving 37 patients with FMS of using: (1) drugs only (ibuprofen, alprazolam); (2) OMT plus medication; (3) placebo (a dummy medication) plus OMT; and (4) a placebo only. The results showed that drug therapy alone resulted in significantly less tenderness being reported than did drugs and manipulation, or the use of placebo and OMT, or placebo alone. Patients receiving placebo plus manipulation reported significantly less fatigue than the other groups. The group receiving medication and OMT showed the greatest improvement in their quality of life (Rubin et al 1990).

As with chiropractic evidence it appears that osteopathic manipulation offers relative benefits to patients with FMS, especially when combined with other modalities.

Massage and FMS

- *Myoglobin levels reduced following massage*: Several studies of massage therapy indicate that plasma myoglobin concentration, which is positively correlated with muscle pain and tension, increases after massage due to the release of myoglobin from the muscles (Danneskiold-Samsoe et al 1986). A gradual decline in the increased myoglobin concentration was observed over repeated massage treatments as self-reported muscle tension decreased over time.
- *Connective tissue massage and FMS*: Two trials of massage therapy have reported improvements among patients with FMS. In the first, 48 patients received either connective tissue massage or a control condition consisting of no intervention or a discussion group (Brattberg 1999). The 15 massages resulted in a self-

reported reduction in pain in 85% of the patients and a reduction in analgesic use by 30% of subjects. Depression and self-rated quality of life improved but no improvements were observed in sleep, ability for activities and anxiety.

- *Swedish massage and FMS*: A second study showed that Swedish massage was associated with improved mobility and a trend for decreased perceived helplessness when compared with two control conditions consisting of medical care from the clinic nurse or physician (Alnigenis et al 2001). However, no impact on pain, depression, well-being and other functioning was noted, and all effects became non-significant after 28 weeks.
- *Massage and FMS*: Research from the Touch Research Institute, University of Miami Medical School, indicates benefits from appropriate forms of massage in treatment of FMS (Sunshine et al 1996).
- *Massage and movement and FMS*: When massage and movement treatment was compared with relaxation and movement in treatment of FMS patients, there were markedly more benefits in the group receiving massage as well as movement therapy. The greatest benefits were noted in areas of mood and depression, as well as in reduced pain levels (Field et al 2003).

Avoid deep tissue with FMS?

While many FMS patients frequently request deep work, this is contraindicated, based on what is known of the mechanisms involved in FMS. The most useful manual methods seem to involve non-specific wellness massage and manual lymphatic drainage (see below), plus finely targeted specific interventions using aspects of soft tissue manipulation, most specifically positional release and vibrational methods.

The removal or deactivation of myofascial trigger points and other local dysfunction by minimally invasive methods, combined with homeostatic enhancing approaches (nutrition, relaxation methods, hydrotherapy, etc.), appear to be additionally useful strategies.

Manual lymphatic drainage and FMS

A pilot study evaluated the benefits of very light massage (manual lymphatic drainage) on pain and stiffness, sleep and sleepiness, and well-being in 17 women with long-standing fibromyalgia (Asplund 2003).

All symptoms showed favorable progress during a 4-week period with manual lymph drainage therapy. The degree of sustained pain relief 3 and 6 months after the start of the treatment among the women (26% and 9%) was comparable to that described in a report on treatment with connective tissue massage (30% and 10%).

One of the main findings in this pilot study of women with initially severe pain due to long-standing and incapacitating fibromyalgia was that they experienced a substantial reduction in their pains during treatment with very light massage in accordance with the technique of manual lymph drainage therapy (Kasseroller 1998).

Although the results of the present study must be interpreted with caution, the extent of the pain relief was surprising. Previously, it has been reported in a double-blind study of 48 women with fibromyalgia that connective tissue massage gives pain relief in one-third of the treated women (Brattberg 1999).

Low levels of oxytocin have been found in women with fibromyalgia with high pain scores and in children with recurrent abdominal pain of non-organic origin (Alfven et al 1994, Anderberg & Uvnas-Moberg 2000). Human infants use their hands to stimulate their mother's breast during breast-feeding, resulting in an increase in the maternal oxytocin level (Matthiesen et al 2001). Oxytocin has an antinociceptive effect (Lundeberg et al 1994), as discussed earlier in this chapter. The pain reduction during lymph therapy in the present study may therefore partly be explained by increased oxytocin release (Lund et al 2002).

Exercise and fibromyalgia

Cardiovascular exercise is stated to be helpful in rehabilitation from FMS. The guidelines most commonly given involve the patient performing active aerobic exercise three times weekly (some say four times) for at least 20 (some say 15) minutes, during which time they are required to achieve between 60 and 85% of their maximum predicted heart rate. The methods of exercise best suited to FMS patients are said to be cycling (static cycle), walking or swimming (McCain et al 1988, Richards & Scott 2002).

Strength training and FMS

Hakkinen et al (2002) have shown that it is possible for strength training exercise to enhance growth hormone production in premenopausal women with FMS. They found that the strength training induced adaptation of the endocrine system, and conclude that the positive growth hormone (GH) response may become systematic following strength training in women with FMS. Since GH deficiency is considered to be a feature of fibromyalgia, this evidence should encourage graded strength training for FMS patients.

Supervised and graduated exercise and FMS

Patients with fibromyalgia often experience increased pain after exertion due to a combination of tight muscles and being less aerobically fit overall. Fibro-myalgia patients who attempt to begin an exercise program often experience an increase in muscle pain which may discourage them from continuing to work on improving their level of fitness. Pellegrino (1997) notes that a prescribed, supervised exercise program is beneficial for fibromyalgia patients, and helps them achieve a gradual increase in overall physical fitness, flexibility and functional ability. The key features of a successful exercise program appear to be:

1. emphasis on stretching and flexibility exercises of all major muscle groups and focus on a warm-up period that consists of stretching only

2. regular performance of a low impact, aerobic-type program which may be referred to as a 'light conditioning' program. Such a program can include walking, water aerobics, using an exercise bicycle, or performing a low impact aerobic program

3. gradually progressing in an exercise program as tolerated. The goal is to achieve improvement, but also to achieve a stable baseline

4. continuation of a regular exercise program – at least three times a week, even on days when there is increased pain

5. following proper posture and body mechanics to minimize strain of the muscles and joints.

Graduated cardiovascular exercise, relaxation and flexibility activities – and FMS

McCain et al (1988), in a randomized controlled trial lasting 12 weeks and involving 136 patients with FMS (male and female, age range 18–70 years), evaluated the effect on their conditions of either graded cardio-vascular fitness exercise or relaxation and flexibility activities, to which they were randomly assigned. Exercise classes, led by qualified personal trainers, took place twice weekly and lasted 1 hour. The aerobic exercise classes are described as follows.

Exercise therapy comprised an individualized aerobic exercise program, mostly walking on tread-mills and cycling on exercise bicycles. Each individual was encouraged to increase the amount of exercise steadily as tolerated. When people first started classes they usually did two periods of exercise per class lasting 6 minutes. By 12 weeks they were doing two periods of 25 minutes at an intensity that made them sweat slightly while being able to talk comfortably in complete sentences.

Relaxation and flexibility comprised upper and lower limb stretches and relaxation techniques. As the classes continued, more techniques were introduced, progressing through progressive muscle relaxation, release-only relaxation and visualization, cue-controlled relaxation and differential relaxation. This occupied the whole 1-hour class.

Outcomes were measured using self-assessment of improvement, tender point count, impact of condition measured by fibromyalgia impact questionnaire, and short form McGill Pain Questionnaire. Compared with relaxation and flexibility exercises, aerobic (car-diovascular) exercise led to significantly more partici-pants rating themselves as much, or very much, better at 3 months. It is worth noting, however, that in both groups the tender point counts had fallen significantly at 3 months and that this was maintained or improved at 1-year follow-up.

After 12 months fewer participants in the aerobic exercise group fulfilled the criteria for fibromyalgia; by this time only 75 (55%) participants still met these diagnostic criteria.

The researchers conclude that:

For people with fibromyalgia prescribed graded aerobic exercise is an effective treatment that leads to improvements in self reported health status. Prescribed exercise can be undertaken effectively in the community by personal trainers previously inexperienced in management of people with ill health.

However, adherence remains an issue. Exercise treatment has limitations. Compliance is a consider-able problem, giving high dropout rates. Reasons include the initial increases in pain and stiffness immediately after exercise and patients believing that exercise worsens the condition. Future strategies to increase the efficacy of exercise as an intervention should confront the issue of compliance. Potential strategies include additional cognitive behavioral therapy and providing physiological explanations for symptoms.

Comment: There is much to learn from this study. Both forms of intervention helped a good number of participants, although clearly aerobic activity pro-duced the most benefit. Over 50% of patients reached a stage where they no longer met the criteria for an FMS diagnosis, suggesting that this low-tech, low-cost, high-benefit outcome should be seen as offering a beacon for individuals in chronic pain. And yet adherence remains a major problem. Sadly, despite obvious benefits, individuals commonly slip back into old habits, abandon exercise regimes and return to their pain condition over time.

Educational lectures, physical training and FMS

Swedish research (Burckhardt et al 1994) compared groups of FMS patients who, over a 6-week period, were given six 1-hour educational lectures about their condition and how to manage it, with a group who attended these same lectures but who also received six 1-hour sessions of physical training. A further group (used to compare the effect of doing something with doing nothing in similar patients) were untreated during this entire study but received treatment after it was over. The results (86 patients completed the study) demonstrated that both the lecture and the lecture plus exercise groups showed a positive impact on their quality of life as well as their pain levels. However, it was those who performed the active exercises who were shown to maintain the benefits more effectively long term – 87% reported that they were still exercising at least three times weekly for 20 minutes or more, about 70% were practicing relaxation techniques, and a number had been able to return to work as a result of the program.

Fitness, flexibility and strengthening compared with relaxation for FMS

In another study (Martin et al 1996) the benefits of exercise (fitness, flexibility and strengthening) programs were compared with relaxation exercises in a group of 60 FMS patients over a 6-week period at the Medical School of the University of Calgary, Canada. Both groups of patients (those doing active exercise, and those doing relaxation) met three times a week for 6 weeks to carry out their routines under supervision. At the start, both groups had the same amount of pain, stiffness, etc. Of the 30 people starting the exercises, 18 completed the course, along with 20 (of the 30) in the relaxation group. Both groups showed an improvement in the number and sensitivity of tender points but those doing the active training exercises were much improved compared with the relaxation group. What this study shows is that a number of people (about a third) fall out of such programs for one reason or another. Those that complete their assignments usually benefit, and exercising appropriately seems to be very beneficial in FMS.

Six-minute walk test and FMS

Gowans et al (1999a) discuss the use of the 6-minute walk test. This involves noting the distance comfortably covered by someone with (for example) FMS, in 6 minutes of walking. It is used in their work as one of the means of evaluating the benefits of interventions such as hydrotherapy pool work: 'We believe the 6-minute walk test is an outcome measure that may be useful in directly assessing physical function' (Gowans et al 1999b).

Cautions: Reactions to any treatment should be particularly carefully observed where exercise is being suggested. Exercise routines should be introduced gradually – see the protocol used by Richards & Scott (2002) described above (page 458) – with caution and patience in individuals with FMS, and even more so with CFS. Unsupervised home exercising is probably unwise until the individual has attended classes where the degree, intensity and timing of exercise can be learned.

Hydrotherapy and fibromyalgia

- *Balneotherapy and FMS*: Evcik et al (2002) report a Turkish study in which 42 primary fibromyalgia patients, diagnosed according to American College of Rheumatology criteria, ages ranging between 30 and 55 years, were randomly assigned to two groups. Group 1 (n = 22) received 20 minutes of bathing once a day, five times per week. Patients participated in the study for 3 weeks (total of 15 sessions). Group 2 (n = 20) was accepted as the control group. Patients were evaluated by the number of tender points, visual analog scale for pain, Beck's Depression Index and Fibromyalgia Impact Questionnaire for functional capacity. Measurements were assessed initially, after the therapy and at the end of the sixth month. In group 1, there were statistically significant differences in number of tender points, visual analog scores, Beck's Depression Index and Fibromyalgia Impact Questionnaire scores after the therapy program (p <0.001). Six months later, in group 1, there was still an improvement in the number of tender points (p <0.001), visual analog scores and Fibromyalgia Impact Questionnaire (p <0.005). However, there was no statistical difference in Beck's Depression Index scores compared to the control group (p >0.05). 'Patients with FMS mostly complain about pain, anxiety, and the difficulty in daily living activities. This study shows that balneotherapy is effective and may be an alternative method in treating fibromyalgia patients.'
- *Underwater exercise and FMS*: In another Turkish study (Cimbiz et al 2005), 470 patients with fibromyalgia and other conditions received spa therapy twice a day (with underwater exercise in the spa pool), 20 minutes total duration per day in the first week and 30 minutes for the

following weeks. Results showed a significant decrease in pain and high blood pressure without hemodynamic risk. The conclusion was that a combined spa and physical therapy program may help to decrease pain and improve hemodynamic response in patients with irreversible pathologies.

- *Sulfur baths and FMS*: Israeli research was conducted to evaluate the effectiveness of balneotherapy on patients with FMS in the Dead Sea (Buskila et al 2001). Forty-eight patients with FMS were randomly assigned to either a treatment group receiving sulfur baths or a control group. All participants stayed for 10 days at a Dead Sea spa. Physical functioning, FMS-related symptoms and tenderness measurements were assessed prior to arrival at the Dead Sea, after 10 days of treatment, and 1 and 3 months after leaving the spa. Physical functioning and tenderness moderately improved in both groups. With the exception of tenderness threshold, the improvement was especially notable in the treatment group and it persisted even 3 months after leaving the spa. Relief in the severity of FMS-related symptoms (pain, fatigue, stiffness and anxiety) and reduced frequency of symptoms (headache, sleep problems and subjective joint swelling) were reported in both groups, but lasted longer in the treatment group. The conclusion was that balneotherapy treatment of FMS is effective and safe.
- *Dead Sea balneotherapy and FMS*: A further study was conducted to assess the effectiveness of balneotherapy in the Dead Sea area (Sukenik et al 2001) in the treatment of patients suffering from both fibromyalgia and psoriatic arthritis. Twenty-eight patients with both psoriatic arthritis and fibromyalgia were treated with various methods of balneotherapy in the Dead Sea area. Clinical indices were assessed and the results showed that the number of active joints was reduced as were the number of tender points. A significant improvement was found in dolorimetric threshold readings after the treatment period in women. The conclusion was that balneotherapy appears to produce a statistically significant, substantial improvement in the number of active joints and tender points in both male and female patients.
- *Pool exercise and FMS*: Swedish research evaluated the effects on FMS of 6 months of pool exercise (temperate temperature)

combined with six sessions of education (Mannerkorpi et al 2000). Fifty-eight individuals were randomized to a treatment and a control group. The treatment group was advised to 'match the pool exercise to their threshold of pain and fatigue'. The educational component comprised discussion of coping strategies and encouragement to physical activity. The outcome was that significant differences were observed and noted on the Fibromyalgia Impact Questionnaire and the 6-minute walk test (see above). There were also improvements in the treatment group, to a significant degree, in physical function, grip strength, pain severity, social functioning, psychological distress and quality of life.

- *Watsu and FMS*: Pool-based Watsu (WATer shiatSU) (Dull 1997) – in which the patient floats in warm water sourced from hot springs (35°C) while having the moves and stretches of Zen Shiatsu applied – has been shown to be a highly effective intervention for FMS (Faul 2005).

Comment: Hydrotherapy/balneotherapy appears to offer benefits comparable with those deriving from exercise.

Caution: Although most balneotherapy trials involving rheumatic conditions such as fibromyalgia report positive findings, many of the studies have been assessed as being methodologically flawed. Therefore, the reported 'positive findings' should be interpreted with caution (Verhagen et al 2003).

Magnets and fibromyalgia

A study was undertaken to determine whether chronic pain and sleep disturbance in FMS patients could be improved by sleeping on magnetic mattress pads. The double-blind, placebo-controlled trial involved 35 female patients diagnosed with FMS (Colbert et al 1999).

The patients using the magnetic pads slept (for 16 weeks) on a surface 'magnetized at a magnet surface field strength of 1100 gauss, delivering 200–600 gauss to the skin surface'. The controls slept on a sham non-magnetized pad. The results showed that patients sleeping on the magnetized pads experienced a significant decrease in overall pain, fatigue and total muscle pain score, and also showed improvement in sleeping patterns and physical functioning. There were no significant changes experienced by the sham/control group. A placebo effect was noted in that both groups reported being less tired on waking.

Physical medicine therapeutic measures for fibromyalgia

- *Manipulation, soft tissue manipulation and massage have all been shown to have beneficial effects on many of the symptoms of fibromyalgia, most effectively when used in combination (massage, movement, relaxation, exercise, etc.).*
- *Manual lymphatic drainage and extremely light massage are more strongly indicated in fibromyalgia than deep tissue methods.*
- *Various forms of exercise (aerobic, graduated weight training, etc.) have all been shown to effectively improve well-being and reduce symptoms in patients with FMS.*
- *Balneotherapy and pool-based exercise and treatments such as Watsu have all been shown to be both safe and relatively effective, particularly in reducing pain levels.*
- *Use of magnets may offer symptomatic relief in FMS, particularly relating to enhanced sleep.*

Note: Additional aspects of management of the pain aspects of FMS are to be found later in this chapter under the subheading 'Pain'.

Gynecological disorders: menstrual and premenstrual irregularities

Dysmenorrhea refers to the occurrence of painful menstrual cramps of uterine origin, a common gynecological condition. One possible treatment is spinal manipulative therapy, the hypothesis being that mechanical dysfunction in certain vertebrae involving decreased spinal mobility could affect the sympathetic nerve supply to the blood vessels supplying the pelvic viscera, leading to dysmenorrhea as a result of vasoconstriction. Manipulation of these vertebrae may therefore improve pelvic blood supply. Another hypothesis is that dysmenorrhea is referred pain arising from musculoskeletal structures that share the same pelvic nerve pathways. The character of pain from musculoskeletal dysfunction can be very similar to gynecological pain, and can present as cyclic pain as it can also be altered by hormonal influences associated with menstruation.

Premenstrual syndrome symptoms include:

- tenderness and/or lumpiness of the breasts
- a feeling of being bloated, caused by fluid retention
- mood changes, including irritability, depression, anxiety and fatigue
- difficulty concentrating and making decisions
- headaches, including migraine headaches

- backache and muscle stiffness
- disrupted sleep
- unusual food cravings.

Symptoms vary among women, and for some the symptoms vary from month to month. Symptoms may begin just before menstruation starts or as long as 2 weeks beforehand. In most women, symptoms disappear by the time menstruation has finished.

Chiropractic and menstrual/premenstrual symptoms

Positive study chiropractic and PMS

A trial found that women who received chiropractic treatment, consisting of spinal manipulation, reported significant reductions in back pain and menstrual distress (Kokjohn et al 1992).

On the first day of their period, the 38 women participating in the trial received either spinal manipulation or a 'sham' adjustment that did not have a therapeutic effect on the spine. The women were asked to fill out a menstrual distress questionnaire and rate their pain on a visual analog scale. The results of the questionnaires showed the greatest reduction in perceived pain among the women receiving spinal manipulation when compared to the women who received sham adjustments. Visual analog scale scores indicated that both abdominal and back pain decreased almost twice as much in the spine manipulated group compared to the sham group.

Other similar studies have shown positive benefits (Walsh & Polus 1998).

Negative review of chiropractic and PMS: a Cochrane Review of trials (Proctor et al 2004)

Four trials of high velocity, low amplitude manipulation (HVLA) and one of the Toftness manipulation technique were evaluated in relation to treatment of primary and secondary dysmenorrhea.

Quality assessment and data extraction were performed independently by two reviewers. Meta-analysis was performed using odds ratios for dichotomous outcomes and weighted mean differences for continuous outcomes. The outcome measures were pain relief or pain intensity (dichotomous, visual analog scales, descriptive) and adverse effects. Results from the four trials of HVLA suggest that the technique was no more effective than sham manipulation for the treatment of dysmenorrhea, although it was possibly more effective than no treatment.

Three of the smaller trials indicated a difference in favor of HVLA; however, the one trial with an adequate sample size found no difference between HVLA and sham treatment. There was no difference in adverse effects experienced by participants in the HVLA or sham treatment. The Toftness technique was shown to be more effective than sham treatment by one small trial, but no strong conclusions could be made due to the small size of the trial and other methodological considerations. The conclusion was that overall there is no evidence to suggest that spinal manipulation is effective in the treatment of primary and secondary dysmenorrhea.

Example: One of these reviewed studies involved 138 women, ages 18–45, with primary dysmenorrhea diagnosed by participating gynecologists. The women were randomly assigned to either spinal manipulative therapy (SMT) or a low-force mimic (LFM) maneuver in a randomized, observer-blinded, clinical trial designed to evaluate the efficacy of SMT in the treatment of women with primary dysmenorrhea (Hondras et al 1999).

No treatment occurred at menstrual cycle 1. Treatment for both groups took place on day 1 of cycles 2, 3 and 4, and prophylactic treatment of three visits took place during the 7 days before cycles 3 and 4.

Although a wide range of measurements and assessments were made during the four consecutive menstrual cycles, no clinically meaningful changes were observed. It was therefore concluded that the postulated superior benefit of high-velocity, short-lever, low-amplitude, high-force spinal manipulation compared to a low-force maneuver is not supported by the results of this study.

Note: It is suggested that the notes under the subheading 'What should we believe?' (below) should be considered when contradictory evidence such as this is presented.

Massage and premenstrual symptoms

Twenty-four women with a history of severe PMS were divided into two groups, one to receive massage (twice weekly for 30 minutes for 5 weeks) with the other group given instruction in the use of progressive muscle relaxation methods, to be applied for 30 minutes, twice weekly for 5 weeks. The results showed that the massage group demonstrated significantly reduced anxiety levels, improved mood and reduction in pain and fluid retention levels, compared with the relaxation group (Hernandez-Reif et al 2000b).

Reflexology and premenstrual symptoms

Oleson & Flocco (1993), in their reflexology study involving 32 women with PMS, compared the benefits, in half of the women, of reflexology treatment (using specific reflex points on the feet, hands and ears) while the remaining 16 women received sham (placebo) treatment, involving 'very light or very rough' massage of points not related to reflex effects. Symptom records were kept daily for the week prior to the next period. The results are described as follows: 'At the end of the study the reflexology group reported a 45% decrease in both somatic and psychological symptoms, compared with a 20% reduction in the placebo group.'

Yoga, exercise and menstrual symptoms

Chen (2005) compared the effect of yoga with aerobic and walking exercise on menstrual disorders. Sixty-nine female university students with menstrual disorders were divided into three groups, and performed aerobics, walking and yoga, respectively, for 18 months. *Results*: The effective rate in the yoga group (78%, 18/23) was significantly higher than those in the aerobics group (57%, 13/23) and the walking group (65%, 15/23) ($\chi^2 = 6.468$, $p < 0.05$). *Conclusion*: Yoga has better therapeutic effects on menstrual disorders as compared with other forms of exercise, although all methods produced benefit in a significant number of participants.

Physical medicine therapeutic measures for menstrual and premenstrual conditions

- *Evidence for the use of chiropractic manipulation (HVLA) in these conditions is equivocal, with some studies showing benefit and others not.*
- *Massage and reflexology appear to be helpful, most probably as a result of reduced levels of anxiety and sympathetic arousal.*
- *All forms of exercise appear to offer benefit to a high proportion of women with menstrual and premenstrual symptoms, with yoga appearing to be more efficacious than aerobics or walking.*

Headache and migraine

Hilton described the concept of headaches originating from the cervical spine in 1860 (Pearce 1995). In 1983, Sjaastad et al introduced the term 'cervicogenic headache' (CGH). Diagnostic criteria have been established by several expert groups, with agreement that these headaches start in the neck or occipital region and are associated with tenderness of cervical paraspinal tissues. Prevalence estimates range from 0.4 to 2.5% of the general population to 15–20% of patients with chronic headaches. CGH affects patients with a mean age of 42.9 years, has a 4 : 1 female disposition, and tends to be chronic. Almost any pathology affecting the cervical spine has been implicated in the genesis of CGH as a result of convergence of sensory input from the cervical structures within the spinal nucleus of the trigeminal nerve. The main differential diagnoses are tension-type headache and migraine headache, with considerable overlap in symptoms and findings between these conditions. No specific pathology has been noted on imaging or diagnostic studies which correlates with CGH (Haldeman & Dagenais 2001).

Despite having many of the same symptoms as true migraine (such as nausea, vomiting, sensitivity to light), many headaches are in fact not migraines at all, but arise from neural irritation, or trigger point activity, in the neck. It is also not uncommon for a person to suffer both migraine headaches and severe headaches that derive from the neck (Bono et al 1998, Sjaastad et al 1990).

One study of patients with neck injuries reported that 35% suffered from headaches deriving from their necks, while another 11% had both neck-related headaches and migraines (Bono et al 2000).

The many different causes of headache obviously require different treatment approaches. Some will need to focus on posture, some on neck restrictions, some on trigger points and others on imbalances affecting the temporomandibular joint (Dworkin & LeResche 1991).

Standing or sitting with the head forward of the body, in a slouched posture, puts a great deal of stress on the muscles and joints of the upper back and neck, which can lead on to formation of trigger points, nerve irritation and headaches (Simons et al 1999b).

Posture, chiropractic and migraine

Analyzing and correcting posture-related muscle imbalances, as well as vertebral restrictions, appears to increase the effectiveness of chiropractic treatment for cervicogenic headache (Moore 2004).

Correcting posture takes time, and requires regular exercising of taught procedures, so that what feels uncomfortable at first (such as holding the head in its correct position) gradually becomes comfortable and starts to 'feel right'. Teachers of Alexander technique have perfected a gradual rehabilitation program which should ideally be accompanied by treatment (and self-treatment) aimed at stretching and releasing tight muscles and joints, and at toning and balancing the body as a whole (Wilson 2002).

It is always worth exploring the possibility that a patient suffering from headache, whether diagnosed as migraine or not, may be helped by appropriate treatment of the neck muscles and joints. Such treatment might involve mobilization or manipulation of restricted joints, release of excessive tension in muscles of the region, or deactivation of trigger points that are capable of feeding pain into the head/neck region (Edeling 1997, Herzog 1999, Simons et al 1999b, Zwart 1997).

Trigger points and headache

Headaches that appear to benefit most from trigger point treatment are those where there is tenderness of the muscles attaching to the head (Fernández-de-las-Peñas et al 2006a). Fernández-de-las-Peñas et al (2007) also caution that although 'myofascial trigger points in the suboccipital muscles might contribute to the origin and/or maintenance of headache a comprehensive knowledge of the role of these muscles in tension-type headache awaits further research'.

In another study (Fernández-de-las-Peñas et al 2006b), trigger points in the upper trapezius muscle showed referred pain patterns in both chronic tension-type headache patients as well as in healthy subjects. In chronic tension-type headache patients, the evoked referred pain and its sensory characteristics shared similar patterns to the patient's habitual headache pain.

Migraine and chiropractic

In a 6-month randomized controlled trial, 127 patients with a diagnosis of migraine made on the basis of the International Headache Society standard, with a minimum of at least one migraine per month, received 2 months of chiropractic spinal manipulative treatment (SMT) focused on vertebral fixations determined by the practitioner (maximum of 16 treatments) (Tuchin et al 2000).

The average response of the treatment group ($n = 83$) showed statistically significant improvement in migraine frequency ($p < 0.005$), duration ($p < 0.01$), disability ($p < 0.05$) and medication use ($p < 0.001$) when compared with the control group. Twenty-two percent of participants reported more than a 90% reduction of migraines as a consequence of the 2 months of SMT. Approximately 50% more participants reported significant improvement in the morbidity of each episode.

Massage and migraine and tension-type headache

Forty-seven migraine sufferers were randomly assigned to massage or control conditions, and completed daily assessments of migraine experiences and sleep patterns for 13 weeks. Massage participants attended weekly massage sessions during weeks 5–10. State anxiety, heart rates and salivary cortisol were assessed before and after the sessions. Perceived stress and coping efficacy were assessed at weeks 4, 10 and 13. *Results*: Compared to control participants, massage participants exhibited greater improvements in migraine frequency and sleep quality during the intervention weeks and the three follow-up weeks (Lawler & Cameron 2006).

Massage and non-migrainous headache

Quinn et al (2002) investigated the effect of massage therapy on chronic non-migraine headache. *Method*: Chronic tension headache sufferers received structured massage therapy treatment directed toward neck and shoulder muscles. Headache frequency, duration and intensity were recorded and compared with baseline measures. *Results*: Compared with baseline values, headache frequency was significantly reduced within the first week of the massage protocol. The reduction of headache frequency continued for the remainder of the study ($p = 0.009$). The duration of headaches tended to decrease during the massage treatment period ($p = 0.058$); however, headache intensity was unaffected by massage ($p = 0.19$).

Exercise and headache

Evidence suggests that deficits in muscle performance of the deep neck flexor muscles may be linked to cervicogenic headache, and that specific exercise prescription utilizing a pressure biofeedback device may play an important treatment role, in conjunction with manipulation treatment (Eldridge & Russell 2005).

Noting that pain symptoms are a major work-related health problem in many countries, even in sedentary occupations, and that therapeutic exercise can decrease the intensity of pain in the neck area (Ylinen et al 2003), Sjögren et al (2005) designed a study to examine the effects of a workplace physical exercise program, consisting of light resistance training and guidance, on the perceived intensity of headache and the intensity of neck and shoulders symptoms, as well as the muscular strength of the upper extremities. The training consisted of six dynamic symmetrical movements: upper extremity extension, upper extremity flexion, trunk rotation to the right, trunk rotation to the left, knee extension and knee flexion. The training movements were carried out 20 times with a 30-second pause between the training movements. Physical exercise intervention resulted in a slight, but statistically significant, decrease in the intensity of headache and neck symptoms, as well as an increase in the extension strength of the upper extremities.

Physical medicine therapeutic measures for migraine and tension-type headache

- *Vertebral manipulation, improved posture, removal of active trigger points, use of massage and of specific exercises to tone weakness in deep neck flexors, all appear to offer benefits to patients who suffer migraine and/or tension-type headaches.*
- *Focused physical exercise to retrain cervical muscles offers some benefits in treatment of headache.*

Hypertension

Hypertension is one of the most pervasive disease processes in the developed world. It can lead to target organ damage, and although there is no one cause of primary hypertension, the theory of an unchecked long-term stress response continues to be a valid argument. Conversely, eliciting a relaxation response may alter the course of the unchecked stress response.

High blood pressure increases with age and is more common in men than in women. It seems to run in families and is more common in people of African–Caribbean descent. Risk factors for the condition include stress, a high alcohol intake, a diet high in salt and excess weight.

Chiropractic and hypertension

There have been both negative and positive studies:

- A randomized clinical trial (Goertz et al 2002) compared the effects of chiropractic spinal manipulation and diet with diet alone for lowering blood pressure in participants with high-normal blood pressure or stage I hypertension. Results showed that for patients with high-normal blood pressure or stage I hypertension, chiropractic spinal manipulation in conjunction with a dietary modification program offered no advantage in lowering either diastolic or systolic blood pressure, compared to diet alone.
- Other studies (Yates et al 1988) suggest beneficial influences of manipulation on hypertensive patients, but no large-scale controlled studies have been carried out.
- There is some evidence that osteopathic manipulation, focused on those spinal areas from where the nerve supply to the kidneys emerges, may be of benefit in reducing hypertension (Johnston & Kelso 1995, Johnston et al 1995).

Massage and hypertension

- *Massage lowers diastolic blood pressure*: Noting that high blood pressure is associated with elevated anxiety, stress and stress hormones, hostility, depression and catecholamines, massage therapy and progressive muscle relaxation were evaluated as treatments for reducing blood pressure and these associated symptoms. Adults who had been diagnosed as hypertensive received ten 30-minute massage sessions over 5 weeks, or were given progressive muscle relaxation instructions (control group). Sitting diastolic blood pressure decreased after the first and last massage therapy sessions, and reclining diastolic blood pressure decreased from the first to the last day of the study. Although both groups reported less anxiety, only the massage therapy group reported less depression and hostility and showed decreased urinary and salivary stress hormone levels (cortisol). The results suggest that massage therapy may be effective in reducing diastolic blood pressure and symptoms associated with hypertension (Hernandez-Reif et al 2000a).

- *Hypertension reduced by massage*: A preliminary study (Olney 2005) tested the effects of a regularly applied back massage on the blood pressure (BP) of patients with clinically diagnosed hypertension. In this experimental, pretest/post-test study, a 10-minute back massage was given to the experimental group ($n = 8$), three times a week for 10 sessions. The control group ($n = 6$) relaxed in the same environment for 10 minutes, three times a week for 10 sessions. Analysis of variance-determined systolic BP changed significantly between groups over time as did the diastolic BP. This preliminary study suggested that regular massage may lower BP in hypertensive persons.

Exercise and hypertension

- *Vigorous exercise and short-term reduction in hypertension*: Research has shown that after women with mild levels of hypertension exercised vigorously (i.e. aerobically) for 30 minutes, using static bicycles, all aspects of their blood pressure reduced, and stayed reduced for up to 7 hours. The researchers conclude that: 'The magnitude and duration of post-exercise hypotension may be sufficient to normalise the blood pressure of certain hypertensive women throughout most of the day' (Pescatello et al 1999).
- *Long-term non-compliance despite benefits*: Aerobic exercise (e.g. jogging, biking, swimming) has been widely studied for its beneficial effects on hypertension (Higashi et al 1999, Moreira et al 1999). However, despite the success of aerobic exercise in reducing blood pressure, most studies show that 50% of adults who begin an

aerobic exercise program drop out within 3–6 months and fewer than 20% continue exercising after 24 months (Dishman 1994).

- *Endurance exercise not beneficial for black women*: There is a major variation in different ethnic groups, relative to high blood pressure. In the first place, black (non-Hispanic) people appear to have a greater tendency to hypertension than whites or Hispanics, although in all groups those with 'higher rates of physical inactivity' have higher blood pressure (Bassett 2002). Additionally, the response of achieving significantly lower blood pressure after aerobic exercise in white women differs markedly from the response in black women, where it rises, or stays the same. The conclusion (Pescatello et al 2003) is that: 'Endurance exercise may adversely affect the blood pressure of black women.'
- *'White-coat' effect reduces over time*: Between 20 and 45% of people suffer from what is known as 'white coat hypertension' – their blood pressure rises when it is tested by a physician or nurse. Research has shown that this tendency improves markedly when regular exercise is taken: '12 weeks of exercise training can result in successful reduction of blood pressure . . . that would be beneficial to patients with white coat hypertension' (Tsai et al 2002).
- *Exercise for weight loss and antihypertensive effects*: Where weight is a major part of a person's high blood pressure, a question is often asked as to which is more important in lowering blood pressure – diet or exercise. This has now been partially answered by Japanese research. The researchers conclude that their results demonstrate that aerobic exercise is much more effective for weight loss, and weight loss-induced blood pressure reduction, than a low caloric diet alone (Masuo 2001).
- *Multiple benefits of modified diet, exercise and education*: A randomized trial (Aldana et al 2005) has clearly demonstrated improvements in resting heart rate, total cholesterol, low-density lipoprotein cholesterol, and systolic and diastolic blood pressure at 6 weeks after a 40-hour educational program on diet and exercise.
- *Moderate exercise and hypertension*: It is now known that one session of exercise can lower blood pressure acutely for up to 24 hours, requiring only 40% of maximal capacity or moderate pace walking, and that after three

consecutive episodes of exercise, blood pressure is reduced for longer but returns to pre-exercise levels by 1–2 weeks of no exercise (Thompson et al 2001).

- *Hypertensives benefit more from exercise*: It is also known that blood pressure falls more in hypertensive than in normotensive people. In fact, regular exercise lowers blood pressure in 75% of hypertensive people, with average systolic and diastolic reductions of 11 and 8 mmHg, respectively. Exercise can reduce 10-year cardiovascular risk by at least 25% in the average hypertensive patient, because of the effect on blood pressure and other cardiovascular risk factors (Hagberg et al 2000).
- *Exercising three times weekly as effective as five times*: Blood pressure reduction is as effective with exercise three times as five times a week. The exercise can be anywhere between 30 and 60 minutes a day, and, perhaps surprisingly, there seems to be little difference in blood pressure reductions achieved between doing 363 and 1866 kcal a week of exercise (e.g. three times 30 minutes of moderate walking a week compared with 60 minutes of brisk walking five times a week). Additionally, low-to-moderate intensities of exercise are as effective at lowering blood pressure, if not more effective, than vigorous exercise (Fagard 2001).

Other factors relative to exercise and hypertension include the following (Elley & Arrol 2005):

- Many cardiovascular effects, such as cardiovascular fitness and serum lipid profiles, can be improved by accumulating the required exercise in brief episodes or 10-minute sessions throughout the day.
- Whilst reductions in blood pressure have not been shown with 10-minute exercise sessions in normotensive people, they are effective in hypertensive people.
- Aerobic exercise appears to be more effective at lowering blood pressure than resistance exercise.
- Any aerobic activity seems to work, including walking, jogging or cycling, although cycling seems the most effective.
- Blood pressure reduction with exercise is independent of weight loss, which typically needs about twice the energy expenditure to achieve.
- Low-to-moderate intensities of exercise are as effective at lowering blood pressure, if not more effective, than vigorous exercise, and are

associated with fewer cardiovascular and musculoskeletal adverse effects.

Yoga and hypertension

- *Yoga breathing and hypertension*: When different methods of stress reduction were compared, it was found that the fastest and most effective way of lowering blood pressure after a stressful episode was to use simple yoga-type breathing methods (Sung et al 2000). Slowing the rate of breathing has been shown to be effectual in lowering blood pressure in people with mild hypertension, where it can be as effective as the use of medication (Sydorchuk & Tryniak 2005).
- *Yoga movement and postures and hypertension*: Apart from the breathing benefits of yoga, there seems to be evidence that the movements and postures of traditional yoga can produce a significant lowering of blood pressure, often sufficient to allow a reduction in medication (Patel 1973, Patel & North 1975).

Physical medicine therapeutic measures for hypertension

- *There is limited evidence suggesting manipulation to be valuable in reducing hypertension.*
- *Massage therapy has been shown to effectively reduce both anxiety levels and hypertension.*
- *Active exercise (moderate aerobic) has been demonstrated to provide major benefits in lowering elevated blood pressure, but not in black women.*
- *Yoga breathing methods are effective in reducing hypertension.*

Hospitalized patients

See discussion in Chapter 8 regarding general techniques and postsurgical care of such patients.

Examples of the efficacy of osteopathic methods used in hospital settings (Dickey 1989, Schwartz 1986, Stiles 1976)

OMT and hospitalized patients with pancreatitis and pneumonia

Osteopathic manipulative treatment has been widely used in hospital settings as an adjunctive treatment for patients with congestive heart failure, respiratory failure, pneumonia, bronchitis and asthma.

In an outcomes research study, Radjieski et al (1998) randomly assigned six patients with pancreatitis to receive standard care plus daily osteopathic manipulative treatment (comprising myofascial release, soft tissue, and strain/counterstrain techniques) for the duration of their hospitalization or to receive only standard care (eight patients). Osteopathic treatment involved 10–20 minutes daily of a standardized protocol, with attending physicians blinded as to group assignment.

Results indicated that patients who received osteopathic attention averaged significantly fewer days in the hospital before discharge (mean reduction 3.5 days) than control subjects, although there were no significant differences in time to food intake or in use of pain medications.

See also details of research by Noll et al (2000), involving hospitalized elderly pneumonia patients, in the next section (Infection).

Can acutely ill patients' hospital stay be shortened?

Schwartz (1986) suggests that:

> Literally thousands of hospital days could be saved by judicious osteopathic examination for interspace dysfunction and appropriate positional release treatment. It may be used on patients with fractures, as well as on post-surgical patients who have pain at the site of incision. It may also be used on patients who have osseous metastatic disease. If the part of the body that is to be treated can be moved by the patient it can safely be treated with SCS.

Results are claimed to be lasting and repetitive treatment is needed (in hospital settings) only if there is ongoing neurosensory reflex activity or if the condition which produced the dysfunction in the first place is repeated or ongoing.

Shorter hospitalization and duration of intravenous antibiotics for elderly pneumonia patients

Noll and colleagues (2000) conducted a randomly controlled study involving elderly patients hospitalized with acute pneumonia. Patients were recruited and randomly placed into two groups: 28 in the treatment group and 30 in the control group. The treatment group received a standardized osteopathic attention protocol (including SCS and functional methods), while the control group received a light touch protocol. There was no statistical difference between groups for age, gender or simplified acute physiology scores. The treatment group had a significantly shorter duration of intravenous antibiotic treatment and a shorter hospital stay.

Osteopathic treatment during acute respiratory failure

As noted in Chapters 7 and 8, and in this chapter, osteopathic manipulation has been used to treat a wide range of diseases in largely outpatient settings. There also exists an emergent use of osteopathic manipulative treatment to improve respiratory mechanics in a critically ill patient with acute respiratory failure. High-velocity mobilization of cervical and thoracic dysfunctions has been shown to result in improved breathing, improved arterial oxygenation, resolution of tachycardia, and an overall improvement in the patient's clinical condition (Stretanski & Kaiser 2001).

Postoperative uses of positional release techniques

Postsurgical OMT care of median sternotomy patients

Dickey (1989) has focused attention on the particular needs of the many thousands of people undergoing surgery each year via median sternotomy, in which the rib cage is opened anteriorly to allow access to the heart and other thoracic structures.

In the USA alone, more than 250 000 patients undergo coronary artery bypass graft surgery annually. This surgery is accomplished via a median sternotomy incision, an approach that has been gaining widespread acceptance.

- In this form of surgery an incision is made from the suprasternal notch to below the xiphoid process.
- The soft tissues below the skin are treated with diathermy to stem bleeding and the sternum is divided by an electric bone saw, the exposed edges being covered with bone wax.
- The sternum is then retracted with the upper level being placed at the level of the 2nd rib.
- Following whatever surgical intervention is involved, the sternal margins are brought together and held by stainless steel sutures.
- There are often drainage tubes exiting from below the xiphoid following surgery.

The degrees of stress and injury endured by all the tissues of the region are clearly of major dimensions, especially considering that the open-chest situation may have been maintained for many hours. The sequelae to this trauma are many and varied, and may include 'dehiscence, substernal and pericardial infection, non-union of the sternum, pericardial constriction, phrenic nerve injuries, rib fractures and brachial plexus injuries'.

Fully 23.5% of patients undergoing these procedures develop brachial plexus injuries.

Dickey reports on this surgical procedure being carried out experimentally on 10 cadavers, of which seven sustained 1st rib fractures, with the fractured ends often impaling the lower trunks of the brachial plexus.

While such negative effects are usually noted immediately postoperatively, many problems do not emerge until later, and these might include structural and functional changes in chest mechanics that do not become evident for weeks or months, particularly restrictions affecting thoracic vertebrae and the rib cage, as well as fascial and diaphragmatic changes.

Dickey (1989) has outlined a number of appropriate manual methods for helping in recovery. He stresses the importance of structural evaluation and treatment, both before and after surgery, involving manual therapeutic methods of various types. However, it is specifically the positional release approaches (Chaitow 2007) that are advocated for treating this type of postsurgical trauma (see Chapter 7 for detail of positional release methods).

Postoperative OMT care following coronary artery bypass surgery

O-Yurvati et al (2005) documented the physiological effects of postoperative osteopathic manipulative treatment (OMT) following a coronary artery bypass graft (CABG) to determine the effects on cardiac hemodynamics. Ten subjects undergoing CABG surgery were recruited for postoperative OMT. The primary assessment compared pre-OMT versus post-OMT, measurements of thoracic impedance, mixed venous oxygen saturation and cardiac index. Immediately following CABG surgery OMT was provided to alleviate anatomic dysfunction of the rib cage caused by median sternotomy, and to improve respiratory function. This adjunctive treatment occurred while subjects were completely anesthetized. Results suggested improved peripheral circulation and increased mixed venous oxygen saturation after OMT. These increases were accompanied by an improvement in cardiac index ($p \leq 0.01$). The authors conclude that OMT has immediate, beneficial hemodynamic effects after CABG surgery when administered while the patient is sedated and pharmacologically paralyzed.

A prospective, match-controlled postoperative outcome study

As noted above, osteopathic manipulative treatment has been reported to relieve a variety of conditions, but no studies have examined the outcome effects of osteopathic manipulative treatment as a complementary modality for treating musculoskeletal problems during postoperative recovery.

In order to assess osteopathic manipulative treatment as a complementary therapy for patients undergoing elective knee or hip arthroplasty, Jarski et al (2000) designed a prospective, single-blinded, two-group, match-controlled outcome study. Of 166 eligible patients, 38 were assigned to a treatment group and matched with 38 control subjects. The treatment group received osteopathic manipulative treatment on postoperative days 2–5. The main outcome showed that, compared to control subjects, the intervention group negotiated stairs 20% earlier (mean = 4.3 postoperative days, SD = 1.2; control subjects 5.4, SD = 1.6, $p = 0.006$) and ambulated 43% farther on the third postoperative day (mean = 24.3 m, SD = 18.3; controls = 13.9, SD = 14.4, $p = 0.008$). The intervention group also required less analgesia, had shorter hospital stays and ambulated farther on postoperative days 1, 2 and 4. The conclusion is that patients receiving osteopathic manipulative treatment in the early postoperative period negotiated stairs earlier and ambulated greater distances than did control group patients.

A single case example of the need for a holistic perspective in a patient following surgery for torn anterior cruciate ligament

Increasing instability of the knee developed in a 27-year-old man who had torn his anterior cruciate ligament (ACL) approximately 10 years prior to surgical intervention (Gugel & Johnston 2006). After initial conservative treatment, including use of a functional brace for activity, the patient opted for surgical reconstruction with a patellar tendon graft.

Preoperative examinations were conducted to assess the condition of the patient's musculoskeletal system. These revealed somatic dysfunction in the lumbopelvic region. In addition, there was extension of muscular tension from the injured left knee and ankle into the lower thorax and ribs 6–9.

During the postoperative rehabilitation process, examination at regular intervals included documentation of somatic dysfunction and osteopathic manipulative treatment (OMT). Following ACL reconstruction and OMT, the patient showed increasingly stable mobility in the lumbopelvic region. Furthermore, episodic new dysfunctions readily resolved with OMT. The patient returned to his regular sports activities 6 months after surgery.

This example highlights the adaptive changes in spine and thorax that evolved following lower limb injury, and how the opportunity to normalize these changes arose when the knee damage was repaired.

Physical medicine therapeutic measures for hospitalized patients

These have been shown to:

- *reduce postoperative complications*
- *induce greater comfort*
- *reduce length of stay*

- *speed ambulation*
- *improve overall recovery time*
- *improve function (breathing, cardiac index, etc.).*

Infection, including respiratory tract infections (pneumonia)

See discussion in Chapter 7 regarding general physical medicine techniques and infection.

Pneumonia and mobilization

Noll et al (1999, 2000) applied osteopathic manual mobilization methods to elderly hospitalized patients with pneumonia, which resulted in a reduction in the length of hospital stay from a mean of 8.6 days without OMT, to 6.6 days with OMT. Additional benefits in this study, for those receiving OMT, included reduced length of use of intravenous antibiotics.

Immune function and physical medicine

- *Immune function markers and physical methods*: Research evidence suggests that both osteopathic and chiropractic methods, as well as massage, can increase levels of the immune system's defensive agents (including natural killer cells, B and T lymphocytes) for many hours after the treatment, improving the body's ability to fight infection (Brennan et al 1991, Lovas et al 2002, Paul et al 1986).
- *Massage and HIV+ patients*: One massage study involved treating HIV-positive individuals with massage therapy (45 minutes of massage five times weekly for 1 month). Not only were stress hormones (cortisol) much lower, together with feelings of anxiety, but natural killer cells, and their activity were significantly increased as a result (Ironson et al 1996).
- *Massage and recurrent respiratory tract infection*: Massage was employed to treat and prevent recurrent respiratory tract infection in children. Susceptible and healthy children of the same age were used as controls. The therapeutic effect of the treatment group was shown to be significantly better ($p < 0.01$) than that of the controls, with all of the immunological indices being approximately normal when the patients were re-examined 3 and 6 months after the massage intervention. Massage was shown to be helpful in enhancing immune function, preventing and treating the condition (Zhu et al 1998).

- *OMT and immune response*: Osteopathic 'pump' techniques have been shown to encourage more effective immune system responses when influenza and hepatitis B immunizations were given (Breithaupt et al 2001, Jackson et al 1998).
- *OMT and pancreatitis*: When OMT was applied to hospitalized patients with acute pancreatitis, along with their regular medical treatment, the results showed that the patients receiving both OMT (10–20 minutes daily) plus standard medication, compared with patients receiving standard medical treatment only, recovered more rapidly and were able to leave hospital on average 3.5 days sooner (Radjieski et al 1998).

Although the ways in which these methods improve immune function are not fully understood, the theories are that the osteopathic method stimulates production, or release from storage sites, of helpful immune substances, while the effect of massage seems to relate to reduction of 'stress hormone' levels. Chiropractic treatment seems to achieve its effect via mediation of the nervous system.

See Chapter 7 for discussion of potential benefits of general manual treatment.

Hydrotherapy, immune function and the common cold

Taking a cold shower regularly has been shown to improve immune function quite dramatically, over a period of months. German research showed that the regular (daily) use of a cold shower had a progressively beneficial effect on immune system efficiency. Medical students were divided into two groups. For 6 months one group took a graduated cold shower (i.e. ending a hot shower with a brief cold shower application, increasing the length of the cold application to tolerance up to 2 minutes), while the other group took a warm shower.

After 6 months those taking the cold shower were found to be having half the number of colds compared with those having warm showers. The cold shower group's colds lasted for approximately half as long as those having warm showers, and were accompanied by far less mucus production (measured by weighing the used paper handkerchiefs of cold sufferers). Cold showers were avoided during, and for 1 week after, experiencing a cold.

The various protective benefits did not become apparent until almost 3 months of regular cold showering (Ernst 1990).

Otitis media and osteopathic manipulation (Degenhardt & Kuchera 2006)

OMT and otitis media

A referred and volunteer sample of pediatric patients ranging in age from 7 months to 35 months, with a history of recurrent otitis media ($n = 8$) all received weekly osteopathic structural examinations and osteopathic manipulative treatment. This intervention was performed concurrently with traditional medical management. Five (62.5%) subjects had no recurrence of symptoms. Of the three remaining subjects in this cohort, one had a bulging tympanic membrane, another had four episodes of otitis media, and the last underwent surgery after recurrence at 6 weeks post-treatment. Closer analysis of the post-treatment course of the last two subjects indicates that there may have been a clinically significant decrease in morbidity for a period of time after intervention. This pilot study indicates that osteopathic manipulative treatment may change the progression of recurrent otitis media, a finding that supports the need for additional research.

OMT and recurrent acute otitis media

A study evaluated the effects of osteopathic manipulative treatment as an adjuvant therapy to routine pediatric care in children with recurrent acute otitis media (AOM) (Mills et al 2003). Patients aged 6 months to 6 years, with three episodes of AOM in the previous 6 months or four in the previous year, who were not already surgical candidates, were placed randomly into two groups: one receiving routine pediatric care, the other receiving routine care plus osteopathic manipulative treatment. Both groups received an equal number of study encounters to monitor behavior and obtain tympanograms. Clinical status was monitored with review of pediatric records. The pediatrician was blinded to patient group and study outcomes, and the osteopathic physician was blinded to patient clinical course.

A total of 57 patients (25 intervention patients and 32 control patients) met criteria and completed the study. Adjusting for the baseline frequency before study entry, intervention patients had fewer episodes of AOM (mean group difference per month, -0.14 (95% confidence interval, -0.27 to 0.00); $p = 0.04$), fewer surgical procedures (intervention patients, 1; control patients, 8; $p = 0.03$), and more mean surgery-free months (intervention patients, 6.00; control patients, 5.25; $p = 0.01$). Baseline and final tympanograms showed an increased frequency of more normal tympanogram types in the intervention group, with an adjusted mean group difference of 0.55 (95% confidence interval, 0.08 to 1.02; $p = 0.02$). No adverse reactions were reported.

The results of this study suggest a potential benefit of osteopathic manipulative treatment as adjuvant therapy in children with recurrent AOM; it may prevent or decrease surgical intervention or antibiotic overuse.

Otitis media and chiropractic manipulation

A number of studies involving chiropractic care of juveniles with otitis media have demonstrated promising outcomes (Sawyer et al 1999). Spinal manipulation and manual lymphatic drainage massage are reported to be the preferred forms of treatment (together with nutritional strategies) used by approximately 75% of a group of 33 chiropractors when treating pediatric otitis media patients (Vallone & Fallon 1997).

Examples of good results with such methods are reported following a study involving over 300 children with otitis media (Fallon 1997), and in five successive cases (Fysh 1996).

Glue ear and chiropractic and massage

Most glue ear problems get better on their own whatever treatment is used: 'About 30% of OME resolves in several weeks *without treatment*, rising to about 90% spontaneous resolution in several months' (Rosenfeld 1997, Zielhuis et al 1990). This makes it difficult to be sure whether treatment, such as massage or chiropractic, helps or not, despite many parents (Spigelblatt et al 1994) and practitioners (Sawyer et al 1999) claiming that these methods have improved the children's glue ear problem.

Tonsillitis and manual methods of treatment

- *Physical medicine manipulation and tonsillitis*: A Czech study (Lewit & Abrahamovic 1975) offers some support for the use of mobilization and manipulation of neck structures, associated (via the nerve supply) to the tonsils, in cases of chronic tonsillitis. This study evaluated the possible connection, in 46 patients, between chronic tonsillitis and dysfunction involving the vertebral joints of the neck. In only in five (11%) of the people examined was there found to be no restriction of the topmost joint of the spine, between the first vertebra (the atlas) and the occiput. The atlanto-occipital joint was the most frequently affected segment (identified by motion palpation) affecting fully 36 patients. Twenty-eight of the patients were treated surgically, and in these the vertebral restriction disappeared spontaneously in only four, but remained in the others. Ten of the patients were treated only by manipulation of the neck vertebrae, and during a 9-month follow-up period no relapse of joint blockage or tonsillitis was observed in these individuals.

- *Combined physical medicine modalities and tonsillitis*: German research suggests that in appropriate cases of chronic tonsillitis a combination of hydrotherapy, electrotherapy and physiotherapy (including massage) may offer benefits (Krahl 1973).

Physical medicine therapeutic measures for immune enhancement in relation to infection

- *A variety of physical medicine approaches, deriving from osteopathy, chiropractic, massage and hydrotherapy, have all been demonstrated either to enhance immune function or to offer benefit in other ways towards prevention and treatment of a variety of upper respiratory and respiratory-related infections, ranging from the common cold, through otitis media and tonsillitis to pneumonia.*

Irritable bowel, including constipation

Many factors have been associated with the occurrence of constipation, particularly poor diet and lack of exercise (although this feature remains unproven, see below). However, the importance of medications and general medical illnesses in constipation remains more uncertain (Zernike & Henderson 1999).

Constipation is a common problem in the community; the symptoms vary from a relatively mild bowel habit disturbance to rare serious sequelae, including bowel obstruction and fecal impaction (Heaton et al 1992a). Population-based studies have estimated that approximately 10–20% of otherwise healthy people report one or more symptoms of chronic constipation, including infrequent stools (<3 bowel movements per week) and excessive straining or hard stools, although the exact rates vary depending on the definition applied (Dent et al 1986, Heaton et al 1992b). Only a minority with constipation seek health care but this represents a substantial health burden – for example, in the United States, constipation accounted for 2.5 million doctor visits per year (Sonnenberg & Koch 1989). The high prevalence and chronicity of constipation is an important public health issue because of its effects on patient well-being and lost productivity, in addition to the costs of medical consultation (Locke et al 2000).

Constipation is a heterogeneous disorder, with multiple causes, including an inadequate diet, medication use, concurrent diseases, and disorders of bowel structure or function. However, the relative importance of these causes in the community remains inadequately documented. In particular, drugs are a recognized cause, but their relevance has been poorly quantified (Drossman et al 2000).

Breathing pattern disorders and colon spasm

- A common side-effect of a rapid upper-chest breathing pattern (hyperventilation, see above, in this chapter) is closely linked to feelings of anxiety (see earlier this chapter), as is elimination of excessive amounts of carbon dioxide in relation to the individual's current metabolic requirements. This causes respiratory alkalosis, one of the effects of which is to encourage the smooth muscles that surround the digestive tract (as well as blood vessels) to contract excessively (Levitsky 1995).
- Research conducted to assess the effects of such a pattern of overbreathing on the behavior of the smooth muscles of the intestinal tract, during deliberate upper chest breathing, showed a significant increase in the tension in the smooth muscles, as well as in their contractility, especially in the regions of the colon. This suggests that hyperventilation alters the way the nervous system controls the colon, and this tendency may be a feature of irritable bowel syndrome in many cases (Ford et al 1995).
- Research has shown that practicing very slow breathing techniques (based on yoga principles) is 'associated with the normally functioning gut' and that breathing retraining can offer a simple, safe and effective way of easing this problem (Grove 1988).

Chiropractic and IBS

Chiropractic manipulation of the spine and neck has been shown in some cases to be able to beneficially change bowel behavior, often in chronic conditions of constipation, and sometimes after just one treatment (Eriksen 1994, Falk 1990, Wagner 1995).

Myofascial trigger points and IBS

Trigger points are local sensitized areas in muscles that can cause pain or discomfort, not only where they are situated but also in target areas some distance away. The effects of trigger point activity can spread far beyond obvious muscle and joint pain, being capable of producing altered function, for example, of the bowel itself. Trigger points lying in the superficial muscle wall of the lower abdomen have been shown to be capable of producing symptoms such as diarrhea (Simons et al 1999c). Trigger points can usually be deactivated by acupuncture, as well as by manual pressure and stretching techniques (see Chapter 7).

Massage of levator ani and coccygeus muscles and IBS

The link between high tone internal pelvic muscles and interstitial cystitis is described elsewhere in this chapter, as are methods used to massage internal pelvic muscles in such cases.

A French osteopathic study involving over 100 patients has shown that similar attention to internal pelvic muscles, specifically levator ani and coccygeus, as well as pelvic manipulation, can assist in normalizing many cases of irritable bowel syndrome (Riot et al 2004). One hundred and one patients (76 females and 25 males; mean age 54 years) with a diagnosis of levator ani syndrome (LVAS) were studied prospectively over 1 year. Massage was given with the patient lying on the left side. Physical treatment of associated pelvic joint disorders was given at the end of each massage session. *Results*: 47 patients (46.5%) suffered from both LVAS and IBS. A mean of less than two sessions of treatment was necessary. At 6 months, 69% of the patients were LVAS-free (p <0.0001) and 10% were improved. At 12 months, 62% were still free of symptoms and 10% improved (p = 0.37). A comparable trend was found in the IBS group: 53% IBS-free initially, 78% at 6 months (p = 0.00001) and 72% at 12 months (p = 1). There was a significant correlation between the favorable outcome of IBS and LVAS at 6 and 12 months. All IBS-free patients were LVAS-free at 6 months. *Conclusion*: At 12 months LVAS may be cured or alleviated in 72% of the cases with one to two treatments. The results suggest a muscular and osteo-ligamentary etiology in LVAS.

Exercise, constipation and IBS

- *Exercise and constipation*: A review of the empirical research on the link between exercise and constipation concludes that whilst 'inactivity may be associated with constipation, exercise has not clearly been shown to be an effective treatment' (Locke et al 2000).
- A review of pertinent scientific research reports that a link has not been proven between exercise and constipation, although there is some evidence that colonic motility may be increased with vigorous exercise such as running and fast walking (possibly due to stimulation by biomechanical bouncing of the gut and compression of the colon by abdominal musculature) (Peters et al 2001).
- *Lack of exercise and IBS*: A survey of over 1000 individuals with IBS has concluded that 'there was a trend towards the higher prevalence of IBS with fewer hours of exercise' although the difference when compared with non-IBS individuals was not significant (Kim & Ban 2005).
- *IBS symptoms reduced by exercise*: A study was conducted to attempt to establish whether physical activity moderates chronic functional gastrointestinal (GI) disorders such as irritable bowel syndrome, and to test whether active women with irritable bowel syndrome had less severe GI symptoms than inactive women with irritable bowel syndrome. Questionnaires were used to measure GI and psychological distress and somatic symptoms in 89 women. A daily symptom and activity diary was kept for one menstrual cycle. Women with IBS were significantly less likely to be active (48%) than control women (71%) (χ^2 = 3.4, p = 0.05). Within the IBS group, active women were less likely to report a feeling of incomplete evacuation following a bowel movement than inactive women (p <0.04), yet active women did not have less severe recalled psychological or somatic symptoms than inactive women. Active women with IBS reported less severe daily somatic symptoms, which were accounted for by a lower level of fatigue (p = 0.003) (Lustyk et al 2001).

Yoga and IBS

A study was conducted to evaluate the comparative effect of yogic and conventional treatment in diarrhea-predominant irritable bowel syndrome (IBS) in a randomized control design. The patients were 22 males, aged 20–50 years, with confirmed diagnosis of diarrhea-predominant IBS. The conventional group (n = 12, 1 dropout) was given symptomatic treatment with loperamide 2–6 mg/day for 2 months, and the yogic intervention group (n = 9) consisted of a set of 12 asanas (yogic poses) along with Surya Nadi pranayama (right-nostril breathing) twice a day for 2 months. All participants were tested at three regular intervals – at the start of the study and at 1 month and 2 months of receiving the intervention – and were investigated for bowel symptoms, autonomic symptoms, autonomic reactivity (five standard tests), surface electrogastrography, and anxiety profile by Spielberger's self-evaluation questionnaire which evaluated trait and state anxiety. Two months of both conventional and yogic intervention showed a significant decrease in bowel symptoms and state anxiety. This was accompanied by an increase in electrophysiologically recorded gastric activity in the conventional intervention group and enhanced parasympathetic reactivity, as measured by heart rate parameters, in the yogic intervention group. The study indicates a beneficial effect of yogic intervention over conventional treatment in diarrhea-predominant IBS (Taneja et al 2004).

Physical medicine therapeutic measures for irritable bowel symptoms, including constipation

- *The benefit of manipulation, while clearly helpful in some cases, remains unproven in these conditions as being universally applicable.*
- *If active myofascial trigger points are identified and deactivated, this may offer rapid relief of IBS symptoms.*
- *In cases where increased pelvic floor tone is a feature, internal massage has been shown to be very helpful.*
- *In cases where breathing pattern imbalances prevail, restoration of normal respiratory function is helpful in IBS.*
- *Yoga therapy appears to offer benefits that are at least as effective in symptom control as medication in diarrhea-predominant IBS, without side-effects.*
- *Exercise as a therapy appears to offer little benefit in regard to specific gastrointestinal symptoms; however, general health benefits make this a reasonable addition to prescribed behavior/lifestyle modification.*

Insomnia

Insomnia is a worldwide problem with more than 1 in 20 individuals experiencing chronic and/or severe insomnia during their lifetime, and around 1 in 3 adults having difficulty sleeping in any one year (Ohayon 2002).

Common complaints are difficulty getting to sleep, staying asleep and non-restorative sleep (Ohayon & Partinen 2003). Short-term insomnia is commonly related to psychosocial stress or environmental disturbances. Causes of chronic insomnia may range from psychophysiological disorders to various medical problems. Nervousness and tension are factors significantly associated with insomnia (Martikainen et al 2003). Sleep disorders are also commonly reported by people complaining of pain (Lobbezoo et al 2004), and

insomnia is in turn associated with increased pain and distress (Wilson et al 2002). Although the poor sleep quality experienced by patients with chronic pain can at times be an expression of depression or anxiety, rather than the intensity of the pain (Sayar et al 2002), painful disorders do interfere with sleep; however, disturbances in sleep also contribute to the experience of pain. There is a clear reciprocal relationship between sleep quality and pain. For example, noise stimuli that disrupt slow-wave sleep lead to unrefreshing sleep and fatigue, as well as widespread musculoskeletal pain and tenderness, even in normal healthy individuals (Moldofsky 2001).

Chiropractic and insomnia associated with pain (Jamison 2005)

Although many patients perceive that chiropractic care offers temporary respite from insomnia problems, when changes have been objectively monitored improvements are seen to be erratic, with no consistent trends detectable. Researchers conducting a pilot study noted that:

Although pain relief would be expected to increase the probability of restful sleep, and a number of subjects did appear to fall asleep more readily and awake less frequently than usual, no clear temporal patterns between the chiropractic consultation and sleep behaviors emerged.

Yoga and insomnia

- *Yoga and insomnia in the elderly*: Manjunath & Telles (2005) designed a study to compare the effects of yoga and Ayurveda on sleep in a geriatric population. Of the 120 residents from a home for the aged, 69 were stratified based on age (5-year intervals) and randomly allocated to three groups, i.e. yoga (physical postures, relaxation techniques, voluntarily regulated breathing and lectures on yoga philosophy), Ayurveda (a herbal preparation) and Wait-list control (no intervention). The groups were evaluated for self-assessment of sleep over a 1-week period at baseline, and after 3 and 6 months of the respective interventions. The yoga group showed a significant decrease in the time taken to fall asleep (approximate group average decrease: 10 minutes, $p < 0.05$), an increase in the total number of hours slept (approximate group average increase: 60 minutes, $p < 0.05$) and in the feeling of being rested in the morning based on a rating scale ($p < 0.05$) after 6 months. The other groups showed no significant change. Similar benefits in improved sleep have been shown resulting from yoga use in cancer patients (Cohen et al 2004).

- *Yoga eye exercises and sleep*: Traditional Hatha yoga eye movement exercises appear to effectively induce a sense of relaxation to assist in sleep acquisition (Hedstrom 1991). The eye exercise consists of 'drawing' a vertical line, with the head held still, for 10 or 15 repetitions, by moving the eyes up and down as far as they will go. The procedure is repeated making a repetitive horizontal line (side to side), and then two diagonal lines, relaxing the eyes in their normal posture in between exercises. These linear exercises are followed by describing two 180° arcs, upper and lower, with the eyes, making a clockwise and a counterclockwise circle. By the time the latter part of the exercise is being performed, 90% of individuals report sleep to be rapidly approaching.

- *Yoga and melatonin production*: The practice of yoga meditation has been shown to effectively increase the levels of melatonin which may assist in normalizing sleep patterns (Tooley et al 2000).

Acupressure and insomnia in end-stage renal disease

Sleep disturbance is common in patients with end-stage renal disease but no intervention studies have addressed this problem. The purpose of a randomized control trial (Tsay et al 2003) was to test the effectiveness of acupoint massage for patients with end-stage renal disease who were experiencing sleep disturbance and diminished quality of life. A total of 98 end-stage renal disease patients with sleep disturbance were randomly assigned into an acupressure group, a sham acupressure group and a control group. Acupressure and sham acupressure group patients received acupoint or no acupoint massage, three times a week during hemodialysis treatment for a total of 4 weeks. The measures included the Pittsburgh Sleep Quality Index, Sleep Log, and the Medical Outcome Study Short Form 36. Acupressure involved consistent pressure applied to Shenmen (HT7) in the ears and hands, and Yungchuan (KI1) in both feet. The degree of finger pressure varied from 3.56 to 3.88 kg. Accuracy of acupoints selection was evaluated and was confirmed to be 100%. Interventions were limited to 14 minutes, consisting of 5 minutes of massage to relax the person and 9 minutes of acupoint massage. Intervention took place on three days per week for four consecutive weeks.

The results indicated significant differences between the acupressure group and the control group in subscale scores of subjective sleep quality, sleep duration, habitual sleep efficiency, sleep sufficiency and global Pittsburgh Sleep Quality Index scores. Sleep Log data revealed that the acupressure group significantly decreased wake time and experienced an improved quality of sleep at night over the control group.

Massage, sleep disturbance and low back pain

A randomized between-groups design was used to evaluate massage therapy versus relaxation therapy effects on chronic low back pain (Field et al 2005). Treatment effects were evaluated for reducing pain, depression, anxiety and sleep disturbances, for improving trunk range of motion (ROM) and for reducing job absenteeism and increasing job productivity. Thirty adults (mean age 41 years) with low back pain with a duration of at least 6 months participated in the study. The groups did not differ in age, socioeconomic status, ethnicity or gender. Sessions were 30 minutes long, twice a week, for 5 weeks. On the first and last day of the 5-week study participants completed questionnaires and were assessed for ROM. By the end of the study, the massage therapy group, as compared to the relaxation group, reported experiencing less pain, depression, anxiety and sleep disturbance. They also showed improved trunk and pain flexion performance.

Low birth weight infant massage and sleep behavior

A Russian study (Kelmanson & Adulas 2006) attempted to evaluate the impact of massage therapy on sleep behavior in infants born with low birth weight (LBW).

Fifty infants (22 boys, 28 girls) born between 2000 and 2002 and defined as LBW babies (<2500 g at birth) were enrolled onto the study at the age of 2 months.

The control group consisted of 50 healthy infants born with LBW who were cross-matched with an experimental group of babies and controlled for gender, gestational age, weight and date of birth. The groups were also matched for proximal geographical distribution. Babies in the experimental group were assigned massage intervention therapy that included gentle rubbing, stroking, passive movements of the limbs and other means of kinesthetic stimulation, performed by professionals until the infant was 8 months old.

The findings suggest that 8-month-old LBW infants who received massage intervention were less likely to snore during sleep, required less feeding on waking up at night, and appeared more alert during the day. These apparent correlations remained significant after adjustment was made for major potential confounders. No statistically significant difference was found in sleep behavior between LBW infants exposed to massage therapy who were either born preterm or at term. The results suggest that massage may be a valuable approach to improve quality of sleep and reduce sleep-disordered breathing in infants born with LBW.

Exercise and sleep (poor correlation)

1. Research studies (Youngstedt et al 2003) examined associations between daily amounts of physical activity and sleep.
   - Study 1 examined self-reported exercise durations and sleep diaries for 105 consecutive days in 31 college students who were normal sleepers.
   - Study 2 examined 71 physically active adults ($n = 38$, ages 18–30 years; and $n = 33$, ages 60–75 years), the majority of whom were normal sleepers.

     No significant associations between physical activity and sleep were found in the main analyses of either study. These results fail to support epidemiological data on the value of exercise for sleep, but are consistent with experimental evidence showing only modest effects of exercise on sleep.

2. Noting that sleep problems become more common with age, affect quality of life for individuals and their families, and can increase health care costs, and that older people are often prescribed a range of drugs for such problems, many of which have side-effects, a systematic review (Montgomery & Dennis 2004) considered the effectiveness of three non-drug interventions – cognitive behavioral therapy (CBT), bright light, and *physical exercise* on sleep quality, duration and efficiency.

     Randomized controlled trials were evaluated where 80% or more of participants were over 60 and had a diagnosis of primary insomnia, and where investigators had taken care to screen participants for dementia and/or depression.

     The data suggest:
   - a mild effect of CBT for sleep problems in older adults, best demonstrated for sleep maintenance insomnia

   - evidence of the efficacy of bright light and exercise was so limited that no conclusions about them could be reached.

3. Differences in the exercise protocols studied (e.g. aerobic or anaerobic, intensity, duration) and interactions between individual characteristics (e.g. fitness, age and gender) cloud the current experimental evidence supporting a sleep-enhancing effect of exercise (Driver & Taylor 2000). In addition, the tendency to study changes in small groups of good sleepers may also underestimate the efficacy of exercise for promoting sleep. Although only moderate effect sizes have been noted, meta-analytical techniques have shown that exercise increased total sleep time and delayed REM sleep onset (10 minutes), increased slow-wave sleep (SWS) and reduced REM sleep (2–5 minutes). The sleep-promoting efficacy of exercise in normal and clinical populations has yet to be established empirically.

Strength training and sleep in older adults

A review of the current research on strength training and older adults evaluated exercise protocols in a variety of populations (Seguin & Nelson 2004). It demonstrated that a variety of strength-training prescriptions, ranging from highly controlled laboratory-based to minimally supervised home-based programs, have the ability to elicit meaningful health benefits in older adults. Research has demonstrated that strength-training exercises have the ability to combat weakness and frailty and their debilitating consequences. Done regularly (e.g. 2–3 days per week), such exercises build muscle strength and muscle mass and preserve bone density, independence and vitality with age. In addition, strength training has the ability to reduce the risk of osteoporosis and the signs and symptoms of numerous chronic diseases such as heart disease, arthritis and type 2 diabetes, while also improving sleep and reducing depression.

Physical medicine therapeutic measures for insomnia and disturbed sleep

- *There is limited evidence of benefit in enhancing sleep from either chiropractic intervention or various forms of exercise, apart from strength training.*
- *Massage assists sleep behavior in low birth weight infants, as well as adults with concurrent low back pain.*

- *Yoga therapy assists sleep patterns in geriatric individuals, as well as cancer patients.*
- *Melatonin levels are shown to increase following yoga meditation.*
- *Yoga eye exercises encourage more rapid sleep acquisition.*
- *Acupressure massage has a positive influence on sleep in patients with advanced renal disease.*

Interstitial cystitis (and associated non-infectious pelvic problems including dyspareunia, prostatitis and pelvic pain)

- Chronic pelvic pain (CPP) is common in women and presents a diagnostic challenge.
- The most common disorders associated with CPP are endometriosis, interstitial cystitis (IC) and irritable bowel syndrome (IBS).
- Between 38 and 85% of women presenting to a gynecologist for CPP may have IC.
- CPP involves non-cyclic pain of 6 or more months' duration that localizes to the anatomic pelvis, abdominal wall, at or below the umbilicus, lumbosacral back or the buttocks, and is of sufficient severity to cause functional disability or lead to medical care (ACOG 2004).

According to the European Association of Urology (2003), the commonest symptoms of CPP are:

- generalized pelvic pain (e.g. lower abdomen, urethra, perineum, medial thighs)
- pain with intercourse (dyspareunia)
- pain on bladder filling
- voiding symptoms (frequency, urgency, nocturia)
- premenstrual exacerbations
- exacerbations after sexual intercourse.

Structural and functional considerations

The functional integrity of the bladder, bladder neck, urethra and rectum are dependent on the interconnecting structural support of the (1) arcus tendineus fasciae pelvic, (2) levator ani muscles, and (3) endopelvic fascia around the urethra and vagina (DeLancey 1990).

Voluntary bladder control requires intact structural support, functional neuromodulatory mechanisms and urethral sphincter competency. The striated muscles of the pelvic floor play an integral role in closure of the urethral lumen and maintenance of continence.

Continence is maintained by contraction of the pelvic floor muscles (PFM), the levator ani, providing stabi-

lization of the fascial layer against which the urethra is compressed.

In women with genuine stress urinary incontinence (GSUI), ineffective contraction of the PFM allows descent of the bladder neck and inadequate occlusion of the urethra, resulting in leakage of urine. Pelvic floor muscle training may be used to strengthen the supportive pelvic floor musculature, often enabling individuals to attain continence and thus reverse or avoid the potential physical, emotional and social sequelae of urinary incontinence (Johnson 2001).

Comment: While Kegel-type exercises are commonly appropriate and helpful for low tone pelvic floor situations (Kegel 1948), if high tone exists in these muscles, such toning exercises would be useless at best, and possibly counterproductive at worst; hence the need for means of releasing/relaxing them when hypertonic (see below).

Note: There is no suggestion intended that chronic pelvic pain, interstitial cystitis and associated symptoms can always be successfully treated via physical medicine methods – whether employing pelvic floor muscle training (Kegel & Powell 1950, Verheul & Dougherty 1990) or reduction in tone of these muscles (Moldwin & Mendelowitz 1994); however, as reported below, a good proportion can be.

Kegel-type pelvic floor exercises for incontinence

In 1996, Nygaard et al conducted a prospective randomized trial involving exercises for weak pelvic floor muscles with 71 women seen for treatment of urinary incontinence in two tertiary care center referral clinics (in the departments of gynecology and urology). The primary outcome measure was the number of incontinent episodes, as documented with a 3-day voiding diary. Forty-four percent of all enrollees had a ~50% improvement in the number of incontinent episodes per day. This increased to 56% of those who completed the treatment course. Six months after completing the course of exercises, approximately one-third of all participants reported that they continued to note good or excellent improvement, and needed no further treatment.

Thiele massage and pelvic symptoms deriving from hypertonia

Some time before the Second World War a physician named Thiele developed a technique in which coccygeal prostate problems were treated by means of massage of specific muscles, mainly levator ani (Thiele 1937). This approach (see description below) is used currently in major centers in the USA to treat prostate pain and high-tone pelvic floor problems (Oyama et al 2004). Examples include the following.

Thiele massage and IC

The effectiveness of transvaginal Thiele massage has been shown (Holzberg et al 2001) on high-tone pelvic floor musculature in 90% of patients with interstitial cystitis (IC). Describing the technique, the researchers note:

> Subjects underwent a total of 6 intravaginal massage sessions using the Thiele 'stripping technique'. This technique encompasses a deep vaginal massage via a 'back and forth' motion over the levator ani, obturator internus, and piriformis muscles as well as a myofascial release technique whereas a trigger point was identified, pressure was held for 8 to 12 seconds and then released.

As to the mechanisms involved, they report:

> As a result of the close anatomic proximity of the bladder to its muscular support, it appears that internal vaginal massage can lead to subjective improvement in symptoms of IC.

Direct myofascial release of pelvic floor muscles, joint mobilization and MET in treatment of IC, dyspareunia and SI joint dysfunction

A link between the sort of symptoms treated in the previous examples, as well as painful intercourse (dyspareunia), together with sacroiliac dysfunction, was noted in a study conducted in Philadelphia (Lukban et al 2001). Sixteen patients with interstitial cystitis were evaluated for: (1) increased pelvic tone and trigger point presence; and (2) sacroiliac dysfunction. The study reports that in all 16 cases SI joint dysfunction was identified. Treatment comprised direct myofascial release, joint mobilization, muscle energy techniques, strengthening, stretching, neuromuscular re-education, and instruction in an extensive home exercise program.

The outcome was that there was a 94% improvement in problems associated with urination; 9 of the 16 patients were able to return to pain-free intercourse. The greatest improvement seen related to frequency symptoms and suprapubic pain. There was a lesser improvement in urinary urgency and nocturia.

Thiele massage and pelvic pain associated with chronic prostatitis

Pelvic pain associated with chronic prostatitis involving non-bacterial urinary difficulties, accompanied by chronic pelvic pain (involving the perineum, testicles and penis), has been shown in a study at Stanford University Medical School to be capable of being effectively treated using trigger point deactivation together with relaxation therapy (Anderson et al 2005). The researchers point out that 95% of chronic cases of prostatitis are unrelated to bacterial infection, and that myofascial trigger points, associated with abnormal muscular tension in key muscles, are commonly responsible for the symptoms. The 1-month study involved 138 men, and the results produced marked improvement in 72% of the cases, with 69% showing significant pain reduction and 80% improvement in urinary symptoms. The study noted that:

> TrPs in the anterior levator ani muscle often refer pain to the tip of the penis. The levator endopelvic fascia lateral to the prostate represents the most common location of TrPs in men with pelvic pain . . . myofascial TrPs were identified and pressure was held for about 60 seconds to release [described as **myofascial trigger point release technique – MFRT**]. Specific physiotherapy techniques used in conjunction with MFRT were voluntary contraction and release/hold-relax/contract-relax/reciprocal inhibition, and deep tissue mobilization, including stripping, strumming, skin rolling and effleurage.

(See Fig. 10.3 and Box 10.9.)

Further reading

1. Lee D 2004 The pelvic girdle, 3rd edn. Churchill Livingstone, Edinburgh
2. Wise D, Anderson R 2003 A headache in the pelvis. National Center for Pelvic Pain Research, Occidental, California

Physical therapy, the pelvic floor and pelvic dysfunction

- *Low-tone pelvic floor muscles involved in interstitial cystitis and other chronic pelvic problems (including dyspareunia) respond well to Kegel-type toning exercises.*
- *High-tone pelvic floor muscles involved in interstitial cystitis and other chronic pelvic problems (including dyspareunia) respond well to Thiele-type massage.*
- *Many chronic pelvic pain and functional problems, including interstitial cystitis and stress incontinence, respond well to deactivation of myofascial trigger points residing on the inner thigh muscles, lower abdominal muscles and internally in pelvic floor muscles.*

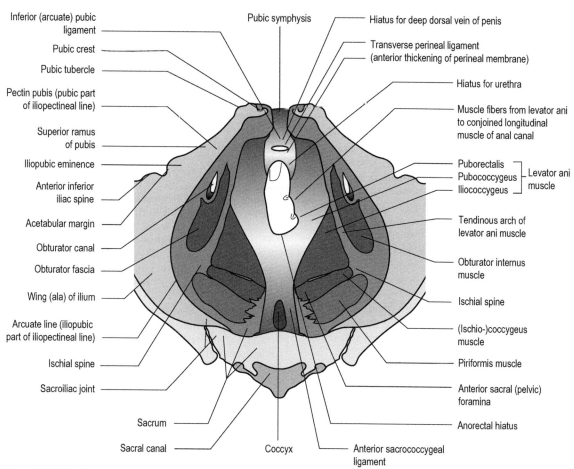

Inferior (arcuate) pubic ligament

Pubic crest

Pubic tubercle

Pectin pubis (pubic part of iliopectineal line)

Superior ramus of pubis

Iliopubic eminence

Anterior inferior iliac spine

Acetabular margin

Obturator canal

Obturator fascia

Wing (ala) of ilium

Arcuate line (iliopubic part of iliopectineal line)

Ischial spine

Sacroiliac joint

Sacrum

Sacral canal

Pubic symphysis

Coccyx

Hiatus for deep dorsal vein of penis

Transverse perineal ligament (anterior thickening of perineal membrane)

Hiatus for urethra

Muscle fibers from levator ani to conjoined longitudinal muscle of anal canal

Puborectalis
Pubococcygeus   Levator ani
Iliococcygeus   muscle

Tendinous arch of levator ani muscle

Obturator internus muscle

Ischial spine

(Ischio-)coccygeus muscle

Piriformis muscle

Anterior sacral (pelvic) foramina

Anorectal hiatus

Anterior sacrococcygeal ligament

Figure 10.3 Internal pelvic musculature and digital myofascial release technique. Reproduced with permission from Anderson et al (2005)

Box 10.9 Physical therapies in the treatment of IC

Manual physical therapy of external pelvis (6–12 weeks)

- Direct myofascial release
- Joint mobilization
- Muscle energy
- Strengthening and stretching
- Neuromuscular re-education
- Home exercise

Intravaginal Thiele massage (6 weeks)

- Intravaginal myofascial release
- Home exercise

Biofeedback/electrical stimulation (6–12 weeks)

- Neuromuscular re-education
- Electrical stimulation frequency, 25 and 50 Hz
- Home exercise

Pain, including musculoskeletal pain and dysfunction (see also discussion of comprehensive rehabilitation in Chapter 9)

Manipulation: What should we believe?

Ernst (2004) reports on six systematic reviews, four of chiropractic and two relating to massage therapy in relation to pain.

He notes that although promising evidence emerged from some, 'there was no fully convincing evidence for effectiveness in controlling musculoskeletal or other pain' as a result of chiropractic or massage.

Flying as it does in the face of the individual clinical and personal experience of tens of thousands of physical therapists, osteopaths, naturopaths, chiropractors and massage therapists, it is important to evaluate this type of negative reporting that bases its findings on meta-analysis of systematic reviews (a 'review of reviews').

- There is a built-in presumption of uniformity of symptoms – 'musculoskeletal and other pain', and of treatment approach – 'chiropractic or massage'. Both these assumptions are false.
- Each painful condition has multiple possible etiologies and no single therapeutic approach could be expected to produce positive outcomes.
- In any case, massage and chiropractic are not terms that define anything other than a broad generic source of treatment, and in no way do these terms specify whether what is being compared in one study is similar to, or entirely different from, what is being considered in another.
- Was the massage gentle or deep tissue?
- Did it involve attention to, and treatment of, myofascial trigger points?
- Did it address abdominal or spinal or whole body tissues?
- Did the chiropractic treatment involve HVLA manipulation or more subtle (e.g. BEST, or Activator) forms of chiropractic, or a soft-tissue variation?
- Was treatment performed daily, weekly, for seconds or minutes or longer?

What is being evaluated when a review is conducted of reviews or multiple studies assumes homogenization of both the symptom ('pain') and treatment method ('massage/chiropractic'), when plainly neither is uniform.

The 'systematic review' process, in such situations, is a seriously flawed model incapable of being a sound basis for any judgment of efficacy.

In other words, what is being analyzed in such reviews is virtually guaranteed in advance to deliver an outcome that states precisely what Ernst pronounces, that 'there is no fully convincing evidence for effectiveness [of massage or chiropractic] in controlling musculoskeletal or other pain'.

These issues are discussed in Chapter 7 under the heading 'Caution over evidence', where an almost identical negative finding (Ernst & Canter 2006) is made in relation to 'manipulation' in treatment of 'back pain' – as though these two terms (manipulation and back pain) have uniformity in all the studies analyzed.

It may be useful to consider an example from a different setting.

Example

Let us imagine that symptom alleviation is being assessed in a group of patients with 'chest pain',

some with reflux symptoms and some with angina symptoms.

If the methods of treatment being assessed involved use of two pharmaceutical drugs specific for the relief of either reflux symptoms or angina-like cardiovascular symptoms, and if the 'appropriate' drug were administered to the appropriate patient, symptom relief would be high.

On the other hand, imagine a study in which such patients were 'homogenized' – since they all have 'chest pain' – and were randomly assigned to just one of these two classes of drug. Apart from a placebo effect, only those receiving the appropriate symptom-relieving medication would demonstrate perceived benefit, and as a result both drugs would be labeled as useless, with no more than a placebo level of symptom reduction, unless the recipient happened to be someone for whom the randomly prescribed drug was appropriate. The person with angina symptoms would not benefit from the reflux medication, and vice versa.

Similarly, in cases of menstrual pain, if a patient receives appropriate treatment to relieve anxiety (e.g. massage, if anxiety had been evaluated as an etiological feature) or to help normalize spasm (e.g. by means HVLA appropriately administered to the lumbar spine, if this was judged to be appropriate), or if treatment was offered to deactivate identified active trigger points in the lower abdomen that were firing painful impulses into the lower pelvis, results would be more likely to be positive.

If, however, the patient with menstrual pain, deriving from, or being aggravated by, any of these causes, received *inappropriate manual treatment*, results would inevitably be poor, and it would be labeled as an ineffective form of treatment.

From a naturopathic perspective, manual (or any other) methods of treatment need to match the needs of the individual in order to achieve one or other of two primary goals – to reduce the adaptive demands that are being responded to, and/or to enhance functionality so that self-regulation can operate more effectively.

As Cleland et al (2006) succinctly explain in regard to low back pain (LBP):

Given that LBP is a heterogeneous condition, it does not seem reasonable to expect that all patients will benefit from a single treatment approach. Rather, the key is to identify subgroups of patients with a high probability of achieving a successful outcome with a particular intervention. Evidence suggests that short- and longterm outcomes are improved when a classification-based approach is used compared to decision-making based on clinical practice guidelines

(Fritz et al 2003). To date, evidence for several subgroups of LBP exist, such as patients likely to benefit from manipulation (Childs et al 2004, Flynn et al 2002), lumbar stabilization (O'Sullivan et al 1997) and specific directional exercise (Long et al 2004).

Manipulation, when this is not required, or massage when this is inappropriate, or exercise when this is contraindicated will never produce optimally desirable outcomes. But when they are appropriate, outcomes will reflect this, and will confound negative reviews that are almost always going to produce findings such as those suggested by Ernst, unless built-in bias is eliminated by avoiding unrealistic assumptions, such as those outlined above.

In Chapter 7, as well as in Chapter 9, ample evidence has been offered as to the value of a variety of manual and rehabilitation methods in treatment of musculoskeletal and other sources of pain of various types. A few additional research-based examples are given below.

Musculoskeletal pain

Essential information relating to pain

If pain is involved as a presenting symptom, the information that can be gleaned by careful questioning is of considerable importance. Interpreting the real meaning of answers is a skill that needs to be developed.

Examples are given in Tables 10.6A and 10.6B of questions to patients without chronic pain syndromes, and with chronic pain syndromes (Wittink & Michel 2002).

Making sense of the answers that result from these questions is part of the process of arriving at a differential diagnosis, and some possible 'meanings' are offered in these tables. In a naturopathic setting these questions should help to identify some of the context out of which painful symptoms are emerging – so that a therapeutic plan can be developed.

Manipulation and exercise strategies for low back pain

Exercise and manipulation strategies have been successfully employed in treatment and rehabilitation of low back pain.

- *Low back pain and exercise*: 12 weeks of structured exercise, using a Swiss ball, by patients with chronic non-specific low back pain, produced significant improvements in pain and disability that was maintained up to 3 months of follow-up (Marshall & Murphy 2006). The exercises were progressed based on

measured EMG activity of the abdominal and back muscles, with lower relative intensity exercises in the first 4 weeks and higher relative intensity exercises in the last 4 weeks. There were significant changes in perceptions of physical and mental well-being, erector spinae fatigue and flexion relaxation measures (Fig. 10.4).

- *Benefits of categorization of back pain patients*: Categorizing low back pain patients into those with pain of less than 16 days' duration, and those whose symptoms did not extend below the knee, has been shown to be a major indicator of benefit if both appropriate exercise as well as manipulation are used (Childs et al 2006). The authors conclude with a comment that could be designed to be read by naturopathic practitioners:

  Manipulation in general remains underutilized by some practitioners whose scope of practice includes manipulation (Armstrong et al 2003), with concern regarding the risks being offered as the most common reason for infrequent utilization (Adams & Sim 1998). However, the risk of serious complication from manipulation of the lumbar spine is extremely low, with estimates suggesting the risk of cauda equina syndrome is less than 1 per 100 million lumbar spine manipulations (Assendelft et al 1996). In light of this information, combined with the recent data from the UK BEAM trial (2004) and data from our study (Childs et al 2004), an overly cautious position regarding the use of spinal manipulation for patients with back pain is not supported by the evidence.

- *Manipulation, exercise and low back pain*: In a randomized controlled trial, 120 patients with chronic low back pain responded better to a combination of manipulation (rotational high velocity thrust, average of four treatments; see Fig. 10.5) and exercise (appropriate for each individual patient's condition) than to a combination of ultrasound (1 MHz, 1.5–2.5 W/cm^2, for 5–10 minutes, for an average of six sessions) and exercise, although both forms of treatment combination offered significant benefit in terms of spinal mobility and pain intensity (Mohseni-Bandpei et al 2006). The authors further noted that: 'A significant difference was also found between the two groups in favor of the manipulation/exercise group at 6-month follow-up.'

- *Slump stretching and centralization of low back pain*: Low back pain with possible neural

0-4 weeks (isometric focus)	4-8 weeks (controlled concentric/eccentric)	8-12 weeks (dynamic exercises)

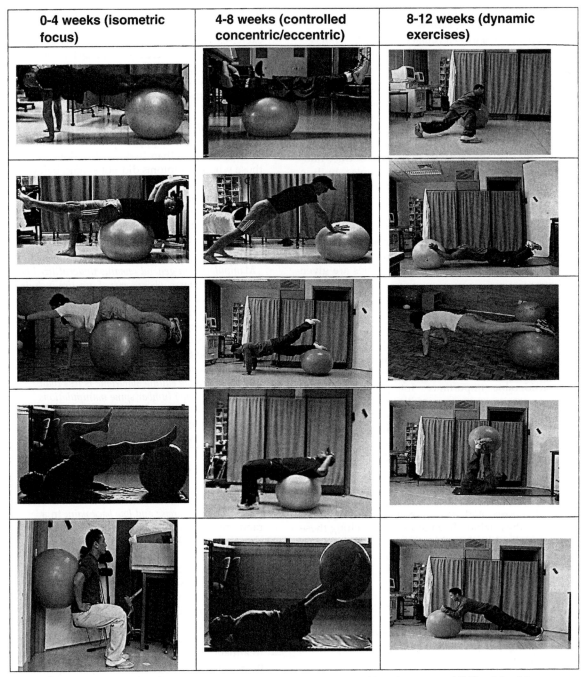

Figure 10.4 Exercises used in the 12-week intervention. The exercises were progressed based on measured EMG activity of the abdominal and back muscles, with lower relative intensity exercises in the first 4 weeks and higher relative intensity exercises in the last 4 weeks. Reproduced with permission from Marshall & Murphy (2006)

Table 10.6A The patient interview: chronic pain in a patient without chronic pain syndrome

Question to patient	Examples of possible answers	Interpretation
When did your pain start?	In an accident 2 years ago – my car was struck from the rear	This is a common injury
Where is your pain?	In my neck, shoulders, and hips. I also feel numbness in both legs when I lie down	This makes no anatomic sense. Be suspicious that this chronic pain has a major psychological component
On a scale of 0–10, how would you rate your pain?	0/10 up to 8/10. I have episodes of no pain, and some very bad days	It is good that he reports episodes of no pain. He may not be a chronic pain patient
How do you describe your pain?	Aching and pulling	–
How often do you get this pain?	I was fine until 2 weeks ago when it started again. It's been constant since then	Is this recurrent pain or reinjury?
What makes your pain worse?	All physical activity, mostly with my arms	This pattern could lead to avoidance of all activity
What makes your pain better?	Heat, massage and physical therapy	These may be passive-role therapies
How often have you had physical therapy treatment?	I have had three separate therapists	He is seeking complete relief
What treatments?	Ice, ultrasound, massage, exercise. Every time I exercised I felt better	This is a very good sign
Are you exercising on your own?	No, I am afraid I will hurt myself. I have five kids to look after when I get home from work	He does not follow through on a home program and takes a passive role for pain relief. He is looking for a complete cure. He uses family and work as an excuse to avoid his responsibility for caring for himself
What is your work?	I am a salesman. I spend 40–50 hours per week driving in my car	This is a very inactive job
Is your sleep interrupted?	Yes, I have trouble falling asleep	This is probably anxiety and is very common in chronic pain patients
Your F-6 shows that your physical functioning is severely limited with severe pain and low vitality. Your mental health score is low enough to suspect depression. Are you depressed?	No, only because of the pain I have. Without pain my life would be perfect. I have wonderful children, my wife loves me, my business is fine	Be suspicious of depression
What are you most afraid that the pain will do to you?	That it will get worse and worse and I will end up in a wheelchair. I would not be able to provide for my family	He is catastrophizing and exaggerating what could happen

Table 10.6B The patient interview: chronic pain syndrome patient

Question to patient	Examples of possible answers	Interpretation
When did your pain start?	My pain started approximately 3 years ago, when I had an accident at work	This is chronic pain. Healing of tissues is finished
Where is your pain?	In my back and down both legs	This pattern of pain is plausible and warrants further questioning
On a scale of 0–10, how would you rate your pain?	10 out of 10	A maximal pain rating is suspicious for chronic pain syndrome
What makes your pain worse?	Everything I do makes it worse	He is catastrophizing. With deconditioning and secondary joint pathologies, his pain response to all activities seems likely
What makes your pain better?	Medication and lying down make it better	He has a passive lifestyle, is displaying avoidance behavior and is dependent on medication
How many hours do you lie down?	21 out of 24	He is deconditioned and severely disabled
How is your sleep?	I cannot sleep; I am too tense	He is anxious and irritable. His waking up at night may be due to depression
What can you now not do because of your pain that you used to do? General activities: bending, lifting. stooping, carrying, sitting, standing	I used to walk 20 minutes every day. Now I can't do anything. I never bend, lift, stoop, carry, sit, stand or walk. My sitting tolerance is 10 minutes. I can walk 5 minutes. I can stand for 6 minutes	He has fear avoidance, fear of pain and fear of reinjury. His sitting tolerance could be misinterpretation of tolerance. His answers could be litigation driven and could be based on his low expectation for function
What activities do you do outside of work?	I used to go bowling and socialize every weekend. Now I do not bowl, I never go out, and I watch TV	This activity tolerance could be depression or fear avoidance based on low self-esteem and low self-efficacy
Can you climb stairs?	No, I sleep on the sofa. I never have sex	He demonstrates fear avoidance
Can you grocery shop? Can you perform housework?	I never used to need any help. Now I can't shop, cook or clean. I get help from my mother or someone else	His dependency on his family may be meeting his unmet dependency needs. There may be disturbed role functioning
Do you live alone?	Yes	–
Who does chores for you?	Now my ex-wife or mother comes over to do everything	The patient's family may contribute to his illness behavior
Do you work?	No	He does not perceive a need to work
Do you like your job?	My job is too demanding. I hate my boss	Apparent job dissatisfaction is a common problem contributing to disability
How long were you working at this job?	6 months	He does not have a stable work pattern
Are you now receiving worker's compensation?	No, but I have a lawyer	There are likely to be employer conflicts. This predicts a poor outcome in rehabilitation
Are you thinking of going back to your job?	No, I am applying for disability benefits	This answer demonstrates passive dependence and probable secondary gains

Table 10.6B The patient interview: chronic pain syndrome patient continued

Question to patient	Examples of possible answers	Interpretation
Are you planning to go back to work at any time?	I will go back to work when my pain is gone	This is pain-contingent behavior and is not realistic
It sounds like the pain that you have has had a great impact on your life	[Patient bursts into tears.] Yes, I am worthless; I cry all the time. I can't live like this. I hate my life; if only something could be done for my pain	Depression is very common in chronic pain patients. It is helped a lot by medications. Make use of psychiatric expertise for assistance. Check his MPI scores for dysfunctional profile and MMPI for depression scores
Do you have a psychiatric diagnosis?	No	Depression can run in families. If never diagnosed in the patient, find out about the family
What would you do a year from now if you had no pain?	All my problems would be solved. I'd be just fine	The patient has unrealistic expectations for treatment. Pain is the scapegoat for all of the patient's problems

MMPI, Minnesota Multiphasic Personality Inventory; MPI, Multidimensional Pain Inventory.

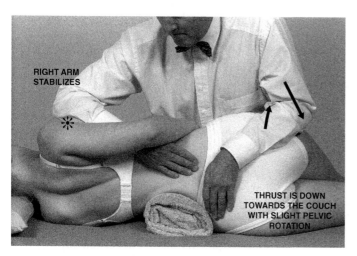

RIGHT ARM STABILIZES

THRUST IS DOWN TOWARDS THE COUCH WITH SLIGHT PELVIC ROTATION

Figure 10.5 HVLA thrust technique. Reproduced with permission from Gibbons & Tehan (2000)

mechanosensitivity. Cleland et al (2006) conducted a study to determine whether low back pain and disability improved, together with centralization of symptoms, when slump stretching was used, in addition to spinal mobilization. Thirty consecutive patients referred to physical therapy by their primary care physician for LBP who met all eligibility criteria including a positive slump test but who had a negative straight leg raise test (SLR) agreed to participate in the study. All patients were treated in physical therapy twice weekly for 3 weeks for a total of six visits. At discharge, patients who received slump stretching demonstrated significantly greater improvements in disability, pain, and centralization of symptoms than patients who did not (see Fig. 10.6 and Box 10.10).

• *Manipulation and back pain with disc protrusion*: Acute back pain with disc protrusion, accompanied by sciatica, has been shown in a randomized, double-blind trial, involving over 100 patients aged between 19 and 63, to respond more effectively to active manipulation than to dummy (simulated) manipulation (Santilli et al 2006).

• *Manipulation for neck pain*: In a randomized controlled trial 70 patients with mechanical

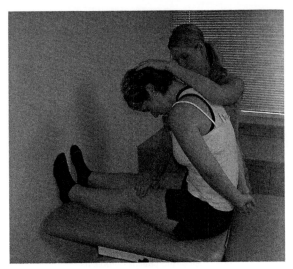

Figure 10.6 Slump stretching technique utilized in the clinic. Reproduced with permission from Cleland et al (2006)

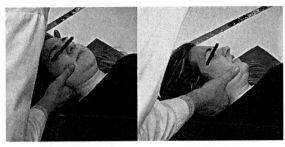

Figure 10.7 High-velocity, low-amplitude procedure. Reproduced with permission from Martínez-Segura et al (2006)

Box 10.10 Summary of slump test procedure

1. Patient was instructed to sit erect with knees in 90° of flexion. The presence or absence of symptoms was recorded.

2. Patient was instructed to 'slump' shoulders and lower back while maintaining the cervical spine in neutral. The presence or absence of symptoms was recorded.

3. While maintaining the position described in step 2, the patient was instructed to tuck their chin to the chest and the clinician applied overpressure into cervical flexion. The presence or absence of symptoms was recorded.

4. While maintaining the overpressure into cervical flexion the patient was instructed to extend the knee. The presence or absence of symptoms was recorded.

5. Position 4 was maintained while the patient was instructed to actively dorsiflex the ankle. The presence or absence of symptoms was recorded.

6. Overpressure of the cervical spine was released and the patient was instructed to return the neck to a neutral position. The presence or absence of symptoms was recorded.

The slump test is considered positive if the patient's symptoms were reproduced in position 5 but alleviated when overpressure of the cervical spine was released.

neck pain received either a single HVLA manipulation (C3–C5 levels) or neck placebo mobilization (Martínez-Segura et al 2006) (see Fig. 10.7). Results suggest that a single cervical HVLA manipulation was more effective in reducing neck pain at rest, and in increasing active cervical range of motion, than a control mobilization procedure in subjects suffering from mechanical neck pain. 'Effect sizes in the manipulative group were large, suggesting a strong clinical effect, whereas the effect size of the mobilization group was small.'

- *Manipulation and thoracic pain*: In a randomized clinical trial the effects were evaluated of thoracic manipulation, compared to placebo manipulation, in patients with neck pain (Cleland et al 2005). The results suggest that high velocity thoracic spine manipulation (Fig. 10.8) produces immediate analgesic effects in patients with mechanical neck pain and improvements in their symptoms.

- *Exercise, advice for chronic whiplash symptoms*: Chronic whiplash pain, and associated disorders, that persist beyond 3 months following the trauma are not commonly responsive to treatment (Scholten-Peeters et al 2003). A randomized, assessor-blinded, controlled trial was conducted at two centers in Australia (Stewart et al 2006). All 132 participants received three advice sessions; in addition, the experimental group participated in 12 exercise sessions over 6 weeks. The exercise program was an individualized, progressive, submaximal program designed to improve participants' ability to complete functional activities specified by the participant as being difficult because of whiplash. As well as a home exercise program, each participant carried out a form of aerobic exercise (e.g. a walking or cycling program), stretches, functional activities, activities to build speed,

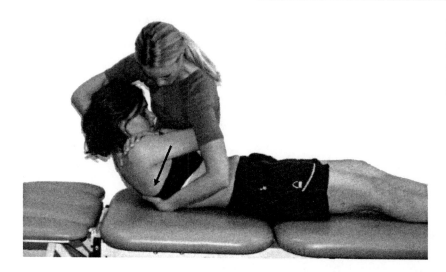

Figure 10.8 Manipulation technique for a flexion restriction. High velocity, small amplitude thrust performed in the direction of the arrow. Reproduced with permission from Cleland et al (2005)

endurance and coordination, and trunk and limb strengthening exercises. Primary outcomes were pain intensity, pain bothersomeness and function, measured at 6 weeks and 12 months. High levels of baseline pain intensity were associated with greater treatment effects at 6 weeks, and high levels of baseline disability were associated with greater treatment effects at 12 months. In the short term, exercise and advice are slightly more effective than advice alone for people with persisting pain and disability following whiplash. Exercise is more effective for subjects with higher baseline pain and disability. The authors note that: 'The small, short-term effect of exercise should be interpreted in light of the fact that there are very few treatments known to be effective for this treatment-resistant patient group.' By implication this suggests that exercise is of particular value in such cases, especially when compared to other approaches/modalities which yield little that is effective – according to these authors.

- *Combined (lymph drainage, heat application, TheraBand exercise) and post whiplash symptoms*: Prevention of chronic whiplash syndrome was evaluated by comparing 7 days of immobilization with a soft collar with 14 days (10 sessions) of heat application (5 minutes), lymph drainage (10 minutes), massage (10 minutes) and an active TheraBand exercise regime, both under supervision and for 20 minutes at home daily (Vassiliou et al 2006). Soft collar usage was allowed on request for the first 2 days in the treatment group. Two

hundred patients were enrolled in a prospective, randomized, controlled trial. In the standard group, treatment consisted of immobilization with a soft collar over 7 days. In the physical therapy group, patients were scheduled for 10 physical therapy appointments including active exercises within 14 days after enrolment. Ninety-seven patients were randomly assigned to the standard treatment group and 103 to the physical therapy group. After 6 weeks, mean pain intensity was significantly ($p = 0.002$) lower in the physical therapy group (1.49 ± 2.26 vs 2.7 ± 2.78). Similarly, after 6 months, significantly ($p < 0.001$) less pain was reported in the physical therapy group (1.17 ± 2.13) than in the standard treatment group (2.33 ± 2.56). The conclusion was that a physical therapy protocol that includes active exercises is superior in reducing pain 6 weeks and 6 months after whiplash injury, compared to the current standard treatment with a soft collar.

- *Different models of care for sacroiliac joint pain*: The different models of care include the McKenzie method, a model of sacroiliac joint (SIJ) dysfunction care in which directional movement preference is used as a guide to rehabilitation exercises (Horton & Franz 2007) (see Fig. 10.9). The approach is in contrast to testing procedures that aim to assess the position of bony landmarks and motion abnormalities of the SIJ using palpation and observation. These SIJ disorders are then named according to the findings (subluxation, upslip, downslip, posterior or anterior fixed

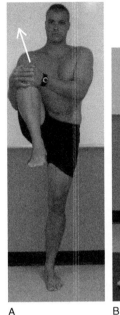
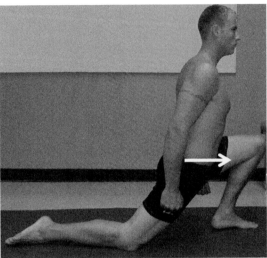

Figure 10.9 **A** Repeated posterior SIJ rotation. Arrow depicts direction of force. **B** Repeated anterior SIJ rotation with self-overpressure. Arrow depicts direction of force by right hand. Reproduced with permission from Horton & Franz (2007)

A   B

innominate) and may be treated by manipulation or mobilization (including muscle energy techniques) (Walker 1992). Alternatively, Lee (2004) has proposed a complex classification system based on an integrated model of function. Treatment techniques proposed to correct 'biomechanical dysfunctions' include belt fixation, mobilization and manipulation procedures. Stretching and massage are also purported to correct muscle imbalance together with a corrective exercise program to restore joint position, including the hip joint. If manual techniques fail to resolve the pain, then prolotherapy injection therapy may prove useful.

• *Graduated exercise and pubic/groin pain*: Use of graduated exercises in the treatment of young athletes (soccer players) with pubic and groin pain (osteitis pubis) helps to demonstrate the need for clinical and functional outcome measures to be features of successful rehabilitation (Wollin & Lovell 2006) (see Chapter 9). The clinical outcome measures included strong effort pain-free hip adduction, with no tenderness over the pubic symphysis, bone or adductor complex. The functional outcome measure involved a pain-free completion of a running program based on average distances covered by players in a game. The performance markers used in this

case study (20 m shuttle run, 20 m and 5 m sprint tests) are frequently employed in football to measure player performance. All players were commenced on a conservative rehabilitation program involving abdominal and pelvic strengthening exercises in a graduated format and successfully achieved this outcome between 10 and 16 weeks after diagnosis. Rehabilitation included completion of a running program consisting of durations and elements specific to football. During their rehabilitation a consistent pattern of clinical milestones emerged that coincided with the players' readiness to return to football. The players were able to perform 5 minutes of skating on a 3 m slide board and three sets of 12 repetitions of adductor exercises against 6 kg of resistance.

• *Prolotherapy for chronic groin strain in athletes*: Topol et al (2005) designed a study to determine the efficacy of simple dextrose prolotherapy in elite kicking-sport athletes with chronic groin pain from osteitis pubis and/or adductor tendinopathy. Twenty-two rugby and two soccer players with chronic groin pain that prevented full sports participation and who were non-responsive both to therapy and to a graded reintroduction into sports activity received monthly injections of 12.5% dextrose and 0.5% lidocaine into the thigh adductor origins, suprapubic abdominal insertions and symphysis pubis, depending on palpation tenderness. Injections were given until complete resolution of pain or lack of improvement for two consecutive treatments. The final data collection point was 6–32 months after treatment (mean, 17 months). A mean of 2.8 treatments were given. The mean reduction in pain during sports, as measured by the visual analog scale, improved from 6.3 ± 1.4 to 1.0 ± 2.4 ($p <0.001$), and the mean reduction in neuropathic pain scale (NPPS) score improved from 5.3 ± 0.7 to 0.8 ± 1.9 ($p <0.001$). Of the 24 patients, 22 had no pain and 22 of 24 were unrestricted with sports at final data collection. *Conclusion*: Dextrose prolotherapy showed marked efficacy for chronic groin pain in this group of elite rugby and soccer athletes.

- *Postural correction and neck pain*: Correction of poor posture was studied in relation to the effects on neck and shoulder pain syndromes (McLean 2005). In this study correct posture was based on the guidelines provided by Kendall et al (1993). The author states:

  *As chronic static muscle use is thought to be associated with the onset of some neck and shoulder pain syndromes, it is important to understand the impact a postural correction program might have on muscle activation amplitudes in the neck and shoulder regions. Normalized surface electromyographic data were recorded from the levator scapulae, upper trapezius, supraspinatus, posterior deltoid, masseter, rhomboid major, cervical erector spinae, and sternocleidomastoid muscles of the dominant side of each of 18 healthy subjects. Subjects performed five repetitions of each of four seated typing postures (habitual, corrected, head-forward and slouched) and four standing postures (habitual, corrected, head-forward and slouched). Repeated-measures analysis . . . revealed that in sitting postural correction tended to decrease the level of muscle activation required in all muscles studied during seated computer work, however this finding was not statistically significant. Corrected posture in sitting did, however, produce a statistically significant reduction in muscle activity compared to forward head posture. Corrected posture in standing **required more** muscle activity than habitual or forward head posture in the majority of cervicobrachial and jaw muscles, suggesting that a graduated approach to postural correction exercises might be required in*

*order to train the muscles to appropriately withstand the requirements of the task. A surprising finding was that muscle activity levels and postural changes had the largest impact on the **masseter** muscle, which demonstrated activation levels in the order of 20% maximum voluntary electrical activation.*

Comment: These findings highlight the need for postural re-education tasks to be graduated and ideally to be accompanied by physical medicine approaches that encourage flexibility and stability (see Fig. 10.10).

- *Trigger point deactivation method*: Treatment of myofascial (trigger point) pain was evaluated in a study that compared a single application of ischemic compression technique with transverse friction massage (Fernández-de-las-Peñas et al 2006b). Forty subjects (17 men and 23 women, aged 19–38) presenting with mechanical neck pain, and diagnosed with myofascial trigger points (MTrPs) in the upper trapezius muscle, participated. Subjects were divided randomly into two groups, one of which was treated with the ischemic compression technique (see Fig. 10.11A), while the other was treated with a transverse friction massage (see Fig. 10.11B). The outcome measures were the pressure pain threshold (PPT) in the MTrP, and a visual analog scale assessing local pain evoked by a second application of 2.5 kg/cm^2 of pressure on the MTrP. The results showed a significant improvement in the PPT ($p = 0.03$), and a significant decrease in the visual analog scores ($p = 0.04$) within each group. Ischemic compression technique and transverse friction massage were equally effective in reducing tenderness in MTrPs.

The pain of fibromyalgia (FMS) and chronic fatigue syndromes (CFS)

Note: The topics of FMS and CFS have been considered in more detail earlier in this chapter.

The pain experienced by people with FMS has been widely researched, with a variety of opinions and conclusions emerging. Several of these are summarized below.

It has been suggested that the origin of the pain noted in fibromyalgia may also derive in large part from muscular ischemia (Henriksson 1999). The rationale for this observation can be summarized as follows:

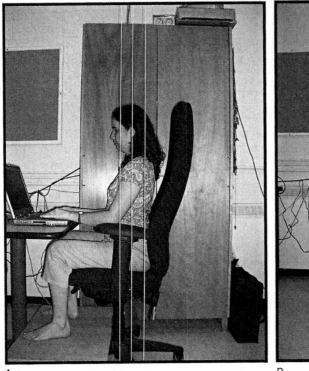
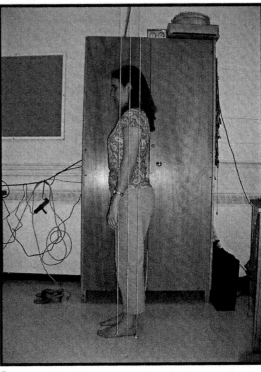

A   B

Figure 10.10 **A** Correct sitting posture according to Kendall et al (1993). The external auditory meatus, the lateral acromion and the greater trochanter should lie along a plumb line. **B** Correct standing posture according to Kendall et al (1993). The external auditory meatus, the lateral acromion, the greater trochanter and the lateral malleolus should lie along a plumb line. Reproduced with permission from McLean (2005)

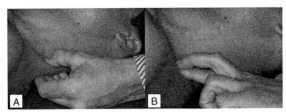

Figure 10.11 The ischemic compression technique and transverse friction massage over myofascial trigger point in the upper trapezius muscle: **A** ischemic compression technique; **B** transverse friction massage. Reproduced with permission from Fernández-de-las-Peñas et al. *Journal of Bodywork and Movement Therapies* 2006;10:3–9

- The pathophysiology of the chronic muscular pain and tenderness of FMS is not fully understood, but seems to involve complex interactions between peripheral and central nervous system mechanisms, with evidence of abnormal processing of somatosensory input (Kosek & Hansson 1997).

- Morphological abnormalities have long indicated that ischemia is a feature of these muscles (Bennett 1989).
- Many FMS patients report a sensation of muscle 'feeling swollen' during exercise.
- The circulatory dysfunction evident in muscles of FMS in relation to exercise (e.g. reduced muscle perfusion) appears to be accentuated by the relative deconditioned status of people with FMS (McCain et al 1988).
- Elvin et al (2006), in a study of this phenomenon, found that contrast enhanced ultrasound was useful in the real-time study of muscle vascularity during and following standardized, low-intensity exercise in fibromyalgia patients and healthy controls (see Fig. 10.12).
- FMS patients had a reduced increase in muscular vascularity following dynamic exercise and during, but not following, static exercise compared to controls.

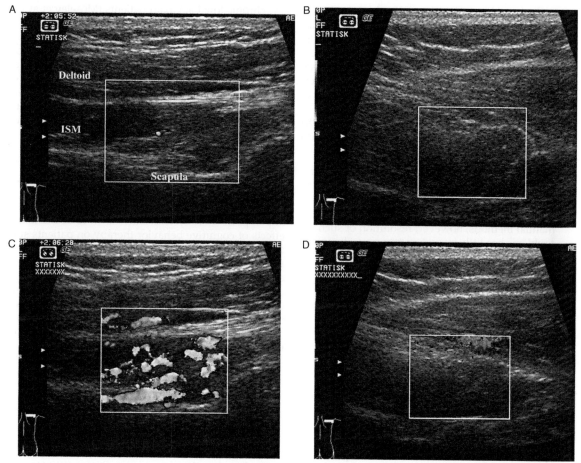

Figure 10.12 Doppler evaluation of infraspinatus muscle (ISM) during static contraction in (**A**) a healthy control subject and (**B**) an FMS patient, showing typical no or small vessel perfusion. In (**C**) after the administration of US contrast media the muscular tissue vascularity is clearly seen in the control subject. Differently in (**D**) the ISM of an FMS patient shows no detectable flow during contraction. Note, however, that normal muscular vascularity is seen in the non-contracting deltoideus muscle in the upper right-hand corner. Reproduced with permission from Elvin et al (2006)

• The results support the suggestion that muscle ischemia contributes significantly to pain in fibromyalgia, possibly by maintaining central sensitization/disinhibition.

A protocol for managing CFS pain and dysfunction

Nijs et al (2006) have evaluated the processes involved in the musculoskeletal pain experienced by patients with CFS, which is almost identical with that experienced by FMS patients, with some subtle differences. Generalized *joint hypermobility* and *benign joint hypermobility syndrome* (BJHS) appear to be highly prevalent among CFS and FMS sufferers, but that 'this does not seem to be of any obvious clinical importance'.

Note: See the comments on hypermobility in relation to trigger points in Chapter 2, and in relation to prolotherapy in Chapter 7, for different perspectives on this opinion. For details of palpation/assessment of hypermobility, see Chapter 6.

A worsening of symptoms (pain, fatigue) is typically experienced by CFS patients after previously well-tolerated levels of exercise/physical activity, whereas in healthy subjects a substantial increase in pain threshold in response to exercise is typically observed.

It is of importance to note that *pain catastrophizing* has been identified as a major predictor of exercise performance in female CFS patients experiencing chronic widespread pain. In addition, pain catastrophizing was found to predict bodily pain, even after controlling for depression. From previous studies, it is concluded that fear of movement ('kinesiophobia') is not related to exercise performance in CFS patients. In addition, kinesiophobia in general (fear of an exercise-triggered increase in general symptom severity), rather than pain-related fear of movement, was related to self-reported disability in CFS patients (Nijs et al 2004).

The suggestions for CFS (and by implication FMS) patient care offered by Nijs et al (2006) encompass both manual and behavioral features:

- Local musculoskeletal problems such as thoracic outlet compression syndrome, low back pain, and neck pain, often noted in CFS patients, can usefully be treated by appropriate manual methods; however, resolution of such problems has little impact on the general symptoms.
- For the main condition (CFS/FMS), where central sensitization has taken place, *cognitive behavioral* treatment strategies (i.e. graded exercise used to diminish avoidance behavior towards physical activity) and pain neurophysiology education are often – but by no means always – useful (Prins et al 2001).
- *Pacing* (Shepherd 2001) – a strategy where patients are encouraged to achieve an appropriate balance between activity and rest in order to avoid exacerbation, and to set realistic goals for increasing activity – is a useful alternative to the cognitive behavioral approach. The aim is to enable the CFS patient to manage daily activities in a way that ensures that fluctuations in symptoms are avoided (stabilization phase).
- Pacing takes into account the considerable fluctuations in symptom severity and the delayed recovery from exercise that typically occur in patients with CFS. The pacing approach slowly moves towards inclusion of graded activity and exercise levels, and is consistent with the recent observations regarding the interactions between malfunctioning of the immune system, physical activity and musculoskeletal pain in CFS patients (CFS/ME Working Group 2001).
- *Pain neurophysiology education* might be indicated for CFS patients with musculoskeletal pain. Patients learn that pain processing is likely to be abnormal in CFS and that evidence shows that pain catastrophizing accounts for a substantial portion of musculoskeletal pain. Pain neurophysiology education was found to be effective in reducing pain catastrophizing in

chronic low back pain patients (Moseley et al 2004).

Comment: This protocol for CFS – which takes account of local musculoskeletal symptoms that are treated appropriately, and which also ensures that rehabilitation is achieved at a pace that matches the adaptation exhaustion apparent in CFS patients, while also offering educational input regarding the processes that are causing the symptoms – can be seen to be naturopathically sound.

Pain associated with cancer

Cognitive and physiotherapy intervention

A prospective study was undertaken to evaluate the effects of cognitive behavior therapy on patients suffering pain as a result of cancer and its treatment, including radiation, surgery and chemotherapy – chronic cancer treatment-related pain (CCTRP). A combination of physical (see below) and psychological techniques was employed. All patients had a positive outcome (Robb et al 2006).

Key elements of the protocol included focus on the following.

- *Meaning of the pain*: This can affect the intensity and distress associated with the experience. Patients may feel angry, believing their pain was an unnecessary result of treatment (Maher Committee 1995). Clinical experience suggests that anger can be associated with a lack of information before treatment on potential pain and/or functional problems. Cancer patients often fear a recurrence of their disease (Ahles et al 1983, Lee-Jones et al 1997) and the presence of a chronic treatment-related pain can act as a constant reminder of their cancer history. The meaning of changes in pain can, therefore, be extremely frightening for cancer patients.
- *Sense of control*: The combined effect of a cancer diagnosis and a chronic pain condition can result in patients experiencing a loss of control. Treatments aimed at empowering patients (i.e. encouraging them to regain control and be actively involved in treatment) appear to be effective (Meyer & Mark 1995), but more research is needed.
- *Communication*: Patients with cancer are often reluctant to disclose their concerns about treatment (Maguire et al 1996). This may be exacerbated by poor communication by medical personnel (Maguire & Pitceathly 2002). A combination of poor communication skills by

health care professionals and lack of disclosure by cancer patients may lead to confusion, misconceptions and heightened anxiety in many patients.

The comorbidity of psychological and physical health problems in chronic illness is well documented, and it is now widely acknowledged that the management of chronic pain requires approaches that address all aspects of the pain experience, such as the sensory, affective and cognitive dimensions.

Example

An example of a physiotherapy intervention – based on clinical findings and associated treatment plans, involving a single patient (patient X) – is summarized below.

- *Clinical finding*: Complete lack of understanding of the causes of her pain; confusion over explanations and advice given to her. *Treatment plan*: Explanation of her reconstructive surgery, the side-effects of radiation and the theory of chronic pain.
- *Clinical finding*: General physical deconditioning secondary to depression, avoidance behavior and underactivity. *Treatment plan*: Introduction of an exercise regime with walking and pacing of activities previously enjoyed (e.g. line dancing).
- *Clinical finding*: Decreased functional use of her left arm secondary to avoidance behavior and underactivity. *Treatment plan*: Graded exercise program, including stretches and strengthening exercises for left arm; pacing of domestic chores.
- *Clinical finding*: Altered posture secondary to pain and muscle spasm. *Treatment plan*: Postural advice and correction of muscle imbalance; advice on relaxation.

Physical outcome measures included:

- a 5-minute walk test (distance walked in 5 minutes)
- sit-to-stand test (number of repetitions in 1 minute)
- arm endurance test (arm outstretched at 90° abduction and small movements, endurance in minutes)
- range of movement: flexion and abduction of the affected shoulder measured with a goniometer.

Comment: From a naturopathic perspective these educational and rehabilitation strategies appear to offer optimal opportunities for recovery of function and reduction of pain and pain behavior. Additional hydrotherapy, acupuncture and nutritional approaches (for example) might add to benefits gained.

Six-week multidimensional intervention

During the 6-week multidimensional intervention (exercise, massage, relaxation, visualization and behavioral methods) for side-effect symptoms of cancer patients undergoing chemotherapy, 12 possible symptoms/side-effects were registered daily: lack of appetite, nausea, vomiting, diarrhea, paresthesia, constipation, physical fatigue, mental fatigue, treatment-related fatigue, muscle pain, arthralgia and other pain (Andersen et al 2006).

Methods included:

- *High-intensity physical training*: In groups, 1.5 hours, three times weekly. Physical training comprised three components: warm-up exercises, heavy resistance training and fitness.
- *Low-intensity physical training*: In groups, 0.5 hour, four times weekly. Groups of patients were instructed in the use of relaxation techniques, using principles of progressive relaxation.
- *Massage*: Individual, 0.5 hour, twice weekly. Massage could be relaxing, facilitative or therapeutic. Classic, scar tissue and venous pump massages were administered as well as ultrasound and exercise therapy
- *Body-awareness training*: In groups, 1.5 hours a week focused on balance/coordination; grounding and integration of the senses.

During the 6-week intervention a decrease in the scoring for 10 out of the 12 side-effects was noted (Ownby 2006).

The results of the study indicate that 6 weeks of a multidimensional exercise intervention for cancer patients, with or without disease, and who are undergoing chemotherapy, can lead to a reduction in symptoms and side-effects. As such, the total burden of pain, including myalgia, arthralgia, paraesthesia and other pain was reduced significantly

Patients with evidence of residual disease scored higher in some symptoms/side-effects compared with patients without evidence of disease. However, both groups responded positively to the intervention as indicated from the sum of symptoms and side-effect scores.

Comment: Use of relaxation and visualization, as well as aerobic exercise and massage, incorporate mind–body elements of care that would fit well in a naturopathic setting.

Pain associated with chronic disease

A variety of chronic diseases are associated with pain. Examples are given of the potential role of physical medicine (e.g. massage, cryotherapy, exercise, yoga) in care of patients with conditions including AIDS, those undergoing dialysis, or with rheumatoid arthritis or vulvodynia.

Ice massage and neuropathic pain of AIDS

Peripheral neuropathic pain is a unique form of chronic pain that afflicts up to 50% of persons with AIDS. The purpose of this pilot study (Chin 2001) was to examine the effects of ice massage to reduce neuropathic pain and improve sleep quality, and to determine the feasibility of a larger study. A repeated measures design was used. The three treatments consisted of ice massage, dry-towel massage and presence. Consecutive sampling was used to select 33 persons with AIDS who had neuropathic pain. Although the results of the study were negative, there was a decrease in pain intensity over time with both the ice massage and towel massage, suggesting that the intervention has some clinical benefit.

The author of the research notes:

An ice massage produces intense sensory input and anesthetizes the area. The theorized mechanism underlying ice massage is that it is a counterirritant. Ice massage may activate nerve fibers responsible for carrying the sensation of cold to the spinal cord. The central nervous system is plastic, and a barrage of nociceptive input conceivably changes the response properties of the dorsal horn neurons. Although neuropathic pain may be exacerbated by cold, allodynia related to postherpetic neuralgia may be decreased with regular applications of cold packs.

The author cautions:

A limitation of the study is that each intervention was applied once. A one-time application of ice or dry-towel massage may not have provided enough tactile stimulation to modulate sensory input to the dorsal horn neurons.

Yoga and end-stage renal disease dialysis patients

The objective of a study by Yurtkuran et al (2007) was to evaluate the effects of a yoga-based exercise program on pain, fatigue, sleep disturbance and biochemical markers in hemodialysis patients.

Yoga-based exercises were done in groups for 30 minutes a day, twice a week, for 3 months. All of the patients in the yoga and control groups were given an active range of motion exercises to do for 10 minutes at home. After a 12-week intervention, significant improvements were seen in the variables: pain −37%, fatigue −55%, sleep disturbance −25%, grip strength +15%, urea −29%, creatinine −14%, alkaline phosphatase −15%, cholesterol −15%, erythrocyte +11%, and hematocrit count +13%; no side-effects were seen. *Conclusion*: A simplified yoga-based rehabilitation program is a complementary, safe and effective clinical treatment modality in patients with end-stage renal disease.

Physical medicine and early rheumatoid arthritis (RA) (Gossec et al 2006)

This comprehensive review offers guidelines that are helpful in approaching acute systemic inflammatory conditions, from the perspective of physical modalities. Quoted extracts are offered below of the findings in relation to physical medicine and early RA.

Physical exercise and sports can be recommended to patients with early RA; muscle strength exercises are advisable.

The role for physical treatment was evaluated separately for physical therapy and exercise programs. In patients with established RA, physical therapy has produced conflicting results (Brosseau et al 2000, 2002, Casimiro et al 2002, Robinson et al 2002, Verhagen et al 2003).

- *Occupational therapy and early RA*: A complex combination of occupational therapy and education with hand exercises was evaluated; none of the outcome measures (pain, function) was influenced by the program (Hammond et al 2004). The other three studies used aerobic exercise in patients with semi-early RA or strength training in patients with early RA.
- *Aerobic exercise and early RA*: One hundred and thirty-six patients with disease durations of 5–7 years followed a program of high-intensity exercise during 75-minute group sessions twice a week for 2 years. The exercises included aerobics, strength training, flexibility exercises, cycling and ball games. The control group (*n* = 145) received usual care. Compliance and patient satisfaction were excellent. In the intervention group, improvements occurred in muscle strength, aerobic capacity, emotional status and quality of life. No consistent improvements in functional ability were obtained (de Jong et al 2004).
- *Strength training and early RA*: Strength training within the first 2 years of RA onset was

investigated in Finnish studies (Hakkinen et al 1999). Seventy RA patients with a mean disease duration of 10 months and no history of disease-modifying antirheumatic drug therapy or systemic glucocorticoid therapy were recruited. Among these patients, 35 followed a strength training program designed to strengthen the major muscle groups in the upper and lower limbs and trunk via exercises against gravity or various loads. The patients exercised at home for 45 minutes twice a week. Exercises were adjusted during supervised sessions at 2-month intervals. Patients in the control group performed flexibility and range-of-motion exercises.

Strength training produced lasting improvements in muscle strength, aerobic capacity and pain. Bone mineral density was not significantly improved. No effects on work disability or functional ability were noted. The exercise program had no adverse effects on disease activity or radiographic progression. The experts felt that these data warranted a recommendation to encourage exercising in patients with early RA.

Conclusion

The multiple examples of a variety of modalities, many of them offering benefit in treatment of patients with a huge range of conditions, provide validation for their employment within the context of naturo-pathic health care.

Naturopathic physical medicine, complementing as it does all the other measures of health promotion that naturopathy encompasses, can be seen to be based on a sound evidence base.

The conclusions that can be drawn from the evidence contained in this and previous chapters suggest that:

- individuals who are ill, virtually irrespective of the named conditions from which they are suffering, are capable of receiving benefit from appropriately applied physical medicine modalities that encourage self-regulation and/or reduce adaptive demands
- manipulation, mobilization, massage or other forms of applied manual therapy (see Chapters 7 and 8) can be modulated and refined to meet individual needs, sometimes removing obstacles to recovery, sometimes enhancing functionality, of patients of all ages, and almost any degree of ill-health – in ways that do not

overwhelm already distressed adaptive potentials
- exercise (see Chapter 9) – taking into account type, intensity, duration and degree, whether involving aerobics, weight training, yoga, breathing retraining, stretching or some other form of physical activity – can be tailored appropriately to assist in health enhancement for most people
- hydrotherapy (see Chapter 11), in one form or another, can be precisely adjusted to achieve a variety of health-enhancing effects in treatment of almost all individuals, whatever the current level of wellness or illness
- constitutional measures – whether involving hydrotherapy (Chapter 11), general (universal) mobilization methods (Chapter 8) or exercise forms including tai chi, yoga and breathing/relaxation approaches (Chapter 9) – are intrinsically naturopathic in that they avoid forcing change, but rather offer the potential for self-generated change.

Naturopathy demands that the individual's innate healing potentials are encouraged, that no harm is done (by omission or commission) and that the individual is taught health-promoting measures.

Within the framework of choices outlined in this and other chapters the tools for achieving these ends are clearly present. All that is required is attention to the reality of the patient's needs while maintaining awareness of the tenets of naturopathic care.

In combination with lifestyle modification, dietary excellence, psychological and spiritual balance, and the repertoire of naturopathic botanical, homeopathic and nutritional modalities, physical medicine has a foundational presence in naturopathic medical care.

References

ACOG 2004 Practice Bulletin No. 51. American College of Obstetricians and Gynecologists. Obstetrics and Gynecology 103:589–605

Adams G, Sim J 1998 A survey of UK manual therapists' practice of and attitudes towards manipulation and its complications. Physiotherapy Research International 3(3):206–227

Ahles T, Blanchard E, Ruckdeschel J 1983 The multidimensional nature of cancer-related pain. Pain 17:277–288

Aksenova AM, Teslenko OI, Boganskaia O 1999 [Changes in the immune status of peptic ulcer patients after combined treatment including deep massage] [article in Russian]. Voprosy Kurortologii, Fizioterapii, Lechebnoi Fizicheskoi Kultury 2:19–20

Aldana S, Greenlaw R, Diehl H et al 2005 Effects of an intensive diet and physical activity modification program on the health risks of adults. Journal of the American Diet Association 105:371–381

Alfven G, de la Torre B, Uvnas-Moberg K 1994 Depressed concentrations of oxytocin and cortisol in children with recurrent abdominal pain of non-organic origin. Acta Paediatrica 83:1076–1080

Alnigenis M, Bradfley J, Wallick J et al 2001 Massage therapy in the management of fibromyalgia: a pilot study. Journal of Musculoskeletal Pain 9:55–67

Anderberg U, Uvnas-Moberg K 2000 Plasma oxytocin levels in female fibromyalgia syndrome patients. Zeitschrift fur Rheumatologie 59:373–379

Andersen C, Adamsen L, Moeller T et al 2006 The effect of a multidimensional exercise programme on symptoms and side-effects in cancer patients undergoing chemotherapy: the use of semi-structured diaries. European Journal of Oncology Nursing 10(4):247–262

Anderson R, Wise D, Sawyer T et al 2005 Integration of myofascial trigger point release and paradoxical relaxation training treatment of chronic pelvic pain in men. Journal of Urology 174(1):155–160

Angst J, Volrath M 1991 The natural history of anxiety disorders. Acta Psychiatrica Scandinavica 84:446–452

Armstrong MP, McDonough S, Baxter GD 2003 Clinical guidelines versus clinical practice in the management of low back pain. International Journal of Clinical Practice 57(1):9–13

Ascensão A, Ferreira R, Magalhãesa J 2007 Exercise-induced cardioprotection – biochemical, morphological and functional evidence in whole tissue and isolated mitochondria. International Journal of Cardiology 17(1):16–30

Asmundson G, Stein M 1994 A preliminary analysis of pulmonary function in panic disorder: implications for the dyspnea-fear theory. Journal of Anxiety Disorders 8:63–69

Asplund R 2003 Manual lymph drainage therapy using light massage for fibromyalgia sufferers: a pilot study. Journal of Orthopaedic Nursing 7(4):192–196

Assendelft WJ, Bouter LM, Knipschild P 1996 Complications of spinal manipulation: a comprehensive review of the literature. Journal of Family Practice 42(5):475–480

Audette J, Jin Y, Newcomer R et al 2006 Tai chi versus brisk walking in elderly women. Age and Ageing 35(4):388–393

Aust G, Fischer K 1997 Changes in body equilibrium response caused by breathing. A posturographic study with visual feedback. Laryngorhinootologie 76(10):577–582

Bachman T, Lantz C 1991 Management of pediatric asthma and enuresis. In: Proceedings of the National Conference on Chiropractic Pediatrics. International Chiropractic Association, Arlington, VA, p 14

BACR 2000 Phase IV exercise instructor manual, 2nd edn. British Association for Cardiac Rehabilitation, London

Balaban C, Thayer J 2001 Neurological bases for balance–anxiety links. Journal of Anxiety Disorders 15(1–2):53–79

Balon J, Mior S 2004 Chiropractic care in asthma and allergy. Annals of Allergy, Asthma and Immunology 93(2 Suppl 1):S55–S60

Basaran S, Guler-Uysal F, Ergen N et al 2006 Effects of physical exercise on quality of life, exercise capacity and pulmonary function in children with asthma. Journal of Rehabilitation Medicine 38(2):130–135

Bassett D 2002 Physical activity and ethnic differences in hypertension prevalence in the United States. Preventive Medicine 34(2):179–186

Bazelmans E, Bleijenberg G, Van Der Meer J et al 2001 Is physical deconditioning a perpetuating factor in chronic fatigue syndrome? A controlled study on maximal exercise performance and relations with fatigue, impairment and physical activity. Psychological Medicine 3:107–114

Beal M 1983 Palpatory testing for somatic dysfunction in patients with cardiovascular disease. Journal of the American Osteopathic Association 82(11):73–82

Beales D, Dolton R 2000 Eating disordered patients: personality, alexithymia, and implications for primary care alexithymia. British Journal of General Practice 50:21–26

Bechgaard P 1981 Segmental thoracic pain in patients admitted to a medical department and a coronary unit. Acta Medica Scandinavica 644(suppl):87

Bei Y 1993 Clinical observations on the treatment of 98 cases of peptic ulcer by massage. Journal of Traditional Chinese Medicine 13(1):50–51

Bennett R 1989 Physical fitness and muscle metabolism in the fibromyalgia syndrome: an overview. Journal of Rheumatology 16(Suppl 19):28–29

Bensoussana A, Myers S, Wua S, O'Connor K 2004 Naturopathic and Western herbal medicine practice in Australia – a workforce survey. Complementary Therapies in Medicine 12:17–27

Berger B, Owen D 1988 Stress reduction and mood enhancement in four exercise modes: swimming, body conditioning, Hatha yoga and fencing. Research Quarterly for Exercise and Sport 59:148–159

Bhole M 1983 Gastric tone as influenced by mental states and meditation. Yoga Mimansa 22(1–2):54–58

Bishop E, McKinnon E, Weir E, Brown DW 2003 Reflexology in management of encopresis and chronic constipation. Paediatric Nursing 15:20–21

Blunt K, Moez H, Rajivani D, Guerriero R 1997 Effectiveness of chiropractic management of fibromyalgia patients: pilot study. Journal of Manipulative and Physiological Therapeutics 20(6):389–399

Boal R, Gillette R 2004 Central neuronal plasticity, low back pain and spinal manipulative therapy. Journal of Manipulative and Physiological Therapeutics 27:314–326

Bockenhauer SE, Julliard KN, Lo KS, Huang E, Sheth AM 2002 Quantifiable effects of osteopathic manipulative techniques on patients with chronic asthma. Journal of the American Osteopathic Association 102(7):371–375

Boesler D, Warner M, Alpers A et al 1993 Efficacy of high velocity, low amplitude manipulative technique in subjects with low back pain during menstrual cramping. Journal of the American Osteopathic Association 93:203–214

Bolton P 2000 Reflex effects of vertebral subluxations: the peripheral nervous system. An update. Journal of Manipulative and Physiological Therapeutics 23:101–103

Bono G, Antonaci F, Ghirmai S et al 1998 The clinical profile of cervicogenic headache as it emerges from a study based on the early diagnostic criteria. Functional Neurology 13(1):75–77

Bono G, Antonaci F, Ghirmai S et al 2000 Whiplash injuries: clinical picture and diagnostic work-up. Clinical and Experimental Rheumatology 18(2 Suppl 19):S23–S28

Boon HC, Cherkin D, Erro J et al 2004 Practice patterns of naturopathic physicians: results from a random survey of licensed practitioners in two US States. BMC Complementary and Alternative Medicine 4:14

Booth R, Rothman R 1976 Cervical angina. Spine 1:28–32

Bowler S, Green A, Mitchell C 1998 Buteyko breathing techniques in asthma: a blinded randomised controlled trial. Medical Journal of Australia 169:575–578

Brattberg G 1999 Connective tissue massage in the treatment of fibromyalgia. European Journal of Pain 3:235–244

Breier A, Charney D, Heninger G 1986 Agoraphobia with panic attacks: development, diagnostic stability, and course of illness. Archives of General Psychiatry 43:1029–1036

Breithaupt T, Harris K, Ellis J et al 2001 Thoracic lymphatic pumping and the efficacy of influenza vaccination. Journal of the American Osteopathic Association 101(1):21–25

Brennan PC, Triano JJ, McGregor M et al 1991 Enhanced neutrophil respiratory burst as a biological marker for manipulation forces: duration of the effect and association with substance P and tumor necrosis factor. Journal of Manipulative and Physiological Therapeutics 14(7):399–408

Briggs L, Boone W 1988 Effects of a chiropractic adjustment on changes in pupillary diameter: a model for evaluating somatovisceral response. Journal of Manipulative and Physiological Therapeutics 11:181–189

Bronfort G, Evans R, Kubic P 2001 Chronic pediatric asthma and chiropractic spinal manipulation: a prospective clinical series and randomised clinical pilot study. Journal of Manipulative and Physiological Therapeutics 24(6):369–377

Brosseau L, Welch V, Wells G et al 2000 Low level laser therapy (classes I, II and III) in the treatment of rheumatoid arthritis. Cochrane Database of Systematic Reviews (2):CD002049

Brosseau LU, Pelland LU, Casimiro L et al 2002 Electrical stimulation for the treatment of rheumatoid arthritis. Cochrane Database of Systematic Reviews (2): CD003687

Brostoff J 1992 Complete guide to food allergy. Bloomsbury, London

Brüggemann W 1986 Hydrotherapie. Springer, Berlin, p 8–36

Buchmann J, Wende W, Kundt G et al 2005 Manual treatment effects to the upper cervical apophysial joints before, during, and after endotracheal anesthesia: a placebo-controlled comparison. American Journal of Physical Medicine and Rehabilitation 84:251–257

Budgell B 2000 Reflex effects of subluxation: the autonomic nervous system. Journal of Manipulative and Physiological Therapeutics 23(2):104–106

Budgell B, Sato A 1996 Modulations of autonomic functions by somatic nociceptive inputs. Progress in Brain Research 113:525–539

Budgell B, Hotta H, Sato A 1995 Spinovisceral reflexes evoked by noxious and innocuous stimulation of the lumbar spine. Journal of the Neuromuscular System 3:122–131

Budgell B, Sato A, Suzuki A et al 1997 Responses of adrenal function to stimulation of lumbar and thoracic interspinous tissues in the rat. Neuroscience Research 28:33–40

Budgell B, Hotta H, Sato A 1998 Reflex responses of bladder motility following stimulation of interspinous tissues in the anesthetized rat. Journal of Manipulative and Physiological Therapeutics 21:593–599

Bühring M 1988 Die Kneippsche Hydrotherapie in der Praxis. Therapeutikon 2:80–86

Buratovich N, Cronin M, Perry A et al 2006 AANP Position Paper on Naturopathic Manipulative Therapy. American Association of Naturopathic Physicians, Washington, DC

Burckhardt CS, Mannerkorpi K, Hedenberg L, Bjelle A 1994 Randomized controlled clinical trial of education and physical training for women with fibromyalgia. Journal of Rheumatology 21(4):714–720

Burns L 1943 Preliminary report of cardiac changes following correction of third thoracic lesions. Journal of the American Osteopathic Association 42:3

Buskila D, Abu-Shakra M, Neumann L et al 2001 Balneotherapy for fibromyalgia at the Dead Sea. Rheumatology International 20(3):105–108

Caffarelli C, Bacchini P, Gruppi L et al 2005 Exercise-induced bronchoconstriction in children with atopic eczema. Pediatric Allergy and Immunology 16(8):655–661

Caldirola D, Perna G, Arancio C et al 1997 The 35% CO_2 challenge test in patients with social phobia. Psychiatry Research 71:41–48

Cappo B, Holmes D 1984 Utility of prolonged respiratory exhalation for reducing physiological and psychological arousal. Journal of Psychosomatic Research 28(4):265–273

Casimiro L, Brosseau L, Robinson V et al 2002 Therapeutic ultrasound for the treatment of rheumatoid arthritis. Cochrane Database of Systematic Reviews (3): CD003787

Castro P, Larrain G, Pérez O 2000 Chronic hyperventilation syndrome, associated with syncope and coronary vasospasm. American Journal of Medicine 109(1):78–80

CFS/ME Working Group 2001 Report to the Chief Medical Officer of an independent working group. Department of Health, London

Chaitow L 2007 Positional release techniques, 3rd edn. Churchill Livingstone, Edinburgh

Chaitow L, Bradley D, Gilbert C 2002 Multidisciplinary approaches to breathing pattern disorders. Churchill Livingstone, Edinburgh

Chen L-X 2005 Curative effect of yoga exercise prescription in treating menstrual disorders. Chinese Journal of Clinical Rehabilitation 9(4):164–165

Childs J, Fritz J, Flynn T et al 2004 A clinical prediction rule to identify patients with low back pain most likely to benefit from spinal manipulation: a validation study. Annals of Internal Medicine 141:920–928

Childs J, Flynn T, Fritz J 2006 A perspective for considering the risks and benefits of spinal manipulation in patients with low back pain. Manual Therapy 11(4):316–320

Chin K 2001 Clinical management of neuropathic pain. Hong Kong Practitioner 23:439–448

Cho Y, Tsay S 2004 The effect of acupressure with massage on fatigue and depression in patients with end-stage renal disease. Journal of Nursing Research 12:51–59

Cider A, Sveälv B, Täng M et al 2006 Immersion in warm water induces improvement in cardiac function in patients with chronic heart failure. European Journal of Heart Failure 8(3):308–313

Cimbiz A, Bayazit V, Hallaceli H et al 2005 The effect of combined therapy (spa and physical therapy) on pain in various chronic diseases. Complementary Therapies in Medicine 13(4):244–250

Cleland JA, Child JD, McRae M, Palmer JA, Stowell T 2005 Immediate effects of thoracic manipulation in patients with neck pain: a randomized clinical trial. Manual Therapy 10:127–135

Cleland JA, Childs JD, Palmer JA, Eberhart S 2006 Slump stretching in the management of non-radicular low back pain: a pilot clinical trial. Manual Therapy 11(4):279–286

Cohen L, Warneke C, Fouladi R et al 2004 Psychological adjustment and sleep quality in a randomized trial of the effects of a Tibetan yoga intervention in patients with lymphoma. Cancer 100:2253–2260

Colbert A, Markov M, Banerji M 1999 Magnetic mattress pad use in patients with FMS: a double blind pilot study. Journal of Back and Musculoskeletal Rehabilitation 13(1):19–31

Cole C, Blackstone E, Pashkow F et al 1999 Heart-rate recovery immediately after exercise as a predictor of mortality. New England Journal of Medicine 341:1351–1357

Cole C, Foody J, Blackstone E et al 2000 Heart rate recovery after submaximal exercise testing as a predictor of mortality in a cardiovascularly healthy cohort. Annals of Internal Medicine 132:552–555

Coplan J, Goetz R, Lein D et al 1998 Plasma cortisol concentrations preceding lactate-induced panic.

Psychological, biochemical and physiological correlates. Archives of General Psychiatry 55:130–136

Crawford J, Hickson G, Wiles M 1986 The management of hypertensive disease: a review of spinal manipulation and the efficacy of conservative therapeutics. Journal of Manipulative and Physiological Therapeutics 9:27–32

Damas-Mora J, Davies L, Taylor W, Jenner F 1980 Menstrual respiratory changes and symptoms. British Journal of Psychiatry 136:492–497

Danneskiold-Samsoe B, Christiansen E, Lund B, Andersen R 1986 Myofascial pain and the role of myoglobin. Scandinavian Journal of Rheumatology 15:174–178

Davis D 1948 Spinal nerve root pain (radiculitis) simulating coronary occlusion: a common syndrome. American Heart Journal 35:70–80

De Guire S, Gervitz R, Kawahara Y, Maguire W 1992 Hyperventilation syndrome and the assessment and treatment for functional cardiac symptoms. American Journal of Cardiology 70:673–677

de Jong Z, Munneke M, Zwinderman A et al 2004 Is a long-term high-intensity exercise program effective? Arthritis and Rheumatism 50:1066–1076

Degenhardt B, Kuchera M 2006 Osteopathic evaluation and manipulative treatment in reducing the morbidity of otitis media: a pilot study. Journal of the American Osteopathic Association 106(6):327–334

DeLancey J 1990 Anatomy and physiology of urinary incontinence. Clinical Obstetrics and Gynecology 33:298–307

Delaney J, Leong K, Watkins A et al 2002 Short-term effects of myofascial trigger point massage therapy on cardiac autonomic tone in healthy subjects. Journal of Advanced Nursing 37:364–371

Dempsey J, Sheel A, St Croix C 2002 Respiratory influences on sympathetic vasomotor outflow in humans. Respiratory Physiology and Neurobiology 130(1):3–20

Dent O, Gouston K, Zubrzycki J et al 1986 Bowel symptoms in an apparently well population. Diseases of the Colon and Rectum 29:243–247

Dhabhar F, Viswanathan K 2005 Stress-induced enhancement of leukocyte trafficking to sites of surgery or immune activation. Brain, Behavior, and Immunity 19(4 Suppl 1):e15

Dickey J 1989 Postoperative osteopathic manipulative management of median sternotomy patients. Journal of the American Osteopathic Association 89(10):1309–1322

Diego M, Field T, Hernandez-Reif M 2002 Aggressive adolescents benefit from massage therapy. Adolescence 37:597–607

DiMatteo M, Hays R, Prince L 1986 Relationship of physicians' nonverbal communication skill to patient satisfaction, appointment noncompliance, and physician workload. Health Psychology 5(6):581–594

Dishman JD, Dougherty PE, Burke JR 2005 Evaluation of the effect of postural perturbation on motoneuronal activity following various methods of lumbar spinal manipulation. Spine 5:650–659

Dishman R 1994 Advances in exercise adherence. Human Kinetics, Champaign, IL, p 2–14

Dratcu L 2000 Panic, hyperventilation and perpetuation of anxiety. Progress in Neuro-Psychopharmacology and Biological Psychiatry 24(7):1069–1089

Driscoll M, Hall M 2000 Effects of spinal manipulative therapy on autonomic activity and the cardiovascular system: a case study using the electrocardiogram and arterial tonometry. Journal of Manipulative and Physiological Therapeutics 23(8):545–550

Driver H, Taylor S 2000 Exercise is a complex activity that can be beneficial to general well-being but may also stress the body. Sleep Medicine Reviews 4(4):387–402

Drossman D, Corazziaria E, Talley N et al 2000 The functional gastrointestinal disorders. Degnon, McLean, VA, p 351–432

Dubois J 1973 Hydrotherapy and climatic treatment of depressive states. Les Cahiers de Médecine 14(7):591–595

Dubois J, Arnaud A 1983 Quantitative study on course of anxiety and depressive states during spa cure at Saujon. Presse Thermale et Climatique 120(3):132–136

Dull H 1997 Watsu: freeing the body in water, 2nd edn. Harbin Springs Publishing, Harbib, CA

Dunne K 2004 Grief and its manifestations. Nursing Standard 18(45):45–51

Dworkin S, LeResche L 1991 Assessing clinical signs of temporomandibular disorders. Journal of Prosthetic Dentistry 63:574–579

Edeling J 1997 Manual therapy rounds. Cervicogenic, tension-type headache with migraine: a case study. Journal of Manual and Manipulative Therapy 5(1):33–38

Edrya J, Barnesa V, Jeratha V 2006 Physiology of long pranayamic breathing: neural respiratory elements may provide a mechanism that explains how slow deep breathing shifts the autonomic nervous system. Medical Hypotheses 67(3):566–571

Eisenberg D, Davis R, Ettner S et al 1998 Trends in alternative medicine use in the United States. Journal of the American Medical Association 280:1569–1575

Eldridge L, Russell J 2005 Effectiveness of cervical spine manipulation and prescribed exercise in reduction of cervicogenic headache pain and frequency: a single case study experimental design. International Journal of Osteopathic Medicine 8(3):106–113

Elley C, Arrol B 2005 Refining the exercise prescription for hypertension. Lancet 366(9493):1248–1249

Elvin A, Siösteen AK, Nilsson A, Kosek E 2006 Decreased muscle blood flow in fibromyalgia patients during standardised muscle exercise: a contrast media enhanced colour Doppler study. European Journal of Pain 10(2):137–144

Emtner M, Hedin A 2005 Adherence to and effects of physical activity on health in adults with asthma. Advances in Physiotherapy 7(3):123–134

Epstein S, Gerber L 1979 Chest wall syndrome – a common cause of unexplained cardiac pain. Journal of the American Medical Association 241:2793–2797

Eriksen K 1994 Effects of upper cervical correction on chronic constipation. Chiropractic Research Journal 3:19–22

Ernst E 1990 Hydrotherapy. Physiotherapy 76(4):207–210

Ernst E 1999 Massage therapy for low back pain: a systematic review. Journal of Pain and Symptom Management 17:65–69

Ernst E 2004 Manual therapies for pain control: chiropractic and massage. Clinical Journal of Pain 20(1):8–12

Ernst E, Canter P 2006 A systematic review of systematic reviews of spinal manipulation. Journal of the Royal Society of Medicine 99:189–193

Erwin W, Jackson P, Homonko D 2000 Innervation of the human costovertebral joint: implications for clinical back pain syndromes. Journal of Manipulative and Physiological Therapeutics 23(6):395–403

Escalona A, Field T, Singer-Strunk R et al 2001 Improvement in behavior of children with autism. Journal of Autism and Developmental Disorders 31:513–516

European Association of Urology 2003 Guidelines on chronic pelvic pain. EUA, Arnhem, The Netherlands

Evcik D, Kizilay B, Gokcen E 2002 The effects of balneotherapy on fibromyalgia patients. Rheumatology International 22(2):56–59

Fagard R 2001 Exercise characteristics and the blood pressure response to dynamic physical training. Medicine and Science in Sports and Exercise 33(Suppl 6):S484–S492

Faling L 1986 Pulmonary rehabilitation physical modalities. Clinical Chest Medicine 7:599–618

Falk J 1990 Bowel and bladder dysfunction secondary to lumbar dysfunctional syndrome. Chiropractic Technique 2:45–48

Fallon J 1997 The role of chiropractic adjustment in the care and treatment of 332 children with otitis media. Journal of Clinical Chiropractic Pediatrics 2(2):167–183

Fallon J, Lok B 1994 Assessing efficacy of chiropractic care in pediatric cases of pyloric stenosis. In: Proceedings of the National Conference on Chiropractic Pediatrics. International Chiropractic Association, Arlington, VA, p 72

Faul K 2005 A pilot study of the comparative effectiveness of two water-based treatments for fibromyalgia syndrome: Watsu and Aix massage. Journal of Bodywork and Movement Therapies 9(3):202–210

Feijó L, Hernandez-Reif M, Field T et al 2006 Mothers' depressed mood and anxiety levels are reduced after massaging their preterm infants. Infant Behavior and Development 29(3):476–480

Fernández-de-las-Peñas C, Alonso-Blanco C, Cuadrado ML, Pareja JA 2006a Myofascial trigger points in the suboccipital muscles in episodic tension-type headache. Manual Therapy 11(3):225–230

Fernández-de-las-Peñas C, Alonso-Blanco C, Fernandez-Carnero J 2006b The immediate effect of ischemic compression technique and transverse friction massage on tenderness of active and latent myofascial trigger points. Journal of Bodywork and Movement Therapies 10(1):3–9

Fernández-de-las-Peñas C, Ge H, Arendt-Nielsen L et al 2007 Referred pain from trapezius muscle trigger points shares similar characteristics with chronic tension type headache. European Journal of Pain 11(4):475–482

Field T, Hernandez-Reif M 1997 Juvenile rheumatoid arthritis benefits from massage therapy. Journal of Pediatric Psychology 22:607–617

Field T, Henteleff T, Hernandez-Reif M 1997a Children with asthma have improved pulmonary functions after massage therapy. Journal of Pediatrics 132:854–858

Field T, Sunshine W, Hernandez-Reif M 1997b CFS: massage therapy affects depression and somatic symptoms. Journal of Chronic Fatigue Syndrome 3:43–51

Field T, Hernandez-Reif M, LaGreca A et al 1997c Massage therapy lowers blood glucose levels in children with diabetes mellitus. Diabetes Spectrum 10:237–239

Field T, Schanberg S, Kuhn C et al 1998 Bulimic adolescents benefit from massage therapy. Adolescence 33:555–563

Field T, Cullen C, Diego M et al 2001 Leukemia immune changes following massage therapy. Journal of Bodywork and Movement Therapies 5:271–274

Field T, Diego M, Cullen C et al 2002 Fibromyalgia pain and substance P decrease and sleep improves after massage therapy. Journal of Clinical Rheumatology 8:72 76

Field T, Delage J, Hernandez-Reif M 2003 Movement and massage therapy reduce fibromyalgia pain. Journal of Bodywork and Movement Therapies 7(1):49–52

Field T, Diego M, Hernandez-Reif M et al 2004 Massage therapy effects on depressed pregnant women. Journal of Psychosomatic Obstetrics and Gynecology 25(2):115–122

Field T, Hernandez-Reif M, Diego M et al 2005 Cortisol decreases and serotonin and dopamine increase following massage therapy. International Journal of Neuroscience 115(10):1397–1413

Flynn T, Fritz J, Whitman J et al 2002 A clinical prediction rule for classifying patients with low back pain who demonstrate short term improvement with spinal manipulation. Spine 27:2835–2843

Forchuk C, Baruth P 2004 Postoperative arm massage. Cancer Nursing 27:25–33

Ford MJ, Camilleri MJ, Hanson RB 1995 Hyperventilation, central autonomic control, and colonic tone in humans. Gut 37:499–504

Foster G, Vaziri N, Sassoon C 2001 Respiratory alkalosis. Respiratory Care 46(4):384–391

Fritz J, Delitto A, Erhard R 2003 Comparison of classification-based physical therapy with therapy based on clinical practice guidelines for patients with acute low back pain: a randomized clinical trial. Spine 28:1363–1371

Fujimoto T, Budgell B, Uchida S et al 1999 Arterial tonometry in the measurement of the effects of innocuous mechanical stimulation of the neck on heart rate and blood pressure. Journal of the Autonomic Nervous System 75:109–115

Fysh P 1996 Chronic recurrent otitis media: case series of five patients. Journal of Clinical Chiropractic Pediatrics 1:66–78

Gabrielsen A, Sorensen V, Pump B et al 2000 Cardiovascular and neuroendocrine responses to water immersion in compensated heart failure. American Journal of Physiology. Heart and Circulatory Physiology 279(4):H1931–H1940

Galantino M, Bzdewka T, Eissler-Russo J et al 2004 The impact of modified hatha yoga on chronic low back pain: a pilot study. Alternative Therapies in Health and Medicine 10(2):56–59

Gamber R, Shores J, Russo D et al 2002 Osteopathic manipulative treatment in conjunction with medication relieves pain associated with fibromyalgia syndrome. Results of a randomized clinical pilot study. Journal of the American Osteopathic Association 102(6):321–326

Gatterman M et al 1990 Muscle and myofascial pain syndromes. In: Gatterman M (ed) Chiropractic management of spine-related disorders. Williams & Wilkins, Baltimore

Gemmell H, Jacobson B 1989 Chiropractic management of enuresis: a time-series descriptive design. Journal of Manipulative and Physiological Therapeutics 12:386–389

Gibbons P, Tehan P 2000 Manipulation of the spine, thorax and pelvis: an osteopathic perspective. Churchill Livingstone, Edinburgh

Gibbs A 2005 Chiropractic co-management of medically treated asthma. Clinical Chiropractic 8(3):140–144

Giesen JM, Center DB, Leach RA 1989 An evaluation of chiropractic manipulation as a treatment of hyperactivity in children. Journal of Manipulative and Physiological Therapeutics 12(5):353–363

Goertz C, Grimm R, Svendsen K et al 2002 Treatment of Hypertension with Alternative Therapies (THAT) Study: a randomized clinical trial. Journal of Hypertension 2(10):2063–2068

Gosling C, Kinross T, Gibbons P et al 2005 The short term effect of atlanto-axial high velocity low amplitude manipulation with cavitation on edge light pupil cycle time. International Journal of Osteopathic Medicine 8(3):81–86

Gossec L, Pavy S, Pham T et al 2006 Nonpharmacological treatments in early rheumatoid arthritis: clinical practice guidelines based on published evidence and expert opinion. Joint, Bone, Spine 73:396–402

Gowans S, de Hueck A, Voss S A 1999a Randomized controlled trial of exercise and education for individuals with FMS. Arthritis Care and Research 12(2):120–128

Gowans S, de Hueck A, Voss SA 1999b Six minute walk test: a potential outcome measure for hydrotherapy. Arthritis Care and Research 12(3):208–211

Goyeche J, Ikemi Y 1977 Yoga as potential psychosomatic therapy. Asian Medical Journal 20(2):26–32

Grove D 1988 Digestive physiology and the clinical electrogastrogram. Paper presented at the annual meeting of the Biofeedback Society of America, Colorado Springs, March 25–30, 1988

Gugel M, Johnston W 2006 Osteopathic manipulative treatment of a 27-year-old man after anterior cruciate ligament reconstruction. Journal of the American Osteopathic Association 106(6):346–349

Guillard A 1990 Depressive syndromes and treatment at the Neris-les-Bains thermal spa cure. Presse Thermale et Climatique 127(4):189–198

Guiney P, Chou R, Vianna A et al 2005 Effects of osteopathic manipulative treatment on pediatric patients with asthma: a randomized controlled trial. Journal of the American Osteopathic Association 105(1):7–12

Gutenbrunner C, Ruppel K 1992 Zur Frage der adaptiven Blutdrucknormalisierung im Verlauf von Bäderkuren unter besonderer Berücksichtigung von Homogenisierungseffekten und Lebensalter. Phys Rehab Kur Med 2:58–64

Haboush A, Floyd M, Caron J et al 2006 Ballroom dance lessons for geriatric depression: an exploratory study. Arts in Psychotherapy 33(2):89–97

Häfner S 2005 Georg Groddeck's approach to patients by psychotherapy and massage. Physikalische Medizin Rehabilitationsmedizin Kurortmedizin 15(1):39–43

Hagberg J, Park J, Brown M 2000 The role of exercise training in the treatment of hypertension: an update. Sports Medicine 30:193–206

Hagen EM, Svensen E, Eriksen H et al 2006 Comorbid subjective health complaints in low back pain. Spine 31(13):1491–1495

Hains G, Hains F 2000 Combined ischemic compression and spinal manipulation in the treatment of fibromyalgia: a preliminary estimate of dose and efficacy. Journal of Manipulative and Physiological Therapeutics 23(4):225–230

Hakkinen A, Sokka T, Kotaniemi A et al 1999 Dynamic strength training in patients with early rheumatoid arthritis increases muscle strength but not bone mineral density. Journal of Rheumatology 26:1257–1263

Hakkinen K, Pakarinen A, Hannonen P et al 2002 Effects of strength training on muscle strength, cross-sectional area, maximal electromyographic activity, and serum hormones in premenopausal women with fibromyalgia. Journal of Rheumatology 29(6):1287–1295

Haldeman S, Dagenais S 2001 Cervicogenic headaches. Spine 1(1):31–46

Haltenhof H, Hesse B, Buhler KE 1995 [Evaluation and utilization of complementary medical procedures – a survey of 793 physicians in general practice and the clinic] [article in German]. Gesundheitswesen 57:192–195

Hamberg J, Lindahl O 1981 Angina pectoris symptoms caused by thoracic spine disorders Acta Medica Scandinavica 644(suppl):34

Hamilton K, Powers H, Sugiura T et al 2001 Short-term exercise training can improve myocardial tolerance to I/R without elevation in heat shock proteins. American Journal of Physiology. Heart and Circulatory Physiology 3:H1346–H1352

Hammond A, Young A, Kidao R 2004 A randomised controlled trial of occupational therapy for people with early rheumatoid arthritis. Annals of the Rheumatic Diseases 63:23–30

Han J, Stegen K, De Valck C et al 1996 Influence of breathing therapy on complaints, anxiety and breathing pattern in patients with hyperventilation syndrome and anxiety disorders. Journal of Psychosomatic Research 41(5):481–493

Harinath K, Malhotra AS, Pal K et al 2004 Effects of Hatha yoga and Omkar meditation on cardiorespiratory performance, psychologic profile, and melatonin secretion. Journal of Alternative and Complementary Medicine 10(2):261–268

Harris A, Cronkite R, Moos R 2006 Physical activity, exercise coping, and depression in a 10-year cohort study of depressed patients. Journal of Affective Disorders 93(1–3):79–85

Harris W, Wagnon R 1987 The effects of chiropractic adjustments on distal skin temperature. Journal of Manipulative and Physiological Therapeutics 10:57–60

Hartel U, Volger E 2004 [Use and acceptance of classical natural and alternative medicine in Germany – findings of a representative population-based survey] [article in German]. Forschende Komplementärmedizin und Klassische Naturheilkunde 11:327–334

Hawk C, Long C, Boulanger K 2001 Prevalence of nonmusculoskeletal complaints in chiropractic practice: report from a practice based research program. Journal of Manipulative and Physiological Therapeutics 24(3):157–169

Heaton K, Radvan J, Cripps H et al 1992a Defecation frequency and timing, and stool form in the general population: a prospective study. Gut 33:818–824

Heaton K, O'Donell L, Braddon F et al 1992b Symptoms of irritable bowel syndrome in a British urban community. Consulters and nonconsulters. Gastroenterology 102:1962–1967

Hedstrom J 1991 Eye movements and relaxation. Behavioral and Experimental Psychiatry 22(1):37–38

Henriksson K 1999 Is fibromyalgia a distinct clinical entity? Pain mechanisms in fibromyalgia syndrome. A myologist's view. Baillière's Clinical Rheumatology 13:455–461

Hernandez-Reif M, Field T, Theakston H 1998 Multiple sclerosis patients benefit from massage therapy. Journal of Bodywork and Movement Therapies 2:168–174

Hernandez-Reif M, Field T, Krasnegor J et al 2000a High blood pressure and associated symptoms reduced by massage therapy. Journal of Bodywork and Movement Therapies 4:31–38

Hernandez-Reif M, Martinez A, Field T et al 2000b Premenstrual symptoms are relieved by massage therapy. Journal of Psychosomatic Obstetrics and Gynecology 21:9–15

Hernandez-Reif M, Field T, Largie S et al 2002 Parkinson's disease symptoms reduced by massage therapy. Journal of Bodywork and Movement Therapies 6:177–182

Hernandez-Reif M, Ironson G, Field T et al 2004 Breast cancer patients have improved immune functions following massage therapy. Journal of Psychosomatic Research 57(1):45–52

Herzog J 1999 Use of cervical spine manipulation under anesthesia for management of cervical disk herniation, cervical radiculopathy, and associated cervicogenic headache syndrome. Journal of Manipulative and Physiological Therapeutics 22(3):166–170

Higashi Y, Sasaki S, Kurisu S et al 1999 Regular aerobic exercise augments endothelium-dependent vascular relaxation in normotensive as well as hypertensive subjects: role of endothelium-derived nitric oxide. Circulation 100:1194–1202

Hix E 1976 Reflex viscerosomatic reference phenomena. Osteopathic Annals 4(12):496–503

Hoag J 1977 The musculoskeletal system: a major factor in maintaining homeostasis. AAO Year Book. American Academy of Osteopathy, Colorado Springs, CO, p 5–16

Hoiriis K, Pfleger B, McDuffie F et al 2004 A randomized clinical trial comparing chiropractic adjustments to muscle relaxants for subacute low back pain. Journal of Manipulative and Physiological Therapeutics 27:388–398

Holdcraft L, Assefi N, Buchwald D 2003 Complementary and alternative medicine in fibromyalgia and related syndromes. Best Practice and Research Clinical Rheumatology 17(4):667–683

Holzberg A, Kellog-Spadt S, Lukban J et al 2001 Evaluation of transvaginal Theile massage as a therapeutic intervention for women with interstitial cystitis. Urology 57(6 Suppl 1):120

Hondras M, Long C, Brennan P 1999 Spinal manipulative therapy versus a low force mimic maneuver for women with primary dysmenorrhea: a randomized, observer-blinded, clinical trial. Pain 81(1–2):105–114

Hondras M, Linde K, Jones A 2005 Manual therapy for asthma. Cochrane Database of Systematic Reviews (2): CD001002

Horton SJ, Franz A 2007 Mechanical diagnosis and therapy approach to assessment and treatment of derangement of the sacro-iliac joint. Manual Therapy 12:126–132

Hucho T, Dina OA, Kuhn J, Levine JD 2006 Estrogen controls PKCepsilon-dependent mechanical hyperalgesia through direct action on nociceptive neurons. European Journal of Neuroscience 24(2):527–534

Ironson G, Field T, Scafidi F et al 1996 Massage therapy is associated with the enhancement of the immune system's cytotoxic capacity. International Journal of Neuroscience 84:205–217

Irving R 1981 Pain and the protective reflex generators. Journal of Manipulative and Physiological Therapeutics 4:69–71

Jackson K, Steele TF, Dugan EP et al 1998 Effect of lymphatic and splenic pump techniques on the antibody response to hepatitis B vaccine. Journal of the American Osteopathic Association 98:155–157

Jacobs B 1990 Cervical angina. New York State Journal of Medicine 90:8–11

Jamison J 2005 Insomnia: does chiropractic help? Journal of Manipulative and Physiological Therapeutics 28(3):179–186

Jarmel M 1989 Possible role of spinal joint dysfunction in the genesis of sudden cardiac death. Journal of Manipulative and Physiological Therapeutics 12(6):469–477

Jarmel ME, Zatkin JL, Charuvastra E et al 1995 Improvement of cardiac autonomic regulation following spinal manipulative therapy. In: Cleveland C, Haldeman S (eds) Conference Proceedings of the Chiropractic Centennial Foundation, Davenport, Iowa, p 359

Jarski R, Loniewski E, Williams J et al 2000 The effectiveness of osteopathic manipulative treatment as complementary therapy following surgery: a prospective, match-controlled outcome study. Alternative Therapies in Health and Medicine 6(5):77–81

Jennett S 1994 Control of breathing and its disorders. In: Timmons B, Ley R (eds) Behavioral and psychological approaches to breathing disorders. Plenum Press, New York, p 67–80

Jiminez C et al 1993 Treatment of FMS with OMT and self-learned techniques. Report: Journal of the American Osteopathic Association 93(8):870

Johnson J 2001 How the principles of exercise physiology influence pelvic floor muscle training. Journal of Wound, Ostomy and Continence Nursing 28:150–155

Johnston WL, Kelso AF 1995 Changes in presence of a segmental dysfunction pattern associated with hypertension: part 2. A long-term longitudinal study. Journal of the American Osteopathic Association 95:315–318

Johnston WL, Kelso AF, Babcock HB 1995 Changes in presence of a segmental dysfunction pattern associated with hypertension: part 1. A short-term longitudinal study. Journal of the American Osteopathic Association 95:243–255

Joos S, Rosemann T, Szecsenyi J et al 2006 Use of complementary and alternative medicine in Germany – a survey of patients with inflammatory bowel disease. BMC Complementary and Alternative Medicine 6:19. Online. Available: www.biomedcentral.com/1472-6882/6/19

Kappler R 1996 Osteopathic considerations in diagnosis and treatment. In: Ward R (ed) Fundamentals of osteopathic medicine. Williams & Wilkins, Baltimore

Karason A, Drysdale D 2003 Somatovisceral response following osteopathic HVLAT: a pilot study on the effect of unilateral lumbosacral high-velocity low-amplitude thrust technique on the cutaneous blood flow in the lower limb. Journal of Manipulative and Physiological Therapeutics 26(4):220–225

Kasseroller R 1998 The Vodder school: the Vodder method. Cancer 83(12 Suppl):2840–2842

Katon WJ, Walker EAJ 1998 Medically unexplained symptoms in primary care. Clinical Psychiatry 59(Suppl 20):15–21

Kegel A 1948 Progressive resistance exercise in the functional restoration of the perineal muscles. American Journal of Obstetrics and Gynecology 56:238–248

Kegel A, Powell T 1950 The physiologic treatment of urinary stress incontinence. Journal of Urology 63:808–814

Kelmanson I, Adulas E 2006 Massage therapy and sleep behaviour in infants born with low birth weight. Complementary Therapies in Clinical Practice 12(3):200–205

Kendall F, Kendall E, Kendall-McCreary P 1993 Muscles, testing, and function, 4th edn. Williams & Wilkins, Baltimore

Kessinger R, Boneva D 1998 Changes in visual acuity in patients receiving upper cervical specific chiropractic care. Journal of Vertebral Subluxation Research 2(1):43–49

Khalsa P 2004 Biomechanics of musculoskeletal pain: dynamics of the neuromatrix. Journal of Electromyography and Kinesiology 14:109–120

Khalsa P, Eberhart A, Cotler A et al 2006 The 2005 Conference on the Biology of Manual Therapies. Journal of Manipulative and Physiological Therapeutics 29(5):341–346

Khumar S, Kaur P, Kaur S 1993 Effectiveness of Shavasana on depression among university students. Indian Journal of Clinical Psychology 20(2):82–87

Kim SS, Kaplowitz S, Johnston MV 2004 The effects of physician empathy on patient satisfaction and compliance. Evaluation and the Health Professions 27(3):237–251

Kim Y-J, Ban D 2005 Prevalence of irritable bowel next term syndrome, influence of lifestyle factors and bowel habits in Korean college students. International Journal of Nursing Studies 42(3):247–254

King H, Tettambel M, Lockwood M et al 2003 Osteopathic manipulative treatment in prenatal care. A retrospective case control design study. Journal of the American Osteopathic Association 103(12):577–582

Kirchfield F, Boyle W 1994 Nature doctors. Buckeye Naturopathic Press, East Palestine, OH

Kirkaldy-Willis WH, Wedge J, Yong-Hing K, Reilly J 1984 Lumbar spondylosis and stenosis correlation of pathological anatomy with high resolution computed tomographic scanning. In: Donovan Post MJ (ed) Computed tomography of the spine. Williams & Wilkins, Baltimore

Kjellgren A, Sundequist U, Norlander T et al 2001 Effects of flotation-REST on muscle tension pain. Pain Research and Management 6(4):181–189

Klein D 1993 False suffocation alarms, spontaneous panics, and related conditions. Archives of General Psychiatry 50:306–317

Klougart N, Nilsson N 1989 Infantile colic treated by chiropractors: a prospective study of 316 cases. Journal of Manipulative and Physiological Therapeutics 12:281–291

Kneipp S 1979 My water cure (facsimile edition). Thorsons, Wellingborough, p 194–195. First published 1893

Knutson G 2001 Significant changes in systolic blood pressure post vectored upper cervical adjustment vs resting control groups: a possible effect of the cervicosympathetic and/or pressor reflex. Journal of Manipulative and Physiological Therapeutics 24:101–109

Kokjohn K, Schmid D, Triano J et al 1992 The effect of spinal manipulation on pain and prostaglandin level in women with primary dysmenorrhea. Journal of Manipulative and Physiological Therapeutics 15:279–285

Korr IM 1970 The physiological basis of osteopathic medicine. Postgraduate Institute of Osteopathic Medicine and Surgery, New York

Korr IM 1976 Spinal cord as organiser of disease process. Academy of Applied Osteopathy Yearbook, Newark, OH

Korr I, Buzzell K, Hix E 1970 Physiological basis of osteopathic medicine. Symposium. Post-Graduate Institute of Osteopathic Medicine and Surgery, New York

Kosek E, Hansson P 1997 Modulatory influence on somatosensory perception from vibration and heterotopic noxious conditioning stimulation (HNCS) in fibromyalgia patients and healthy subjects. Pain 70:41–51

Krahl P 1973 [Physiotherapy and otolaryngology] [article in German]. HNO 21(9):277–283

Kuchera M, Kuchera W 1991 Osteopathic considerations in systemic dysfunction. KCOM Press, Kirksville, MO

Kumar P, Clark M 1998 Clinical medicine, 4th edn. WB Saunders, Edinburgh, p 687–668

Kurosawa M, Lundeberg T, Agren G et al 1995 Massage-like stroking of the abdomen lowers blood pressure in anesthetized rats: influence of oxytocin. Journal of the Autonomic Nervous System 56:26–30

Lafferty W, Tyree P, Bellas A et al 2006 Insurance coverage and subsequent utilization of complementary and alternative medicine providers. American Journal of Managed Care 12(7):397–404

Lane R 2000 Chronic fatigue syndrome: is it physical? Journal of Neurology, Neurosurgery and Psychiatry 69:289

Lane T, Matthews D, Manu P 1990 The low yield of physical examinations and laboratory investigations of patients with chronic fatigue. American Journal of Medical Science 299:313–318

Lapp C 1997 Exercise limits in chronic fatigue syndrome. American Journal of Medicine 103:83–84

Latha D, Kaliappan K 1992 Efficacy of yoga therapy in the management of headaches. Journal of Indian Psychology 10:41–47

Lawler S, Cameron L 2006 A randomized, controlled trial of massage therapy as a treatment for migraine. Annals of Behavioral Medicine 32(1):50–59

Lee D 2004 The pelvic girdle. An approach to the examination and treatment of the lumbopelvic–hip region, 3rd edn. Churchill Livingstone, Edinburgh

Lee-Jones C, Humphris G, Dixon R et al 1997 Fear of cancer recurrence – a literature review and proposed cognitive formulation to explain exacerbation of recurrence fears. Psychooncology 6:95–105

Leibetseder V, Strauss-Blaschea G, Holzerb F et al 2004 Improving homocysteine levels through balneotherapy: effects of sulphur baths. Clinica Chimica Acta 343(1–2):105–111

Levine J, Khasarb S, Green P 2006 Neurogenic inflammation and arthritis. Annals of the New York Academy of Sciences 1069:155–167

Levitsky L 1995 Pulmonary physiology, 4th edn. McGraw-Hill, New York

Lewit K 1985 The muscular and articular factor in movement restriction. Manual Medicine 1:83–85

Lewit K 1999 Manipulative therapy in rehabilitation of the locomotor system. Butterworth-Heinemann, Oxford

Lewit K, Abrahamovic M 1975 [Chronic tonsillitis and the upper cervical spine] [article in Czech]. Sbornik Lekarsky 77(1):30–32

Lindlahr H 1988 Philosophy of natural therapeutics. Edited and revised by JCP Proby. CW Daniel, Saffron Wallden, Essex, p 125

Lobbezoo F, Visscher C, Naeije N 2004 Impaired health status, sleep disorders, and pain in the craniomandibular and cervical spinal regions. European Journal of Pain 8:23–30

Locke G, Pemberton J, Phillips S 2000 AGA technical review on constipation. Gastroenterology 119:1766–1778

Loeppky J, Scotto P, Charlton G et al 2001 Ventilation is greater in women than men, but the increase during acute altitude hypoxia is the same. Respiration Physiology 125(3):225–237

Long A, Donelson R, Fung T 2004 Does it matter which exercise? Spine 29:2593–2602

Lovas J, Craig A, Raison E et al 2002 The effects of massage on human immune response in healthy adults (pilot study). Journal of Bodywork and Movement Therapies 6(3):143–150

Lukban J, Whitmore K, Kellog-Spadt S et al 2001 The effect of manual physical therapy in patients diagnosed with interstitial cystitis, high-tone pelvic floor dysfunction, and sacroiliac dysfunction. Urology 57(6 Suppl 1):121–122

Lum C 1996 Hyperventilation and asthma: the grey area. Biological Psychology 43(3):262

Lum L 1984 Hyperventilation and anxiety state [editorial]. Journal of the Royal Society of Medicine, January, p 1–4

Lum L 1987 Hyperventilation syndromes in medicine and psychiatry. Journal of the Royal Society of Medicine 80:229–231

Lum L 1994 Hyperventilation syndromes. In: Timmons B, Ley R (eds) Behavioral and psychological approaches to breathing disorders. Plenum Press, New York, p 113–123

Lund I, Ge Y, Yu L et al 2002 Repeated massage-like stimulation induces long-term effects on nociception: contribution of oxytocinergic mechanisms. European Journal of Neuroscience 16:330–338

Lundeberg T, Uvnas-Moberg K, Agren G et al 1994 Anti-nociceptive effects of oxytocin in rats and mice. Neuroscience Letters 170:153–157

Lustyk M, Jarrett M, Bennett J et al 2001 Does a physically active lifestyle improve symptoms in women with irritable bowel syndrome? Gastroenterology Nursing 24(3):129–137

Madias N, Adrogue H 2003 Cross-talk between two organs: how the kidney responds to disruption of acid–base balance by the lung. Nephron Physiology 93(3):61–66

Maguire P, Pitceathly C 2002 Key communication skills and how to acquire them. British Medical Journal 325:697–700

Maguire P, Faulkner A, Booth K et al 1996 Helping cancer patients disclose their fears. European Journal of Cancer 32A:78–81

Maher Committee 1995 Management of adverse effects following breast radiotherapy. Royal College of Radiologists, London

Malhotra V, Singh S, Singh KP et al 2002 Study of yoga asanas in assessment of pulmonary function in NIDDM patients. Indian Journal of Physiology and Pharmacology 46(3):313–320

Manjunath N, Telles S 2005 Influence of Yoga and Ayurveda on self-rated sleep in a geriatric population. Indian Journal of Medical Research 121(5):683–690

Mannerkorpi K, Nyberg B, Ahlmen M, Ekdahl C 2000 Pool exercise combined with an education program for patients with FMS. A prospective, randomized study. Journal of Rheumatology 27(10):2473–2481

Manocha R, Marks G, Kenchington P et al 2002 Sahaja yoga in the management of moderate to severe asthma: a randomised controlled trial. Thorax 57(2):110–115

Marshall W, Murphy B 2006 Evaluation of functional and neuromuscular changes after exercise rehabilitation for low back pain using a Swiss ball: a pilot study. Journal of Manipulative and Physiological Therapeutics 29:550–560

Martikainen K, Partinen M, Hasan J et al 2003 The impact of somatic health problems on insomnia in middle age. Sleep Medicine 4:201–206

Martin L, Nutting A, McIntosh BR et al 1996 An exercise program in treatment of fibromyalgia. Journal of Rheumatology 23(6):1050–1053

Martínez-Segura R, Fernández-de-las-Peñas C, Ruiz-Sáez M et al 2006 Immediate effects on neck pain and active range of motion after a single cervical high-velocity low-amplitude manipulation in subjects presenting with mechanical neck pain: a randomized controlled trial. Journal of Manipulative and Physiological Therapeutics 29:511–517

Masuo K 2001 Which is more effective on weight loss-induced blood pressure reduction: a low caloric diet or an aerobic exercise? American Journal of Hypertension 14(4 Suppl 1):A214

Matthiesen A, Ransjo-Arvidson A, Nissen E et al 2001 Postpartum maternal oxytocin release by newborns: effects of infant hand massage and sucking. Birth 28:13–19

McCain G, Bell D, Mai F et al 1988 A controlled study of the effects of a supervised cardiovascular fitness training program on the manifestations of primary fibromyalgia. Arthritis and Rheumatism 31:1135–1141

McCully K 1969 Vascular pathology of homocysteinemia: implications for the pathogenesis of arteriosclerosis. American Journal of Pathology 56:111–128

McEwen B, Wingfield J 2003 The concept of allostasis in biology and biomedicine. Hormones and Behavior 43:2–15

McGuiness J, Vicenzino B, Wright A 1997 Influence of cervical mobilisation technique on respiratory and cardiovascular function. Manual Therapy 2:216–220

McLean L 2005 The effect of postural correction on muscle activation amplitudes recorded from the cervicobrachial region. Journal of Electromyography and Kinesiology 15:527–535

Mehling W, Hamel K 2005 Randomized, controlled trial of breath therapy for patients with chronic low-back pain. Alternative Therapies in Health and Medicine 11(4):44–52

Melzack R, Wall P 1989 Textbook of pain, 2nd edn. Churchill Livingstone, London

Messinger-Rapport B, Pothier Snader C, Blackstone E et al 2003 Value of exercise capacity and heart rate recovery in older people. Journal of the American Geriatric Society 51:63–68

Meyer K 2001 Exercise training in heart failure: recommendations based on current research. Medicine and Science in Sports and Exercise 33(4):525–531

Meyer TJ, Mark M 1995 Effects of psychosocial interventions with adult cancer patients: a meta-analysis of randomised experiments. Health Psychology 4:101–108

Michaud C 2004 Osteopathy – a very promising approach to improve the quality of life in persons suffering from panic attacks [Ostheopathie- Ein viel versprechender Ansatz zur Verbesserung der Lebensqualität bei Panikattacken]. Osteopathische Medizin 5(3):9–15

Millenson J 1995 Mind matters – psychological medicine in holistic practice. Eastland Press, Seattle

Mills M, Henley C, Barnes L et al 2003 The use of osteopathic manipulative treatment as adjuvant therapy in children with recurrent acute otitis media. Archives of Pediatrics and Adolescent Medicine 157(9):861–866

Mohammadian P, Gonsalves A, Tsai C et al 2004 Areas of capsaicin-induced secondary hyperalgesia and allodynia are reduced by a single chiropractic adjustment: a preliminary study. Journal of Manipulative and Physiological Therapeutics 27:381–387

Mohseni-Bandpei M, Critchley J, Staunton T et al 2006 A prospective randomised controlled trial of spinal manipulation and ultrasound in the treatment of chronic low back pain. Physiotherapy 92:34–42

Moldofsky H 2001 Sleep and pain. Sleep Medicine Reviews 5:385–396

Moldwin R, Mendelowitz F 1994 Pelvic floor dysfunction and interstitial cystitis. Journal of Urology 15(suppl):285A

Mollet GA, Harrison D 2006 Emotion and pain: a functional cerebral systems integration. Neuropsychology Review 16:99–121

Montgomery P, Dennis J 2004 A systematic review of non-pharmacological therapies for sleep problems in later life. Sleep Medicine Reviews 8(1):47–62

Moore M 2004 Upper crossed syndrome and its relationship to cervicogenic headache. Journal of Manipulative and Physiological Therapeutics 27(6):414–420

Mootz R, Dhami M, Hess J 1994 Chiropractic treatment of chronic episodic type headache in male subjects: a case series analysis. Journal of the Canadian Chiropractic Association 38(3):152–159

Moreira W, Fuchs F, Ribeiro R et al 1999 The effects of two aerobic training intensities on ambulatory blood pressure in hypertensive patients: results of a randomized trial. Journal of Clinical Epidemiology 52:637–642

Moseley G, Nicholas M, Hodges P 2004 A randomized controlled trial of intensive neurophysiology education in chronic low back pain. Clinical Journal of Pain 20:324–330

Müller-Oerlinghausen B, Berg C, Scherer P et al 2004 Effects of slow-stroke massage as complementary treatment of depressed hospitalized patients: result of a controlled study. Deutsche Medizinische Wochenschrift 129(24):1363–1368

Nagarathna R, Nagendra H 1985 Yoga for bronchial asthma – a controlled study. British Medical Journal 291:172–174

Nakao K, Ohgushi M, Yoshimura M et al 1997 Hyperventilation as a specific test for diagnosis of coronary artery spasm. American Journal of Cardiology 80(5):545–549

Nijs J, De Meirleir K, Duquet W 2004 Kinesiophobia in chronic fatigue syndrome: assessment and associations with disability. Archives of Physical Medicine and Rehabilitation 85:1586–1592

Nijs J, Meeus M, Meirleira K 2006 Chronic musculoskeletal pain in chronic fatigue syndrome. Manual Therapy 11:187–191

Nishime E, Cole C, Blackstone E et al 2000 Heart rate recovery and treadmill exercise score as predictors of mortality in patients referred for exercise ECG. Journal of the American Medical Association 284:1392–1398

Nixon P 1989 Hyperventilation and cardiac symptoms. Internal Medicine 10(12):67–84

Nixon P, Andrews J 1996 A study of anaerobic threshold in chronic fatigue syndrome (CFS). Biological Psychology 43(3):264

Noll D, Shores J, Bryman P et al 1999 Adjunctive osteopathic manipulative treatment in the elderly hospitalized with pneumonia: a pilot study. Journal of the American Osteopathic Association 99(3):143–152

Noll D, Shores J, Gamber R et al 2000 Benefits of osteopathic manipulative treatment for hospitalized elderly patients with pneumonia. Journal of the American Osteopathic Association 100(12):776 –782

Nygaard I, Kreder K, Lepic M et al 1996 Efficacy of pelvic floor muscle exercises in women with stress, urge, and mixed urinary incontinence. American Journal of Obstetrics and Gynecology 174(1):120–125

Ohayon M 2002 Epidemiology of insomnia: what we know and what we still need to learn. Sleep Medicine Reviews 6:97–111

Ohayon M, Partinen P 2003 Insomnia and global sleep dissatisfaction in Finland. Journal of Sleep Research 11:339–346

Oken B, Kishiyama S, Zajdel D et al 2004 Randomized controlled trial of yoga and exercise in multiple sclerosis. Neurology 62:2058–2064

Oleson T, Flocco W 1993 Randomised controlled study of pre-menstrual symptoms treated with ear, hand and foot reflexology. Obstetrics and Gynaecology 82(6):906–911

Olney C 2005 The effect of therapeutic back massage in hypertensive persons: a preliminary study. Biological Research for Nursing 7(2):98–105

O'Sullivan P, Phyty G, Twomey L et al 1997 Evaluation of specific stabilizing exercise in the treatment of chronic low back pain with radiologic diagnosis of spondylolysis or spondylolisthesis. Spine 22:2959–2967

Ownby K 2006 Effects of ice massage on neuropathic pain in persons with AIDS. Journal of the Association of Nurses in AIDS Care 17(5):15–22

Oyama I, Rejba A, Lukban A et al 2004 Modified Thiele massage as therapeutic intervention for female patients with interstitial cystitis and hightone pelvic floor dysfunction. Urology 64(5):862–865

O-Yurvati AH, Carnes MS, Clearfield MB et al 2005 Hemodynamic effects of osteopathic manipulative treatment immediately after coronary artery bypass graft surgery. Journal of the American Osteopathic Association 105(10):475–481

Pal G, Velkumary S 2004 Effect of short-term practice of breathing exercises on autonomic functions in normal human volunteers. Indian Journal of Medical Research 120(2):115–121

Panjwani U, Gupta HL, Singh SH et al 1995 Effect of Sahaja yoga practice on stress management in patients of epilepsy. Indian Journal of Physiology and Pharmacology 39:111–116

Paroo Z, Haist J, Karmazyn M et al 2002 Exercise improves postischemic cardiac function in males but not females: consequences of a novel sex-specific heat shock protein 70 response. Circulation Research 8:911–917

Patel C 1973 Yoga and biofeedback in the management of hypertension. Lancet 10:1053–1055

Patel C, North W 1975 Randomised controlled trial of yoga and biofeedback in management of hypertension. Lancet 2:93–95

Paul RT, Stomel RJ, Broniak FF, Williams BB 1986 Interferon levels in human subjects throughout 24 hour period following thoracic lymphatic pump manipulation. Journal of the American Osteopathic Association 86:92–95

Pearce J 1995 Cervicogenic headache: an early description. Journal of Neurology, Neurosurgery and Psychiatry 58(6):698

Pedersen B, Saltin B 2006 Evidence for prescribing exercise as therapy in chronic disease. Scandinavian Journal of Medicine and Science in Sports 16(Suppl 1):3–63

Pellegrino M 1990 Atypical chest pain as an initial presentation of primary fibromyalgia. Archives of Physical Medicine and Rehabilitation 71:526–528

Pellegrino MJ 1997 Fibromyalgia: managing the pain, 2nd edn. Anadem Publishing, Columbus, OH, Ch 20

Perrin R 1993 Chronic fatigue syndrome: a review from the biomechanical perspective. British Osteopathic Journal XI:15–23

Perrin R 2007 Lymphatic drainage of the neuraxis in chronic fatigue syndrome: a hypothetical model for the cranial rhythmic impulse. Journal of the American Osteopathic Association 107(6):218–224

Perrin R, Edwards J, Hartley P 1998 Evaluation of the effectiveness of osteopathic treatment on symptoms associated with myalgic encephalomyelitis. A preliminary report. Journal of Medical Engineering and Technology 22(1):1–13

Pescatello LS, Miller B, Danias PG et al 1999 Mildly hypertensive premenopausal women. American Heart Journal 138(5 pt 1):916–921

Pescatello LS, Bairos L, Vanheest JL et al 2003 Postexercise hypotension differs between white and black women. American Heart Journal 145(2):364–370

Petajan J, Gappmaier E, White A et al 1996 Impact of aerobic training on fitness and quality of life in multiple sclerosis. Annals of Neurology 39:432–441

Peters H, DeVries W, Vanberge-Henegouwen G 2001 Potential benefits and hazards of physical activity and exercise on the gastrointestinal tract. Gut 48(3):435–439

Pickar J 2002 Neurophysiological effects of spinal manipulation, Spine 2:357–371

Pickar J, Wheeler J 2001 Response of muscle proprioceptors to spinal manipulative-like loads in the anesthetized cat. Journal of Manipulative and Physiological Therapeutics 24:2–11

Pikalov A, Kharin V 1994 Use of spinal manipulative therapy in treatment of duodenal ulcer. Journal of Manipulative and Physiological Therapeutics 17:310–313

Pilkington K, Kirkwood G, Rampe H 2005 Yoga for depression: the research evidence. Journal of Affective Disorders 89(1–3):13–24

Pioro-Boisset M, Esdaile J, Fitzcharles M 1996 Alternative medicine use in fibromyalgia syndrome. Arthritis Care and Research 9:13–17

Price DD, Craggs J, Verne GN et al 2007 Placebo analgesia is accompanied by large reductions in pain-related brain activity in irritable bowel syndrome patients. Pain 127:63–72

Prins J, Bazelmans E, Elving L et al 2001 Cognitive behaviour therapy for chronic fatigue syndrome: a multicentre randomised controlled trial. Lancet 357:841–847

Proctor M, Hing W, Johnson T et al 2004 Spinal manipulation for primary and secondary dysmenorrhoea. Cochrane Database of Systematic Reviews (3):CD002119

Pryor J, Prasad S 2002a Physiotherapy for respiratory and cardiac problems, 3rd edn. Churchill Livingstone, Edinburgh

Pryor J, Prasad S 2002b Physiotherapy for respiratory and cardiac problems, 3rd edn. Churchill Livingstone, Edinburgh, p 353

Quinn C, Chandler C, Moraska A 2002 Massage therapy and frequency of chronic tension headaches. American Journal of Public Health 92(10):1657–1661

Radjieski J, Lumley M, Cantieri M 1998 Effect of osteopathic manipulative treatment on length of stay for pancreatitis: a randomized pilot study. Journal of the American Osteopathic Association 98(5):264–272

Ram F, Robinson S, Black P, Picot J 2005 Physical training for asthma. Cochrane Database of Systematic Reviews (4):CD001116

Ramaratnam S, Sridharan R 2000 Yoga for epilepsy. Cochrane Database of Systematic Reviews (1): CD001524

Reid S, Wessely S, Crayford T, Hotopf M 2001 Medically unexplained symptoms in frequent attenders of secondary health care: retrospective cohort study. British Medical Journal 322:767–769

Reynolds WJ, Scott B 1999 Empathy: a crucial component of the helping relationship. Journal of Psychiatric and Mental Health Nursing 6(5):363–370

Rhudy J, Meagher M 2000 Fear and anxiety: divergent effects on human pain thresholds. Pain 84:65–75

Rhudy J, Williams A 2005 Gender differences in pain: do emotions play a role? Gender Medicine 2(4):208–226

Richards S, Scott D 2002 Prescribed exercise in people with fibromyalgia: parallel group randomised controlled trial. British Medical Journal 325:185

Riot F, Goudet P, Mouraux J-P et al 2004 Levator ani syndrome, functional intestinal disorders and articular abnormalities of the pelvis: the place of osteopathic treatment. Presse Medicale 33(13):852–857

Ritter R 2005 Naturopathic scope of practice gap analysis: a report to the British Columbia Ministry of Health Services by the British Columbia Naturopathic Association. Supporting material collated by King C, Swetlikoff G (Manipulation segment: Brown H.)

Robb K, Williams J, Duvivier V, Newham D 2006 A pain management program for chronic cancer-treatment-related pain. Journal of Pain 7(2):82–90

Robinson V, Brosseau L, Casimiro L et al 2002 Thermotherapy for treating rheumatoid arthritis. Cochrane Database of Systematic Reviews (2):CD002826

Romero L 2004 Physiological stress in ecology: lessons from biomedical research. Trends in Ecology and Evolution 19(5):249–255

Rosenfeld R 1997 Amusing parents while nature cures otitis media with effusion. International Journal of Pediatric Otorhinolaryngology 43(2):189–192

Rowane W, Rowane M 1999 A osteopathic approach to asthma. Journal of the American Osteopathic Association 99(5):259–264

Rowe M, Alfred D 1999 Effectiveness of slow-stroke massage in diffusing agitated behaviours in individuals with Alzheimer's disease. Journal of Gerontology and Nursing 25:22–34

Rubin B et al 1990 Treatment options in fibromyalgia syndrome. Report. Journal of the American Osteopathic Association 90(9):844–845

Rupert R, McKinzie C, Monter M Jr et al 2005 Treatment of chronic nonresponsive patients with a non-force technique. Journal of Manipulative and Physiological Therapeutics 28(4):259–264

Santilli V, Beghi E, Finucci S 2006 Chiropractic manipulation in the treatment of acute back pain and sciatica with disc protrusion: a randomized double-blind clinical trial of active and simulated spinal manipulations. Spine 6:131–137

Sathyaprabha T, Murthy H, Murthy B 2001 Efficacy of naturopathy and yoga in bronchial asthma – a self controlled matched scientific study. Indian Journal of Physiology and Pharmacology 45(1):80–86

Sato A, Swenson R 1984 Sympathetic nervous system response to mechanical stress of the spinal column in rats. Journal of Manipulative and Physiological Therapeutics 7:141–147

Sawyer CE, Evans RL, Boline PD et al 1999 A feasibility study of chiropractic spinal manipulation versus sham spinal manipulation for chronic otitis media with effusion in children. Journal of Manipulative and Physiological Therapeutics 22(5):292–298

Sayar K, Arikan M, Yontem T 2002 Sleep quality in chronic pain patients. Canadian Journal of Psychiatry 47:844–848

Scholten-Peeters G, Verhagen A, Bekkering G et al 2003 Prognostic factors of whiplash associated disorders: a systematic review of prospective cohort studies. Pain 104:303–322

Schwartz H 1986 The use of counterstrain in an acutely ill in-hospital population. Journal of the American Osteopathic Association 86(7):433–442

Seguin R, Nelson M 2004 The benefits of strength training for older adults. American Journal of Preventive Medicine 25(3 Suppl 2):141–149

Selvamurthy W 1994 Yoga and stress management: physiological perspective. Indian Journal of Physiology and Pharmacology 38:46–47

Selye H 1946 The general adaptation syndrome and the diseases of adaptation. Journal of Clinical Endocrinology 6:117–230

Selye H 1971 Hormones and resistance. Journal of Pharmaceutical Sciences 60:1

Selye H 1976 Stress in health and disease. Butterworths, Reading, MA

Shambaugh P 1987 Changes in electrical activity in muscles resulting from chiropractic adjustment. Journal of Manipulative and Physiological Therapeutics 10:300–304

Shepherd C 2001 Pacing and exercise in chronic fatigue syndrome. Physiotherapy 87:395–396

Shetler K, Marcus R, Froelicher V et al 2001 Heart rate recovery: validation and methodologic issues. Journal of the American College of Cardiology 38:1980–1987

Shulman K, Jones G 1996 Effectiveness of massage therapy intervention on reducing anxiety in the work place. Journal of Applied Behavioral Science 32:160–173

Simons J, Travell J, Simons L 1999a Myofascial pain and dysfunction: the trigger point manual, vol 1: upper half of body, 2nd edn. Williams & Wilkins, Baltimore, p 829–830

Simons J, Travell J, Simons L 1999b Myofascial pain and dysfunction: the trigger point manual, vol 1: upper half of body, 2nd edn. Williams & Wilkins, Baltimore

Simons J, Travell J, Simons L 1999c Myofascial pain and dysfunction: the trigger point manual, vol 1: upper half of body, 2nd edn. Williams & Wilkins, Baltimore, p 941

Singh A 2006 Role of yoga therapies in psychosomatic disorders. International Congress Series 1287:91–96. Psychosomatic Medicine – Proceedings of the 18th World Congress on Psychosomatic Medicine, Kobe, Japan, August 21–26, 2005

Singh S, Malhotra V, Singh K et al 2004 Role of yoga in modifying certain cardiovascular functions in type 2 diabetic patients. Journal of the Association of Physicians of India 52:203–206

Sjaastad O, Saunte C, Hovdahl H et al 1983 'Cervicogenic' headache. An hypothesis. Cephalalgia 3(4):249–256

Sjaastad O, Fredriksen TA, Pfaffenrath V 1990 Cervicogenic headache: diagnostic criteria. Headache 301(1):725–726

Sjögren T, Nissinen K, Järvenpää S et al 2005 Effects of a workplace physical exercise intervention on the intensity of headache and neck and shoulder symptoms and upper extremity muscular strength of office workers: a cluster randomized controlled cross-over trial. Pain 116(1–2):119–128

Sonnenberg A, Koch T 1989 Physician visits in the United States for constipation: 1958–1986. Digestive Diseases and Sciences 34:606–611

Sorrell M, Flanagan W, McCall J 2003 The effect of depression and anxiety on the success of multidisciplinary treatment of chronic resistant myofascial pain. Journal of Musculoskeletal Pain 11(1):17–20

Spigelblatt L, Laîné-Ammara G, Pless IB, Guyver A 1994 The use of alternative medicine by children. Pediatrics 96:811–814

Squier R 1990 A model of empathic understanding and adherence to treatment regimens in practitioner–patient relationships. Social Science and Medicine 30(3):325–339

Sridevi K, Krishna-Rao P 1996 Yoga practice and menstrual distress. Journal of the Indian Academy of Applied Psychology 22:47–54

Stanford K, Mickleborough T, Ray S et al 2006 Influence of menstrual cycle phase on pulmonary function in asthmatic athletes. European Journal of Applied Physiology 96(6):703–710

Stathopoulou G, Powers M, Berry A et al 2006 Exercise interventions for mental health: a quantitative and qualitative review. Clinical Psychology: Science and Practice 13(2):179–193

Sterling M, Jull G, Wright A 2001 Cervical mobilisation: concurrent effects on pain, sympathetic nervous system activity and motor activity. Manual Therapy 6:72–78

Stewart M, Maher C, Refshauge K et al 2006 Randomized controlled trial of exercise for chronic whiplash-associated disorders. Pain 128(1–2):59–68

Stiles E 1976 Osteopathic manipulation in a hospital environment. Journal of the American Osteopathic Association 76:243–258

Stiles E 1977 Osteopathic manipulation in a hospital environment. Yearbook of the American Academy of Osteopathy, Colorado Springs, CO, p 18–19

Stoltz A 1993 Effects of OMT on the tender points of FMS. Report. Journal of the American Osteopathic Association 93(8):866

Stretanski M, Kaiser G 2001 Osteopathic philosophy and emergent treatment in acute respiratory failure. Journal of the American Osteopathic Association 101(8):447–449

Sukenik S, Baradin R, Codish S et al 2001 Balneotherapy at the Dead Sea area for patients with psoriatic arthritis and concomitant fibromyalgia. Israeli Medical Association Journal 3(2):147–150

Sung B et al 2000 Effectiveness of various relaxation techniques in lowering blood pressure associated with mental stress. American Journal of Hypertension 13(4 Suppl 1).S185

Sunshine W, Field T, Quintino O et al 1996 Fibromyalgia benefits from massage therapy and TENS. Journal of Clinical Rheumatology 2:18–22

Sydorchuk L, Tryniak M 2005 Effect of voluntary regulation of the respiration on the functional state of the autonomic nervous system. Lik Sprava 1–2:65–68

Szentivaneji A, Goldman A 1997 Vagotonia and bronchial asthma. Chest 111(1):8–11, 65–70

Tanaka S, Martin C, Thibodeau P 1998 Clinical neurology. In: Anrig C (ed) Pediatric chiropractic. Williams & Wilkins, Baltimore, p 608

Tanasescu M, Leitzmann M, Rimm E et al 2002 Exercise type and intensity in relation to coronary heart disease in men. Journal of the American Medical Association 288:1994–2000

Taneja I, Deepak K, Poojary G et al 2004 Yogic versus conventional treatment in diarrhea-predominant irritable bowel syndrome: a randomized control study. Applied Psychophysiology Biofeedback 29(1):19–33

Tanizak Y, Kitani H, Okazaki M et al 1993 Clinical effects of complex spa therapy on patients with steroid dependent intractable asthma (SDIA). Japanese Journal of Allergology 42(31):219–227

Telles S, Nagarathna R, Nagendra H 1994 Breathing through a particular nostril can alter metabolism and autonomic activities. Indian Journal of Physiology and Pharmacology 38(2):133–137

Thiele G 1937 Coccygodynia and pain in the superior gluteal region. Journal of the American Medical Association 109:271–1275

Thompson P, Crouse S, Goodpaster B et al 2001 The acute versus the chronic response to exercise. Medicine and Science in Sports and Exercise 33(Suppl 6): S438–S445

Thorpe R 1971 An analysis of the central nature of the musculoskeletal system in the development, function, design and biological ecology of homo sapiens. American Academy of Osteopathy Yearbook, Colorado Springs, CO, p 40–50

Tisp B, Burns M, Kro D 1986 Pursed lip breathing using ear oximetry. Chest 90:218–221

Tiukinhoy S, Beohar T, Hsie M 2003 Improvement in heart rate recovery after cardiac rehabilitation. Journal of Cardiopulmonary Rehabilitation 23:84–87

Tooley GA, Armstrong SM, Norman TR, Sali A 2000 Acute increases in night-time plasma melatonin levels following a period of meditation. Biological Psychology 53(1):69–78

Topol G, Reeves K, Hassanein K 2005 Efficacy of dextrose prolotherapy in elite male kicking sport athletes with chronic groin pain. Archives of Physical and Medical Rehabilitation 86:697–702

Triano J 2001 Biomechanics of spinal manipulative therapy. Spine 1(2):121–130

Tsai JC, Liu JC, Kao CC et al 2002 Beneficial effects on blood pressure and lipid profile of programmed exercise training in subjects with white coat hypertension. American Journal of Hypertension 15(6):571–576

Tsay S-L, Rong J-R, Lin P-F 2003 Acupoints massage in improving the quality of sleep and quality of life in patients with end-stage renal disease. Journal of Advanced Nursing 42(2):134–142

Tuchin PJ, Pollard H, Bonello R 2000 A randomized controlled trial of chiropractic spinal manipulative therapy for migraine. Journal of Manipulative and Physiological Therapeutics 23(2):91–95

UK Beam Trial Team 2004 United Kingdom back pain exercise and manipulation (UK BEAM) randomised trial: effectiveness of physical treatments for back pain in primary care. British Medical Journal 329:1381

Upledger J 1978 The relationship of craniosacral examination findings in grade school children with developmental problems. Journal of the American Osteopathic Association 77(10):760–776

Vallone S, Fallon J 1997 Treatment protocols for the chiropractic care of common pediatric conditions: otitis media and asthma. Journal of Clinical Chiropractic Pediatrics 2:113–115

Van Dieën J, Selen L, Cholewicki J 2003 Trunk muscle activation in low-back pain patients, an analysis of the literature. Journal of Electromyographic Kinesiology 13:333–351

Van Dixhoorn J, Duivenvoorden H 1985 Efficacy of Nijmegen questionnaire in recognition of the hyperventilation syndrome. Journal of Psychosomatic Research 29:199–206

Vansteenkiste J, Rochette F, Demedts M 1991 Diagnostic tests of hyperventilation syndrome. European Respiratory Journal 4:393–399

Vassiliou T, Kaluz G, Putzke C 2006 Physical therapy and active exercises – an adequate treatment for prevention of late whiplash syndrome? Randomized controlled trial in 200 patients. Pain 124:69–76

Verhagen AP, Bierma-Zeinstra SM, Cardoso JR et al 2003 Balneotherapy for rheumatoid arthritis. Cochrane Database of Systematic Reviews (4):CD000518

Verheul J, Dougherty M 1990 Stress urinary incontinence: effect of pelvic muscle exercise. Obstetrics and Gynecology 75:671–675

Verhoef M, Boon H, Mutasingwa D 2006 The scope of naturopathic medicine in Canada: an emerging profession. Social Science and Medicine 63(2):409–417

Vernon H, Dhami M, Howley T et al 1986 Spinal manipulation and beta-endorphin: a controlled study of the effect of a spinal manipulation on plasma beta-endorphin levels in normal males. Journal of Manipulative and Physiological Therapeutics 9:115–123

Vicenzino B, Collins D, Wright A 1996 The initial effects of a cervical spine manipulative physiotherapy treatment on the pain and dysfunction of lateral epicondylalgia. Pain 68:69–74

Vicenzino B, Collins D, Wright A 1998a Cardiovascular and respiratory changes produced by lateral glide mobilization of the cervical spine. Manual Therapy 3:67–71

Vicenzino B, Collins D, Benson H, Wright A 1998b An investigation of the interrelationship between manipulative therapy-induced hypoalgesia and sympathoexcitation. Journal of Manipulative and Physiological Therapeutics 21:448–453

Wagner T 1995 Irritable bowel syndrome and spinal manipulation. Chiropractic Technique 7:139–140

Walach H, Guthlin C, Konig M 2003 Efficacy of massage therapy in chronic pain – a pragmatic randomized trial. Journal of Alternative and Complementary Medicine 9:837–846

Walker J 1992 The sacroiliac joint: a critical review. Physical Therapy 72(12):903–916

Walsh M, Polus B 1998 A randomized placebo controlled clinical trial on the efficacy of chiropractic therapy on premenstrual syndrome. In: Proceedings of the International Conference on Spinal Manipulation, Vancouver, BC, July 16–19, 1998

Wells M, Giantonoto S, D'Agate D et al 1999 Standard osteopathic manipulative treatment acutely improves gait performance in patients with Parkinson's disease. Journal of the American Osteopathic Association 99(2):92–98

White P, Naish V 2001 Graded exercise therapy for chronic fatigue syndrome: an audit. Physiotherapy 87(6):285–288

Wikstrom S, Gunnarsson T, Nordin C 2003 Tactile stimulus and neurohormonal response: a pilot study. International Journal of Neuroscience 113:787–793

Wilson A 2002 Effective management of musculoskeletal injury. Churchill Livingstone, Edinburgh

Wilson K, Eriksson M, D'Eon J et al 2002 Major depression and insomnia in chronic pain. Clinical Journal of Pain 18:77–83

Wittink H, Michel T 2002 Chronic pain management for physical therapists, 2nd edn. Butterworth-Heinemann, Boston, p 80–83

Wolfe F 1986 The clinical syndrome of fibrositis. American Journal of Medicine 81:7–14

Wollin W, Lovell G 2006 Osteitis pubis in four young football players: a case series demonstrating successful rehabilitation. Physical Therapy in Sport 7:153–160

Wright D, Khan K, Gossage E et al 2001 Assessment of a low-intensity cardiac rehabilitation programme using the six-minute walk test. Clinical Rehabilitation 15:119–124

Wyke B 1975 Morphological and functional features of the innervation of the costovertebral joints. Folia Morphologica 23:296–305

Xi L 2002 Exercise does not protect the female heart: an unconvincing conclusion? Circulation Research 3:e2

Yates H, Vardy T, Kuchera M et al 2002 Effects of osteopathic manipulative treatment and concentric and eccentric maximal effort exercise on women with MS: a pilot study. Journal of the American Osteopathic Association 102(5):267–275

Yates RG, Lamping DL, Abram NL, Wright C 1988 Effects of chiropractic treatment on blood pressure and anxiety. A randomized controlled trial. Journal of Manipulative and Physiological Therapeutics 11:484–488

Ylinen J, Takala E-O, Nykänen M et al 2003 Active neck muscle training in the treatment of chronic neck pain in women. A randomized controlled trial. Journal of the American Medical Association 289(19):2509–2516

Yokota S, Mifune T, Mitsunobu F et al 1997 Psychological investigation on spa therapy in patients with bronchial asthma. Japanese Journal of Allergology 46(6):511–519

Youngstedt S, Perlis M, O'Brien P 2003 No association of sleep with total daily physical activity in normal sleepers. Physiology and Behavior 78(3):395–401

Yurtkuran M, Alp A, Yurtkuran M et al 2007 A modified yoga-based exercise program in hemodialysis patients: a randomized controlled study. Complementary Therapies in Medicine 15(3):164–171. Available online ScienceDirect 22 August 2006

Zernike W, Henderson A 1999 Evaluation of a constipation risk assessment scale. International Journal of Nursing Practice 5(2):106–109

Zhang J, Dean D, Nosco D et al 2006 Effect of chiropractic care on heart rate variability and pain in a multisite clinical study. Journal of Manipulative and Physiological Therapeutics 29(4):267–274

Zhu S, Wang N, Wang D et al 1998 A clinical investigation on massage for prevention and treatment of recurrent respiratory tract infection in children. Journal of Traditional Chinese Medicine 18(4):285–291

Zielhuis GA, Straatman H, Rach GH, van den Broek P 1990 Analysis and presentation of data on the natural course of otitis media in children. International Journal of Epidemiology 19:1037–1044

Zwart J 1997 Neck mobility in different headache disorders. Headache 37(1):6–11

11

Eric Blake ND

With contributions from:

Leon Chaitow ND DO

Douglas C. Lewis ND

Benjamin Lynch ND

Les Moore ND

Naturopathic Hydrotherapy

Naturopathic medical hydrotherapy is the application of water in any form, either externally or internally, for the treatment of disease and the maintenance of health, that is applied in accordance with the principles and practice of the naturopathic sciences. The modern field of hydrotherapy is sometimes referred to as medical hydrology. Balneology or balneotherapy is a branch of the science that studies baths and their therapeutic uses. Crenology or crenotherapy is the science and use of waters from mineral springs (Boyle & Saine 1988a). Today, we use the terms hydrotherapy and medical hydrology interchangeably, with medical hydrotherapy indicating all uses of water therapeutically (Bender 2006).

History of hydrotherapy in relation to naturopathy

Medical hydrology has a rich history. Water was used for healing in Biblical records and by the ancient Greeks and Romans. Hippocrates (460 BC), the father of systematic medicine, who practiced much as a 19th century naturopath would, applied water for healing, along with diet, exercise, manipulation and herbs. In his tract on the use of fluids he laid down rules for the treatment of acute and chronic diseases by water, which were followed by the hydropaths in the 19th century and which, together with subsequent developments, place hydrotherapy among orthodox and scientific methods of treatment. Galen (AD 129), Celsus (25 BC) and Asclepiades (100 BC) also used water therapeutically (Baruch 1892).

Asclepiades popularized balneology throughout Rome. He relied on diet, massage, exercise and baths for his marvelous cures and to build his medical reputation. Asclepiades was the philosophical founder of the school from which sprang Cornelius Celsus and Coelius Aurelianus (5th century AD). Cornelius Celsus, called the Latin Hippocrates, prescribed water freely in acute and chronic disease. Coelius Aurelianus was the originator of the abdominal compress for hypochondriacs. Galen was an able and judicious advocate of cold-water baths, and advised cold effusions upon the head while the body was immersed in warm water (Baruch 1892).

King Henry's Herbalists Charter points to the use of water in diseases in the 16th century. The charter firmly legitimized the populist herbal health movement in the Western world. It was frequently referred to by the early 20th century naturopathic profession as the common law that legalized naturopathic practice in the United States.

The modern history of medical hydrology begins with Floyer, an educated English physician who wrote a book on hydrotherapy, published in 1697, which passed through six editions and was translated into German 40 years later.

Vincent Priessnitz (1829), a Silesian peasant, did more to popularize hydropathy than any other single person. He is recognized as the progenitor of the 19th century nature cure and modern naturopathic movement. His success was great and he was known as a careful observer and a good judge of human nature, and his mechanical skill enabled him to invent various technical modifications of hydrotherapy, many of which are still in use today (Priessnitz 1843).

John Wesley, the founder of Methodism, wrote and published *Primitive Physick* (1747), a book of hydrotherapy and herbal and folk remedies. It was a bestseller and was reprinted 19 times during his lifetime. It is still available today. Many of these evangelists/ ministers were traveling preachers at night and itinerant doctors during the day, curing both the body and the soul.

Wilhelm Winternitz was a Viennese physician who wrote over 200 articles and books on hydrotherapy and trained hundreds of doctors and nurses in his techniques and treated thousands of patients. His scientific hydrotherapy techniques and approaches influenced both Simon Baruch and John Harvey Kellogg (Boyle & Saine 1988b).

Russell Thatcher Trall (1812–1877) was a very influential hydropathist of the mid-19th century when the first wave of hydrotherapy was coming into the United States. Trall had a water-cure sanitarium as early as 1844 in New York City. Trall wrote over 25 books and published the *Hydropathic Encyclopedia* in 1853 which influenced the entire hydropathic medical profession in America.

Dr Henry Foster founded Clifton Springs Water Cure Sanitarium in 1850 in Clifton Springs, New York. He had been trained as a physician at Case Western in Cleveland and had previously worked at New Grafenburg Sanitarium in Utica, New York, where he was also involved in the *Water-Cure Reporter*. Dr Foster combined allopathy (which was botanical medicine then), homeopathy, hydropathy, hygienic reforms, dietary therapy, mental therapy, and pastoral and spiritual care all under the same roof, being one of our first models of integrative medicine. His hospital, Clifton Springs Hospital, still exists today, and was the first place to offer pastoral and spiritual care on a full-time basis with a chaplain available full time; the first place to have an open-floor psychiatric ward (where the term sanitarium became associated with mental health); the second place in the country to have an x-ray machine (quite progressive); and the place where the American Occupational Medicine Association began (Adams 1921).

Dr Foster employed Cordelia Greene as a hydropathic physician in 1853. This was the first female physician to work in a hospital setting. She spent 6 years working with Dr Foster as his right-hand person until, at the bequest of her brother, she came to run her father's water cure sanitarium in Castile, New York. She treated Susan B. Anthony at Clifton Springs and was instrumental in providing the first donation to the women's rights movement. She wrote three books and was considered by Spitler in *Basic Naturopathy* (1948) as one of the pillars of naturopathy and one of three people responsible for the natural medicine movement in the United States.

James Caleb Jackson ran a colorful water cure sanitarium in Dansville, New York. In 1874 he wrote *How to Treat the Sick Without Medicine* and believed that hydrotherapy was most effective when used with fresh air, simple foods, water, sunlight, dress, exercise, sleep, rest, social influence and mental and moral forces in a system he termed 'Psycho-Hygienic'. He was the first one to prepare, box and sell dry cereal to be used, which he called granula. The sanitarium was eventually purchased by the famous naturopath and founder of physcultopathy, Bernarr Macfadden.

Simon Baruch is considered by some as the 'Father of Scientific Hydrotherapy' and considered himself a balneologist. He taught, practiced and conducted research on hydrotherapy in New York, practicing at Saratoga Springs. He wrote *The Principles and Practice of Hydrotherapy* (1898) and *An Epitome of Hydrotherapy* (1920). He was, however, firmly opposed to the populist nature cure movement and criticized his medical colleagues for neglecting the field and allowing nonmedical practitioners to dominate the field.

The 'nature cure' was born from the larger 'wasser kur' or 'water cure' movements of the 19th century. For example, Russell Trall MD had used the term 'naturepathy' in the *Water Cure Journal* published in the 1850s. Sebastian Kneipp trained several early leaders of naturopathy, including Benedict Lust and Henry Lindlahr. Sebastian Kneipp was the most famous nature doctor of the time, treating emperors, popes, archdukes and tens of thousands of patients. His book *My Water Cure* (1894) was a bestseller and was translated into numerous languages. His brand of hydrotherapy was combined with diet, exercise, botanical medicine and massage.

O.G. Carroll ND SP developed the system of constitutional hydrotherapy in the first half of the 20th century. He systematically combined various electrotherapy treatments with a refined approach to hydrotherapy. Dr Carroll was first treated and then trained by the New Orleans physician Dr Ledoux, who had in turn been taught by Father Kneipp. Dr Carroll also collaborated with Dr Lindlahr when living in the Chicago area. He was encouraged to move to the Western United States and establish a school.

O.G. Carroll did establish a very large clinical practice in Spokane, Washington, and instead of a physical school, he developed what eventually became a 'school of naturopathic medicine'. While the school of practice centered about clinical 'constitutional hydrotherapy' treatments, it also included dietetics, herbal therapeutics, spinal adjustment and Schussler tissue salts. Combining electrophysiotherapy with the Kneipp understanding of hydrotherapy, a new clinical approach to hydrotherapy evolved. He also developed the food intolerance test based on work developed by Albert Abrams MD (Boyle & Saine 1988c).

Dr Carroll trained many other doctors in the mid-20th century, including Dr Bastyr. He trained three other Spokane doctors – his son Dr Carroll, Dr Leo Scott and Dr Harold Dick. The latter two also opened constitutional hydrotherapy treatment clinics in Spokane. These doctors carried this clinical knowledge to the resurgent US naturopathic profession in the latter half of the 20th century. It continues to be taught, practiced and developed in naturopathic colleges as a relevant approach to whole-body constitutional naturopathic physical medicine clinical practice. Constitutional hydrotherapy will be described in more detail later in this chapter as a representative example of the evolution of a modern clinical naturopathic method that employs a constitutional approach.

Physiological responses to hydrotherapy application

Water is universally required for life and health. Water also has unique physical properties which render it a valuable therapeutic agent. Understanding water and its physical characteristics is necessary to effectively apply it as an agent of healing.

Water has unique properties by which it can beneficially affect the body and aid in the prevention and recovery of disease. These unique properties are:

1. the ability of water to communicate and absorb large quantities of heat by contact (specific heat and latent heat)
2. the intensity of temperature impressions obtained by the use of water
3. the fluidity of water, rendering it efficient in applying mechanical stimuli
4. its properties as a solvent and its use in nutritive changes such as improved assimilation and elimination (Abbott 1915a).

It is generally conceded that it is the action of the thermic impression of water that principally produces the therapeutic effect when it is applied to the body. Water has great heat-conveying properties and when used in accordance with naturopathic principles definite and specific results are to be obtained from it (Boyle & Saine 1988d).

Thermic impressions

Whenever a substance whose temperature differs from that of the skin comes into contact with the skin, in the presence of normally functioning temperature receptors in the skin, the impressions of heat or cold are perceived and adapted to rapidly (Moor et al 1964). Nerve transmission impulse is controlled by the sympathetic vasoconstrictor nerve fibers that secrete norepinephrine, with sensitivity due in part to spinal cord reflexes (Prentice 1998) or the sympathetic constriction influences are mediated chemically through neural transmitters, with both norepinephrine and epinephrine involved (Guyton 1991). Water seems hotter or colder than other substances because it stores so much heat and gives it off readily (Giancoli 1995a).

This makes water a most valuable means of applying thermic stimuli to the body (Giancoli 1995b).

Heat is transferred to the body superficially in hydrotherapy primarily by conduction and convection.

- *Conduction* occurs when two or more adjacent bodies (objects) of different temperature are placed in contact and a state of energy exchange affects portions of each. Heat is transferred from the warmer to the cooler body by the process of conduction. The rate of heat exchange depends upon the different properties in heat conductivity of each medium, the difference in temperature of the adjacent bodies, and the length of time the process is allowed to continue. Hot packs, wet packs, hot compresses and fomentations are examples of conductive heating modalities.
- *Convection* involves the exchange of heat between a surface and a fluid (can be liquid or gas; e.g. sauna) moving over that surface. Mineral baths, whirlpool baths, saunas and Hubbard tanks are examples of hydrotherapeutic applications of convection heat (Krusen 1971).

Physical effects of heating

Heat causes a rise in temperature (hyperthermia) in the tissues to which it is applied. The results of this thermal effect vary in proportion to the degree of heat, the duration the heat is applied, the speed in which the thermal effects are dispersed, and the type or source of heat.

Care should always be taken in the application of heat to the body. Heat should never be applied above patient tolerance or in situations where the patient doesn't have the ability to identify or communicate the amount of heat applied, such as with peripheral neuropathy in diabetes or the inability to communicate. It takes time for heat applied via hydrotherapy to penetrate into the body. It takes approximately 30 minutes for the skin temperature to rise from 90 to 110°F (32–43°C), approximately 40 minutes for subcutaneous tissue to rise from 94.2 to 105.5°F (34.5–40.8°C), and approximately 50 minutes for intramuscular temperature to rise from 94.2 to 99.6°F (34.6–37.6°C) (Schafer 1982). A common therapeutic range for heat modalities is from 100 to 115°F, depending on the patient's tolerance level. The maximum safe exposure time for applying heat at 113°F (45°C) at close contact is 30 minutes, although temperatures as low as 107.6°F (42°C) left on for several hours can cause thermal damage (Krusen 1971).

The application of heat initiates a transient vasoconstriction in the circulatory system that is followed by a secondary and sustained hyperemia through vasodilation. Heat will increase the blood flow to and from the area being treated, and initially increases metabolism within the treated area. Heat applied longer than 7 minutes exhausts the vasoconstrictor reflex and leads to vasostasis. This may lead to edema, local congestion and reduced metabolism (Guyton 1996). Care should be taken to avoid increased edema and congestion (Jaskoviak & Schafer 1993a).

Local heat promotes activity of the sweat glands, which may help to promote elimination of toxic wastes. Local heat may also increase the threshold of cutaneous sensory receptors, through enkephalin production, although it is a minor pain control method. Heat also relaxes some patients and the psychological effect can also be noted.

Physical effects of cold application

Cold application initially causes skin vasoconstriction, and if a cold compress covers a large area of the body, a significant amount of blood will be driven into the internal organs. Prolonged cold causes a secondary reaction, inducing vasodilation of the surface skin blood vessels. The time required to qualify as 'prolonged cold' will vary, dependent upon method of application. *This secondary effect, referred to as a reaction, is of significant therapeutic importance in naturopathic hydrotherapy.* Extending the cold application longer will lead to prolonged vasoconstriction and diminished circulation, which is generally avoided in naturopathic hydrotherapy applications. The reaction, or dynamic circulatory response in response to physiological stress, is analogous to the adaptive response of the body to physical exercise. It is a culmination of neurological vasomotor activity mediated via the smooth muscles embedded within the circulatory system. The method of cold water application in naturopathic hydrotherapy, particularly the cold wet pack, exercises this neuromuscular response over time with a constitutional benefit to the organism (Boyle 1988).

Hydrostatic effect on circulation

The hydrostatic effect in hydrotherapy is the shifting of fluid from one part of the body to another. The hydrostatic effect can be used clinically in the treatment of conditions in which it is suspected that there is a locally congested area which is giving rise to symptoms, such as congestive headache, nasal congestion, sinusitis and pulmonary congestion. Derivation, or dilation of the blood vessels of the skin at some area distal and inferior to the area affected, can be effective in relieving congested tissues. This happens because, when a large area of the body is exposed to heat, vasodilation of the skin takes place, which is the body's method of eliminating heat. This process causes a quantity of blood to shift from the interior of the body to the superficial.

Principles of thermic impression

Thermic applications and their influence on circulation and metabolism have been categorized in the following way by naturopaths:

- *Short hot* <5 minutes: Local vasodilation mediated via vasomotors, resulting in increased local circulation and local tissue metabolism
- *Long hot* >5 minutes: Vasodilation becomes vasostasis (*due to vasomotor decompensation*) and local circulation is decreased while local metabolism continues to increase
- *Short cold* <5 minutes: Vasoconstriction followed by active, pulsating dilation, increasing local circulation and local metabolism (note the similar tissue effects of short heat)
- *Long cold* >5 minutes: Vasoconstriction as a protective adaptive effect and depression of metabolism and circulation.

	Circulation	Metabolism
Short hot	↑	↑
Long hot	↓	↑
Short cold	↑	↑
Long cold	↓	↓

These principles of time and temperature effect are assuming no net change in the water temperature during their period of application and *do not take into account convection or conduction*. For example, a bath applied for more than 5 minutes, where the temperature of the water for all purposes remains the same, would be considered a long hot or long cold depending upon the bath temperature. The application of a cold wet pack (Priessnitz/Kneipp/Lindlahr/Carroll method) beyond 5 minutes does not become a long cold application because of the conductive transfer of heat as evidenced in the warming of the cotton towel (Boyle 1988). The wet pack is therefore considered a short cold application. Combination of short hot and short cold (such as contrast hydrotherapy or the towel treatment portion of the constitutional hydrotherapy method) has beneficial additive effects (Abbott et al 1945a) (see Figs 11.1 and 11.2).

Hematological composition and hydrotherapy

The composition of the blood is also affected by hydrotherapy. There is a significant increase in all blood cells in the peripheral circulation following a variety of cold hydrotherapy procedures associated with mechanical stimulation (friction) and after hot applications when followed by cold applications. There is often an increase in peripheral circulation of red blood cells from 20 to 35% and in white blood cells from 200 to 300%. Hemoglobin also shows an increase of 10% or more (see Fig. 11.2).

Local effects of contrast hydrotherapy

Contrast hydrotherapy, or local alternating hot and cold, produces marked stimulation of local circulation. Cold needs to be only long enough to produce vasoconstriction, which has been shown to occur in as little as 20 seconds. Contrasting hydrotherapy is an extremely clinically useful hydrotherapy procedure because of its marked stimulation of local blood flow (Boyle 1988).

Classification of hydrotherapy applications

Naturopathic hydrotherapy applications are commonly classified according to technique, temperature, medication and area of application. Classifying the almost infinite variety of treatments available with hydrotherapy, due to the plasticity of water, is well served through such a schematic approach. The various parameters can then be combined based upon condition, part affected, physiological impression desired, reflex effects, etc. These combinations can then be grouped practically for their therapeutic effects such as peptogenic, diuretic, tonic, stimulant, etc.

Technique of application

- *Ablutions* are the application of water to the body with the hands. A light rubbing technique accompanies.
- *Affusions* are the application of water in the form of a gentle pouring. Father Kneipp developed a whole series of affusions using a simple garden watering can.
- *Douches* are the application of falling water at a higher velocity than the affusion so that mechanical pressure effects are also elicited. The Kneipp and the Scott douche are examples of this approach.
- *Showers* are the application of falling water at an intermediate velocity compared to the affusion (negligible velocity) and the douche (high velocity).
- *Sprays* involve the addition of a diffuser head to an affusion, shower or douche.

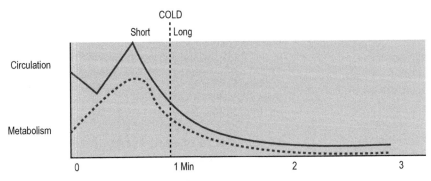

Short cold stimulates and long cold depresses both the circulation and metabolism as reflected by the basically parallel curves in the above graph

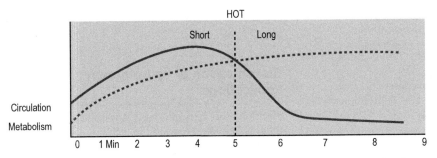

A short hot application stimulates the circulation and metabolism similarly, but if the heat is prolonged, the circulation is depressed to a point which may not be able to adequately support the increased metabolism

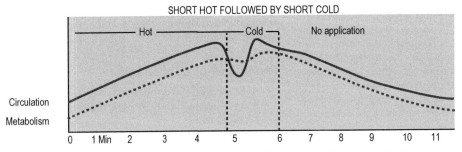

Short hot followed by short cold yields no significant depressive phase for either the circulation or the metabolism. Note the heightened metabolism and circulation is maintained well after such a treatment is terminated

Figure 11.1 Time and temperature influence on metabolism and circulation. Redrawn from Boyle & Saine (1988)

- *Wet packs* are the application of cool to cold wet toweling surrounded by an insulating layer such as wool or vellux.
- *Fomentations* are the application of warm to hot wet toweling surrounded by an insulating layer such as wool or vellux.

- Wet packs and fomentations are also commonly referred to as *compresses*.
- *Baths* are the submersion of some part of the body in water of various temperatures.
- *Steam vapors* are the exposure of some part or all of the body to steam.

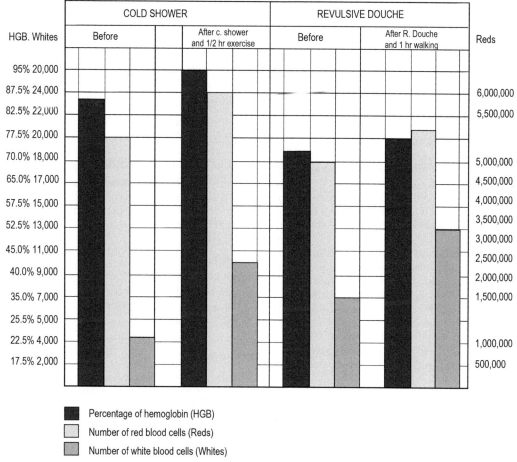

| HGB. Whites | COLD SHOWER | | | | REVULSIVE DOUCHE | | | | Reds |
| | Before | | | After c. shower and 1/2 hr exercise | Before | | | After R. Douche and 1 hr walking | |

Figure 11.2 Peripheral blood values after a short hot followed by a short cold application. Redrawn from Abbott et al (1945a)

Legend:
- Percentage of hemoglobin (HGB)
- Number of red blood cells (Reds)
- Number of white blood cells (Whites)

Left axis (HGB. Whites): 95% 20,000 / 87.5% 24,000 / 82.5% 22,000 / 77.5% 20,000 / 70.0% 18,000 / 65.0% 17,000 / 57.5% 15,000 / 52.5% 13,000 / 45.0% 11,000 / 40.0% 9,000 / 35.0% 7,000 / 25.5% 5,000 / 22.5% 4,000 / 17.5% 2,000

Right axis (Reds): 6,000,000 / 5,500,000 / 5,000,000 / 4,500,000 / 4,000,000 / 3,500,000 / 3,000,000 / 2,500,000 / 2,000,000 / 1,500,000 / 1,000,000 / 500,000

Temperature classifications

Temperature classifications can be made according to the following useful categories:

- *Hot*: above 104°F (40°C)
- *Warm*: 99–104°F (37.2–40°C)
- *Neutral*: 93–99°F (33.9–37.2°C)
- *Tepid*: 70–93°F (21.1–33.9°C)
- *Cold*: 40–70°F (4.4–21.1°C).

Contrast alternating, or *revulsive* is the application of alternating temperature combinations.

Medicated applications

Certain applications such as baths, fomentations and packs lend themselves to the delivery of medications through the skin – for example, Nauheim baths, Epsom baths, herbal fomentations, etc.

Area of application

- Whole body
- Face
- Neck
- Shoulder
- Elbow
- Arm
- Hand
- Chest
- Abdomen
- Back
- Spine
- Sitz
- Hip
- Leg
- Foot

Practical effects of hydrotherapeutic applications

There are two general classes of effect produced by hydrotherapeutic applications: tonic and stimulant, and depressant and sedative (Scott 1990).

Tonic and *stimulant* effects yield a strengthening (tonic) or increase (stimulant) of vital activity and metabolism. They are similar, but differ in degree. The intensity of the effect will be greater or less according to the intensity of the hydrotherapy application. A very brief intense application stimulates, while one less intense and of longer duration may produce tonic effects *if a reaction is obtained*.

Depressant and *sedative* effects are due to a decrease of vital activity. They also differ as to the extent of the decrease, with a depressant being more intense than a sedative.

Not only does hydrotherapy change the cellular composition of the blood but also it changes the chemical reaction of the blood. Blood is normally alkaline, but during diseases, infections, fevers, etc., this alkalinity is decreased (though the blood never becomes acid) due to the accumulation of acid waste products which partially neutralize the normal alkalinity. The *reaction* obtained through cold applications *increases* the alkalinity of the blood, restoring it to normal by oxidation of waste products.

Tonics and stimulants

Stimulant treatments bring forth energy that the body is unable to replace while a tonic makes the body better able to perform its usual work. An analogous relationship is found in phytotherapy in comparison of stimulants (such as coffee) and tonic adaptogens (such as *Eleuthrococcus senticoccus*).

Hydrotherapeutic tonics are mild in action and heighten body functions within normal limits. Their after-effects improve adaptive processes of the body. Tonic effects are derived mainly from cold applications or alternate hot and cold applications. Tonic hydrotherapy techniques increase the speed and force of circulation, increase muscular activity, heighten nerve sensitivity, improve immune function and increase heat production. Tonic hydrotherapeutic measures can be used in practically all diseases, but are particularly indicated for anemia, fatigue, digestive disorders, insomnia, arthritis, obesity and flaccid paralysis.

Abbott (1915a) lists the hydrotherapeutic tonic treatments in order of their intensity as follows:

- Wet hand rub
- Cold mitten friction
- Cold towel rub
- Salt glow
- Pail pour
- Cold douche
- Wet sheet rub
- Dripping sheet rub
- Shallow bath
- Cold plunge.

The towel treatment of constitutional hydrotherapy should also be classified as a tonic treatment.

Sedative effects of hydrotherapy

Hydrotherapy can also be used to bring about a sedative effect. A sedative effect was classically referred to as a nerve sedative in hydrotherapeutic literature. The principal hydrotherapy sedatives as classified by Abbott (1915a) are:

- cold sitz bath
- hot foot bath with cold to the head
- alternate hot and cold foot bath
- neutral or warm bath (94–98°F/34.4–36.7°C)
- neutral wet sheet pack
- sponge baths (cool, tepid or warm)
- warm or hot shower, spray, douche or affusion.

Pure sedative techniques are indicated in nervous disorders, mania, chorea, insomnia, spasticity, spinal paralysis and epilepsy.

Expectorant effects

Naturopathic hydrotherapy can be used to induce expectoration. Hydrotherapy can have a beneficial effect upon the respiratory tract and increase the flow and secretion of mucus, generally resulting in decreased cough and pain. In order to increase the flow of mucous secretions during a respiratory tract infection and relieve the symptoms, generally hot, moist applications are used. Hot, moist applications will generally increase mucous secretions, improve breathing and decrease pain. These may be steam inhalations, fomentations to the chest and throat, hot water drinking, or sweating hydrotherapeutic techniques. The wet packs applied so successfully by naturopaths in the 1918 flu epidemic take advantage of the rewarming process of the packs to achieve this effect, simultaneously yielding a dynamic circulatory reaction. The towel portion of the constitutional hydrotherapy further combines the wet pack with a preceding warm compress and will be found very effective in respiratory infections, particularly in combination with diathermy and high frequency. Once the symptoms have been relieved, mild tonic hydrotherapy techniques such as the cold mitten friction or wet hand rub can be employed.

Diaphoretic effects

Diaphoresis (sweating) can be induced by naturopathic hydrotherapy techniques. Diaphoretic hydrotherapy techniques increase perspiration, increase catabolic changes, relieve internal congestion, improve the nutrition of the skin, increase elimination of toxins directly through the skin and indirectly through the kidneys, and prepare the patient for cold treatment. Such treatments can be used for colds and congestion, obesity, gout and other metabolic diseases. The chief naturopathic hydrotherapy techniques to induce diaphoresis are Russian bath, full hot tub bath, hot blanket pack, heating wet sheet pack, hot foot bath, hot sitz bath, Turkish bath, fomentations to the spine, hot water drinking and heliotherapy (sun bath) (Abbott et al 1945b).

Excessively hot systemic applications used to induce diaphoresis – as in fever therapy – *do not follow the general principles of thermic impression* previously outlined because the temperature input is so great that it stimulates total metabolism of the organism.

Clinical observations of systemically applied heat are as follows:

1. *Tachycardia*: Increased circulation created by applications of heat has an effect on pulse rate. For every 1°F of temperature increase, there is generally a rise in the pulse rate of approximately 10 beats. This is often observed when noting the pulse rate during febrile episodes.
2. *Hypotension*: Blood pressure gradually lowers as more blood flows from the central venous system toward the body part being treated with heat.
3. *Increased oxidation*: The rate of oxidation is increased two to three times for every temperature rise of 18°F (Van't-Hoff Law) (Abramson et al 1964). Even slight increases in temperature can have a profound effect on cellular oxidates and on systemic physiology. Hydrotherapy, which can increase temperature by about 8°F, substantially affects oxidation, membrane permeability and metabolic activity (Abramson et al 1961).
4. *Tachypnea*: The respiratory rate increases in response to the above factors.
5. *Alkalemia*: Heat slightly increases alkalinity in the blood of the treated area.
6. *Polyuria*: Heat triggers an increase in urine formation, with its constituent water, urea, nitrogenous waste and salts.
7. *Increased plasma blood volume and oxygen consumption*: When a patient is treated within heated water, increased plasma blood volume and oxygen consumption occur because there is no fluid loss due to perspiration evaporation (Jaskoviak & Schafer 1993b).

Diuretic effects

Diuretic effects are indicated in decreased kidney function, uremia, toxicity, colds, nephritis and gout. The hydrotherapy techniques that increase diuresis are hot fomentations to the lumbar spine, heating trunk pack, full warm tub bath, Russian bath and full hot blanket pack. Clinical laboratory observations of the influence of constitutional hydrotherapy towel treatments on improving kidney function are detailed in the section on treatment description.

Peptogenic effects

Naturopathic hydrotherapy also has a direct peptogenic effect, increasing the function of the digestive system. Tonic effects in general will increase the muscular and glandular activity of the stomach and intestines and liver, but a specific peptogenic effect upon the digestive organs and functions causing an increase in digestive activity can be induced by naturopathic hydrotherapy. Peptogenic effects are indicated in atonic indigestion, chronic congestion of the liver, hypochloridia, gastric prolapse, decreased gastric motility and hyperacidity. The hydrotherapeutic techniques indicated are fomentations to the abdomen, hot trunk pack (Winternitz pack), hot and cold to the spine, hot and cold douche to the abdomen, liver or spine, or constitutional hydrotherapy.

Reflex effects of external hydrotherapy application

Virtually every part of the body may be influenced by hydrotherapeutic applications to the skin surface. The skin has at times been referred to as the 'peripheral heart' (Abbott 1915b) and the 'third kidney' (Jensen 1946) due to its ability to improve circulation and assist in detoxification.

The epidermis of the skin contains both nerves and blood vessels. The connective tissue of the dermis contains smooth muscles in connection with hair follicles, which, when contracted, move the blood out of the vessels. Since the capillary blood vessels do not possess a muscular coat, the muscles of the skin help to perform the work for the capillaries that the muscular coat performs in the larger blood vessels. The venules of the skin are much wider and are capable of holding much more blood than the arterioles. The skin blood vessels are a reservoir capable of holding

30% of the total blood volume (Thrash & Thrash 1981a).

The skin also contains an enormous network of lymphatic vessels, and the application of hydrotherapy to the skin can stimulate the lymph that bathes each cell to move nutrients to cells and wastes towards elimination from the body (Starkey 1999) as well as enhance the immune status of the body (Thrash & Thrash 1981b).

Circulation-reflex effects

It has been postulated that the neurological connections of the sympathetic ganglia, and the efferent sympathetic nerves connected to blood vessels of internal organs and muscles and glands, allows for functions of the body to be tonified, stimulated or depressed by influences arising in the skin. When a hydrotherapeutic application to the skin affects a body part through nerve connection, it produces a reflex effect. A reflex effect is an indirect effect that produces activity at a location distal to the application site via neurological pathways (Dittmar 1960).

Beginning with the skin, stimulation produced by heat or cold is conveyed to the spinal cord by sensory nerves. The impulse is conveyed upward or downward in the spinal cord to various levels by these sensory nerves, which also communicate with cells in the spinal cord that provide spinal level and ascending influence over internal organ function. These impulses pass over nerves that enter the chain of sympathetic ganglia, and pass with the sympathetic nerves to the internal organs. These efferent sympathetic nerves are connected not only with the blood vessels of the internal organs but also with their muscles and glands. Because of these connections, it has been proposed that every function of the body may be stimulated or depressed by influences arising in the skin. When an application to the skin affects a part of the body through nerve connection, it produces a reflex effect. A reflex effect is an indirect effect produced through nerve connection (Engel et al 1950). More research is required to clarify and more completely document these observations.

The following are examples of reflex areas employed in hydrotherapy (Fig. 11.3):

- The back of the neck is reflexively related with the mucous membrane of the nose.
- The skin areas of the face, scalp and back of the neck are reflexively related with the brain. (Treatment of hemorrhage or congestion of the mucous membranes of the nasopharynx, or swelling or congestion of the cranial tissues, are therefore affected through applications to the back of the neck.)
- The lower lumbar and sacral spine, with the pelvic organs (uterus, ovaries, bladder and rectum). (Treatment of the lumbar and sacral spine will therefore affect the pelvic organs.)

Reflex effects of short cold applications

Short cold applications to a reflex area produce tonic and stimulating effects in the deep part by virtue of the reaction which soon follows.

- Short, intense cold (as brief as 30 seconds) will cause a general peripheral vasoconstriction.
- Short cold applications to the face and head stimulate mental activity and alertness.
- A short cold application to the chest, as a cold rub, friction or cold douche, at first increases the respiration rate. It soon results in deeper respiration with a somewhat slowed rate.
- A very short cold percussion douche to a reflex area causes active dilation of the blood vessels in the related viscera. For example, a short cold percussion douche to the sacrum or feet causes a dilation of the vessels of the uterus (Abbott et al 1945b).
- A short very cold douche to the liver causes active dilation of its vessels, and increases its activity.

Reflex effects of hot applications

- Prolonged hot application to a reflex area produces passive vasodilation of the related organ.
- Prolonged heat to one extremity causes vasodilation in the contralateral extremity.
- Hot, moist applications to the chest facilitate respiration and expectoration.
- Prolonged hot applications to the abdomen lessen peristalsis, decrease intestinal blood flow, diminish intestinal motility and decrease secretion of stomach acid (Fischer & Solomon 1958).
- A large hot application to the trunk, as a hot trunk pack in biliary or renal colic, relaxes the muscles of the bile ducts, gall bladder or ureters, and aids in relieving the pain due to spasm.

Selected clinical hydrotherapy research

Laboratory and clinical research on hydrotherapy has been ongoing for well over 150 years. Awareness of the current terminology for the terms hydrotherapy, balneotherapy and spa therapy are useful for proper interpretation of the literature.

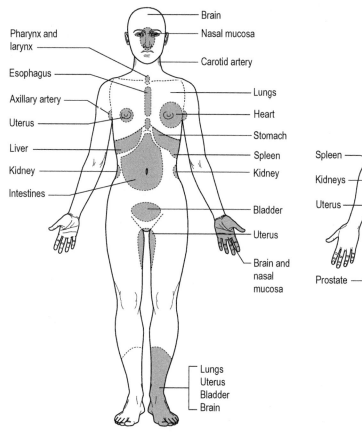

Reflex areas of the skin (Anterior)

Reflex areas of the skin (Posterior)

Figure 11.3 Reflex areas of the skin

- Hydrotherapy generally refers to plumbed water applied at various temperatures, aquatic therapy, and therapeutic rehabilitation methods.
- Balneotherapy is the therapeutic use of bathing agents such as mineral and thermal waters, muds and gases.
- Spa therapy combines hydrotherapy, balneotherapy and drinking cures in an inpatient setting.

The naturopathic professional literature of the 20th century has utilized a slightly different classification:

- Hydrotherapy is the use of water in all its forms.
- Baths and mud packs are considered one of the branches of hydrotherapy.
- Sanitarium care describes comprehensive inpatient care that would include various hydrotherapy methods.

Hydrotherapy systematic review

Geytenbeek (2002) conducted a systematic review using 10 medical and allied health databases from which studies relevant to hydrotherapy as used in physiotherapy practice were retrieved. The trials were critically appraised for research merit using recognized published guidelines and the results were collated into clinical, functional and affective outcomes. *Results*: 17 randomized controlled trials, 2 case-control studies, 12 cohort studies and 2 case reports were included in the appraisal. Two trials achieved appraisal scores indicating high-quality evidence in a subjectively evaluated merit categorization; 15 studies were deemed to provide moderate quality evidence for the effectiveness of hydrotherapy. *Discussion*: Flaws in study design and reporting attenuated the strength of the research evidence. Recommendations were made for the future direction of clinical hydrotherapy research. Randomized controlled trials with larger sample sizes, assessor blinding and the use of validated and reliable outcome measures in subjects with neurological conditions and acute orthopedic injuries are particularly required. *Conclusion*: The balance of high- to moderate-quality evidence supported benefit from hydrotherapy in pain, function, self-efficacy and affect, joint mobility, strength and balance, particularly among older adults, subjects with rheumatic conditions and chronic low back pain.

Hydrotherapy, immune function and the common cold

Taking a cold shower regularly has been shown to improve immune function quite dramatically, over a period of months. German research (Ernst 1990) showed that the regular (daily) use of a cold shower had a progressively beneficial effect on immune system efficiency. Medical students were divided into two groups. For 6 months one group took a graduated cold shower (i.e. ending a hot shower with a brief cold shower application, increasing the length of the cold application to tolerance up to 2 minutes). The other group took a warm or hot shower.

After 6 months those taking the cold shower were found to be having half the number of colds compared with those having warm showers. The cold shower group's colds lasted for approximately half as long as those having warm showers, and were accompanied by far less mucus production (measured by weighing the used paper handkerchiefs of cold sufferers). Cold showers were avoided during, and for 1 week after, experiencing a cold. The various protective benefits did not become apparent until almost 3 months of regular cold showering (see Fig. 11.2 for the basic science observations that provide insight to account for this phenomenon).

Hydrotherapy and fibromyalgia

A Brazilian study (Vitorino 2006) compared the treatment effects of hydrotherapy versus physiotherapy on fibromyalgia syndrome (FMS). Fifty female outpatients were divided into two groups. After 3 weeks of treatment, the hydrotherapy group improved total sleep time and decreased total nap time as compared to the subjects receiving physiotherapy. There was no difference reported in quality of life (both improved). *Note*: The form of hydrotherapy was not reported.

Aquatic therapy and fibromyalgia

Swedish research evaluated the effects on FMS of 6 months of pool exercise combined with six sessions of education (Mannerkorpi et al 2000). Fifty-eight individuals were randomized to a treatment and a control group. Those in the treatment group were advised to 'match the pool exercise to their threshold of pain and fatigue'. The educational component comprised discussion of coping strategies and encouragement to physical activity. The outcome was that significant differences were observed and noted on the Fibromyalgia Impact Questionnaire and the 6-minute walk test. There were also improvements in the treatment group, to a significant degree, in physical function, grip strength, pain severity, social functioning, psychological distress and quality of life.

A follow-up study to the one above was done at 24 months. Symptom severity, physical and social function parameters were still improved at 24 months.

Hydrotherapy and cardiovascular health

Treatment of cardiovascular disease and dysfunction by means of hydrotherapy has a long tradition.

Kneipp (1979; first published in 1893) described his treatment of a young man with 'head and heart complaints' as follows:

Every morning the young gentleman walked for half an hour in the wet dewy grass, and daily stood in the water up to the pit of his stomach, with a lavation of the upper body . . . later on, by way of strengthening, he received frequent upper affusions daily, one or two, in alternation with semi-baths. Head and heart complaints soon vanished with the gradual increase of his general strength.

Over 100 years later researchers in Germany evaluated Kneipp's empirical approach. They explain:

*In central-European physical therapy, warm-water baths and sauna are commonly supplemented by repeated cold water stimuli with peripheral cold water immersions and cold water pourings (hydrotherapy according to Kneipp) (Bühring 1988). Serial hydrotherapeutic cold- and warm-water applications are also used as a supportive treatment for patients with coronary artery disease and patients with CHF in cardiological rehabilitative facilities. The beneficial effects of hydrotherapy in patients with chronic heart failure (CHF), hypertension, and coronary artery disease have been described in some empirical and observational reports (Brüggemann 1986, Gutenbrunner & Ruppel 1992). However, its efficacy has never been tested in controlled trials. **The current study was designed to test whether a specific and intensive home-based hydrotherapeutic treatment program, consisting of a structured combination of warm and cold thermal applications, can induce improvements** *in exercise performance, quality of life (QOL), and heart-failure-related symptoms in patients with mild CHF.*

The home-based hydrotherapy is described as follows:

Patients were advised to practice warm and cold applications at least three times a day to a total maximum of 30 minutes daily. Warm thermal applications consisted of peripheral warm water baths (arm baths, foot baths) with incremental temperature (maximum 40°C) and warm sheet packs. For cold applications, short-term arm or foot baths and peripheral water pourings with a water temperature below 18°C were taught. Patients were instructed to apply the hydrotherapeutic applications long enough to induce a postprocedural reactive feeling of warmth with respective mild redness of the treated skin area, but no longer than 15 minutes for baths and 5 minutes for cold pourings.

After the 6-week study the researchers noted:

Our findings imply that an appropriately performed home-based hydrotherapeutic program may provide a practical, salutary, nonpharmacological therapy for patients with CHF without the need for expensive rehabilitation facilities. Furthermore, this therapy approach may be applicable in patients who are unable to participate in exercise training. We conclude that a simple, home-based, hydrotherapeutic program is feasible and effective in improving symptoms, QOL, and hemodynamics of patients with non-severe CHF. Further studies are needed to investigate the effects of hydrotherapy in patients with larger populations and more severe heart failure, and to clarify the mechanisms behind this non-pharmacological therapy approach.

Aquatic therapy and cardiovascular disease

Low workload exercises for mobility, strength and cardiovascular fitness, when immersed (standing) in warm (33–34°C) water, induce beneficial hemodynamic effects in patients with chronic heart failure. There were no signs of adverse reactions. The findings indicate that an increased venous return is balanced by a reduction of heart rate and a probable decrease in afterload, promoting an increase in left ventricular output. These positive hemodynamic effects of short-term immersion support previous evidence of positive effects during training in warm water (Cider et al 2006). This evidence is supported by other studies (Gabrielsen et al 2000, Meyer 2001).

Balneotherapy and chronic low back pain

A meta-analysis (Pittler et al 2006) of randomized trials of the use of spa and balneotherapy in treatment of low back pain has shown favorable, if not conclusive, results:

- The data for spa therapy, assessed on a 100 mm visual analogue scale (VAS), suggest significant beneficial effects compared with waiting list control groups (weighted mean difference 26.6 mm, 95% confidence interval 20.4–32.8, $n = 442$) for patients with chronic low back pain.
- For balneotherapy the data, assessed on a 100 mm VAS, also suggest beneficial effects compared with control groups.
- Conclusions: Even though the data are scarce, there is encouraging evidence suggesting that spa therapy and balneotherapy may be effective for treating patients with low back pain. These data are not compelling but warrant rigorous large-scale trials.

Batsialou (2002) describes the elements that might be involved in balneotherapy when treating chronic back pain:

Balneotherapy represents a therapy by various hot or warm baths in natural mineral waters of specific physical and chemical characteristics. When used externally, they have mechanical, chemical and thermic effects. Balneotherapy of lumbar syndrome includes: individual baths, swimming in the pool, hydrokinesitherapy, underwater massage, underwater extension, mud therapy, mud baths.

Balneotherapy and ankylosing spondylitis

A prospective study (Yurtkuran et al 2005) evaluated the efficacy of balneotherapy and balneotherapy plus non-steroidal anti-inflammatory drug (NSAID) use in 61 ankylosing spondylitis (AS) patients. The 21 patients on balneotherapy received treatment for 20 minutes daily, five days a week for 3 weeks. Results were compared with 20 patients receiving identical balneotherapy as well as NSAID medication (1000 mg naproxen) A further 20 patients received only NSAID medication. All of the participants did respiratory and postural exercises for 20 minutes a day for the whole study period. Each patient was evaluated on admission (before treatment), at the end of the therapy and 6 months after the treatment.

At the end of the study, statistically significant improvement was observed in all the clinical parameters of the patients receiving balneotherapy, balneotherapy plus NSAID, and in the NSAID only group. Improvements in chest expansion and morning stiffness were, however, better in the two groups receiving balneotherapy, as were measures of morning pain, nocturnal pain, global well-being of the patient and various functional indicators. The conclusion was that balneotherapy can be suggested as an effective symptomatic treatment modality in patients with AS.

Balneotherapy and chronic heart failure

In order to assess the acute hemodynamic response of immersion and peripheral muscle training in elderly patients with chronic heart failure (CHF), 13 patients and 13 healthy subjects underwent echocardiography on land and in a temperature-controlled swimming pool (91.4–93.2°F/33–34°C) (Cider et al 2006). A general increase in early diastolic filling was accompanied by a decrease in heart rate, leading to an increase in stroke volume and ejection fraction in most patients with CHF during warm water immersion. These beneficial hemodynamic effects might be the reason for the previously observed good tolerability of exercises for mobility, strength and cardiovascular fitness when performed in water. The results support those of previous studies (Gabrielsen et al 2000).

Changes in homocysteine levels following balneotherapy (Leibetseder 2004)

Researchers observed that plasma homocysteine (tHcy) is a risk factor for cardiovascular disease, and that it has been associated with anti-oxidative status. Forty patients with degenerative osteoarthrosis were randomized into a treatment group receiving stationary spa therapy plus daily sulfur baths (sulfur group) and a control group receiving spa therapy alone (control group). The results support the findings of previous investigations that therapeutic sulfur baths have clear effects on biochemical parameters: in particular, that they positively influence plasma tHcy.

Balneotherapy research and fibromyalgia

Although most balneotherapy trials involving rheumatic conditions such as fibromyalgia report positive findings, many studies have been assessed as being methodologically flawed. Therefore, the reported 'positive findings' should be interpreted with caution (Verhagen et al 2003). Improved studies are needed.

- Israeli research was conducted to evaluate the effectiveness of balneotherapy on patients with FMS in the Dead Sea (Buskila et al 2001). Forty-eight patients with FMS were randomly assigned to either a treatment group receiving sulfur baths or a control group. All participants stayed for 10 days at a Dead Sea spa. Physical functioning, FMS-related symptoms and

tenderness measurements were assessed prior to arrival at the Dead Sea, after 10 days of treatment, and 1 and 3 months after leaving the spa. Physical functioning and tenderness moderately improved in both groups. With the exception of tenderness threshold, the improvement was especially notable in the treatment group and it persisted even 3 months after leaving the spa. Relief in the severity of FMS-related symptoms (pain, fatigue, stiffness and anxiety) and reduced frequency of symptoms (headache, sleep problems and subjective joint swelling) were reported in both groups, but lasted longer in the treatment group. The conclusion was that balneotherapy treatment of FMS is effective and safe.

- A study was conducted to assess the effectiveness of balneotherapy in the Dead Sea area in the treatment of patients suffering from both fibromyalgia and psoriatic arthritis (Sukenik et al 2001). Twenty-eight patients with both psoriatic arthritis and fibromyalgia were treated with various methods of balneotherapy in the Dead Sea area. Clinical indices were assessed and the results showed that the number of active joints was reduced as were the number of tender points. A significant improvement was found in dolorimetric threshold readings after the treatment period in women. The conclusion was that balneotherapy appears to produce a statistically significant, substantial improvement in the number of active joints and tender points in both male and female patients.

- Evcik et al (2002) report a Turkish study in which 42 primary fibromyalgia patients, diagnosed according to American College of Rheumatology criteria, ages ranging between 30 and 55 years, were randomly assigned to two groups. Group 1 ($n = 22$) received 20 minutes of bathing once a day, five times per week. Patients participated in the study for 3 weeks (total of 15 sessions). Group 2 ($n = 20$) was accepted as the control group. Patients were evaluated by the number of tender points, visual analog scale for pain, Beck's Depression Index and Fibromyalgia Impact Questionnaire for functional capacity. Measurements were assessed initially, after the therapy, and at the end of the sixth month. In group 1, there were statistically significant differences in the number of tender points, visual analog scores, Beck's Depression Index and Fibromyalgia Impact Questionnaire scores after the therapy program (p <0.001). Six months later, in group 1, there was still an improvement in the number of tender points (p <0.001), visual analog scores and Fibromyalgia Impact Questionnaire (p <0.005). However, there was no statistical difference in Beck's Depression Index scores compared to the control group (p >0.05). 'Patients with FMS mostly complain about pain, anxiety, and the difficulty in daily living activities. This study shows that balneotherapy is effective and may be an alternative method in treating fibromyalgia patients.'

• Pool-based Watsu (WATer shiatSU) (Dull 1997) – in which the patient floats in warm water sourced from hot springs (35°C) while having the moves and stretches of Zen Shiatsu applied – has been shown to be a highly effective intervention for FMS (Faul 2005).

Spa therapy

As spa therapy is typically practiced in a health resort, it is sometimes called health resort medicine. Spa therapy combines hydrotherapy, balneotherapy, patient education, nutrition and physical therapy as the main modalities used. In combination, spa therapy has been shown to be clinically beneficial for a variety of common health conditions. Studies (Van Tubergen et al 2002) show that spa therapy is cost-effective as compared to standard treatment alone, for example in treatment of osteoarthritis of the knee.

Spa therapy and fibromyalgia

In a Turkish study (Cimbiz et al 2005), 470 patients with fibromyalgia and other conditions received spa therapy twice a day (with underwater exercise in the spa pool), 20 minutes total duration per day in the first week and 30 minutes for the following weeks. Results showed a significant decrease in pain and high blood pressure without hemodynamic risk. The conclusion was that a combined spa and physical therapy program may help to decrease pain and improve hemodynamic response in patients with irreversible pathologies.

Spa therapy and breast cancer

A 2005 Austrian study by Strauss-Blasche and colleagues investigated the changes of quality of life, mood, and the tumor marker CA 15-3 associated with a 3-week inpatient breast cancer rehabilitation program incorporating spa therapy. There were 149 women, aged 32–82 years, who participated in the study 3–72 months after breast cancer surgery. Quality of life, anxiety and depression were measured 2 weeks before, at the end, and 6 months after rehabilitation; CA 15-3 at the beginning, end, and at 6 months follow-up. Patients received an individualized rehabilitation program incorporating manual lymph drainage, exercise therapy, massages, psychological counseling, relaxation training, carbon dioxide baths and mud packs.

Quality of life and mood improved significantly, the greatest short-term improvements found for mood-related aspects of quality of life, the most lasting improvements found for physical complaints (e.g. fatigue). Tumor marker CA 15-3 declined significantly to follow-up. Older patients, non-obese patients, patients with a greater lymphedema and patients with an active coping style showed slightly greater improvements. *Hot mud packs inducing hyperthermia did not affect CA 15-3.*

The combination of inpatient rehabilitation with spa therapy provides a promising approach for breast cancer rehabilitation (Van Tubergen et al 2006).

Spa therapy and depression

There is a modest degree of support for the value of spa therapy in the treatment of moderate depression. The majority of spas do not accept individuals with serious behavioral problems or those who are at risk of suicide. Thus, this form of therapeutic intervention has only limited evidence of value in these conditions due to the lack of research (Dubois 1973, Dubois & Arnaud 1983, Guillard 1990). While spas may not accept serious behavioral problems, it is important to consider chronic pain or other medical conditions as causes for depression or thoughts of suicide. The evaluation of the depressed patient and determination of a positive treatment outcome is based on the cause of depression. Given that chronic pain and other medical conditions may seriously affect the activities of daily living, it is plausible that hydrotherapy, balneotherapy or spa therapy may improve these medical conditions, thereby diminishing depression.

Flotation tank treatment (restricted environmental stimulation technique – REST)

REST has been shown to reduce anxiety and depression in patients with chronic pain treated in this way (Kjellgren et al 2001). Treatment comprised a procedure in which the individual is immersed in a tank filled with water of an extremely high salt concentration. Thirty-seven patients (14 men and 23 women) suffering from chronic pain participated in the study. They were randomly assigned to either a control group (17 participants) or an experimental group (20 participants).

The experimental group received nine flotation-REST treatments over a 3-week period. The results indicated that the most severe perceived pain intensity was significantly reduced, whereas low perceived pain intensity was not influenced. Flotation-REST treatment elevated the participants' optimism, reduced the degree of anxiety or depression, and improved the sleep pattern.

Current (2006) calls for continued and expanded research are occurring at an international level by the Cochrane Library and the International Society of Medical Hydrology and Climatology (Bender 2006). Ongoing hydrotherapy research, especially research that appreciates the multivariant approach of clinical naturopathic approaches, will continue to clarify the possibilities of hydrotherapy application in a wide variety of conditions.

Naturopathic applications and the role of constitutional hydrotherapy

A large number of health care practitioners apply various hydrotherapy modalities in practice. Unique naturopathic approaches have also been developed. One such approach is the constitutional hydrotherapy system developed by Dr O.G. Carroll in the first half of the 20th century. Dr Carroll developed a flexible clinical system that combined Kneipp hydrotherapy methods with a variety of physiotherapy modalities. These included most commonly the low volt alternating current, low volt galvanic, shortwave diathermy and high frequency. Relative to the terminology of his day, as described in Chapter 3, Dr Carroll would have been considered not in the nature curist camp but in the physiotherapist camp of the naturopathic profession due to his wide inclusion of electrotherapy modalities.

Dr Carroll also incorporated irisdiagnosis, heart tone diagnosis, food intolerance evaluation and physiomedicalist botanical prescriptions, and used the Schuessler Biochemic minerals in a systematic approach to naturopathic clinical practice. As mentioned above, Dr Carroll was trained by Dr Ledoux of New Orleans and Dr Henry Lindlahr of Chicago. Dr Carroll was encouraged to move to the American West and establish a naturopathic college. While he was unable to do that, he did operate a very busy and well-known clinic until his death in 1962.

The standard constitutional hydrotherapy treatment combines a modified Kneipp torso pack with the spondylotherapy methods of Dr Abrams (see Chapter 12). The spondylotherapy levels in the standard treatment are T5–T8 and T11–L2. This treatment could be modified in a number of ways with various physiotherapy modalities to direct treatment to appropriate organs or to treat particular pathology. The overarching goal of the treatment system is to 'improve the quality of the circulating blood'. This uniquely naturopathic concept was espoused by Kuhne, Kneipp and Lindlahr, and virtually all of the early 20th century naturopathic profession.

In the words of the developer of constitutional hydrotherapy, Dr O.G. Carroll:

Health must at all times come from and be maintained by digested foods. Naturopathic Physicians understand this principle and use it to repair the damage done to organs, tissues and cells, which have become depleted of the necessary constructive elements. These necessary elements can come only from digested foods. After a food is digested, it goes through a process of assimilation which converts it into nutrition [that] is carried by the circulation to every organ, tissue, and cell. Remember this process begins first with the digestion of food, and no drug yet offered can rectify damage done by failure of digestion. (Boyle & Kirchfield 1995)

The strategy of application within the constitutional hydrotherapy system is to then harness the improved blood supply and direct it towards the pathology to be treated. The tactic of how to direct the circulation is determined by the pathology and the physical effects of the modality chosen. For example, in upper respiratory infection such as pneumonia, the standard constitutional treatment with the addition of 10 minutes of shortwave diathermy to the portion of the respiratory tree affected is a very common modification. Or, in the case of osteoarthritis of the knee, a standard constitutional treatment with the addition of 10 minutes of constant low voltage alternating current to the limb affected is a very common modification (Boyle & Saine 1988e).

The standard treatment is a tonification of the organism and as such represents the basic treatment of the system. The approach is constitutional in nature, treating the whole organism to enhance general adaptation mechanisms particularly relevant to circulatory distribution and metabolic function. The treatment was developed during the 1920s, which was a particularly fruitful period for the profession. During this period the whole-body constitutional approach that utilized physical medicine for a wide variety of complaints was widely lauded by the profession. It was during this period that the general naturopathic tonic treatment was originally developed, as well as the basic spinal and abdominal treatments of neuromuscular technique.

Constitutional hydrotherapy treatments are still widely taught, applied and researched because of their reliably beneficial outcomes as observed by a large number of clinicians. The system of constitutional hydrotherapy represents the clinical evolution of an eclectic, flexible, constitutional and uniquely naturopathic approach to comprehensive physiotherapy treatment for a general clinical setting.

Representative treatment descriptions

Standard constitutional hydrotherapy

As previously discussed in the naturopathic applications section, constitutional hydrotherapy is a systematic approach to physiotherapy that is constitutionally applied. The treatment described below is the 'standard treatment', the representative treatment and cornerstone of the system.

Indications

The standard constitutional treatment is designed to tonify digestion, enhance appropriate immune function, improve intestinal flora balance and gently detoxify the body. Modifications of the physiotherapy modalities allow for a flexible application to a large variety of clinical conditions such as inflammatory bowel disease, asthma, upper respiratory infection, dermal infections, organ specific infections, endocrine dysfunction, cancer, musculoskeletal injury and/or disease, metabolic diseases as well as cardiac conditions (Blake 2006b, Boyle & Saine 1988e, Scott 1992).

Methodology

Patient supine, undressed from the waist up, covered with a vellux blanket.

1. Two Turkish towels, each folded in half, well wrung from hot water (130–140°F/54–60°C; note the relatively high temperature of the compress) are applied covering chest and abdomen, from clavicle to anterior superior iliac spine (ASIS). Fold the lateral edges of the towel as needed so that they do not lie beyond the anterior axillary line. Cover the patient with a blanket. (*Note*: If a cotton sheet is used to separate the patient and the blanket, as is common for sanitation reasons, an impermeable barrier (such as a thin rubber mat) should be placed over wet towels so as to avoid wetting the cotton sheet and thus fundamentally changing the treatment impression and outcome.)

2. At the 5-minute mark one Turkish towel, folded in half, well wrung from hot water,

replaces the two Turkish towels previously applied.

3. Ask patient to arch the back or roll onto one shoulder. Slide two 4-inch electrode pads underneath the patient, *one from each side*, so that each is on one side of the spine with the upper edge of the electrode approximately level with the fifth thoracic vertebra. This is referred to as the 5–5 treatment.

4. Replace the hot towel with one Turkish towel well wrung from cold water from the faucet (40–55°F/4–12°C; note this does not include iced or especially cold water) and folded in half. The application should cover the same area as the hot towels, from clavicle to ASIS, bordered at the anterior axillary lines. Again cover the patient with the blanket.

5. Place the low volt alternating current sine wave unit within reach of the patient and instruct the patient to adjust the intensity. The current output should be on the surge (massage) setting with a low duty cycle of 6–10 cycles each minute. Current intensity is adjusted by the patient, and the following levels are noted in this order:

   a. The patient will feel a tingling on the back.

   b. The patient will feel a gentle contraction somewhere in the abdomen, usually under the costal margin on the right, but not always. This is the ideal setting.

   c. The patient will feel strong contractions of the muscles of the upper back. This is unnecessary and counterproductive.

6. At the 10-minute mark (approximately 15 minutes of total treatment time have elapsed), check the center of the towel over the solar plexus to see if the patient has warmed the towel to at least body temperature. If the patient has warmed the towel, then remove the towel and proceed. If the patient has not, then cover the patient again with the blanket, wait 2 minutes, then remove the towel.

7. Ask the patient to arch the back or lift the shoulder in order to move the sine wave pads from the upper back to the abdomen. One pad is placed on the back and will be *centered* over the spine at the thoracolumbar junction, the top edge at approximately the 11th thoracic vertebra. The second pad is placed on the abdomen overlying the stomach, i.e. the epigastric region (directly superior to the umbilicus on adults). Place a bean bag on top

of the abdominal pad. This is referred to as the stomach treatment.

8. Instruct the patient to adjust the sine wave intensity until a gentle contraction at one or both pads is felt. The sine wave output remains on the surge (massage) cycle at the same low duty cycle.

9. At the 10-minute mark (approx 25 minutes total), remove the sine wave pads. Ask the patient to turn over onto the abdomen.

Repeat the towel treatment, this time applied to the back:

10. Place two Turkish towels (the same as previously used), freshly well wrung from hot water, each folded in half, on the patient's back. The towels should cover from the superior edge of the scapula to the posterior superior iliac spine (PSIS). The lateral towel edges are folded up so as not to lie beyond the posterior axillary line.

11. At the 5-minute mark (approx 30 minutes total), replace the two towels with one fresh towel wrung from hot water. Quickly replace this towel with a towel well wrung from cold water. The towels should cover from the superior edge of the scapula to the PSIS. The lateral towel edges are folded up so as not to lie beyond the posterior axillary line.

12. At the 10-minute mark (approximately 40 minutes), check the center of the towel to see if the patient has warmed the towel to at least body temperature. If the patient has warmed the towel, then remove the towel and proceed. If the patient has not, then cover the patient again with the blanket, wait 2 minutes, then remove the towel.

Finish with a dry friction rub to the back:

13. Use a fresh dry towel to give a 5–20 second dry friction rub to the patient's back.

Safety issues

Care should be taken when applying any thermal modality not to burn the patient. Regardless of the relatively high temperature of the constitutional towel application, the temperatures are *usually* well tolerated by patients. Appropriate knowledge of physiotherapy modality application is necessary.

Validation of efficacy = 2 (see Table 7.2)

The standard constitutional treatment has been in continuous and widespread clinical use since the 1920s. Numerous clinicians have observed significant beneficial clinical outcomes, and a number of cases have been described in the literature (Blake 2006b, Watrous 1996).

Alternatives

Standard constitutional hydrotherapy is a broadly applicable modality for a wide variety of clinical complaints. Internal medications (e.g. homeopathic and botanical) may provide an alternative for portions of the treatment in certain circumstances. Internal medications do not supply the same physiological responses though, and application of constitutional hydrotherapy in combination with internal medications will have additive effect.

Physiological effects

There have been a number of preliminary investigations into clinical and laboratory effects of the 'standard constitutional hydrotherapy'. Since 2006 research has been conducted at the National College of Naturopathic Medicine to investigate the blood count parameters and to identify if heat shock proteins are involved in any changes observed. Results are not available at the time of this printing. Previous investigation has identified that post-treatment core temperature is more likely to show a net increase than a decrease, or no change (55% of patients). Additionally, peripheral temperatures likewise are more likely to show a net increase (91% of patients) (Wickenheizer et al 1995).

Unpublished research conducted at the Southwest College of Naturopathic Medicine by Mark Carney ND and Bryan McConnell ND demonstrated increased vitality, physical role, decreased pain (SF-36 subjective form), decreased body fat, increased total body water (bioelectrical impedance), increased T3, T4, T7, decreased alkaline phosphatase, decreased cholesterol (triglycerides, high-density and low-density lipoproteins), a slight increase in oral temperature and a slight decrease in mean arterial pressure.

Unpublished research at the National College of Naturopathic Medicine by Kate Wiggin ND showed a post-treatment increase in leukocyte circulation that remained elevated for 2 hours (longest point of observation), particularly the monocyte levels.

Drs Carroll and Scott regularly observed a decreased urinary indican level following a course of treatments, as compared to before the treatment series (Boyle & Saine 1988e). Simultaneously, after completing a course of treatments, the urine specific gravity has been observed to increase post treatment (Boyle & Saine 1988e). These two observational trends suggest improved intestinal flora balance and improved kidney function. It should be understood that during a serial course of treatments, variations from the 'standard' are commonly employed on an as-indicated basis.

Naturopathic perspectives

The constitutional hydrotherapy system is a uniquely naturopathic approach to clinical physiotherapy treatments. The overarching goal of the treatment is detoxification of the system, immune enhancement and improved digestive function. There are also focused treatments for addressing regional functional and pathological conditions.

Urinary indican levels are a measure of intestinal putrefaction (Yarnell 2000). Intestinal putrefaction by-products that are excreted via the kidneys are presumably absorbed via intestinal circulation. All intestinal circulation enters into portal circulation prior to entrance into pulmonary and then systemic circulation (Guyton 2000). Presumably liver detoxication pathways are required for oxidation/reduction and conjugation of certain putrefaction by-products.

An increased urine specific gravity is indicative of an increased urine concentrating capacity of the kidneys (Fischbach 2004). The observation of improved urinary indican levels and increased kidney concentrating capabilities point to the adaptation benefits of the treatment and the overarching global benefits to the organism.

Further reading

For more information on the system of constitutional hydrotherapy, see:

1. Blake E 2006 Constitutional hydrotherapy: a workbook of clinical lessons. Holistic Health Publications, Portland, OR
2. Boyle W, Saine A 1988 Naturopathic hydrotherapy. Eclectic Medical Publications, Sandy, OR
3. Scott L 1992 Clinical hydrotherapy. Leo Scott, Spokane, WA

The following are of historical interest:

- The books by Dr John Harvey Kellogg MD provide further clinical evidence for hydrotherapy. Dr Kellogg's main works on hydrotherapy are *Rational Hydrotherapy* and *Rational Hydrotherapy Part II*.
- Father Kneipp authored *My Water Cure*, which was the most popular book of the day second to the Bible. This book provides further clinical case evidence of hydrotherapy.

- *The Water Cure in America: Over 300 Cases of Various Diseases Treated with Water* by Wesselhoeft et al, published in 1856 by Fowlers & Wells, New York, contains numerous cases from a number of water cure doctors of the era. The cases include pneumonia, tuberculosis and various other acute and chronic diseases, including appendicitis, peritonitis and salpingitis. The cases document the potential usefulness of a simple yet effective naturopathic approach to hydrotherapy.

Hyperthermia

Douglas C. Lewis ND

Indications/description

Hyperthermia is the increase of body temperature above 'normal', utilizing a triggering agent to induce fever or an outside source of heating to produce a tissue temperature rise (TTR). Hyperthermia treatments may be used in the prevention or treatment of disease. Treatment with hyperthermia is based on the concept that fever is a normal, constructive response to illness, and where fever does not naturally occur, it can be created. Hyperthermia treatments may be applied locally, regionally or to the whole body.

In 500 BC the Greek physician Parmenides argued that if only he had the means to create fever, he could cure all illness. This was an echo of the maxim of Hippocrates. Hydropathic physicians of the 19th century, the early 20th century naturopathic physicians, and doctors such as Dr Henry Lindlahr and Dr O.G. Carroll endorsed a similar tenet, even anticipating the evolution of a naturally occurring febrile process (healing crisis or healing reaction) in the course of taking serial treatments (Constitutional Hydrotherapy is NOT a clinical fever treatment.) There are many historical examples of the application of external sources of heating for the purpose of improving health. These include the Roman baths, the Finnish sauna, the Russian and Turkish steam, and the Native American sweat lodge.

Hyperthermia may be used as an adjunct in the removal of toxic elements from body tissues (Gard & Brown 1992). It has been used in the treatment of both bacterial and viral infections and in cancer treatment (Park et al 1990, Spire et al 1985, Toffoli et al 1989, Tyrrell et al 1989). It has shown benefits in improving immune function (Konings 1988, Neville & Sauder 1988) and is useful in the treatment of insulin resistance (Baron et al 1994, Hooper 1999, Petrofsky et al 2003), hypertension (Biro et al 2003, Reaven et al 1996), congestive heart failure (Kihara et al 2002) and endothelial damage associated with atherosclerosis (Imamura et al 2001).

Methodology

Fever may be induced by the introduction of a pyretic agent into the body. This method is difficult to control and runs a greater risk of doing harm to the patient. It is not commonly (if ever) utilized by naturopathic physicians and will not be discussed in this section.

Exogenous heating to produce a fever is more commonly employed but has the limitation of being difficult to use to produce an even, consistent TTR. Various methods have been attempted. Arrays of ultrasound or diathermy (shortwave/microwave) have been utilized with mixed results in clinical settings. Infrared heating has been used and found to be quite successful. Hot air (sauna), steam, and immersion baths are common tools used in the production of elevated tissue temperature.

Safety issues

The most obvious safety issue with hyperthermia is the avoidance of burns. It is common knowledge that foods can be cooked 'fast and hot' or 'low and slow'. The same can be said for hyperthermia applications. In general, the 'low and slow' approach to hyperthermia treatment provides plenty of leeway for its safe application and is much more appropriate clinically.

There are those for whom additional care should be taken when applying hyperthermia treatments. These include persons with anemia, heart disease, hypertension and diabetes. In fact, these conditions may be specific indicators for the use of hyperthermia with appropriate care.

Persons with advanced liver disease (Skibba et al 1991) and women who are or may be pregnant may need to avoid hyperthermia treatment altogether (Sedgwick et al 1981).

Hyperthermia is known to potentiate the effects of radiation therapy in cancer treatment (Thomas et al 2006). It also increases intracellular drug accumulation through alteration of cell membrane transfer (Toffoli et al 1989). Therefore, it is important that if a patient is receiving radiation therapy or chemotherapy, their oncologist is aware of and approves the use of hyperthermia.

Hyperthermia is a very safe treatment when appropriately monitored, and is useful especially as an adjunctive treatment.

Validation of efficacy = 3 (see Table 7.2)

Most of the studies on hyperthermia reviewed included small numbers of participants and have the typical limitations of such studies. However, considering the evidence (see studies cited above) of improvement in the chronic lifestyle diseases (e.g. diabetes, hypertension and chronic heart failure), balanced against the low-cost/low-risk aspects of treatment, its measure of efficacy should be recognized.

Alternatives

While there are alternative methods for increasing body temperature (e.g. exercise or chemically induced methods), the only alternative to the production of hyperthermia is to not artificially raise the body temperature.

Physiological effects

Hyperthermia produces a number of physiological effects. With a TTR comes an increased metabolic rate. According to Guyton (1981), the metabolic rate would increase 100% for every 10°C rise in temperature. This increased metabolic rate no doubt accounts for some of the enhanced immune activity.

Spire et al (1985) and Tyrrell et al (1989) describe the thermal inactivation of viruses. Many viruses, including HIV, are heat labile. Hyperthermia treatments therefore may be beneficial in reducing viral load.

Toffoli et al (1989) discuss the effect of hyperthermia on increased cell membrane permeability and the subsequent intracellular uptake of drugs, while Konings (1988) discusses *membranes as targets for hyperthermic cell killing*.

Thomas et al (2006) state that: 'Hyperthermia is known to be synergistic or supra-additive with radiation therapy.' They go on to say that: 'The mechanism of action of combined hyperthermia and ionizing radiation involves heat-inhibited repair of radiation-induced single-strand DNA breaks and radiation-induced chromosomal aberrations.'

Park et al (1990) reported on the increase in immune cell activity of cancer patients following hyperthermia treatment, while in 1988 Neville & Sauder reported on the induction of interleukin-1 production in vivo from whole-body hyperthermia at 41–42°C.

In 1999, Hooper asked if 'partial immersion in a hot tub [would] simulate the effects of exercise?' with regard to the benefits for type 2 diabetes. They found that after 30 minutes of immersion to the shoulders, 6 days per week for 3 weeks, a group of eight patients (five men and three women) saw a mean fasting plasma glucose decline from 182 ± 37 mg/dL to 159 ± 42 mg/dL, and a mean glycosylated hemoglobin decrease from 11.3 ± 3.1% to 10.3 ± 2.6%.

Kihara (2002) sought 'to determine whether sauna therapy . . . improves endothelial function in patients with coronary risk factors'. Twenty patients (62 ± 15 years) in New York Heart Association (NYHA) functional class II or III CHF were treated in a dry sauna at 60°C for 15 minutes and then kept on bed rest with a blanket for 30 minutes, once a day for 2 weeks. They concluded after extensive evaluation that: 'Repeated sauna treatment improves vascular endothelial function, resulting in an improvement in cardiac function and clinical symptoms.'

Cautions

See 'Safety issues', above.

Naturopathic perspectives

Hyperthermia appears to be an efficacious, cost-effective treatment for many of today's chronic diseases. It may have limited use as a stand-alone treatment, but appears to be quite useful in a multi-modality treatment approach. In association with few side-effects, low cost (depending on application), possibilities for home treatment and supportive benefits with other treatments, it appears to be a particularly useful and safe treatment from a naturopathic perspective.

References

Abbott G 1915a Elements of hydrotherapy for nurses. Reprinted by Leaves-of-Autumn Books, Payson, AZ

Abbott G 1915b Elements of hydrotherapy for nurses. Reprinted by Leaves-of-Autumn Books, Payson, AZ, p 28

Abbott GK, Moor FB, Jensen-Nelson KL 1945a Physical therapy in nursing care. Review and Herald Publishing, Washington, DC. Clinical observations provided by Winternitz.

Abbott GK, Moor FB, Jensen-Nelson KL 1945b Physical therapy in nursing care. Review and Herald Publishing, Washington, DC

Abramson DI, Mitchell RE, Tuck S, Bell Y, Zays AM 1961 Changes in blood flow, oxygen uptake, and tissue temperatures produced by the topical application of wet heat. Archives of Physical Medicine and Rehabilitation 42:305–318

Abramson DI, Tuck S, Chu LS, Agustin C 1964 Effect of paraffin bath and hot fomentation on local tissue temperatures. Archives of Physical Medicine and Rehabilitation 45:87–94

Adams S 1921 Life of Henry Foster, MD. Rochester Times-Union, Rochester, NY

Baron AD, Steinberg H, Brechtel G, Johnson A 1994 Skeletal muscle blood flow independently modulates insulin-mediated glucose uptake. American Journal of Physiology 266(2 Pt 1):E248–253

Baruch S 1892 The uses of water in modern medicine. GS Davis, Detroit, MI, p 2–22

Baruch S 1898 The principles and practice of hydrotherapy. William Wood, New York

Baruch S 1920 An epitome of hydrotherapy for physicians, architects, and nurses. WB Saunders, Philadelphia

Batsialou I 2002 Balneotherapy in the treatment of subjective symptoms of lumbar syndrome. Medicinski Pregled 55(11–12):495–499

Bender T 2006 International Society of Medical Hydrology and Climatology. www.ismh-direct.net

Biro S, Masuda A, Kihara T, Tei C 2003 Clinical implications of thermal therapy in lifestyle-related diseases. Experimental Biology and Medicine 228:1245–1249

Blake E 2006a Constitutional hydrotherapy: a workbook of clinical lessons. Holistic Health Publications, Portland, OR, p 33–34

Blake E 2006b Constitutional hydrotherapy: a workbook of clinical lessons. Holistic Health Publications, Portland, OR

Boyle W 1988 Lectures in naturopathic hydrotherapy. Buckeye Naturopathic Press, East Palestine, OH

Boyle W, Kirchfield F 1995 Nature doctors. Buckeye Naturopathic Press, East Palestine, OH, p 251

Boyle W, Saine A 1988a Lectures in naturopathic hydrotherapy. Buckeye Naturopathic Press, East Palestine, OH, p 19

Boyle W, Saine A 1988b Lectures in naturopathic hydrotherapy. Buckeye Naturopathic Press, East Palestine, OH, p 8

Boyle W, Saine A 1988c Lectures in naturopathic hydrotherapy. Buckeye Naturopathic Press, East Palestine, OH, p 135

Boyle W, Saine A 1988d Lectures in naturopathic hydrotherapy. Buckeye Naturopathic Press, East Palestine, OH, p 23

Boyle W, Saine A 1988e Naturopathic hydrotherapy. Eclectic Medical Publications, Sandy, OR

Brüggemann W 1986 Hydrotherapie. Springer, Berlin, p 8–36

Bühring M 1988 Die Kneippsche Hydrotherapie in der Praxis. Therapeutikon 2:80–86

Buskila D, Abu-Shakra M, Neumann L et al 2001 Balneotherapy for fibromyalgia at the Dead Sea. Rheumatology International 20(3):105–108

Cider A, Sveälv B, Täng M et al 2006 Immersion in warm water induces improvement in cardiac function in patients with chronic heart failure. European Journal of Heart Failure 8(3):308–313

Cimbiz A, Bayazit V, Hallaceli H et al 2005 The effect of combined therapy (spa and physical therapy) on pain in various chronic diseases. Complementary Therapies in Medicine 13(4):244–250

Dittmar F 1960 Viscerocutaneous and cutivisceral reflexes and their importance for physical and neurological medicine. Wiener Medizin Wochenschrift 110:840

Dubois J 1973 Hydrotherapy and climatic treatment of depressive states. Les Cahiers de Médecine 14(7):591–595

Dubois J, Arnaud A 1983 Quantitative study on course of anxiety and depressive states during spa cure at Saujon. Presse Thermale et Climatique 120(3):132–136

Dull H 1997 Watsu: freeing the body in water, 2nd edn. Harbin Springs Publishing, Harbib, CA

Engel J, Wakim KG et al 1950 The effect of contrast baths on the peripheral circulation of patients with rheumatoid arthritis. Archives of Physical Medicine and Rehabilitation 31:135–144

Ernst E 1990 Hydrotherapy. Physiotherapy 76(4):207–210

Evcik D, Kizilay B, Gokcen E 2002 The effects of balneotherapy on fibromyalgia patients. Rheumatology International 22(2):56–59

Faul K 2005 A pilot study of the comparative effectiveness of two water-based treatments for fibromyalgia syndrome: Watsu and Aix massage. Journal of Bodywork and Movement Therapies 9(3):202–210

Fischbach F 2004 A manual of laboratory and diagnostic tests. Lippincott Williams & Wilkins, Philadelphia

Fischer E, Solomon S 1958 Physiological responses to heat and cold. In: Licht S (ed) Therapeutic heat. Elizabeth Licht, New Haven, CT

Gabrielsen A, Sorensen V, Pump B et al 2000 Cardiovascular and neuroendocrine responses to water immersion in compensated heart failure. American Journal of Physiology. Heart and Circulatory Physiology 279(4):H1931–H1940

Gard ZR, Brown EJ 1992 Literature review and comparison studies of sauna/hyperthermia in detoxification. Townsend Letter for Doctors 107:470–478

Geytenbeek J 2002 Evidence for effective hydrotherapy. Physiotherapy 88(9):514–529

Giancoli D 1995a Physics: principles with applications, 4th edn. Prentice Hall, Englewood Cliffs, NJ, p 404

Giancoli D 1995b Physics: principles with applications, 4th edn. Prentice Hall, Englewood Cliffs, NJ, p 412

Guillard A 1990 Depressive syndromes and treatment at the Neris-les-Bains thermal spa cure. Presse Thermale et Climatique 127(4):189–198

Gutenbrunner C, Ruppel K 1992 Zur Frage der adaptiven Blutdrucknormalisierung im Verlauf von Bäderkuren unter besonderer Berücksichtigung von Homogenisierungseffekten und Lebensalter. Phys Rehab Kur Med 2:58–64

Guyton A 1981 Textbook of medical physiology, 6th edn. WB Saunders, Philadelphia

Guyton A 1991 Medical physiology. WB Saunders, Philadelphia

Guyton A 1996 Textbook of medical physiology, 9th edn. WB Saunders, Philadelphia

Guyton A 2000 Textbook of medical physiology, 10th edn. WB Saunders, Philadelphia, p 724–725

Hooper PL 1999 Hot tub therapy for type 2 diabetes mellitus. New England Journal of Medicine 341:924–925

Imamura M, Biro S, Kihara T et al 2001 Repeated thermal therapy improves impaired vascular endothelial function in patients with coronary risk factors. Journal of the American College of Cardiology 38(4):1083–1088

Jackson J 1874 How to treat the sick without medicine. Jackson, Dansville, NY

Jaskoviak P, Schafer R 1993a Applied physiotherapy. American Chiropractic Association, Arlington, VA, p 132–136

Jaskoviak P, Schafer R 1993b Applied physiotherapy. American Chiropractic Association, Arlington, VA, p 136

Jensen B 1946 The joy of living and how to attain it. B. Jensen, Los Angeles, CA

Kihara T 2002 Repeated sauna treatment improves vascular endothelial and cardiac function in patients with chronic heart failure. Journal of the American College of Cardiology 39(5):754–759

Kihara T, Biro S, Imamura M et al 2002 Repeated sauna treatment improves vascular endothelial and cardiac function in patients with chronic heart failure. Journal of the American College of Cardiology 39(5):754–759

Kjellgren A, Sundequist U, Norlander T et al 2001 Effects of flotation-REST on muscle tension pain. Pain Research and Management 6(4):181–189

Kneipp S 1894 My water cure. Koesel, Kempten, Bavaria

Kneipp S 1979 My water cure (facsimile edition). Thorsons, Wellingborough, p 194–195. First published 1893

Konings AWT 1988 Membranes as targets for hyperthermic cell killing. Recent Results in Cancer Research 109:9–21

Krusen F 1971 Handbook of physical medicine and rehabilitation. WB Saunders, Philadelphia, p 262

Leibetseder V 2004 Improving homocysteine levels through balneotherapy: effects of sulphur baths. Clinica Chimica Acta 343(1–2):105–111

Mannerkorpi K, Nyberg B, Ahlmen M, Ekdahl C 2000 Pool exercise combined with an education program for patients with FMS. A prospective, randomized study. Journal of Rheumatology 27(10):2473–2481

Meyer K 2001 Exercise training in heart failure: recommendations based on current research. Medicine and Science in Sports and Exercise 33(4):525–531

Moor FB, Peterson SC, Manwell EM et al 1964 Manual of hydrotherapy and massage. Pacific Press Publishing Association, Boise, ID

Neville AJ, Sauder DN 1988 Whole body hyperthermia (41–42°C) induces interleukin-1 in vivo. Lymphokine Research 7(3):201–206

Park MM, Hornback NB, Endres S, Dinarello CA 1990 The effect of whole body hyperthermia on the immune cell activity of cancer patients. Lymphokine Research 9(2):213–223

Petrofsky JS, Besonis C, Rivera D et al 2003 Does local heating really help diabetic patients increase circulation. Journal of Neurological and Orthopaedic Medicine and Surgery 21:40–46

Pittler MH, Karagulle MZ, Karagulle M et al 2006 Spa therapy and balneotherapy for treating low back pain: meta-analysis of randomized trials. Rheumatology 45(7):880–884

Prentice W 1998 Therapeutic modalities for the allied health professionals. McGraw-Hill, New York, p 207

Priessnitz V 1843 The cold water cure. Reprinted by Kessinger Publishing, Whitefish, MT

Reaven GM, Lithell H, Landsberg L 1996 Hypertension and associated metabolic abnormalities – the role of insulin resistance and the sympathoadrenal system. New England Journal of Medicine 334:374–382

Schafer R 1982 Chiropractic management of sports and recreational injuries. Williams & Wilkins, Baltimore, p 199

Scott L 1990 Clinical hydrotherapy. Leo Scott, Spokane, WA

Scott L 1992 Clinical hydrotherapy. Leo Scott, Spokane, WA

Sedgwick H, McRorie MM, Smith DW 1981 Suggested limits to the use of the hot tub and sauna by pregnant women. CMA Journal 125:50–53

Skibba JL, Powers RH, Stadnicka A et al 1991 Oxidative stress as a precursor to the irreversible hepatocellular injury caused by hyperthermia. International Journal of Hyperthermia 7(5):749–761

Spire B, Dormont D, Barre-Sinoussi F et al 1985 Inactivation of lymphadenopathy-associated virus by heat, gamma rays, and ultraviolet light. Lancet i:188–189

Spitler H 1948 Basic naturopathy. American Naturopathic Association, New York

Starkey C 1999 Therapeutic modalities. FA Davis, Philadelphia, p 123

Strauss-Blasche G, Gnad E, Ekmekcioglu C et al 2005 Combined inpatient rehabilitation and spa therapy for breast cancer patients: effects on quality of life and CA 15-3. Cancer Nursing 28(5):390–398

Sukenik S, Baradin R, Codish S et al 2001 Balneotherapy at the Dead Sea area for patients with psoriatic arthritis and concomitant fibromyalgia. Israeli Medical Association Journal 3(2):147–150

Thomas CT, Ammar A, Farrell JJ, Elsaleh H 2006 Radiation modifiers: treatment overview and future investigations. Hematology/Oncology Clinics of North America 20(1):119–139

Thrash A, Thrash C 1981a Home remedies: hydrotherapy, massage, charcoal, and other simple treatments. Thrash Publications, Seale, AL, p 17

Thrash A, Thrash C 1981b Home remedies: hydrotherapy, massage, charcoal, and other simple treatments. Thrash Publications, Seale, AL, p 13

Toffoli G, Bevilacqua C, Franceschin A, Boiocchi M 1989 Effect of hyperthermia on intracellular drug accumulation and chemosensitivity in drug-sensitive and drug-resistant P388 leukaemia cell lines. International Journal of Hyperthermia 5(2):163–172

Trall RT 1853 The hydropathic encyclopedia: a system of hydropathy and hygiene. Fowlers & Wells, New York

Tyrrell D, Barrow I, Arthur J 1989 Local hyperthermia benefits natural and experimental common colds. British Medical Journal 298:1280–1283

Van Tubergen A, Boonen A, Landewe R 2002 Cost effectiveness of combined spa-exercise therapy in ankylosing spondylitis: a randomized controlled trial. Arthritis and Rheumatology 47(5):459–467

Van Tubergen A et al 2006 Therapeutic effect of spa therapy and short wave therapy in knee osteoarthritis. Rheumatology International Nov

Verhagen AP, Bierma-Zeinstra SM, Cardoso JR et al 2003 Balneotherapy for rheumatoid arthritis. Cochrane Database of Systematic Reviews (4):CD000518

Vitorino D 2006 Hydrotherapy and conventional physiotherapy improve total sleep time and quality of life of fibromyalgia patients: randomized clinical trial. Sleep Medicine 7(3):293–296

Watrous L 1996 From nature cure to advanced naturopathic medicine. Journal of Naturopathic Medicine 7(2):72–79

Wesley J 1747 Primitive physick. Thomas Trye, London

Wickenheizer D, Bettenburg R, Landi K al 1995 Constitutional hydrotherapy research paper. National College of Naturopathic Medicine, Portland, OR

Yarnell E 2000 Naturopathic gastroenterology. Naturopathic Medical Press, Sisters, OR, p 22–25

Yurtkuran M, Ay A, Karakoc Y 2005 Improvement of the clinical outcome in ankylosing spondylitis by balneotherapy. Joint, Bone, Spine 72(4):303–308

12

Eric Blake ND

With contributions from:

Carolyn McMakin DC

Douglas C. Lewis ND

Nick Buratovich ND

Dean E. Neary Jr ND

Electrotherapy Modalities

Chapter objectives

This chapter provides an overview of the role of representative electrotherapy modalities in naturopathic practice. These modalities are commonly applied for a wide variety of reasons such as musculoskeletal dysfunction, rehabilitation, pain management, infection or specific localized tissue effect. They may be utilized individually or in combination with one another depending upon therapeutic strategy and desired outcome.

Naturopathic clinical strategies

In the broadest sense, all physiotherapy and associated modalities should be seen as a branch of naturopathic therapeutics. The history chapter (Chapter 3) reviews in detail the overlap of the early naturopathic and physiotherapy professions and the significant role of physical modalities in the early 20th century naturopathic professions. The rehabilitation focus of modern conventional physiotherapy practice is a valuable adjunct that may play a beneficial role for the patients of all physicians, naturopathic and allopathic. Familiarity and awareness of the proper scope of conventional physiotherapy is presumed and is not the focus of this chapter. The focus of this chapter is the role of the application of electrical physiotherapy modalities in general clinical practice for the naturopathic doctor. For that reason, both older sources of clinically reported applications that are in concert with the mechanism of action of the modality, as well as modern research which has a more limited musculoskeletal rehabilitation focus, have been incorporated into the chapter.

Clinical goals and treatment strategies, as well as the anticipated clinical outcome, all play a large role in selecting appropriate interventions. For these reasons, understanding of current and past models of the process of healing from a naturopathic perspective is fundamental. Consideration should be given to the models outlined in Chapters 1, 7, 8 and 10. Constitutional approaches, regional approaches, or a combination of the two, will influence selection of physiotherapy modality. Additionally, an understanding of the general adaptation syndrome (GAS) – see Chapter 2 – and the physiological processes that coordinate homeodynamics is important to modality selection.

The hallmark of electrical physiotherapeutic modalities is that they elicit predictable physiological responses. The naturopathic principle of the *vis medicatrix naturae* guides the naturopathic doctor to identify which physiological mechanisms should be augmented or inhibited, in an effort to facilitate self-regulating mechanisms. Efforts may be directed to enhance the function of a particular organ or group of organs, or techniques may be applied for the benefit of the local tissue effect of the modality itself. For example, diathermy application methods demonstrate these different clinical strategies.

Diathermy application over the low back to enhance tissue perfusion and metabolism of the kidneys and adrenal glands has been reported to be of clinical benefit in allergic rhinitis and asthma (Linder 1964). Diathermy directly over the nasal sinuses has been recommended as clinically beneficial in a sinusitis of infectious origin (Poesnecker 1978). In both cases the goal of resolving the sinus inflammation can be achieved; however, the means to the end requires an understanding of the healing processes involved and appropriate strategy selection (localized or indirect). Clinical strategies are, of course, dependent upon the goal of therapeutic impression and the role of the electrotherapy modalities in the comprehensive treatment plan.

Goals of clinical treatments

Goals may include reduction of pain, inflammation, edema or muscular spasm. Likewise, the cumulative effect may include intrinsic antimicrobial activity, enhancement of endogenous antimicrobial activity of the body, improved joint range of motion, improved muscular strength, resorption of scar tissue, increased circulation and quality of tissue repair. Immediate symptom reduction may or may not be one of the goals of the therapy. The principles of treating the whole person and identifying and treating the cause of illness may require indirect strategies to achieve the goal of improved health and reduction of symptoms ('cure'). The ultimate goal of resolution of the patient's complaints is an important overarching outcome that, when possible to achieve, is the important end outcome. In conditions or situations when this is not possible or unlikely to occur, palliative techniques may be all that can be offered.

As detailed in Chapter 3, the role of physical modalities in naturopathic practice is far broader than in conventional physical therapy. The general clinical application of electrotherapy is no exception. While every effort has been made to include recent references as evidence and support for this chapter, we have also included less recent references. These older references are included when they are compatible with the modern understanding of the mechanism of action of the modality.

The hallmark of physical modalities is the *predictable physiological response elicited*. These responses should be considered stable over time. Many of the references included are derived from naturopathic clinician reports and respected educational literature of the early naturopathic profession. The naturopathic profession has long used case evidence and clinic experience to guide clinical practice (case evidence-based naturopathic medicine – CEBM). In many ways, the unique political obstacles to the formation of a stable naturopathic profession have limited naturopathic research agendas, and further research in these areas is warranted.

Electrotherapy modalities

- Low volt alternating current (sine wave)
- Low volt galvanic
- Short wave diathermy
- High frequency Tesla coil
- Microcurrent
- Ultrasound
- Low level laser

(See Table 7.2 in Chapter 7 for an explanation of the validation of efficacy ratings outlined in the following electrotherapy modalities.)

Low volt alternating current (sine wave)

Low voltage alternating current is a biphasic current produced with a low voltage and low amperage. There are a variety of biphasic waveforms such as rectangular, sawtooth and square. However, we will consider the sinusoidal current as representative. The biphasic waveform does not produce any polarity effect. Sinusoidal current has enjoyed a long and popular use in naturopathic practice (Abbott et al 1945a, Post-Graduate Study of Naturopathy 1937b, Starkey 1999a).

Mechanism of action and physiological effects

The sinusoidal current is utilized to depolarize sensory and motor nerves. The depolarization of the sensory nerves is utilized in transcutaneous electrical nerve stimulation for pain control. Muscle stimulators employ the sinusoidal output. The sensory nerves are stimulated in a fashion that disrupts pain perception through gate control or opiate system mechanisms. The stimulation of the motor nerves elicits muscular contractions. The intensity and frequency of the muscular contractions can be utilized to exhaust muscular spasm, exercise muscles and reduce edema (Abbott et al 1945a, Jaskoviak 1993a, Johnson 1946a).

The physiological effects of the sine wave encourage tissue healing by promoting increased tissue perfusion of arterial blood, increased venous return and increased lymphatic circulation. These effects can be utilized to mechanically reduce edema. The sinusoidal current can also be used for muscular re-education, strengthening, and relaxation of muscular spasm by causing muscular fatigue. The sinusoidal current is typically applied in a constant (tetanize), surging or pulsed fashion (Agresta 2004, Jaskoviak 1993a).

Safety and contraindications

Low volt current has a long history of use with a relatively high margin of safety. Implanted neurological devices and cardiac pacemakers or defibrillators should be considered contraindications. Diminished neurological sensation or motor capabilities should be approached with caution. Active contraction of muscular tissue in the vicinity of a thrombotic clot may precipitate emboli. Caution should be exercised in the event of vascular insufficiency (Johnson 1946a, Starkey 1999a).

Indications: validation of efficacy = 5

Low volt sinusoidal current can be utilized to re-educate and rehabilitate the musculoskeletal system. Reduction of edema through muscular pumping, encouraging tissue healing through increased vascular supply and stimulation of local metabolism, and pain relief through enkephalins, endorphin pathways, opiate and gate control strategies are also possible. Diabetic ulcers and stress incontinence have also shown benefit from low volt sinusoidal treatment (Baker et al 1997, Castro et al 2004).

Naturopathic indications and applications: validation of efficacy = 4

Naturopathic clinical application of sinusoidal current includes sinusoidal low volt for musculoskeletal re-education, pain control and edema reduction. It also incorporates sinusoidal low volt for other indications such as re-education of large bowel peristaltic rhythm (Lindquist 1948a) and spinal reflex stimulation (Cordingley 1923, Gregory 1922, Johnson 1946b). The enhanced tissue perfusion, increased lymphatic circulation and improved return of venous blood make the low volt sinusoidal quite a useful modality for indirect treatment that encourages tissue healing through mechanical detoxication and increased exposure to nutrients. Constant tetanizing current through an affected limb, with the other electrode at the spinal dermatomal origin, has been described for sprains, strains, cellulitis or infection of the limb, edema, carpal tunnel syndrome, and other pathologies of the limb that would benefit from enhanced tissue perfusion, and venous and lymphatic drainage (Blake 2006, Boyle 1988, Scott 1990, Watrous 1996).

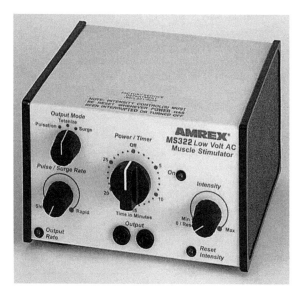

Figure 12.1 Low volt alternating current or 'sine wave'. Photograph courtesy of Amrex-Zetron

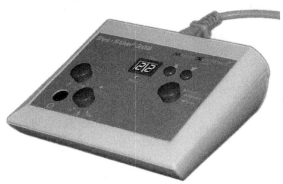

Figure 12.2A Low volt alternating current or 'sine wave'. Photograph courtesy of Mettler Electronics

Naturopathic spinal reflex stimulation: validation of efficacy = 3

Spinal reflex stimulation is largely derived from Abrams' original work on spondylotherapy (Abrams 1912, Puderbach 1925) (see also Chapter 7). Spondylotherapy is analogous to the back shu points of Traditional Chinese Medicine. In spondylotherapy the internal organs are stimulated through the spinal nerves (Blake 2006, Boyle 1988, Johnson 1946b). Surging sine wave application is most often used for this purpose (Cordingley 1925, Gregory 1922). The low volt sinusoidal current is utilized in the system of constitutional hydrotherapy to elicit the abdominal reflexes as described by Abrams (Blake 2006, Boyle 1988, Scott 1990).

Abrams recommended placement of one sacral electrode and a second 'active' electrode at the level of the spine where stimulation was desired. Others recommended side-by-side placement of the electrodes 2 inches (5 cm) lateral from the spinous processes for eliciting these reflexes (Johnson 1946b, Lindquist 1948a). A third method for eliciting the reflexes is one pad placed over the spinal center and the other in close superficial proximity to the organ(s) under treatment (Blake 2006, Boyle 1988, Lindquist 1948a, Scott 1990). The periodic stimulation of spinal centers is recommended to encourage restoration of normal organ functioning in chronic cases and appropriate organ stimulation in acute conditions (see Boxes 12.1 and 12.2).

The sinusoidal current's ability to stimulate spinal reflexes, to enhance tissue perfusion and drainage, and to re-educate muscular contraction pathways has made it quite popular in naturopathic practice. Its use has been described for constipation, enhanced digestive function, sciatica, encouraging circulation to treat local infection, restoring prolapsed arches of the feet, visceroptosis, treatment of intestinal sphincter tone, hepatic drainage through sinusoidal massage, bronchial asthma, encouraging lactation, gastritis, enuresis, hiccough, congested liver, paralysis, low back pain and a large variety of conditions through stimulation of the spinal reflexes. Colson (1953) also lists over 300 indications for applications of spinal reflexes such as Addison's disease, aortic stenosis, aphthous stomatitis, renal calculi, conjunctivitis, dyspnea, glossitis, hernias, lead poisoning, mastoiditis, myocarditis and retinitis.

Low volt galvanic

Galvanism is a direct current with a low voltage and amperage. Galvanic current is one of the oldest forms of therapeutic electricity. The waveform is a continuous or pulsed flow of electrons. The flow of electrons in the direction of the negative pole results in electrochemical effects at the poles of the circuit. The electrochemical effect results in certain physiological alterations to the tissues at the site of application. Eliciting physiological changes of the tissue based upon the effects of the current is referred to as *medical galvanism*. This effect is harnessed for driving ionic medication into tissues in the process of *iontophoresis*. While the local electrochemical and physiological effects are of interest, the naturopathic physician

---

Box 12.1 Spinal levels and associated organ reflexes

C1	Larynx, parotid gland, eyes	T5	Stomach, dilates pylorus, contracts cardia
C2		T6	Stomach and duodenum
C3	Control of the diaphragm via the phrenic nerve	T7	Liver
C4		T8	Diaphragm
C5	Phrenic nerve, trachea, esophagus, bronchial tubes	T9	Pancreas and spleen
		T10	Kidney
C7	Inferior cervical ganglia, increases vagus tone, contracts heart blood vessels, dilates abdominal viscera	T12	Kidney and prostate
		L1	Bladder, peritoneum, scrotum, penis
T1	Bronchial tubes	L2	Bladder, peritoneum, scrotum, penis, cecum (right), sigmoid (left)
T2	Heart, fixates other reflexes elicited	L3	Ovaries and testicles
T3	Lungs, contracts pylorus, dilates cardiac orifice of stomach	L4	Ovaries and testicles, uterus, fallopian tubes
		L5	Uterus, fallopian tubes
T4	Dilates heart blood vessels	Sacral	Bladder and lower bowel

This is a synoptic chart of reflexes based upon Abrams (1912), Colson (1953), Cordingley (1925), Gregory (1922), Johnson (1946b) and Puderbach (1925). Further research to confirm and expand these reflexes and conditions is warranted.

Box 12.2 Naturopathic spinal reflex applications

C4–5	Indications: bronchial asthma, emphysema	T9–12	Heart reflex of dilation. Indications: angina pectoris, dilates thoracic aorta, infantile paralysis of legs and arms
C4–7	Indications: arm paralysis		
C5	*Contraindicated in emphysema*		
C7	Indications: cardiac asthma, tachycardia, palpitations, arrhythmia, migraine, exophthalmic goiter, diabetes mellitus, acute bronchial congestion, pertussis, congestion of orifices of the head, epistaxis. *Contraindicated in angina, bronchial asthma, splenomegaly, hepatic engorgement*	T10	Dilation of the kidneys, relieves pain of duodenal ulcer. Dilates abdominal viscera, contracts and empties appendix. Indications: nephritis, stimulates visceral activity, appendicitis that is not suppurative. *Contraindicated in splanchnoptosis*
T2–3	Reduces high blood pressure, hiccough	T11	Dilation of the intestines, dilates liver and spleen. Indications: spastic constipation, increases red blood cells and hemoglobin, dysmenorrhea due to rigid os. *Contraindicated in atonic constipation*
T3–8	Constricts splanchnic blood vessels. Indications: splanchnic neurasthenia, dilates the lungs		
T2–4	Diminishes vagus tone. Indications: emphysema, cardiotonic, increased mammary gland flow, dysmenorrhea, enuresis, asthma. *Contraindicated in low blood pressure, cardiac dilation, cardiac asthma, arrhythmia, palpitations, hyperthyroidism*	T12	Contracts the kidney. Indications: glomerulonephritis, increases pains with renal calculi, contracts the prostate gland, prostatic hypertrophy
T4–6	Contracts gall bladder and pancreas. Indications: cholecystitis, choledocholithiasis	L1–4	Contracts stomach, intestines, liver, spleen, prostate, uterus. Indications: atonic constipation, meno/metrorrhagia, enlarged spleen, increases leukocyte count, uterine displacement. *Contraindicated in spastic constipation, hepatic cirrhosis, dysmenorrhea due to rigid os*
T5	Dilates pylorus. Indications: headache, nausea, aid in duodenal intubation, gastritis		
T6–7	Dilates the kidneys. Indications: interstitial nephritis		
T7–8	Visceroptosis	L3	Stimulates gonads
T8	*Contraindicated in emphysema*	L5	Contracts urinary bladder. Indications: cystocele, chronic cystitis, enuresis
T9	Dilates gall bladder. Indications: choledocholithiasis. *Contraindicated in cholecystitis*	S2	Contracts inguinal canal. Indications: early hernia

This is a synoptic chart of reflexes based upon Abrams (1912), Colson (1953), Cordingley (1925), Gregory (1922), Johnson (1946b) and Puderbach (1925). Further research to confirm and expand these reflexes and conditions is warranted.

should not overlook the general effects of galvanization which include vasomotor stimulation and therefore influence on the distribution of blood and lymph (Jaskoviak 1993b).

Mechanism of action and physiological effects

The galvanic current produces predictable electrochemical and physiological effects at the site of application (Jaskoviak 1993c, Johnson 1946c) (Table 12.1).

The physiological effects of the positive pole of the galvanic current are somewhat analogous to the effect of cold applications and the negative pole to hot applications.

In order to elicit the polar effect of the galvanic current, two unequally sized electrodes are required. The smaller electrode is the active pad and is typically at most only half the size of the larger 'dispersive' electrode. The milliamp rule limits the amperage density to 1 mA/square inch of the active electrode. The smaller pad will demonstrate stronger polar effects as compared to the larger dispersive pad because, as the size of the electrode decreases, the current density will increase.

A relatively simple means of identifying which lead is negative is to immerse the leads in a glass of salted water and increase the amperage until bubbles are seen forming at the leads. The negative pole will attract the positively charged hydrogen ions in the vicinity. There are twice as many hydrogen ions in a

Table 12.1 Predictable electrochemical and physiological effects produced by galvanic current

Positive pole (anode)	Negative pole (cathode)
Electrochemical effects	
Attracts acids	Attracts bases (alkaloids)
Attracts oxygen	Attracts hydrogen
Physiological effects	
Stops hemorrhage	Increases hemorrhage
Relieves acute inflammation	Relieves chronic inflammation
Dehydrates/hardens tissue	Congests/irritates tissue
Constricts arterioles	Dilates arterioles
Decreases nerve irritability	Increases nerve irritability

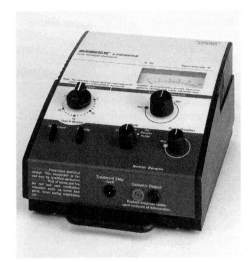

Figure 12.2B Low volt galvanic current. Photograph courtesy of Amrex-Zetron

molecule of water and the hydrogen ion is much smaller than the oxygen. Therefore, more bubbles that are smaller will accumulate at the negative as compared to the positive lead.

The current can be utilized to drive charged ions, ionic medication, into the tissues. As like charges repel one another, positively charged medications will be delivered by the positive pole of the circuit and negative by the negative. The galvanic current penetrates into the corium of the dermis only (about 1 mm), not very deeply into the tissues. The medication is then dispersed via capillary circulation to a larger amount of tissue. While the depth of penetration of the current and the ionic dispersal are shallow, the field effect generated is thought by some to affect ionic molecules at a greater depth.

Safety and contraindications

The galvanic current is relatively safe. Observation of the milliamp rule reduces the likelihood of burning the patient from application of too high amperage. Caution should be observed for allergic sensitivity to ions applied. Electrode pads should not be applied over broken skin. Patients with electronic implants should not be treated with galvanism as there is a risk of interference with the operation of the implant. Tissues that have impaired pain sensation should not have electrodes applied to them (Johnson 1946d, Starkey 1999b).

Indications: validation of efficacy = 4

With the exception of hyperhydrosis, medical galvanism is primarily utilized for musculoskeletal complaints such as adhesions, joint pain, neuritis, myalgia, sprains, strains and arthritic complaints. The modern application of galvanism generally focuses upon the role of iontophoresis. Iontophoresis has been found useful in a variety of conditions such as bursitis, plantar fasciitis, Peyronie's disease, allergic rhinitis, edema, Bell's palsy, frozen shoulder, fibrositis, dissolution of scar tissue, osteoarthritis, muscular spasm, arthritis, tenosynovitis, healing of skin ulcers, lymphedema, carpal tunnel syndrome, epicondylitis and temporomandibular joint disorders (Agresta 2004). The effect of iontophoresis is generally considered dependent upon the ionic medication applied (Starkey 1999c).

Naturopathic indications and application: validation of efficacy = 2

In 1955 the American Association of Naturopathic Physicians (AANP) described an extensive use of medical galvanism and iontophoresis: '(g)alvanism is applicable in proper form in practically every case which enters your office.' Galvanism is described as being clinically applied for hepatic drainage, rhinitis, various forms of hemorrhoid treatment, positive iontophoresis with magnesium sulfate for wart removal and tinea infections, with sodium chloride for corn removal, zinc ionization for indolent ulcers, copper ionization in cervicitis, and positive galvanism for rhinitis, hay fever and otitis media (Cordingley 1937). Adjunctive galvanic treatment is also recommended in dysmenorrhea, abscesses, amenorrhea, adhesion resorption, bronchitis, colitis, emphysema, endometritis, reducing tonsillar swelling, uterine and intestinal hemorrhage, incontinence, inflammation in its second stage, pelvic inflammation, hepatitis, meningitis, menorrhagia, metrorraghia, migraine, neuralgia, orchitis, cardiac palpitation, chronic peritonitis, salpingitis, impotence, urethral stricture and trachoma, and for reducing toothache pain (AANP 1955, Farnsworth & Kirkbride 1959, Post-Graduate Study of Naturotherapy 1939a, Scott 1990).

Cordingley (1937) also discusses two techniques that he describes as 'general' and 'central' galvanization. General galvanization consists of one electrode applied to the sacrum while the other is moved slowly along the spine and extremities. Central galvanization is similar but the stationary pad is placed over the solar plexus rather than the sacrum. General galvanization is applied to enhance lymphatic circulation (Post-Graduate Study of Naturotherapy 1938a).

Short wave diathermy

Diathermy has been in continuous clinical use for over 80 years. Diathermy literally means 'through heat'. The depth of penetration of the therapeutic heat is one of the deepest produced by physiotherapy modalities (Jaskoviak 1993d). The heat is generated by the resistance of the tissues to the passage of the current. The current is an electromagnetic one in the radio wave frequency. The first diathermy units had a relatively long wave and have been superseded by the modern short wave unit for a variety of reason. For a period of time microwave diathermy units were produced but have demonstrated some deleterious health risk; their clinical use is uncommon today, *and their use not the subject of this section* (Prentice 1988a, Starkey 1999d).

Mechanism of action and physiological effects

Short wave diathermy was developed in the 1930s and produces an electromagnetic radio wave. The most common frequency is 27.12 MHz, which produces an 11-meter wavelength. The waveform can be delivered in a constant or pulsed fashion at a variety of intensity settings. The electromagnetic energy is a non-ionizing form of radiation produced at a high frequency with low amplitude. The absorption of the electromagnetic energy by the tissues in the treatment field results in increased kinetic energy and therefore heat. The high frequency of the diathermy wave

(greater than 10 MHz) does not elicit muscular contraction or nerve depolarization (Starkey 1999d).

The absorption of energy increases kinetic energy, and therefore heat increases cellular metabolism in the treatment field. This is considered the primary effect of diathermy treatment (Jaskoviak 1993d). Another type of diathermy application, pulsed short wave diathermy, was developed in the 1960s. This type of application allows a pulsed, non-continuous waveform. The pulsed waveform creates a pulse train whose intensity and frequency can be manipulated. The pulse train allows for a brief pause during which the kinetic energy can be dispersed and distributed by the target tissues. This theoretically creates an athermal treatment where the energy transferred does not appreciably absorb in the target tissues. The effect of the treatment is theorized to be a product of the primary field effect of the energy rather than the secondary effects of the heat produced (Jaskoviak 1993d).

Thermal effects

As the tissues resist the flow of current, the physiological effects of diathermy are mediated through high frequency vibration of molecules in the treatment field. The result of the vibration is friction that creates a heating effect. The heating is to a depth of 1–2 inches (2–5 cm) depending upon type of application. The thermal effects increase tissue perfusion, increase capillary pressure and cell membrane permeability, relax muscles, increase transfer of metabolites across cell membranes, increase local metabolic rate, increase pain threshold, increase range of motion and decrease tension in collagenous tissues, and enhance tissue recovery (Prentice 1998a, Starkey 1999d).

The degree of heat delivered to the tissue by short wave units is not a quantified unit. Heating in tissue occurs as the equivalent of the current density squared multiplied by the resistance. Doses are measured by verbal communication from the patient as to the perceived intensity. Four levels are commonly utilized:

I: No perceived heat
II: Mild heat
III: Moderate heat (described by patients as a comfortable 'velvety warmth')
IV: Vigorous and barely tolerable heat (Agresta 2003).

Athermal effects

A field effect is proposed for pulsed short wave diathermy that is independent of thermal impressions and due solely to the influence of the electromagnetic field. The proposed mechanism of action is via changes in cellular ion levels and cell membrane potential, due

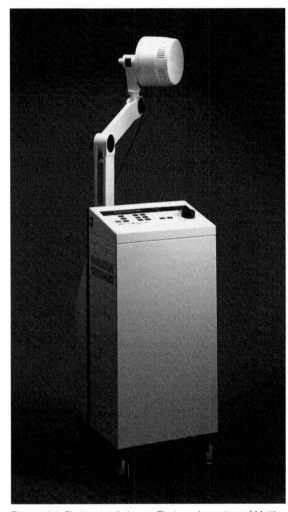

Figure 12.3 Short wave diathermy. Photograph courtesy of Mettler Electronics

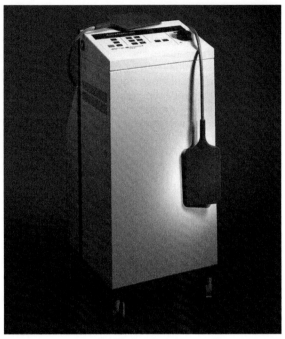

Figure 12.4 Short wave diathermy. Photograph courtesy of Mettler Electronics

to the influence of the wave on the cellular sodium pump that encourages normalization of the cells' ionic balance. This proposed mechanism has not been substantiated (Sanservino 1980).

Observations of the clinical effect (Cameron 1961, Goldin et al 1981, Van den Bouwhuijsen et al 1990) include:

- increased number of white blood cells, histiocytes and fibroblasts in a wound
- improved rate of edema dispersion
- enhanced fat activity
- encouragement of canalization and absorption of hematoma
- reduction of the inflammatory process

- a more rapid rate of fibrin fiber orientation and deposition of collagen
- improvement in collagen formation
- stimulation of osteogenesis
- improved healing of the peripheral and central nervous systems.

Safety and contraindications

Diathermy has been utilized for decades with a relatively strong safety record (Prentice 1998b). Most of the negative reported effects attributed to diathermy were associated with microwave diathermy and not with short wave diathermy (Prentice 1998b, Starkey 1999e). The recent evidence of beneficial tissue effects of pulsed diathermy is not only a validation of the relative safety of the electromagnetic wave field but is also evidence of a positive influence of the field (Gorbunov et al 1995, Hill et al 2002, Kerem & Yigiter 2002).

Diathermy should not be applied, or only cautiously so, directly over most metal implants (dental fillings and bridgework excluded), as metal selectively heats and can burn the patient. Likewise, diathermy should not be used over anything wet, as the water is likely to turn to steam, potentially resulting in a burn. Dry towels should always be used and sensible precautions should be taken to ensure that the area to be treated is dried, so avoiding common clinical errors.

It is best to have patients remove jewelry in the area to be treated. Most dental work is safe and no adverse response to use over fillings or other dental implants has been reported. A Danish study on abdominal diathermy in women with copper IUDs demonstrated no adverse effects and the researchers concluded that it is safe in commonly used dosages (Heick 1991).

Diathermy should not to be used if a patient has a pacemaker or implanted neurological device. Patients with a pacemaker or implanted neurological device should not be allowed within a 25 feet (7.5 m) radius of an active diathermy unit as the waveform can interfere with the functions of these devices.

Diathermy is not used directly over the abdomen of pregnant patients, and generally avoided with pregnancy primarily because of its temperature-elevating ability. The balance of studies on pregnant physiotherapist diathermy operators has shown no consistent significant differences in pregnancy outcomes or newborn health when compared with controls (Guberan et al 1994, Larsen 1991, Lerman et al 2001, Taskinen 1990). Studies and case reports and studies associated with negative outcome appear to involve the microwave forms of diathermy and the high volume of exposure for operators using diathermy (Oullet Hellstrom & Stewart 1993). A study on the mutagenicity for short wave radiofrequency has demonstrated no negative effect (Hamnerius 1985).

When a patient has a temperature elevation over 99.5°F oral, diathermy may only drive the fever higher – perhaps overwhelmingly so – and some advise against its use in these cases (Watrous 1996). However, case reports of patients with pneumonia and high fever receiving diathermy treatments with excellent outcome have been published (Abbott et al 1945b). Diathermy increases heat and therefore blood flow. If there is circulatory insufficiency, caution should be used with local treatment of an affected area.

Diathermy should not be used over an active epiphysis and is generally not advised directly over malignant tissue (Starkey 1999f). However, the latter admonition will probably change in the future because historically it has been used as a treatment for cancer with report of success (Darst 1936) and there is research that supports local hyperthermia and tumor treatment (Connor et al 1977, Hurwitz et al 2005, Laptev 2004, Tilly et al 2005).

Constant short wave indications: validation of efficacy = 5

Diathermy is used wherever deep heating is indicated. Modern physiotherapy application of dia-

thermy treatment is focused primarily upon its musculoskeletal application – subacute musculoskeletal injury, increased tissue circulation, vasodilation, increased local metabolism, muscle relaxation, trigger point relaxation and increased tissue repair, including neurological tissue (Goats 1989). Evidence exists for its application in osteoarthritis (Atamaz 2006, Jan et al 2006), acute soft tissue injury (Shields et al 2002), temporomandibular joint pain (Gray et al 1994) and herpes zoster (Allberry et al 1972, 1974).

Naturopathic indications and applications: validation of efficacy = 2

These previous indications are all quite useful in the daily practice of a naturopathic clinical setting. There are quite a number of other applications for which diathermy has been utilized. Use of diathermy has been reported in a variety of infectious processes and especially various forms of pneumonia (De Groot 1964, Kitaigorodskaia 1956, Ravitskii 1954, Saperov 1974, Sergeev et al 1986, Uglov 1965). Diathermy reduces the viscosity of mucus and is very useful for upper respiratory tract diseases. In an early study of diathermy, its introduction and use in hospitals decreased pneumonia mortality by 50% (Stewart 1923). Naturopathic physicians have reported clinical usefulness of diathermy in all forms of upper respiratory infections for several decades (Abbott et al 1945c, Johnson 1946e, Watrous & Blake 2004, Wolf 1935a).

Initially this usefulness in infectious processes was thought to be due to specific bactericidal effects of the waveform (Lindquist 1948b). Later evaluation of the evidence led to a general consensus that the positive effects were indirect effects primarily of improved circulation (Wolf 1935b). The net result is the observation of the *vis medicatrix naturae* and validation of the naturopathic approach of improving non-specific physiological function, such as increased metabolism and tissue perfusion, by incorporating beneficial natural agents, in this case electromagnetic energy, to enhance the natural resolution of infectious processes.

In 1939, W.H. Allen ND published a treatise on the application of short wave diathermy. He categorized conditions into constitutional, local or infectious, and then described the incorporation of diathermy into each of these three categories. For local conditions such as an ankle sprain in an otherwise healthy individual a short local application was recommended. If there was constitutional weakness then treatment was directed through the liver. Infectious conditions would require a combination of the two strategies – both local and constitutional.

Box 12.3 Naturopathic indications

- Acne (Abbott et al 1945d)
- Angina pectoris (Abbott et al 1945d)
- Appendicitis (chronic) (Wolf 1935c)
- Bronchial asthma (Abbott et al 1945d)
- Bronchiectasis (Wolf 1935d)
- Carbuncles
- Cholecystitis (Abbott et al 1945d)
- Colds (Wolf 1935e)
- Colitis (spastic and ulcerative) (Abbott et al 1945d)
- Cystitis (Abbott et al 1945d)
- Empyema (Wolf 1935f)
- Endocarditis (Wolf 1935c)
- Erysipelas (Wolf 1935c)
- Eyes (inflammation and infection)
- Furunculosis (Abbott et al 1945d)
- Glaucoma (threatening)
- Glomerulonephritis (Wolf 1935g)
- Gonorrhea (Wolf 1935h)
- Hemiplegia (Wolf 1935i)
- Hepatitis (Wolf 1935j)
- Lung abscess (Wolf 1935k)
- Mastitis (Wolf 1935l)
- Migraine (Wolf 1935m)
- Myocarditis (Wolf 1935c)
- Osteomyelitis (Johnson 1946e, Wolf 1935n)
- Otitis media (Wolf 1935o)
- Paronychia (Wolf 1935p)
- Pelvic inflammatory disease (Abbott et al 1945d)
- Perianal abscess (Wolf 1935o)
- Peritonsillar abscess (Wolf 1935o)
- Pleuritis (Abbott et al 1945d)
- Pneumonia (Abbott et al 1945d, Wolf 1935q)
- Poliomyelitis
- Prostatitis (Johnson 1946e)
- Pyelonephritis (Wolf 1935r)
- Sinusitis (Abbott et al 1945d)
- Tonsillitis (Wolf 1935e)
- Tuberculosis (Wolf 1935j)

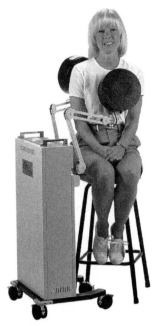

Figure 12.5 Short wave diathermy. Photograph courtesy of International Medical Electronics

A long list of positive clinical outcomes is described in the observational literature on short wave diathermy. Modern evaluation of these individual conditions is strongly recommended. A variety of applicators such as rectal, vaginal and urethral sounds existed for the application of treatment to the various orifices of the body. It will be seen that the majority of the applications involve infectious processes and those that do not would benefit from the predictable physiological response of the body to diathermy application.

An interesting passage from Shriber's (1975) electrotherapy manual states: 'The effective use of antibiotics has eliminated the need to treat infected body cavities with diathermy over lengthy periods.' While the advent of antibiotics may have contributed to the decline of the application and continued evaluation of diathermy in infectious processes, with the modern rise of antibiotic resistance diathermy may have a much larger role to play again in the future.

Pulsed short wave indications: validation of efficacy = 3

Evidence for the benefit of pulsed short wave therapy can be confusing and requires a thorough understanding of the subject to properly evaluate. Post-dental surgical wound recovery (Aronofsky 1971), acute whiplash injury and skin grafts have demonstrated benefit. It is considered safe and has shown no increase in microbial populations of affected tissues (Badea et al 1993). Significant benefit has been demonstrated with a strong recommendation for use in chronic decubitus ulcer treatment (Comorsan et al 1993, Itoh et al 1991, Salzberg et al 1995). Improvement in fibronectin synthesis with both local and hepatic treatment has shown a positive influence in postsurgical healing times (Arghiropol et al 1992). Beneficial application

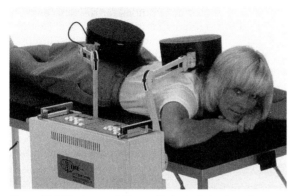

Figure 12.6 Short wave diathermy. Photograph courtesy of International Medical Electronics

for non-union fracture healing is substantiated by the observed positive influence on osteoblast differentiation (Lohmann et al 2000) and a positive influence on growth factor regulation. This result is substantiated by research on liver enzymes that shows a beneficial stimulating effect (Pop et al 1989). These findings have particular relevance for the naturopathic therapeutic approach.

Naturopathic indications and applications: validation of efficacy = 2

The late naturopathic physician Dr Poesnecker described clinical application of pulsed short wave therapy using an indirect approach to enhance organ metabolism and detoxification. His treatment was directed to hepatic, splenic, renal and adrenal tissue, with the goal of enhancing organ metabolism and detoxification. He applied this indirect approach in chronic disorders such as chronic fatigue syndrome and fibromyalgia (Poesnecker 1978).

Pulsed short wave has been recommended at low pulse rate intervals for internal organ stimulation and the higher pulse rates, which have less thermal dispersion due to the increased frequency, for acute infections and inflammations. In acute infection and inflammation a primary local application with a secondary application to the liver and spleen is recommended for stimulation of the reticuloendothelial system (Linder 1964).

Benefit has been shown in osteoarthritis (Thamsborg et al 2005 Trock et al 1994) and chronic tinnitus, and inconsistent results are found with ankle sprains. Beneficial observation in neural tissue repair has been reported consistently in animal models (Raji 1984, Raji et al 1983, Sisken et al 1989). A study on Guillain–Barré syndrome demonstrated enhanced neurological tissue healing with pulsed short wave (Gorbunov et al 1995).

Interestingly, pulsed diathermy applied to metastasizing melanoma cell cultures demonstrated increased cell death for a period of 4 minutes after exposure (Hakkinen et al 1975).

High frequency Tesla coil

High frequency Tesla coil (HFTC) is similar to diathermy but produces less tissue heating. It is one of the oldest physiotherapy devices and has been in use since the end of the 19th century. High frequency is essentially a modified Tesla coil that produces a high frequency, high voltage current at low amperage. The high frequency of the current does not depolarize sensory or motor neurons (Matijaca 1919a).

HFTC currents rapidly oscillate well above 10 000 Hz. The rapidly oscillating currents are applied to the body through vacuum glass electrodes. As the current moves through the electrode, the partially vacuumed atmosphere inside the glass ionizes and assumes color dependent upon the degree of vacuum. The most common color is violet and the units are commonly referred to as 'violet ray' devices. The electrodes do not, however, emit any ultraviolet rays.

Mechanism of action and physiological effects

When the electrode is applied to the body it induces a local current in tissues and creates a local heating effect as the tissues resist the current flow. The increased resistance promotes increased tissue perfusion locally. If the electrode is separated from the body by thin gauze, electrical sparks will shower the skin with a resulting counterirritation effect. If the electrode current is concentrated into a point it can be used for fulguration and is the current used in hyfrecation. The high voltage ionizes the atmosphere immediately around it, resulting in the production of a small amount of ozone, which then has germicidal effects. The effects on tissue have been described as a 'cellular massage' (Hewlett-Parsons 1968). Others consider that the person who has the HFTC applied to them acts as a plate in a condenser and capacitatively stores a charge (Neiswanger 1925a). Interestingly, Edgar Cayce advocated the use of the HFTC and considered that it 'charged the nervous system'.

HFTC has the following effects on tissue. It:

- increases oxidation and local nutrition (Matijaca 1919b)
- produces hyperemia and stimulates circulation in areas to which it is applied (this hyperemia is believed to last from 10 to 24 hours) (Matijaca 1919b)

- adds oxygen to the blood (Matijaca 1919b)
- increases elimination of carbon dioxide
- increases elimination of waste products through the skin
- increases the temperature where applied
- is topically germicidal, encourages leukocytosis and enhances phagocytosis (Matijaca 1919b)
- increases local glandular activity of the skin (Cordingley 1925, Gerson 2002, Neiswanger 1925b, Post-Graduate Study of Naturotherapy 1937a).

Safety and contraindications

The HFTC current has a long history of use with a strong safety record. No adverse effects were identified in a literature search. Caution should be observed with pregnancy due to a lack of research on its effects. Caution should also be observed with flammable lubricants as the sparks may potentially cause ignition. Caution should also be exercised with pacemakers, implanted defibrillators and implanted neurological devices until further research of the safety of HFTC with these devices is known.

Indications: validation of efficacy = 2

Contemporary conventional application of high-frequency current is primarily limited to dermatalogical diseases such as acne and atopic dermatitis, for which it is considered safe and effective. There are numerous electrodes produced for use with the HFTC and a wide variety of therapeutic applications have been recommended. Extensive therapeutic applications were recommended historically by manufacturers of the units until prosecution in the 1950s in the United States for being unable to adequately substan-tiate recommended applications for the devices they produced (Museum of Questionable Medical Devices 2000), resulting in manufacturers' literature limiting recommendations to conditions such as atopic dermatitis and acne. Subsequently we will not rely on historical manufacturers' recommendations and restrict ourselves to independent sources. Bierman & Licht mention the HFTC only briefly in their conventional physical medicine textbook published in 1952 and, while admitting that mild heating and increased local circulation do occur, they consider the method 'obsolete' and recommend 'less spectacular' means.

Naturopathic indications and applications: validation of efficacy = 2

HFTC was advocated for its ability to reduce inflammation in both chronic and acute local inflammatory conditions. The effect of the current is considered soothing and able to reduce inflammation (Boyle 1988, Post-Graduate Study of Naturotherapy 1937b, 1938b), rheumatic pains, eczema, asthma, emphysema (Hewlett-Parsons 1968, Post-Graduate Study of Naturotherapy 1937c, Scott 1990), trachoma (Post-Graduate Study of Naturotherapy 1939b), arthritis (Post-Graduate Study of Naturotherapy 1939c), muscular spasm, torticollis, low back pain, rheumatoid arthritis (Post-Graduate Study of Naturotherapy 1939b), peritonitis, pelvic adhesions, ovarian neuralgia, tic douloureux, neuritis, neuralgia, migraine, recuperation after measles (Post-Graduate Study of Naturotherapy 1938c, Scott 1990), acute and chronic cystitis, chorea (Post-Graduate Study of Naturotherapy 1938d), menstrual cramping, muscle tears, localized pain, fibroids, ovarian cysts (Blake 2006), bronchitis and nephritis (Scott 1990). HFTC is commonly encountered in estheticians' practice where it is used to reduce wrinkles and pore size, and to treat acne and atopic dermatitis (Clayton 1928, Johnson 1946b, Luke 1922, Neiswanger 1925a).

Microcurrent

Carolyn McMakin MA DC

Microcurrent devices provide current in millionths of an ampere to the patient being treated. The current is delivered using adhesive electrode pads or graphite-conducting fabric. An ampere is the rate of movement of electrons past a point in space and one millionth of an ampere is a microamp (μA). The body itself generates microamperage current in every cell and membrane as part of its normal physiological activity. This current flow creates the polarity observed by Becker in the human system in which the body is polarized more positively at the head, negatively at the feet, more positive centrally and more negative distally

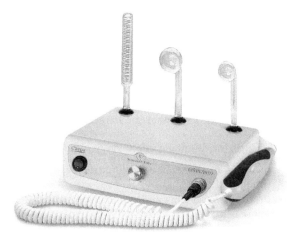

Figure 12.7 High frequency. Photograph courtesy of Silhouet-Tone

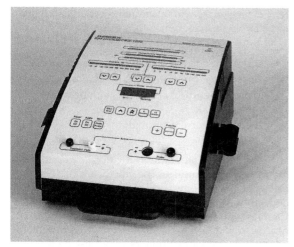

Figure 12.8 Microcurrent. Photograph courtesy of International Medical Electronics

(Becker & Seldon 1985). Most microcurrent devices are battery operated but some are plugged into a wall current source and current levels are stepped down to microamperage.

Microcurrent creates its effects by delivering current within a normal physiological range, making it particularly consistent with naturopathic principles and appropriate to a naturopathic practice. This subsensory physiological current has been demonstrated to increase ATP production, protein synthesis and amino acid transport in rat skin (Cheng 1982). Current levels above 500 µA caused ATP and protein synthesis to level off and current levels above 750 µA caused inhibition and reduction of ATP. Most electrotherapy devices deliver current in the milliamp range, or thousandths of amps, to create their therapeutic effect.

The increased production of ATP is the presumed mechanism of action that facilitates the increased rate of wound, injury and fracture healing and pain reduction seen in the clinical use of microcurrent therapy. Injured tissue loses its ability to hold and carry charge efficiently. It is hypothesized that some of microcurrent's clinical effects are due to its ability to restore normal membrane polarity.

Some microcurrent devices deliver straight DC current but most deliver pulsed DC current, modulated so that it is alternating with a square wave or ramped square wave form. Some devices are very simple, one-channel devices and modulate current with only a few frequencies such as 0.3 Hz, 3 Hz, 30 Hz and 300 Hz. Other devices allow a complex, two-channel frequency choice, accurate to two or three digits.

In 1997 the development of frequency-specific microcurrent (FSM) added the clinical effects of a frequency-specific response to the known effects of the delivery of unmodulated direct current or non-specific frequency choices. The frequencies were resurrected from lists of frequencies used with wall current electrotherapy modalities used from 1914 to 1937. While published clinical outcomes and some preliminary animal research have been performed in order to separate the effects of the microcurrent alone from any additional frequency-specific effect, further research is necessary. The research needed to separate the effects of the current alone from the additional effects of the frequency response is an area of interest but published clinical outcomes and some preliminary animal research are promising.

Validation of efficacy = 4

Microcurrent has documented effects in increasing wound, tissue and fracture healing, decreasing pain and edema and treating myofascial trigger points and neuropathic pain.

- Thirty hospital patients with non-healing ulcers were divided into two groups, one treated with conventional wound dressings and one with microcurrent stimulation at 300–700 µA. The latter group was given two 2-hour stimulation periods per day. After 6 weeks of such treatments, the group treated with microcurrent showed a 150–250% faster healing rate, with stronger scar formation, less pain and lessened infection of the treated area (Carley & Wainapel 1985).

- Researchers applied microcurrent stimulation ranging from 200 to 800 µA to a wide variety of wounds, using negative polarity over the lesions in the initial phase, and then alternating positive and negative electrodes every 3 days. The treated group showed 200–350% faster healing rates than controls, with stronger tensile strength of scar tissue and antibacterial effects in infected wounds in the treated group (Wolcott et al 1969).

- DuPont et al (1999) described techniques for locating and stimulating trigger points (TPs) using a microcurrent stimulator, specifically for the treatment of temporomandibular disorders. They state that electrical conductivity is highest over trigger points, and galvanic skin response (GSR) testing can be used to locate such points. Probe electrodes were used to treat small TPs, and pad electrodes to treat larger ones. Probe treatment was delivered at 0.3 Hz, 20–40 µA, with treatment time of 10–30 seconds per site. These researchers suggest administering treatment in 24- to 48-hour intervals, and state that results should be seen within two to three treatments.

- Bertolucci & Grey (1995) divided 48 patients into three groups, some receiving placebo, some microcurrent and some laser to treat pain of temporomandibular syndrome. Both microcurrent and laser were found to be significantly more effective than placebo, with laser slightly more effective than microcurrent. The author acknowledges that microcurrent's easy accessibility makes it more practical for practitioners here.
- Frequency-specific microcurrent has been shown to be effective in the treatment of myofascial trigger points and pain in the head, neck and face, and low back (McMakin 1998, 2004). The frequency-specific response has been shown to reduce inflammatory cytokines, substance P and pain and increase endorphin levels in fibromyalgia associated with cervical spine trauma using 40 Hz on channel A and 10 Hz on channel B (McMakin 2005).
- In unpublished animal research carried out at the University of Sydney Veterinary Science Department the frequency to reduce inflammation (40 Hz) in the immune system (116 Hz) was shown to reduce lipoxygenase-mediated inflammation in a mouse model by 62% in 4 minutes as compared to no reduction in the placebo group. None of the three other frequency combinations tested had any effects on reducing inflammation. In COX-mediated inflammation, 40 Hz/116 Hz produced a 30% reduction of swelling which was equivalent to that seen with injectable ketorolac (Toradol). Both 40 Hz and 103 Hz reduced COX-mediated inflammation by 30% in the same trial but 40 Hz and 355 Hz had no effect on swelling and was equivalent to placebo. This demonstration of a frequency-specific response is a promising preliminary finding and is awaiting a larger trial for publication (V Reeve, Veterinary Science Department, University of Sydney, personal communication, 2003).

Indications, contraindications and safety

Microcurrent is in an awkward position in the area of indications, contraindications and safety. Microcurrent devices are approved by the FDA in the category of TENS devices even though TENS devices deliver milliamperage current for the control of pain by blocking transmission of pain impulses up the spinal cord and have been shown to reduce the rate of wound healing and ATP production. The device manufacturers can only make claims for the microcurrent device as if it was a TENS device, which it is not. Microcur-

rent devices must carry contraindications as if they were TENS devices, which they are not.

Contraindications to TENS include:

- cannot run current through a pregnant uterus
- cannot run current through the brain
- cannot use current on people with demand-type pacemakers
- cannot run current through the eye.

Microamperage current has been used clinically in 'off label' uses in all of these situations except during pregnancy. In clinical usage, microcurrent is safe to use with plates, pins, artificial joints and implants, and in new injuries, chronic pain and swelling. Caution should be exercised in running current near or through the chest in patients with demand pacemakers and practitioners may best be advised to contact the pacemaker manufacturer's technical support line to ask for guidance about use with the particular unit installed. When in doubt it is best to 'do no harm' and err on the side of caution.

The manufacturers of the devices are limited to claims that can be made for indications as if microcurrent devices are TENS devices, which they are not. The research is clear that the effects of microcurrent and frequency-specific microcurrent are useful in the successful treatment of new injuries, wound healing, fracture repair, myofascial trigger points, neuropathic pain and spinal cord-mediated pain in fibromyalgia due to cervical spine trauma. None of these indications can be claimed by the manufacturers or distributors of the devices.

Therapeutic ultrasound

Douglas C. Lewis ND

Indications/description

Therapeutic ultrasound is the application of acoustic energy to living tissues. Its therapeutic use for the relief of pain and/or the relaxation of soft tissues began in the United States in the early 1950s or late 1940s (Shankar & Randall 2002a). Basic and clinical research in the use of ultrasound began earlier in Europe and especially Germany (Griffin & Karselis 1988).

Ultrasound has been described as a diathermy modality. This is due to its ability to produce a tissue temperature rise (TTR) in the treated tissues. However, the mechanism by which it achieves that action differs dramatically from the TTR achieved by the action of electromagnetic energy when applied to living tissues. In addition, ultrasound produces other effects not generated by electromagnetic energy.

The energy of ultrasound is focused to an area under the ultrasound head. It is therefore well adapted to focused treatment and less well suited to heating large areas.

Therapeutic ultrasound is generally recognized for its use in, or treatment of, the following (Cameron 2003, Griffin & Karselis 1988, Hayes 2000, Shankar & Randall 2002a):

- Relief from pain
- Relief from muscle spasm/trigger points
- Acute, subacute and chronic inflammation of tendons, bursae, etc.
- Joint contracture
- Scar tissue/adhesion remodeling
- Neurofibroma
- Plantar warts
- Carpal tunnel syndrome
- Healing of wounds, tendons and bone
- Organized hematoma
- Abnormal tissue mineralization
- Transdermal drug delivery.

Ultrasound produces its action through the coupling of mechanical energy into tissues. As an alternating current is applied to the piezoelectric crystal in the ultrasound head, the crystal vibrates, producing compression and rarefaction waves. The vibration energy is conducted into the tissues through an elastic coupling medium such as water or a coupling gel. Movement of the molecules of the coupling medium causes movement of the molecules of the tissues. As those molecules move, heat is generated through friction; hence the historical description of ultrasound as a diathermy modality (Griffin & Karselis 1988).

Methodology

Therapeutic ultrasound may be applied with either a continuous or a pulsed output. It may be applied at frequencies between 850 kHz and 3 MHz, with 1 MHz as the most common compromise. The output frequency of each device is fixed and cannot be adjusted. Lower frequencies of ultrasound have a greater depth of penetration into tissues and, conversely, higher frequencies have a shallower depth of penetration. See discussion under 'Physiological effects' below. The intensity of treatment (power) may be varied between 0.25 and 2.0 watts per square centimeter (W/cm^2) of effective crystal size, depending on the desired therapeutic effect.

An ultrasound treatment consists of all of the following:

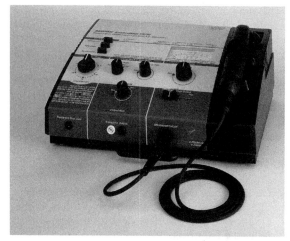

Figure 12.9 Ultrasound. Photograph courtesy of Amrex-Zetron

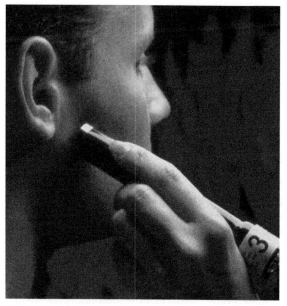

Figure 12.10 Ultrasound application to the temporomandibular joint. Photograph courtesy of Mettler Electronics

- A choice of area to be treated
- A determination of frequency to be used (as stated, a compromise frequency of 1 MHz is common to most ultrasound devices, but some devices are available with interchangeable heads of different frequencies)
- A choice of power level to be applied
- A decision as to whether to use pulsed or continuous output
- The duration of treatment.

The modality must be applied with the use of a coupling medium. Either water or a coupling gel is adequate and appropriate for this use. Most modern ultrasound heads may be immersed in water. Thus underwater treatments are best for areas that are small or uneven, such as the hand, wrist, foot, etc. Large flat areas such as the low back or shoulder are appropriate for the use of a coupling gel.

Once the above decisions are made as to the appropriate treatment parameters, the treatment is performed with a constant motion of the ultrasound head over the desired treatment area for the duration of the treatment.

Each indication suggests its own specific treatment parameters. It is beyond the scope and intent of this text to provide an exhaustive description of each, but consider the following:

1. Pulsed ultrasound will not produce a TTR as readily as continuous ultrasound. It is therefore a more appropriate application in acute inflammatory conditions such as acute sprains and strains or under other circumstances where a TTR is undesirable.
2. Overall TTR is a function of power, time and size of the area treated. To apply the same 'dose' to a larger treatment area, either the duration or the power (intensity) of the treatment must be increased and vice versa.

For more on this subject, see 'Physiological effects' below.

Safety and contraindications

Ultrasound exerts its greatest influence at the interface of different tissue types due to absorption and reflection of its energy at these interfaces. Absorption is greatest in tissues with high collagen content (Cameron 2003, Griffin & Karselis 1988, Hayes 2000, Shankar & Randall 2002a).

For this reason the energy of ultrasound may concentrate in the interfaces of tendon and periosteum. Intense heating may occur in these areas, leading to a pathological temperature increase. The periosteum is richly supplied with sensory receptors, including thermal receptors. Therefore, in persons with a normally functioning sensory nervous system, pain will alert them to danger long before harm is done (Griffin & Karselis 1988).

Other common contraindications to the use of ultrasound (Cameron 2003, Griffin & Karselis 1988, Hayes 2000, Shankar & Randall 2002a) include treatments over:

- the eye
- the open spinal cord (s/p laminectomy)
- the heart
- implanted medical devices (insulin pumps, pacemakers, etc.)
- the pregnant uterus
- malignancies or suspected malignancies
- thrombophlebitis
- the carotid sinus or cervical ganglia.

Special care must be taken when applying ultrasound in the following cases:

- in the presence of orthopedic pins or artificial joints
- in areas of active bleeding
- over areas of hypo- or dysesthesia
- in the presence of vascular insufficiency
- over fractures
- the epiphysis of growing bones
- breast implants.

Validation of efficacy = 4

Ultrasound is very commonly used in clinical practice. This author uses it in practice daily and chooses it over almost any other electrical modality. It has a high degree of safety, and patient response to treatment is generally positive and rarely, if ever, negative.

Cameron (2003) and Griffin & Karselis (1988) cite numerous studies demonstrating the effectiveness of ultrasound in the treatment of soft tissue shortening, pain control, dermal ulcers, surgical skin incisions, tendon injuries, resorption of calcium deposits, bone fractures, carpal tunnel syndrome, plantar warts and herpes zoster.

However, Shankar & Randall (2002a) describe a meta-analysis performed and published by Gam & Johannsen (1995) and a systematic review performed and published by van der Windt et al (1999) in which those authors state that the studies they reviewed were lacking in information that would allow them to be statistically analyzed. Therefore they concluded that there was little evidence to support the use of ultrasound in the treatment of musculoskeletal disorders.

It should be remembered that studies which fail to prove efficacy do not, by default, prove the modality to be ineffective.

Alternatives

Depending on the physiological effect desired, there may be several alternatives to ultrasound. Heating of tissues may be accomplished in many different ways. Hot water immersion, exercise, infrared, short wave or microwave diathermy may all produce a TTR

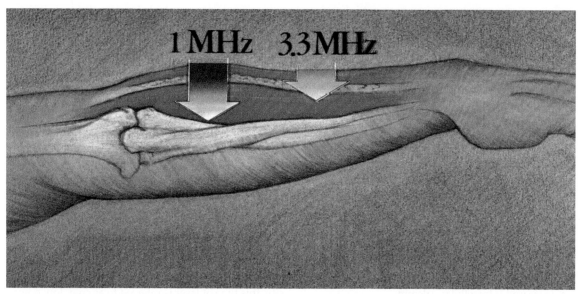

Figure 12.11 Varying depth of ultrasound penetration. Photograph courtesy of Mettler Electronics

though perhaps not as deeply into tissues or as specifically. In the case of diathermy, there is a tendency to heating of subcutaneous fat that does not occur with ultrasound.

Cross-fiber releasing and myofascial release techniques may be useful in the release of scars and adhesions, though again these may not be as effective in deep tissues.

Increasing blood flow to an area may be accomplished perhaps more effectively with the use of contrast hydrotherapy if that is the primary desired effect.

Physiological effects

As stated previously, ultrasound produces an increase in tissue temperature (TTR) when applied continuously for an adequate period of time. The time required to produce a therapeutic TTR depends on the area treated and the intensity of the application. Thus, TTR = area $\times$ W/cm^2 $\times$ duration of treatment. Utilization of ultrasound in a pulsed mode eliminates most of the thermal effects of the modality.

Manipulation of the depth of penetration of ultrasound is accomplished to some extent by the choice of frequency generated by the device. As mentioned, most devices are equipped with a 10 cm effective crystal size operating at a frequency of 1 MHz. As the frequency of ultrasound increases, the depth of penetration decreases. Some manufacturers have released instruments with a 7 cm crystal operating at 1 MHz and others have produced devices with interchange-

able head units producing 3 MHz with a 5 cm crystal and 3.5 MHz with a 1 cm crystal in addition to the standard 10 cm, 1 MHz crystal.

The thermal effects of ultrasound (Cameron 2003, Griffin & Karselis 1988, Hayes 2000, Shankar & Randall 2002a) include:

- increased tissue extensibility (tendon, ligament, etc.)
- altered blood flow
- altered nerve conduction velocity[1]
- increased enzyme activity
- changes in muscle activity.

The vibrations generated by ultrasound also produce mechanical effects from both stable and unstable cavitation as well as acoustic streaming and microstreaming. These are thought to produce the non-thermal effects of ultrasound. Acoustic streaming describes the steady flow of cellular fluids induced by the high frequency sound waves. This is believed to alter cell membrane permeability and facilitate transfer of material from one area to another. Microstreaming describes the eddying that takes place near any

---

[1]Griffin & Karselis report that at ultrasound intensities between 0.5 and 2.0 W/cm^2 nerve conduction velocities decline, whereas at intensities below 0.5 and above 2.0 W/cm^2 nerve conduction velocities increase. They go on to state that where electromagnetic energy is sufficient to produce a TTR, nerve conduction velocity invariably increases.

vibrating object. According to Shankar & Randall, microstreaming may cause 'cell lysis, alteration of cellular function, degradation of DNA, and inactivation of certain enzymes' (Cameron 2003, Shankar & Randall 2002a).

Cavitation is described as the expansion and contraction of gas- or vapor-filled bubbles in blood and tissue fluids. With stable cavitation, bubbles vary in size but do not burst. In unstable cavitation, bubbles grow and implode, which may cause local tissue damage and free radical formation. It is believed that unstable cavitations do not occur at the intensity levels used for therapeutic ultrasound.

The non-thermal effects attributed to ultrasound include the following:

- Increased skin and cell membrane permeability
- Increased mast cell degranulation
- Increased histamine and chemotactic factor release
- Increased intracellular calcium
- Increased macrophage responsiveness
- Increased rate of protein synthesis by fibroblasts leading to increased collagen synthesis and strength
- Changes in electrical activity of nervous tissue
- Increases in enzymatic activity
- Increases in angiogenesis.

Phonophoresis describes the utilization of ultrasound for the localized delivery of medications. Several theories have been presented to explain the phenomenon, but the exact mechanism of action is unknown. It is thought that ultrasound increases both skin permeability and cell membrane permeability, thus increasing the uptake of medications. Unlike the use of iontophoresis for drug delivery, phonophoresis does not require ionization of a medication. Anti-inflammatory agents and analgesics have been commonly used in phonophoresis.

Cautions

See 'Safety and contraindications' above.

Naturopathic perspectives

Ultrasound is a very safe and effective modality that fits well within naturopathic practice. It is certainly agreed that, for purposes of clinical science, additional, well-developed research should be done to determine the efficacy of ultrasound in many of its applications. However, given its low cost, low risk of harm and clinical evidence of efficacy, it would seem likely that ultrasound will remain a useful tool for the naturopathic physician.

Low level laser therapy (LLLT)

Nick Buratovich ND

The concept of therapeutic light, phototherapy, has evolved from the taking of sunbaths (heliotherapy) to the use of infrared, ultraviolet lamps and, since the 1960s, the use of LASER (i.e. Light Amplification by Stimulated Emission of Radiation) light (Belanger 2002a). Laser light is a focused beam of light that emits photon energy. Laser light is therapeutically generated by the gaseous helium-neon (HeNe) laser, the gallium arsenide (GaAs) and the gallium aluminum arsenide (GaAlAs) semiconductor or diode lasers.

Contrary to lasers used in surgery and industry, which are of high power and capable of tissue destruction and thermal effects, those used in physical medicine and rehabilitation are low power (1–20 mW) and athermal. They are capable of cell photobiomodulation and healing. As a result of this low power intensity, this type of laser is referred to as cold, low power or low level laser therapy (LLLT) (Shankar & Randall 2002b).

Lasers characteristically produce light which is monochromatic (a single wavelength and color), coherent (waves travel in highly ordered, parallel wavelengths and frequencies) and collimated (minimal divergence over distance) (Weisberg 1994). Laser light may be generated in the visible spectrum of light (390–770 nm) or in the invisible spectrum in the near infrared band (600–1200 nm). The mode of delivery may be continuous or pulsed through probes or grids applied perpendicularly to the treatment surface, either in direct skin contact or above the skin in a sweeping fashion. The typical application may be from 15 to 30 seconds up to 2 minutes, or longer in certain instances.

Mechanism of action and physiological effects

Like other forms of radiation, laser light can be absorbed, transmitted or reflected by tissue. Penetration of laser light may be direct (absorption) and indirect after refraction, dispersion and reflection up to approximately 2 inches (5 cm) (Saliba & Foremans 1998). Laser light works by initiating athermic photochemical reactions within specific wavelengths and frequencies on dependent tissue chromophores within cell membranes and organelles (mitochondria) (Smith 1991).

The physiological effects of laser therapy are considered to be from a photobiomodulation effect. This effect may be either stimulatory or inhibitory. This photobiomodulation effect is believed to follow the

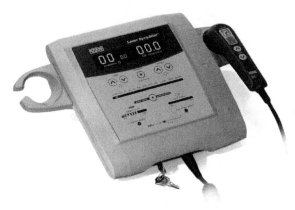

Figure 12.12 Laser. Photograph courtesy of Mettler Electronics

Arndt–Schultz law of biological activation (Baxter et al 1994). This law stipulates a dosage-dependent effect where a lower dosage triggers a biostimulation response and a higher dosage triggers a bioinhibition response. The biostimulation effect will promote tissue healing and repair while the bioinhibitory effect promotes pain management and relief. The reported clinical effects of laser light include marked improvements in wound healing, nerve repair, musculoskeletal pain and various inflammatory processes (Basford 1993).

Safety and contraindications

Laser therapy has a history of a high margin of safety. There is no electrical charge introduced into the body and the effects of laser light are primarily athermal so it will not damage tissue. The main contraindication is direct exposure over the eye. Other significant contraindications and precautions exist for the use over a pregnant uterus, neoplastic lesions and in those patients who are photosensitive or are taking photosensitizing medications (Belanger 2002b, Kahn 2002). Safe, effective and optimal application of laser therapy requires that the clinician go through a systematic set of steps and procedures for each and every application.

Indications: validation of efficacy = 3

The main clinical indications for laser therapy have been for cutaneous wounds and ulcers and pain management for a wide variety of local and systemic clinical disorders primarily of the musculoskeletal system. This would include such conditions as rheumatoid and osteoarthritis, various tendinopathies, trigger points, strains/sprains, neuropathic pain including carpal tunnel syndrome, diabetic neuropathy, radicu-

lopathy, postherpetic neuralgia, occipital neuralgia, oral/facial pain and restricted joint range of motion. Tinnitus and immune modulation have also shown benefit from laser therapy (Basford 1993, Belanger 2002c, Kahn 2000, Shankar & Randall 2002b).

Naturopathic indications and applications: validation of efficacy = 2

Naturopathic clinical application of laser therapy is to stimulate cells and tissues to bring them back to their most natural state by photonic absorption converting into chemical energy which initiates a cascade of events at a cellular level. This is an evolution of the naturopathic therapeutic use of heliotherapy (sunbaths) to stimulate a healing response. In following the principle of 'first do no harm', laser therapy uses athermal light energy and biomodulation to stimulate the healing process and inhibit pain. By this stimulation of cellular tissues, ATP production can be increased, oxygenation available to the cell can be made greater, and the combined result is an increase in lymphatic activity for cellular detoxification.

The living matrix produces coherent or laser-like oscillations. These oscillations serve as signals that integrate processes such as growth, injury repair and the functioning of the organism as a whole. Each molecule, cell, tissue and organ has an ideal resonance or frequency that coordinates its activities. Normally these frequencies are stable. If, for some reason, a sufficient number of cells shift their frequency, the strength of the system's collective vibrations decreases to the point where stability (health) is lost. Loss of coherence can lead to disease or disorder. Hence, laser therapy providing the correct or healing wavelength and frequency may bring the oscillations back to coherence and restore balance and health and relieve pain (Oschman 2000).

References

Abbott GK, Moor FB, Jensen-Nelson KL 1945a Physical therapy in nursing care. Review and Herald Publishing, Washington, DC, p 256–258

Abbott GK, Moor FB, Jensen-Nelson KL 1945b Physical therapy in nursing care. Review and Herald Publishing, Washington, DC, p 336–381

Abbott GK, Moor FB, Jensen-Nelson KL 1945c Physical therapy in nursing care. Review and Herald Publishing, Washington, DC, p 280

Abbott GK, Moor FB, Jensen-Nelson KL 1945d Physical therapy in nursing care. Review and Herald Publishing, Washington, DC, p 281

Abrams A 1912 Spondylotherapy: physiotherapy of the spine based on a study of clinical physiology. Philopolis Press, San Francisco

Agresta J 2003 Physical therapy notes 2. National College of Naturopathic Medicine Course Notes

Agresta J 2004 Physical therapy notes 1. National College of Naturopathic Medicine Course Notes

Allberry J, Manning FR, Smith EE et al 1972 Treatment of herpes zoster with short-wave diathermy to the spinal cord. Practitioner 208(247):687–688

Allberry J, Manning FR, Smith EE 1974 Short-wave diathermy for herpes zoster. Physiotherapy 60(12):386

Allen WH 1939 Short wave therapy. Naturopath and Herald of Health. Benedict Lust Publications, New York

American Association of Naturopathic Physicians 1955 Galvanism. Journal of the American Association of Naturopathic Physicians, December. American Association of Naturopathic Physicians, Washington, DC

Arghiropol M, Jieanu V, Paslaru L et al 1992 The stimulation of fibronectin synthesis by high peak power electromagnetic energy (Diapulse). Revue Roumaine de Physiologie 29(3–4):77–81

Aronofsky DH 1971 Reduction of dental postsurgical symptoms using nonthermal pulsed high-peak-power electromagnetic energy. Oral Surgery, Oral Medicine, Oral Pathology 32(5):688–696

Atamaz F 2006 A comparison of two different intra-articular hyaluronan drugs and physical therapy in the management of knee osteoarthritis. Rheumatology International 26(10):873–878

Badea MA, Vasilco R, Sandru D et al 1993 The effect of pulsed electromagnetic field (Diapulse) on cellular systems. Romanian Journal of Physiology 30(1–2):65–71

Baker LL, Chambers R, DeMuth SK, Villar F 1997 Effects of electrical stimulation on wound healing in patients with diabetic ulcers. Diabetes Care 20(3):405–442

Basford JR 1993 Laser therapy: scientific basis and clinical role. Orthopedics 16:541–547

Baxter GD, Walsh DM, Allen JM et al 1994 Effects of low intensity infrared laser radiation upon conduction in the human median nerve in vivo. Experimental Physiology 79:227–234

Becker RO, Seldon G 1985 The body electric, electromagnetism and the foundation of life. Quill, William Morrow, New York

Belanger A 2002a Evidence-based guide to therapeutic physical agents. Lippincott Williams & Wilkins, Philadelphia, p 191

Belanger A 2002b Evidence-based guide to therapeutic physical agents. Lippincott Williams & Wilkins, Philadelphia, p 211–212

Belanger A 2002c Evidence-based guide to therapeutic physical agents. Lippincott Williams & Wilkins, Philadelphia, p 208–211

Bertolucci LE, Grey T 1995 Clinical comparative study of microcurrent electrical stimulation to mid-laser and placebo treatment in degenerative joint disease of the temporomandibular joint. Journal of Craniomandibular Practice 13(2):116–120

Bierman W, Licht S 1952 Physical medicine in general practice, 3rd edn. Hoeber, New York

Blake E 2006 Constitutional hydrotherapy: a workbook of clinical lessons. Holistic Health Publications, Portland, OR

Boyle W 1988 Lectures in naturopathic hydrotherapy. Buckeye Naturopathic Press, East Palestine, OH

Cameron BM 1961 Experimental acceleration of wound healing. American Journal of Orthopedics 3:336–343

Cameron MH 2003 Physical agents in rehabilitation. WB Saunders, Philadelphia

Carley PJ, Wainapel SF 1985 Electrotherapy for acceleration of wound healing: low intensity direct current. Archives of Physical Medicine and Rehabilitation 66:443–446

Castro RA, Girao MJ, Arruda RM et al 2004 Does electrical stimulation of the pelvic floor make any change in urodynamic parameters? When to expect a cure and improvement in women with stress urinary incontinence? Clinical and Experimental Obstetrics and Gynecology 31(4):274–278

Cheng N 1982 The effect of electric currents on ATP generation, protein synthesis and membrane transport in rat skin. Clinical Orthopedics 171:264–272

Clayton EB 1928 Physiotherapy in general practice, 2nd edn. Wood, New York

Colson T 1953 Spondylotherapy guide. Electronic Medical Digest XXVII(3):third quarter. (Original article published in the November 1942 issue of the Journal of Electronic Medicine, details unknown)

Comorsan S, Vasilco R, Arghiropol M et al 1993 The effect of diapulse therapy on the healing of decubitus ulcer. Romanian Journal of Physiology 30(1–2):41–45

Connor WG, Gerner EW, Miller RC, Boone MLM 1977 Prospects for hyperthermia in human cancer therapy. Radiology 123:497–503

Cordingley EW 1923 Let us standardize the practice of naturopathy. Naturopath and Herald of Health. Benedict Lust Publications, New York, p 687

Cordingley EW 1925 Principles and practice of naturopathy: a compendium of natural healing. O'Fallon, Bazan, CA

Cordingley EW 1937 The galvanic current in naturopathic practice. Naturopath and Herald of Health. Benedict Lust Publications, New York, p 259

Darst WD 1936 Cancer mastered naturopathic way. Naturopath and Herald of Health. Benedict Lust Publications, New York, p 6, 17

De Groot AL 1964 The value of physical therapy in lung diseases. Nederlands Tijdschrift voor Geneeskunde 108:2502–2506

DuPont JS, Graham R, Tidwell JB 1999 Trigger point identification and treatment with microcurrent. Journal of Craniomandibular Practice 17(4):293–296

Farnsworth GR, Kirkbride DJ 1959 Panel Chairmen's Report of the Management of Five Diseases – Asthma, Angina Pectoris, Rheumatoid Arthritis, Herniated Disc Lesions, Diabetes Mellitus. Resulting from the discussion at the Annual Educational Symposium of Association of Naturopathic Physicians of British Columbia, Canada. Held in Nanaimo Bay, BC, 1958. Journal of Naturopathic Medicine, Graham, FL

Gam AN, Johannsen F 1995 Ultrasound therapy in musculoskeletal disorders: a meta-analysis. Pain 63(1):85–91

Gerson J 2002 Skin care: how to save your skin. Delmar Thomson Learning, Albany, New York

Goats GC 1989 Continuous short-wave (radio-frequency) diathermy. British Journal of Sports Medicine 23(2):123–127

Goldin JH, Broadbent NR, Nancarrow JD, Marshall T 1981 The effects of Diapulse on the healing of wounds: a double blind randomised controlled trial in man. British Journal of Plastic Surgery 34:267–270

Gorbunov FE, Vinnikov AA, Strelkova NI, Krupennikov AI 1995 [The use of pulsed and continuous UHF electrical fields in the rehabilitation of patients with the Guillain–Barré syndrome and other peripheral myelinopathies] [article in Russian]. Zhurnal Nevropatologii i Psikhiatrii Imeni S.S. Korsakova 95(5):22–26

Gray RJ, Quayle AA, Hall CA, Schofield MA 1994 Physiotherapy in the treatment of temporomandibular joint disorders: a comparative study of four treatment methods. British Dental Journal 176(7):257–261

Gregory A 1922 Spondylotherapy simplified. Gregory, Oklahoma City

Griffin JE, Karselis TC 1988 Physical agents for physical therapists. CC Thomas, Springfield, IL

Guberan, E, Campana A, Faval P et al 1994 Gender ratio of offspring and exposure to short wave radiation among female physiotherapists. Scandinavian Journal of Work and Environmental Health 20(5):345–348

Hakkinen AM, Blomqvist K, Spring E, Valtonen E 1975 Simultaneous application of pulsed high frequency currents and gamma-rays to cultured melanoma cells. Strahlentherapie 149(2):205–207

Hamnerius Y 1985 Biological effects of high-frequency electromagnetic fields on Salmonella typhimurium and Drosophila melanogaster. Bioelectromagnetics 6(4):405–414

Hayes KW 2000 Manual for physical agents. Prentice Hall Health, Upper Saddle River, NJ

Heick E 1991 Is diathermy safe in women with copper-bearing IUDs? Acta Obstetrica Gynecologica Scandinavica 70(2):153–155

Hewlett-Parsons J 1968 Naturopathic practice: a valuable guide to students and others in the principles and practice of naturopathy. Arco Publishing, New York

Hill J, Lewis M, Mills P et al 2002 Pulsed short-wave diathermy effects on human fibroblast proliferation. Archives of Physical Medicine and Rehabilitation 83(6):832–836

Hurwitz MD, Kaplan ID, Hansen JL et al 2005 Hyperthermia combined with radiation in treatment of locally advanced prostate cancer is associated with a favourable toxicity profile. International Journal of Hyperthermia 21(7):649–656

Itoh M, Montemayor JS, Matsumoto E et al 1991 Accelerated wound healing of pressure ulcers by pulsed high peak power electromagnetic energy (Diapulse). Decubitus 4(1):24–25, 29–34

Jan MH, Chai HM, Wang CL et al 2006 Effects of repetitive short wave diathermy for reducing synovitis in patients with knee osteoarthritis: an ultrasonographic study. Physical Therapy 86(2):236–244

Jaskoviak PA 1993a Applied physiotherapy: practical clinical applications with emphasis on the management of pain and related syndromes. American Chiropractic Association, Arlington, VA, p 281

Jaskoviak PA 1993b Applied physiotherapy: practical clinical applications with emphasis on the management of pain and related syndromes. American Chiropractic Association, Arlington, VA, p 297

Jaskoviak PA 1993c Applied physiotherapy: practical clinical applications with emphasis on the management of pain and related syndromes. American Chiropractic Association, Arlington, VA, p 293

Jaskoviak PA 1993d Applied physiotherapy: practical clinical applications with emphasis on the management of pain and related syndromes. American Chiropractic Association, Arlington, VA, p 183–208

Johnson AC 1946a Principles and practice of drugless therapeutics, 3rd edn. Chiropractic Educational Extension Bureau, Los Angeles, p 41

Johnson AC 1946b Principles and practice of drugless therapeutics, 3rd edn. Chiropractic Educational Extension Bureau, Los Angeles

Johnson AC 1946c Principles and practice of drugless therapeutics, 3rd edn. Chiropractic Educational Extension Bureau, Los Angeles, p 34

Johnson AC 1946d Principles and practice of drugless therapeutics, 3rd edn. Chiropractic Educational Extension Bureau, Los Angeles, p 42–43

Johnson AC 1946e Principles and practice of drugless therapeutics, 3rd edn. Chiropractic Educational Extension Bureau, Los Angeles, p 30

Kahn J 2000 Principles and practice of electrotherapy, 4th edn. Churchill Livingstone, New York, p 39

Kerem M, Yigiter K 2002 Effects of continuous and pulsed short-wave diathermy in low back pain. Pain Clinic 14(1):55–59

Kitaigorodskaia OD 1956 Use of diathermia in complex therapy in of pneumonia in children. Pediatriia 39(1):74–75

Laptev PI 2004 Use of local UHF hyperthermia and CO_2 laser in treatment of cancer of the lip, lingual mucosa, and bottom of the oral cavity. Stomatologiia 83(1):30–32

Larsen AI 1991 Congenital malformations and exposure to high-frequency electromagnetic radiation among Danish physiotherapists. Scandinavian Journal of Work and Environmental Health 17(5):318–323

Lerman Y, Jacubovich R, Green MS 2001 Pregnancy outcome following exposure to short waves among female physiotherapists in Israel. American Journal of Industrial Medicine 39(5):499–504

Linder P 1964 Pulsed short wave therapy. American Naturopath. Naturopathic Physicians Association of California

Lindquist RJ 1948a Approach to electrotherapy. Lindquist, Los Angeles

Lindquist RJ 1948b Approach to electrotherapy. Lindquist, Los Angeles, p 82

Lohmann CH, Schwartz Z, Liu Y et al 2000 Pulsed electromagnetic field stimulation of MG63 osteoblast-like cells affects differentiation and local factor production. Journal of Orthopaedic Research 18(4):637–646

Luke TD 1922 Manual of physiotherapeutics. Wood, New York

Matijaca A 1919a Principles of electromedicine, electrosurgery, and radiology. In: Lust B (ed) The universal naturopathic directory and buyer's guide. Benedict Lust Publications, Butler, NJ, p 606

Matijaca A 1919b Principles of electromedicine, electrosurgery, and radiology. In: Lust B (ed) The universal naturopathic directory and buyer's guide. Benedict Lust Publications, Butler, NJ, p 618

McMakin C 1998 Microcurrent treatment of myofascial pain in the head, neck and face. Topics in Clinical Chiropractic 5:29–35

McMakin C 2004 Microcurrent therapy: a novel treatment method for chronic low back myofascial pain. Journal of Bodywork and Movement Therapies 8:143–153

McMakin C 2005 Cytokine changes with microcurrent treatment of fibromyalgia associated with cervical spine trauma. Journal of Bodywork and Movement Therapies 9:169–176

Museum of Questionable Medical Devices 2000 Violet ray generators. Notices of Judgment: 3458. Misbranding of violet ray device, S. v 2 Cases ***. (F.D.C. No. 30801. Sample no. 3858-L.) Online. Available: www.mtn.org/quack/devices/uv.htm

Neiswanger CS 1925a Electro-therapeutical practice: a ready reference guide for physicians in the use of electricity, 23rd edn. Ritchie, Chicago

Neiswanger CS 1925b Electro-therapeutical practice: a ready reference guide for physicians in the use of electricity, 23rd edn. Ritchie, Chicago, p 238

Oschman J 2000 Energy medicine, the scientific basis. Churchill Livingstone, Edinburgh

Oullet Hellstrom R, Stewart WF 1993 Miscarriages among female physical therapists who report using radio- and microwave-frequency electromagnetic radiation. American Journal of Epidemiology 138(10):775–786. Comment in: American Journal of Epidemiology 1995;141(3):273–274

Poesnecker GE 1978 It's only natural. Ad Ventures, Hatfield, PA

Pop L, Muresan M, Comorosan S, Paslaru L 1989 The effects of pulsed, high frequency radio waves on rat liver (ultrastructural and biomedical observations). Physiological Chemistry and Physics and Medical NMR 21(1):45–55

Post-Graduate Study of Naturotherapy 1937a Naturopath and Herald of Health. Benedict Lust Publications, New York, July, p 202

Post-Graduate Study of Naturotherapy 1937b Naturopath and Herald of Health. Benedict Lust Publications, New York

Post-Graduate Study of Naturotherapy 1937c Naturopath and Herald of Health. Benedict Lust Publications, New York, June

Post-Graduate Study of Naturotherapy 1938a Naturopath and Herald of Health. Benedict Lust Publications, New York

Post-Graduate Study of Naturotherapy 1938b Naturopath and Herald of Health. Benedict Lust Publications, New York, September

Post-Graduate Study of Naturotherapy 1938c Naturopath and Herald of Health. Benedict Lust Publications, New York, October

Post-Graduate Study of Naturotherapy 1938d Naturopath and Herald of Health. Benedict Lust Publications, New York, January

Post-Graduate Study of Naturotherapy 1939a Naturopath and Herald of Health. Benedict Lust Publications, New York

Post-Graduate Study of Naturotherapy 1939b Naturopath and Herald of Health. Benedict Lust Publications, New York, January

Post-Graduate Study of Naturotherapy 1939c Naturopath and Herald of Health. Benedict Lust Publications, New York, February

Prentice W 1998a Therapeutic modalities for the allied health professions. McGraw-Hill, New York, p 169–193

Prentice W 1998b Therapeutic modalities for the allied health professions. McGraw-Hill, New York, p 170

Puderbach P 1925 The massage operator. Benedict Lust Publications, Butler, NJ

Raji AM 1984 An experimental study of the effects of pulsed electromagnetic field (Diapulse) on nerve repair. Journal of Hand Surgery [Br] 9(2):105–112

Raji ARM, Bowden REM 1983 Effects of high-peak pulsed electromagnetic field on the degeneration and regeneration of the common peroneal nerve in rats. Journal of Bone and Joint Surgery 65B(4):478–492

Ravitskii AB 1954 [Results of short-wave therapy of pneumopleuritis] [article in Russian]. Problemy Tuberkuleza 5:61–65

Saliba E, Foremans S 1998 Low level lasers. In: Prentice WE (ed) Therapeutic modalities for allied health professionals. McGraw-Hill, New York, p 313–326

Salzberg CA, Cooper SA, Perez P et al 1995 The effects of non-thermal pulsed electromagnetic energy on wound healing of pressure ulcers in spinal cord-injured patients: a randomized, double-blind study. Ostomy/Wound Management 41(3):42–44, 46, 48

Sanservino E 1980 Membrane phenomena cellular processes under action of pulsating magnetic fields.

Lecture at the 2nd International Congress of Magneto Medicine, Rome, November 1980

Saperov VN 1974 High-frequency electrotherapy in the complex treatment of chronic pneumonia. Klinicheskaia Meditsina 52(8):94–100

Scott L 1990 Clinical hydrotherapy. Leo Scott, Spokane, WA

Sergeev VM, Esipova IK, Manzhos PI et al 1986 [Low-frequency ultrasound in the treatment of acute and chronic suppurative diseases of the lungs and pleura in children] [article in Russian]. Vestnik Khirurgii Imeni I.I. Grekova 137(8):75–80

Shankar K, Randall KD 2002a Therapeutic physical modalities. Hanley & Belfus, Philadelphia

Shankar K, Randall KD 2002b Therapeutic physical modalities. Hanley & Belfus, Philadelphia, p 84–86

Shields N, Gormley J, O'Hare N 2002 Short-wave diathermy: current clinical and safety practices. Physiotherapy Research International 7(4):191–202

Shriber W 1975 A manual of electrotherapy. Lea & Febiger, Philadelphia, p 219

Sisken BF, Kanje M, Lundborg G et al 1989 Stimulation of rat sciatic nerve regeneration with pulsed electromagnetic fields. Brain Research 485(2):309–316

Smith K 1991 The photobiological basis of low-level laser radiation therapy. Laser Therapy 3:19–24

Starkey C 1999a Therapeutic modalities. FA Davis, Philadelphia, p 178–179

Starkey C 1999b Therapeutic modalities. FA Davis, Philadelphia, p 171

Starkey C 1999c Therapeutic modalities. FA Davis, Philadelphia, p 256

Starkey C 1999d Therapeutic modalities. FA Davis, Philadelphia

Starkey C 1999e Therapeutic modalities. FA Davis, Philadelphia, p 156

Starkey C 1999f Therapeutic modalities. FA Davis, Philadelphia, p 163

Stewart HE 1923 Diathermy and its application to pneumonia [with forty-five illustrations and fifteen charts]. PB Hoeber, New York

Taskinen H 1990 Effects of ultrasound, short waves, and physical exertion on pregnancy outcome in physiotherapists. Journal of Epidemiology and Community Health 44(3):196–201

Thamsborg G, Florescu A, Oturai P et al 2005 Treatment of knee osteoarthritis with pulsed electromagnetic fields: a randomized, double-blind, placebo-controlled study. Osteoarthritis and Cartilage 13(7):575–581

Tilly W, Gellermann J, Graf R et al 2005 Regional hyperthermia in conjunction with definitive radiotherapy against recurrent or locally advanced prostate cancer T3 pN0 M0. Strahlentherapie und Onkologie 181(1):35–41

Trock DH, Bollet AJ, Markoll R 1994 The effect of pulsed electromagnetic fields in the treatment of osteoarthritis of the knee and cervical spine. Report of randomized, double blind, placebo controlled trials. Journal of Rheumatology 21(10):1903–1911

Uglov FG 1965 Treatment of postoperative pneumonias in thoracic patients with short-wave diathermy. Klinicheskaia Khirurgiia 6:3–6

Van den Bouwhuijsen F et al 1990 Pulsed and continuous short wave therapy. BV Enhaf-Nonius, Delft, Holland, p 17

van der Windt DA, van der Heijden GJ, van den Berg SG et al 1999 Ultrasound therapy for musculoskeletal disorders: a systematic review. Pain 81(3):257–271

Watrous L 1996 Constitutional hydrotherapy: from nature cure to advanced naturopathic medicine. Journal of Naturopathic Medicine 7(2):72–79

Watrous L, Blake E 2004 Advanced hydrotherapy seminar [video presentation]. Canadian College of Naturopathic Medicine, Toronto

Weisberg J 1994 Lasers. In: Hecox B, Mehretaab TA, Weisberg J (eds) Physical agents: a comprehensive text for physical therapists. Appleton & Lange, Norwalk, CT, p 391–396

Wolcott LE, Wheeler PC, Hardwicke HM, Rowley BA 1969 Accelerated healing of skin ulcers by electrotherapy: preliminary clinical results. Southern Medical Journal 62(7):795–801

Wolf H 1935a Short wave therapy and general electro-therapy. Modern Medical Press, New York, p 28

Wolf H 1935b Short wave therapy and general electro-therapy. Modern Medical Press, New

Wolf H 1935c Short wave therapy and general electro-therapy. Modern Medical Press, New York, p 15. Compilation of successful reports – Schliephake

Wolf H 1935d Short wave therapy and general electro-therapy. Modern Medical Press, New York, p 15. Compilation of successful reports – Schliephake, Laquer, Liebensy, Weissenberg

Wolf H 1935e Short wave therapy and general electro-therapy. Modern Medical Press, New York, p 15. Compilation of successful reports – Schliephake, Weissenberg

Wolf H 1935f Short wave therapy and general electro-therapy. Modern Medical Press, New York, p 15. Compilation of successful reports – Schliephake, Laquer, Liebensy

Wolf H 1935g Short wave therapy and general electro-therapy. Modern Medical Press, New York, p 15. Compilation of successful reports – Raab

Wolf H 1935h Short wave therapy and general electro-therapy. Modern Medical Press, New York, p 15. Compilation of successful reports – Schriber, Bierman & Licht, Neiswanger

Wolf H 1935i Short wave therapy and general electro-therapy. Modern Medical Press, New York, p 15. Compilation of successful reports – Schliephake, Dausset, Laszlo, Weissenberg

Wolf H 1935j Short wave therapy and general electro-therapy. Modern Medical Press, New York, p 15. Compilation of successful reports – Schliephake, Liebensy

Wolf H 1935k Short wave therapy and general electro-therapy. Modern Medical Press, New York, p 15. Compilation of successful reports – Schliephake, Liebensy, Laquer

Wolf H 1935l Short wave therapy and general electro-therapy. Modern Medical Press, New York, p 15. Compilation of successful reports – Laquer, Liebensy, Vaernet

Wolf H 1935m Short wave therapy and general electro-therapy. Modern Medical Press, New York, p 15. Compilation of successful reports – Schliephake, Liebensy, Dausset, Rechou

Wolf H 1935n Short wave therapy and general electro-therapy. Modern Medical Press, New York, p 15. Compilation of successful reports – Schliephake, Liebensy, Laquer, Vaernet

Wolf H 1935o Short wave therapy and general electro-therapy. Modern Medical Press, New York, p 15. Compilation of successful reports – Vaernet

Wolf H 1935p Short wave therapy and general electro-therapy. Modern Medical Press, New York, p 15. Compilation of successful reports – Schliephake, Laquer, Weissenberg

Wolf H 1935q Short wave therapy and general electro-therapy. Modern Medical Press, New York, p 15. Compilation of successful reports – Schliephake, Laquer, Wolfe

Wolf H 1935r Short wave therapy and general electro-therapy. Modern Medical Press, New York, p 15. Compilation of successful reports – Raab, Weissenberg

Index

NB: Page numbers in bold refer to boxes, figures and tables

Printed and bound by CPI Group (UK) Ltd, Croydon, CR0 4YY

08/05/2025

01864672-0002